T0133050

# CRC SERIES IN NUTRITION AND FOOD

Editor-in-Chief

## Miloslav Rechcigl, Jr.

**Handbook of Nutritive Value of Processed Food**
Volume I: Food for Human Use
Volume II: Animal Feedstuffs

**Handbook of Nutritional Requirements
in a Functional Context**
Volume I: Development and Conditions of
Physiologic Stress
Volume II: Hematopoiesis, Metabolic Function, and
Resistance to Physical Stress

**Handbook of Agricultural Productivity**
Volume I: Plant Productivity
Volume II: Animal Productivity

# Handbook
## of
# Nutritive Value
## of
# Processed Food

## Volume I
## Food for Human Use

### Miloslav Rechcigl, Jr., Editor

Nutrition Advisor and Director
Interregional Research Staff
Agency for International Development
U.S. Department of State

CRC Series in Nutrition and Food
Miloslav Rechcigl, Jr., Editor-in-Chief

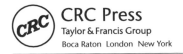

## CRC Press
Taylor & Francis Group
Boca Raton London New York

CRC Press is an imprint of the
Taylor & Francis Group, an **informa** business

CRC Press
Taylor & Francis Group
6000 Broken Sound Parkway NW, Suite 300
Boca Raton, FL 33487-2742

Reissued 2019 by CRC Press

© 1982 by Taylor & Francis Group, LLC
CRC Press is an imprint of Taylor & Francis Group, an Informa business

No claim to original U.S. Government works

A Library of Congress record exists under LC control number:

Publisher's Note
The publisher has gone to great lengths to ensure the quality of this reprint but points out that some imperfections in the original copies may be apparent.

Disclaimer
The publisher has made every effort to trace copyright holders and welcomes correspondence from those they have been unable to contact.

ISBN 13: 978-0-367-25916-7 (hbk)
ISBN 13: 978-0-367-25919-8 (pbk)
ISBN 13: 978-0-429-29052-7 (ebk)

Visit the Taylor & Francis Web site at http://www.taylorandfrancis.com and the
CRC Press Web site at http://www.crcpress.com

# PREFACE
## CRC SERIES IN NUTRITION AND FOOD

Nutrition means different things to different people, and no other field of endeavor crosses the boundaries of so many different disciplines and abounds with such diverse dimensions. The growth of the field of nutrition, particularly in the last 2 decades, has been phenomenal, the nutritional data being scattered literally in thousands and thousands of not always accessible periodicals and monographs, many of which, furthermore, are not normally identified with nutrition.

To remedy this situation, we have undertaken an ambitious and monumental task of assembling in one publication all the critical data relevant in the field of nutrition.

The *CRC Series in Nutrition and Food* is intended to serve as a ready reference source of current information on experimental and applied human, animal, microbial, and plant nutrition presented in concise tabular, graphical, or narrative form and indexed for ease of use. It is hoped that this projected open-ended multivolume compendium will become for the nutritionist what the *CRC Handbook of Chemistry and Physics* has become for the chemist and physicist.

Apart from supplying specific data, the comprehensive, interdisciplinary, and comparative nature of the *CRC Series in Nutrition and Food* will provide the user with an easy overview of the state of the art, pinpointing the gaps in nutritional knowledge and providing a basis for further research. In addition, the series will enable the researcher to analyze the data in various living systems for commonality or basic differences. On the other hand, an applied scientist or technician will be afforded the opportunity of evaluating a given problem and its solutions from the broadest possible point of view, including the aspects of agronomy, crop science, animal husbandry, aquaculture and fisheries, veterinary medicine, clinical medicine, pathology, parasitology, toxicology, pharmacology, therapeutics, dietetics, food science and technology, physiology, zoology, botany, biochemistry, developmental and cell biology, microbiology, sanitation, pest control, economics, marketing, sociology, anthropology, natural resources, ecology, environmental science, population, law politics, nutritional and food methodology, and others.

To make more facile use of the series, the publication has been organized into separate handbooks of one or more volumes each. In this manner the particular sections of the series can be continuously updated by publishing additional volumes of new data as they become available.

The Editor wishes to thank the numerous contributors many of whom have undertaken their assignment in pioneering spirit, and the Advisory Board members for their continuous counsel and cooperation. Last but not least, he wishes to express his sincere appreciation to the members of the CRC editorial and production staffs, particularly President Bernard J. Starkoff, Earl Starkoff, Sandy Pearlman, Pamela Woodcock, Lisa Levine Eggenberger, John Hunter, and Amy G. Skallerup for their encouragement and support.

We invite comments and criticism regarding format and selection of subject matter, as well as specific suggestions for new data which might be included in subsequent editions. We should also appreciate it if the readers would bring to the attention of the Editor any errors or omissions that might appear in the publication.

Miloslav Rechcigl, Jr.
Editor-in-Chief

# PREFACE
## HANDBOOK OF NUTRITIVE VALUE OF PROCESSED FOOD

Industrial as well as home processing can bring about profound changes in the chemical composition of food and its nutritive value. While a variety of treatments may be detrimental, certain modifications of foodstuffs can actually improve their digestibility and biological value. The effect on specific nutrients also varies and may differ depending on the type of treatment and food used. The purpose of this handbook is to provide a systematic and critical treatment of these questions. This publication should be an invaluable tool to food technologists, dieticians, and nutritionists, as well as to livestock producers and persons engaged in production, processing, and formulation of animal feeds. It should also be of great interest to conscientious consumers concerned about the quality and wholesomeness of food products.

Miloslav Rechcigl, Jr.

# THE EDITOR

**Miloslav Rechcigl, Jr.** is a Nutrition Advisor and Chief of Research and Methodology Division in the Agency for International Development.

He has a B.S. in Biochemistry (1954), a Master of Nutritional Science degree (1955), and a Ph.D. in nutrition, biochemistry, and physiology (1958), all from Cornell University. He was formerly a Research Biochemist in the National Cancer Institute, National Institutes of Health and subsequently served as Special Assistant for Nutrition and Health in the Health Services and Mental Health Administration, U.S. Department of Health, Education and Welfare.

Dr. Rechcigl is a member of some 30 scientific and professional societies, including being a Fellow of the American Association for the Advancement of Science, Fellow of the Washington Academy of Sciences, Fellow of the American Institute of Chemists, and Fellow of the International College of Applied Nutrition. He holds membership in the Cosmos Club, the Honorary Society of Phi Kappa Pi, and the Society of Sigma Xi, and is recipient of numerous honors, including an honorary membership certificate from the International Social Science Honor Society Delta Tau Kappa. In 1969, he was a delegate to the White House Conference on Food, Nutrition, and Health and in 1975 a delegate to the ARPAC Conference on Research to Meet U.S. and World Food Needs. He served as President of the District of Columbia Institute of Chemists and Councillor of the American Institute of Chemists, and currently is a delegate to the Washington Academy of Sciences and a member of the Program Committee of the American Institute of Nutrition.

His bibliography extends over 100 publications including contributions to books, articles in periodicals, and monographs in the fields of nutrition, biochemistry, physiology, pathology, enzymology, molecular biology, agriculture, and international development. Most recently he authored and edited *Nutrition and the World Food Problem* (S. Karger, Basel, 1979), *World Food Problem: a Selective Bibliography of Reviews* (CRC Press, 1975), and *Man, Food and Nutrition: Strategies and Technological Measures for Alleviating the World Food Problem* (CRC Press, 1973) following his earlier pioneering treatise on *Enzyme Synthesis and Degradation in Mammalian Systems* (S. Karger, Basel, 1971), and that on *Microbodies and Related Particles, Morphology, Biochemistry and Physiology* (Academic Press, New York, 1969). Dr. Rechcigl also has initiated a new series on *Comparative Animal Nutrition* and was Associated Editor of *Nutrition Reports International*.

# CONTRIBUTORS

Jean Adrian
Professor of Food Science and
  Biochemistry
Conservatoire National des Arts et
  Métiers
Paris, France

Harold R. Bolin, Ph.D.
Research Chemist
Food Technology Research Unit
U.S. Department of Agriculture,
  Science, and Education
  Administration
Western Regional Research Center
Berkeley, California

I.H. Burger, Ph.D.
Animal Studies Centre
Pedigree Petfoods, Melton Mowbray
Leicestershire, England

Elmer De Ritter
Assistant Director (Retired)
Product Development
Hoffman-La Roche, Inc.
Nutley, New Jersey

Paul S. Dimick, Ph.D.
Professor of Food Science
Pennsylvania State University
University Park, Pennsylvania

E. Dworschák, Ph.D.
Head, Department of Protein and
  Vitamin Research
Institute of Nutrition
Budapest, Hungary

Edgar R. Elkins, Jr.
Director, Chemistry Division
National Food Processors Association
Eastern Research Laboratory
Washington, D.C.

John W. Erdman, Jr., Ph.D.
Associate Professor of Food Science
University of Illinois
Urbana, Illinois

Edith A. Erdman, M.S.
Department of Food Science
University of Illinois
Urbana, Illinois

Richard P. Farrow
Senior Vice President and General
  Manager
National Food Processors Association
Western Research Laboratory
Berkeley, California

Owen Fennema, Ph.D.
Chairman, Department of Food
  Science
University of Wisconsin-Madison
Madison, Wisconsin

James M. Flink, Ph.D.
Professor of Plant Product
  Technology
Department for the Technology of
  Plant Food Products
The Royal Veterinary and Agricultural
  University
Copenhagen, Denmark

P. F. Fox, Ph.D.
Professor, Department of Food
  Chemistry
University College
Cork, Ireland

Norman D. Heidelbaugh, VMD,
  MPH, SM, Ph.D.
Professor of Food Science and
  Technology
Head, Department of Veterinary
  Public Health
Texas A & M University
College Station, Texas

Ange A. Joseph
Office de la Recherche Scientifique et
  Technique Outre-Mer
Paris, France
Section Nutrition de l'Orstom
Yaoundé, Cameroon, Africa

Marcus Karel, Ph.D
Professor of Food Engineering
Department of Nutrition and Food
  Science
Massachusetts Institute of Technology
Cambridge, Massachusetts

Barbara P. Klein, Ph.D.
Associate Professor, Department of
  Foods and Nutrition
University of Illinois
Urbana, Illinois

Amihud Kramer, Ph.D.
Professor, Food Science Program
University of Maryland
College Park, Maryland

H. F. Kraybill, Ph.D.
Scientific Coordinator for
  Environmental Cancer
National Cancer Institute
Bethesda, Maryland

Frank C. Lamb
Head, Chemistry Division (Retired)
National Food Processors Association
Western Research Laboratory
Berkeley, California

Daryl Lund, Ph.D.
Professor of Food Science
University of Wisconsin-Madison
Madison, Wisconsin

B. E. March
Professor, Department of Poultry
  Science
University of British Columbia
Vancouver, British Columbia, Canada

J. Mauron
Head, Research Laboratories
Nestlé Products Technical Assistance
  Co., Ltd.
La Tour-de-Peilz, Switzerland

P. A. Morrissey, Ph.D.
Professor, Department of Food
  Chemistry
University College
Cork, Ireland

S. J. Ritchey, Ph.D.
Professor of Human Nutrition
Dean, College of Home Economics
Virginia Polytechnic Institute and
  State University
Blacksburg, Virginia

B. A. Rolls
National Institute for Research in
  Dairying
University of Reading
Shinfield, Reading, England

John T. Rotruck, Ph.D.
The Proctor & Gamble Company
Cincinnatti, Ohio

Bohdan M. Slabyj, Ph.D.
Associate Professor of Food Science
University of Maine
Orono, Maine

Lloyd A. Witting, Ph.D.
Technical Director Biochemical
  Research and Manufacturing
Supelco, Inc.
Bellefonte, Pennsylvania

## DEDICATION

To my inspiring teachers at Cornell University—Harold H. Williams, John K. Loosli, the late Richard H. Barnes, the late Clive M. McCay, and the late Leonard A. Maynard. And to my supportive and beloved family—Eva, Jack, and Karen.

# TABLE OF CONTENTS

## Volume I

# TABLE OF CONTENTS

## Volume II

*Specific Processes*

# EFFECT OF PROCESSING ON NUTRIENT CONTENT AND NUTRITIONAL VALUE OF FOOD: HEAT PROCESSING

## Daryl Lund

Heat processing is one of the most important methods for extending the storage life of foodstuffs. Because of this extended storage life, foods that are abundantly available only during relatively short harvesting periods are made available throughout the year. However, heat processing also has a detrimental effect on nutrients, since thermal degradation of nutrients can and does occur. Therefore, thermal processing makes it possible to extend and increase availability of a foodstuff to the consumer, but it may have a lower nutrient content than the fresh form. The challenge to the food processing industry is to minimize the loss of nutrients during thermal processing while providing an adequate process to insure an extended storage life.

Heat processes that are applied to foods commercially include cooking, blanching, pasteurization, and commercial sterilization. "Cooking" includes baking, broiling, roasting, boiling, frying, and stewing. The duration and severity of these cooking processes are dependent upon individual preference, and consequently, it is difficult at best to quantify or predict the extent of thermal destruction of nutrients in these processes. However, for the other commercial operations in which specific objectives for the process can be established, it is possible to design the process to maximize retention of nutrients. For this, it is necessary to describe quantitatively the effects of heat on nutrients.

The most common method of reporting the effect of heat processing on nutrients has been to express the nutrient content after processing as a percentage of the original amount present. This is obviously the simplest way, since it requires only two analyses: one before and one after the process. Most of the data reported in review articles are in this form.[1-9] These data have also been summarized in handbook form.[10,12]

The problem with reporting data in this manner is that there is no longer a typical or universal thermal process. In canning, for example, there are at least five systems which could be used to produce a canned product.[12] Each of these processes may differ in time/temperature combination, therefore, each will produce differences in nutrient retention. Consequently, the value of reporting nutrient losses for "canning" can be seriously questioned.

The review articles previously mentioned are rather uniform in format, presenting first the positive and then the negative effects of heat processing. The desirable effects of heat may be summarized as follows:

1.  Favorable alteration of the characteristics of the product, e.g., browning reaction, textural changes, increased palatability, etc.
2.  Destruction of microorganisms, e.g., sterilization, pasteurization
3.  Destruction of enzymes, e.g., peroxidase, ascorbic acid oxidase, thiaminase
4.  Improvement in availability of nutrients, e.g., gelatinization of starches and increased digestibility of proteins
5.  Destruction of undesirable food components, e.g., avidin in egg white, trypsin inhibitor in legumes

The undesirable effects of heat processing include changes in proteins and amino acids, carbohydrates, lipids, vitamins, and minerals. Proteins undergo denaturation when heated, which generally enhances their digestibility by proteases.[13] In the presence of reducing sugars, proteins are degraded via the Maillard reaction, the basic amino acids being especially reactive. Lysine and threonine are the most heat labile.

## Table 1
## SUMMARY OF EFFECTS OF BLANCHING ON NUTRIENTS IN VEGETABLES[a]

| Blanching method | Nutrient | %Loss |
|---|---|---|
| Water | Vitamin C | 16—58 |
| | Riboflavin | 30—50 |
| | Thiamin | 16—34 |
| | Niacin | 32—37 |
| Steam | Vitamin C | 16—26 |
| | Vitamin $B_6$ | 21 |

[a]  Although there are other blanching systems available (e.g., hot gas, microwave, and individual quick blanching), data on nutrient retention were not sufficiently complete to allow reporting percentage loss.

## Table 2
## SUMMARY OF EFFECTS OF PASTEURIZATION ON NUTRIENTS IN MILK

| Pasteurization method | Nutrient | %Loss |
|---|---|---|
| High temperature | Thiamin | 10 |
| Short time | Vitamin C | 10 |
| | Vitamin $B_{12}$ | 0 |
| Holder Method | Thiamin | 10 |
| | Vitamin C | 20 |
| | Vitamin $B_{12}$ | 10 |

## Table 3
## SUMMARY OF EFFECTS OF CONVENTIONAL CANNING ON NUTRIENTS IN VEGETABLES

| Nutrient | % Loss |
|---|---|
| Vitamin C | 33—90 |
| Thiamin | 16—83 |
| Riboflavin | 25—67 |
| Niacin | 0—75 |
| Folacin | 35—84 |
| Pantothenic acid | 30—85 |
| Vitamin $B_6$ | 0—91 |
| Biotin | 0—78 |
| Vitamin A | 0—84 |

## Table 4
## KINETIC PARAMETERS FOR THE THERMAL DEGRADATION OF NUTRIENTS

| Nutrient | Medium | pH | Temperature range (°F) | $E_a$ (kcal/mol)[a] | $D_{121}$[b] | Ref. |
|---|---|---|---|---|---|---|
| Thiamin | Whole peas | Nat[c] | 220—270 | 21.2 | 164 min | 19 |
| Thiamin | Carrot puree | 5.9 | 228—300 | 27 | 158 min | 17 |
| | Green bean puree | 5.8 | 228—300 | 27 | 145 min | |
| | Pea puree | 6.6 | 228—300 | 27 | 163 min | |
| | Spinach puree | 6.5 | 228—300 | 27 | 134 min | |
| | Beef heart puree | 6.1 | 228—300 | 27 | 115 min | |
| | Beef liver puree | 6.1 | 228—300 | 27 | 124 min | |
| | Lamb puree | 6.2 | 228—300 | 27 | 120 min | |
| | Pork puree | 6.2 | 228—300 | 27 | 157 min | |
| Thiamin | Phosphate buffer | 6.0 | 250—280 | 29.4 | 156.8 min | 20 |
| | Pea puree | Nat | 250—280 | 27.5 | 246.9 min | |
| | Beef puree | Nat | 250—280 | 27.4 | 254.2 min | |
| | Peas-in-brine puree | Nat | 250—280 | 27.0 | 226.7 min | |
| Thiamin | — | — | — | 20.0 | — | 21 |
| Riboflavin | — | — | — | 23.0 | — | |
| Vitamin B₁ | Pork | — | ?—250 | 19.5 | 6.03 hr | 22 |
| Vitamin B₁ · HCl | Liquid multivitamin preparation | 3.2 | 39—158 | 26 | 1.35 days | 23 |
| D-Pantothenic acid | Liquid multivitamin preparation | 3.2 | 39—158 | 21 | 4.46 days | |
| Vitamin C | Liquid multivitamin preparation | 3.2 | 39—158 | 23.1 | 1.12 days | |
| Vitamin B₁₂ | Liquid multivitamin preparation | 3.2 | 39—158 | 23.1 | 1.94 days | |
| Folic acid | Liquid multivitamin preparation | 3.2 | 39—158 | 16.8 | 1.95 days | |
| Vitamin A | Liquid multivitamin preparation | 3.2 | 39—158 | 14.6 | 12.4 days | |
| Calcium pantothenate | Phosphate buffer | 3.8 | 40—212 | 19.0 | 0.58 days | 24 |

## Table 4 (continued)
## KINETIC PARAMETERS FOR THE THERMAL DEGRADATION OF NUTRIENTS

| Nutrient | Medium | pH | Temperature range (°F) | $E_a$ (kcal/mol)[a] | $D_{121}$[b] | Ref. |
|---|---|---|---|---|---|---|
| Inosinic acid | Buffer solution | 3 | 140—208 | 34.0 | — | 25 |
| | Buffer solution | 4 | 140—208 | 30.4 | — | |
| | Buffer solution | 5 | 140—208 | 28.1 | — | |
| Carotenoids | Paprika | Nat | 125—150 | 34.0 | 0.038 min | 26 |
| Lysine | Soybean meal | — | 212—260 | 30.0 | 13.1 hr | 27 |

[a]   $E_a$ — Arrhenius activation energy.
[b]   $D_{121}$ — Time at 121°C to destroy 90% of the nutrient.
[c]   Nat indicates that the system was at its natural pH.

Table 5

OPTIMIZATION OF THERMAL PROCESSES FOR NUTRIENT
RETENTION

| Process | Method of optimization |
| --- | --- |
| Blanching | Based on considerations other than thermal losses (e.g., leaching losses, oxidative degradation, damage to products) |
| Pasteurization | High temperature-short time (HTST) if heat-resistant enzymes and not present |
| Commercial sterilization | Convection heating foods and aseptic processing — HTST until heat resistant enzymes become important |
| | Conduction heating — generally not HTST; constant steam temperature in range 250—265°F |

Carbohydrates are generally not of concern with respect to optimizing their retention in foods. Of greater consequence and research interest are the products of the degradative reactions. Reducing sugars undergo the carmelization reaction, and products of the reaction have been investigated for their toxic effects. For example, Lang[13] reported that 5-hydroxymethyl-furfural had no adverse effects at levels of 450 mg/kg body weight in a rat diet. Generally, heating of starch in the presence of water increases digestibility because of gelatinization.

Fats, like carbohydrates, are usually not investigated for their retentive properties at elevated temperatures. The degradation products are of interest, however, and have received considerable attention.[13]

Perhaps the most widely studied group of nutrients is the vitamins. Under conditions generally found in foods, ascorbic acid (vitamin C), thiamin (vitamin $B_1$), vitamin D, and pantothenic acid are the most heat labile.

The effect of processing on water-soluble vitamins has been reviewed by Cain.[2] Significant losses of these vitamins occur in the washing and blanching steps[14] during the canning process. Using previously published data, Schroeder[9] has concluded that, during canning operations, vitamin $B_6$ and pantothenic acid are significantly reduced (57 to 77% loss for vitamin $B_6$ and 46 to 78% loss for pantothenic acid). The thermal stability of thiamin has been reviewed by Farrer.[15]

The fat-soluble vitamins are generally less heat labile than the water-soluble vitamins. They are, however, susceptible to degradation at high temperatures in the presence of oxygen.

The effect of heat processing on trace minerals has recently been reviewed by Schroeder.[9] In conventional canning, losses of trace minerals occur in the blanching operation. Zinc, chromium, and manganese retention may be of concern in terms of availability and quantity in foods.

Because there are literally an infinite number of time/temperature combinations that can be used to achieve the objectives of a thermal process, it is difficult to generalize about the effects of thermal processing on nutrients other than to say that nutrients are destroyed. However, Tables 1, 2, and 3 summarize data presented by Lund[16] on the effects of blanching, pasteurization, and commercial sterilization processes, respectively. The wide range of reported losses of nutrients is a result of variability in methods of analysis, biological variability in initial quantity of nutrient, and variability in exact conditions of the process.

Lund[7] reviewed the effects of heat processing on nutrients and discussed recent developments in optimization of thermal processes (blanching, pasteurization, and commercial sterilization). Calculation methods used to predict destruction during these thermal processes require values for kinetic parameters that describe the rate of degradation at a reference temperature ($k_r$ or $D_r$) and the dependence of the reaction rate constant on temperature ($E_a$ or z). Table 4 summarizes available kinetic parameters which were obtained under adquately defined and controlled conditions.

Thiamin has been the most extensively studied vitamin, and Farrer[15] presented an excellent review of the literature. The Arrhenius activation energy ($E_a$) and/or reference reaction rate constant for degradation ($k_r$) appears to be dependent upon the type of product, pH, moisture, buffer salts, and oxygen. Feliciotti and Esselen[17] studied thiamin destruction in pureed meats and vegetables, and their data have been used extensively by other authors who have developed equations for predicting nutrient retention.

These kinetic parameters have been used in conjunction with equations describing the time/temperature history of the food during a thermal process to optimize the thermal process for nutrient retention. Lund[18] reviewed the considerations in optimizing thermal processes for nutrient retention, and a summary is presented in Table 5. The interesting observation is that the food processing industry generally employs thermal processes that result in maximum nutrient retention.

## ACKNOWLEDGMENT

Contribution from the College of Agricultural and Life Sciences, University of Wisconsin, Madison.

## REFERENCES

1. **Bender, A. E.**, Nutritional effects of food processing, *J. Food Technol.*, 1, 261—289, 1966.
2. **Cain, R. F.**, Water soluble vitamins: changes during processing and storage of fruits and vegetables, *Food Technol. (Chicago)*, 21, 998-1007, 1967.
3. **Cameron, E. J. and Esty, J. R.**, Canned Foods in Human nutrition, National Canners Association, Washington, D. C., 1950.
4. **Cameron, E.J., Clifcorn, L. E., Esty, J. R., Feaster, J. F., Lamb, F. C., Monroe, K. H., and Royce, R.**, Retention of Nutrients During Canning, National Canners Association, Washington, D. C., 1955.
5. **DeRitter, E.**, Stability characteristics of vitamins in processed foods, *Food Technol. (Chicago)*, 30(1), 48-51, 54, 1976.
6. **Hartman, A. M. and Dryden, L. P.**, Vitamins in Milk and Milk Products, American Dairy Science Association, Champaign, Ill., 1965.
7. **Hein, R. E. and Hutchings, I. J.**, Influence of processing on vitamin-mineral content and biological availability in processed foods, in *Nutrients in Processed Foods,* Publishing Sciences Group, Acton, Mass., 1974.
8. **Mapson, L. W.**, Effect of processing on the vitamin content of foods, *Br. Med. Bull.*, 12, 73-77, 1956.
9. **Schroeder, H. A.**, Losses of vitamins and trace minerals resulting from processing and preservation of foods, *Am. J. Clin. Nutr.*, 24, 562-573, 1971.
10. **Orr, M.**, Pantothenic acid, vitamin $B_6$ and vitamin $B_{12}$ in foods, *U.S. Dep. Agric. Home Econ. Res. Rep.*, 36, 1, 1969.
11. **Watt, B. K. and Merrill, A. L.**, Composition of Foods, Handbook No. 8, U.S. Department of Agriculture, Agricultural Research Service, Consumer and Food Economics Research Division, Washington, D. C., 1963.
12. **Goldblith, S. A.**, Thermal processing of foods: a review, *World Rev. Nutr. Diet.*, 13, 165-193, 1971.
13. **Lang, K.**, Influence of cooking in foodstuffs, *World Rev. Nutr. Diet.*, 12, 266—317, 1970.
14. **Lee, F. A.**, The blanching process, *Adv. Food Res.*, 8, 63-109, 1958.
15. **Farrer, K. H. T.**, The thermal degradation of vitamin $B_1$ in foods, *Adv. Food Res.*, 6, 257-311, 1955.
16. **Lund, D. B.**, Effects of blanching, pasteurization and sterilization on nutrients, in *Nutritional Evaluation of Food Processing,* Harris, R. S. and Karmas, E., Eds., Avi, Westport, Conn., 1975, 205-240.

17. Feliciotti, E. and Esselen, W. B., Thermal destruction rates of thiamine in pureed meats and vegetables, *Food Technol. (Chicago),* 11, 77-84, 1957.

18. Lund, D. B., Design of thermal processes for maximizing nutrient retention, *Food Technol. (Chicago),* 31 (2), 71-78, 1977.

19. Bendix, G. H., Heberlein, D. G., Ptak, L. R., and Clifcorn, L. E., Thiamine destruction in peas, corn, lima beans, and tomato juice from 104.5 to 132°C (220—270°F), *J. Food Sci.,* 16, 494-503, 1951.

20. Mulley, E. A., Stumbo, C. R., and Hunting, W. M., Kinetics of thiamine degradation by heat. A new method for studying reaction rates in model systems and food products at high temperatures, *J. Food Sci.,* 40, 985-988, 1975.

21. Gillespy, T. G., Principles of heat sterilization, in *Recent Advances of Food Sciences,* Vol. 2, Hawthorn, J. and Leitch, J. M., Eds., Butterworths, London, 1962.

22. Herrmann, J., Berechnung der Chemischen und sensorischen Veränderunger unserer Lebensmittel bei Erhitzungs — und Lagerungsporzessen, *Ernaehrungsforschung,* 15, 279-299, 1970.

23. Garrett, E. R., Prediction of stability in pharmaceutical preparations. II. Vitamin stability in liquid multivitamin preparations, *J. Am. Pharm. Assoc.,* 45, 171-178, 1956.

24. Frost, D. V. and McIntire, F. C., The hydrolysis of pantothenate. A first order reaction. Relation to thiamin stability, *J. Am. Chem. Soc.,* 66, 425—427, 1944.

25. Davidek, J., Velisek, J., and Janicek, G., Stability of inosinic acid, inosine and hypoxanthine in aqueous solutions, *J. Food Sci.,* 37, 789-790, 1972.

26. Ramakrishnan, T. V. and Francis, F. J., Color degradation in paprika, *J. Food Sci.,* 38, 25-28, 1973.

27. Taira, H., Taira, H., and Sukurai, Y., Studies on amino acid contents of processed soybean. VIII. Effect of heating on total lysine and available lysine in defatted soybean flour, *Jap. J. Nutr. Food.* 18, 359, 1973.

# EFFECT OF PROCESSING ON NUTRITIVE VALUE OF FOOD: CANNING

Frank C. Lamb, Richard P. Farrow, and Edgar R. Elkins

## EARLY NUTRITIONAL STUDIES ON CANNED FOOD

From the earliest days of nutritional research, the canning industry has been concerned with the investigation of the effect of canning on the nutritional value of its products. In 1922, Kohman[1] published survey results of the knowledge available at that time. This led to 15 years of extensive scientific investigations on the effect of commercial canning on nutritive value. References to some 17 papers resulting from these collaborative studies are given by Cameron.[2] At the time these studies were conducted, the chemical nature of many of the vitamins had not been established, and chemical and microbiological methods for their determination had not been developed. Results obtained by these early studies, consequently, were based primarily upon animal feeding studies.

Contrary to a prevalent belief at that time, these studies conclusively demonstrated that canning and heat processing did not result in the destruction of major nutrients. Colonies of rats and guinea pigs were raised for several generations on diets consisting entirely of canned foods without any impairment of their growth and longevity.[3] Comparative studies on animals fed diets consisting entirely of raw, home cooked, or canned foods showed remarkably little difference in their growth rate, reproduction, and general health.[4]

Kohman and Eddy found that vitamin C and one member of the B complex of vitamins, later identified as vitamin $B_1$ or thiamin, suffered partial loss during canning. Other vitamins and food nutrients were not found to be affected by canning. It is interesting to note that Kohman and Eddy, at an earlier date established that vitamin C underwent destruction only when oxygen was present and was not affected by heating in the absence of oxygen. Kohman et al.[5] suggested a procedure for canning tomato juice without loss of vitamin C by exclusion of air from the product during preparation. Kohman et al.[6] established that vitamin C in apples was preserved by allowing the oxygen in the tissues to be removed by natural respiration of the raw fruit when immersed in water. Much subsequent work has confirmed the accuracy of these early findings.

At the conclusion of the studies by Kohman and Eddy in 1937, a large body of information had been developed establishing the effects of canning on nutritive value; however, available quantitative analytical procedures for the vitamins did not permit accurate evaluation of the results. Information available at that time was summarized by the American Can Company[7] and revised in 1943 and in 1947.

## NUTRITION PROGRAMS ON EFFECT OF PROCESSING OF CANNED FOODS

Interest in nutritional research received an added stimulus in 1941 as a result of the National Nutrition Conference for Defense called on May 26, 1941 in Washington, D.C. At the advent of World War II the nutritional needs of the nation were brought into clear focus. As a result, a nationwide nutrition program was instituted by the canning industry under the direction of a committee of the National Canners Association and the Can Manufacturers Institute.[2] The program developed by this committee resulted in grants to nine universities that were outstanding for their competence in nutrition investigations. Work was also conducted by the National Canners Association Western Branch Laboratory and the Wisconsin Alumni Research Foundation. Additional studies were conducted by the laboratories of the American and Continental Can Companies and the Washington Laboratory of the National Canners Association.

The work was divided into two phases. Phase one consisted of a study of the nutritional value of canned foods as they were then being produced, with respect to proximate constitutents (carbohydrate, protein and fat), the minerals (calcium, phosphorus, and iron), and the known vitamins for which quantitative assay methods had been developed. The results of these studies were summarized by Cameron and Esty.[8] Phase two consisted of a study of the effect of specific canning operations on the retention of nutrients in a number of canned food products of major interest from the standpoint of their contribution to the nutritional requirements of the consuming public, and a study of possible means of improving these operations from a nutritional standpoint. Included in phase two were studies of the effect of warehouse storage of canned foods on the retention of nutrients. During the period from 1944 to 1953, a total of 45 papers were published on work sponsored by the National Canners Association - Can Manufacturers Institute (NCA-CMI). The phase two results have been summarized[9] and a complete listing of these references is given by Cameron.[2]

Certain operations of food canning such as blanching and heat processing were given special study with the objective of determining how these operations could be modified to produce the maximum retention of nutrients in canned foods. These results are reviewed below.

It also became apparent that much could be accomplished with nutritional enhancement of raw products through improved agricultural practices.[10] This involved encouragement of research on the genetic and ecological factors affecting nutritive value of the crop and improvement in methods of handling the raw product. The effect of holding raw vegetables prior to canning was studied with respect to ascorbic acid,[11] thiamin,[12] riboflavin,[13] and carotene.[14] These studies showed that of the vitamins studied, ascorbic acid was the most adversely affected by holding; the other vitamins were little affected.

Following the work sponsored by the NCA-CMI nutrition program in 1955, little additional work on the nutritional value of canned food was performed and relatively few papers were published until regulations for nutrition labeling were proposed by the U.S. Food and Drug Administration.[15] At about this same time the U.S. Department of Agriculture instituted a program of updating the nutrition information in Handbook No. 8.[16] Efforts are now under way to establish a data bank in which computerized information on nutritive value will be made available.[17,18] Harris and Karmas[19] have updated the book of Harris and Von Loesecke[19a] compiling available information on the nutritional value of processed food.

Since previous studies were performed during the period 1940 to 1955, questions have been raised concerning the effect of technological changes occurring since these studies were completed. Changes in varietal and cultural conditions and the widespread use of mechanical harvesting that have taken place during this period might also be expected to produce changes in the nutritional value of canned foods.[20] Recent surveys have been made of canned tomato juice, whole kernel corn,[21] and green beans, clingstone peaches, and sweet potatoes.[22] Heat processing and storage studies have been performed on green beans,[23] clingstone peaches,[24] and sweet potatoes.[25] In general, these studies do not indicate that significant changes have taken place in the overall nutritional value of canned foods. All studies demonstrate the high degree of variability in the nutritive value of a single product and indicate that varietal, regional, and seasonal variations must be taken into account in assessing nutritive value. As an aid to canners wishing to make voluntary nutrition labeling statements, the National Canners Association[26] has prepared guidelines for a number of canned products.

## EFFECT OF CANNING OPERATIONS ON NUTRITIVE VALUE OF FOOD

### Introduction

The major portion of the work on canned and other processed foods is devoted to the retention of two vitamins, vitamin C (ascorbic acid) and vitamin $B_1$ (thiamin), since these vitamins are the least stable during canning and processing operations. It is reasonable that work should be concentrated on these two nutrients; however, it must be noted that except for minor losses during leaching, the other nutrients are well-retained. It may be assumed that procedures resulting in good retention of ascorbic acid and thiamin will result in uniformly high retention of the other nutrients.

Primary attention will be devoted to studies performed directly on commercial canning operations rather than to laboratory-type experiments. Although useful in establishing principles, the latter experiments generally are difficult to interpret in terms of actual commercial operations.

In evaluating new or modified procedures leading to improved nutrient retention, product acceptability must be kept in mind. The advantages of better nutritional quality are nullified if the product is less acceptable to the consuming public. In many of the studies that have been conducted on improvement of nutritional value, little attention has been devoted to product acceptability.

### Juices

#### Citrus Juice

Since citrus fruits are considered one of the best sources of ascorbic acid, a considerable amount of work has been done on the retention of this vitamin during canning. Retention of ascorbic acid during canning of grapefruit juice has been reported by Moore et al.,[27] Wagner et al.,[28] Lamb,[29] and Krehl and Cowgill.[30] Similar studies on canned orange juice have been reported by Moore et al.[27] Lamb,[29] and Krehl and Cowgill.[30] All of these investigators have reported uniformly high retentions during canning. Overall retention of ascorbic acid in grapefruit juice averaged 97% in a survey of 12 canneries. An average of 98% was obtained in a study of five orange juice canneries in California and 99% at a Florida cannery. Slightly lower results were reported in a few canneries as a result of contact of hot juice with copper alloy fittings, or by holding hot juice in contact with air for a considerable period of time before canning. Studies by Lamb[29] have shown that freshly extracted grapefruit juice can be allowed to stand in contact with air for periods ranging from 2½ to 5 hr without a detectable loss of ascorbic acid. The ascorbic acid content of citrus products generally appears to be little affected by canning and processing operations. Less attention has been devoted to other vitamins in citrus juices; however, Krehl and Cowgill[30] report excellent retention of biotin, folic acid, pryridoxine, and inositol in canned grapefruit and orange juice.

#### Tomato Juice

Tomato juice, although somewhat lower than the citrus juices in vitamin C, is recognized as an important source of this vitamin. It is also an important source of vitamin A (carotene) and certain of the B vitamins. Maximum, minimum, and average retentions of these vitamins in commercially canned tomato juice are shown in Table 1. These results show that thiamin, riboflavin, and niacin are well retained in the canning of tomato juice. The retention of carotene shown by these studies was moderate,

Table 1
RETENTION OF ASCORBIC ACID, THIAMIN,
RIOFLAVIN, NIACIN, AND CAROTENE IN THE
CANNING OF TOMATO JUICE[35]

| | Number of observations | After processing[a] | | |
| --- | --- | --- | --- | --- |
| | | Maximum (%) | Minimum (%) | Mean (%) |
| Ascorbic acid | 90 | 90 | 35 | 67 |
| Thiamin | 18 | 100 | 73 | 89 |
| Riboflavin | 17 | 100 | 86 | 97 |
| Niacin | 17 | 100 | 83 | 98 |
| Carotene | 7 | 74 | 60 | 67 |

[a]    When 30 or more observations were made, the maximum and minimum retentions represent the range within which 90% of the observations were found to fall.

reflecting a loss of carotene resulting from removal of pulp during screening operations.[31] Retention of ascorbic acid was highly variable depending upon the canning procedure employed.

Later investigators have confirmed the finding as originally reported by Kohman et al.,[5] that ascorbic acid is destroyed by heat in the presence of oxygen, and that this loss can be prevented by elimination of air during the canning procedure. Studies reported by Lamb et al.,[32] Clifcorn and Peterson,[33] Clifcorn,[34] and Cameron et al.,[35] have led to the following recommendations for obtaining the maximum retention of ascorbic acid in tomato juice:

1.    Brief steaming of tomatoes prior to extraction
2.    Cold extraction of tomatoes
3.    Elimination of as much air as possible during operations subsequent to extraction
4.    Heating of the juice to its top temperature as quickly as possible
5.    Holding the juice at as low a temperature as possible unless air has been removed from it and contact with air during the holding period is eliminated
6.    Elimination of copper-containing equipment
7.    Avoidance of unnecessary pumping or handling of the juice and simplification of the canning line
8.    Shortening the time between crushing the tomatoes and sealing the juice in the cans

Unlike many other products, enzyme inactivation is not a problem with commercial canning varieties of tomatoes since it has been demonstrated that enzyme systems capable of accelerating the destruction of ascorbic acid are not present in juice extracted from these tomatoes. For purposes of optimum nutrient retention, heating of the juice is not necessary for the inactivation of enzymes. An active enzyme system causing destruction of ascorbic acid has been found in one variety of tomatoes not used for canning.[36] This possibility must be kept in mind when new varieties are introduced for canning purposes.

Practices that incorporate air into juice during the period of manufacture include discharging juice into a tank from above the surface of the juice in the tank and operating centrifugal pumps at less than full capacity. Rapid heating is advantageous in dispelling air from tomato juice before it can oxidase ascorbic acid. Clifcorn and Peterson[33] have shown that the rate of oxidation of ascorbic acid increases with increasing temperature up to about 160 to 180°F, after which it suddenly decreases, reaching zero as the boiling point is reached. Traces of copper have a catalytic effect on the oxidation of ascorbic acid; however, studies have shown that in the absence of air, copper (and other metals) have no effect on the destruction of ascorbic acid.[37,38]

Cold extraction of tomatoes (cold break) is recommended as a means of preserving the maximum amount of ascorbic acid since, even in the presence of air, oxidation takes place at a slower rate at a lower temperature. However, heating tomatoes to a high temperature (hot break) prior to extraction causes inactivation of pectic enzymes along with the production of a more viscous juice that has less tendency to separate into two phases during storage. This type of juice is generally considered to be more acceptable to consumers than a cold-break juice. A compromise must be reached, therefore, between high retention of ascorbic acid and consumer acceptability. Clifcorn and Peterson[33] showed that complete elimination of air during the extraction procedure would prevent destruction of ascorbic acid even when a hot break procedure was used. Hot-break procedures employing temperatures of 180°F or higher and rapid heating rates are now employed almost exclusively for the manufacture of tomato juice. Farrow et al.[21] have shown that a high ascorbic acid content can be obtained using modern canning procedures.

In 1974 the Food and Drug Administration (FDA) standard of identity for tomato juice was amended to permit the addition of ascorbic acid in a quantity such that there would be 10 mg of vitamin C in each fluid ounce of the juice.[39] In response to objections raised, however, the amendment was stayed indefinitely. In announcing the stay,[40] the Commissioner of Food and Drugs expressed an opinion in the *Federal Register* that tomato juice complying with the stayed amendment could be legally marketed as an unstandarized food if labeled as "Enriched with Vitamin C" or "With Added Vitamin C" and bearing a statement of all added ingredients with full nutritional labeling. A 6-oz. serving of such enriched tomato juice would contain 100% of the U.S. recommended daily allowance of vitamin C.

## Fruit

Fruit that is canned without peeling gives high retention of nutrients during canning. Guerrant et al.[41] found an average retention of 96% of the ascorbic acid of cherries and practically complete retention of carotene. Lamb et al.[32] studied the retention of unpeeled apricots canned at four levels of maturity. Ascorbic acid retention varied from 76 to 96% retention with an average of 85%. Carotene varied from 78 to 98% with an average of 89%. Although retentions were comparable between fruit of different maturies, the final concentration of both vitamins was higher in the riper fruit.

Fruit that is peeled prior to canning might be expected to show less complete retention of nutrients than unpeeled fruit. Lamb et al.[32] reported retentions of ascorbic acid, carotene, thiamin, and niacin of clingstone peaches after commercial canning at four canneries. Carotene was well retained, but ascorbic acid and thiamin decreased both after lye peeling and during the time peaches were held prior to processing. Average retentions of 72% ascorbic acid and thiamin and 88% niacin were reported after processing. More recent studies showed overall retentions of ascorbic acid, carotene, thiamin, riboflavin, and niacin of 80, 100, 85, 100, and 95%, respectively.[24] The retentions reported in these later studies did not include losses during lye peeling; however, procedures for lye peeling peaches have changed since the earlier studies were made. Peaches formerly were peeled after pit removal by immersion of the peach halves in a lye bath heated to boiling or near boiling. The modern practice is to spray the outer surfaces of the peach halves with hot, concentrated lye solution as they are passed under the spray on a belt in the cups down position. The excess lye is removed by water sprays following a brief holding period. This procedure is found to remove less of the flesh of the peach under the peel and may consequently remove less nutrients that are concentrated just under the peel.[42] Earlier studies of lye peeling losses, therefore, are not representative of modern canning practices.

Similar data are reported on freestone peaches peeled by hand after steaming.[32] Freestone peaches are no longer peeled by hand, but are lye peeled in a manner similar to clingstone peaches. Data are lacking on the effect of this change in canning procedure on nutrient retentions.

### Vegetables

Retention of nutrients during the canning of vegetables has been given a large amount of study both in the laboratory and pilot plant and in commercial canneries. The results of a number of experiments performed in commercial canneries during the period 1945 to 1950 are summarized in Table 2.

Vegetables are customarily washed and sorted to remove defective units, blanched in hot water or steam, and filled into cans. The cans are then filled with hot brine, closed in such a way as to produce a vacuum in the cans, and heat processed. Separation into various size and/or maturity classifications may be accomplished, usually by mechanical means. Studies have been made of the effect of each of these operations on the retention of nutrients.

### Effect of Blanching

Studies have shown that washing with cold or lukewarm water has little or no effect of the retention of nutrients. When vegetables are exposed to water sufficently warm to cause wilting of the tissues, leaching and oxidation of nutrients may occur.[43] This operation is referred to as blanching and has been the subject of a great deal of investigation from the standpoint of nutrient retention. The purpose of blanching for canning is primarily to drive air from the tissues and to wilt the product sufficiently for it to be filled into cans. Other purposes of blanching are to inactivate enzymes that produce undesirable changes in the vegetable and to produce modifications of color and flavor that are necessary for the production of a suitable canned product. Blanching has proved to be the step in the canning procedure most likely to produce nutrient changes. Retentions after blanching are shown for most of the vegetables in Table 2.

Certain generalizations on the effect of blanching may be made. Products such as asparagus, which have a low surface area in relation to their bulk, are not seriously affected by blanching. Products such as lima beans and peas, which consist of small units, are affected to a much greater extent by blanching. There is a considerable amount of evidence relating the size and maturity of vegetables to the losses incurred during blanching. Guerrant et al.[41] and Wagner et al.[44] have shown that maturity of green beans is the most important factor in retention of ascorbic acid and thiamin; the larger, more mature beans retaining more of these vitamins than the smaller, less mature beans. Similarly with peas, these same investigators present data showing higher retention of these vitamins in mature than in immature peas. Spinach has an extremely large surface area in relation to its mass and consequently might be expected to be affected more seriously by blanching than other products (Table 2). The effect of blanching on spinach has been studied in some detail by Lamb et al.[32]

There are a number of modifications of blanching procedure that have been investigated. Blanching may be accomplished either by immersion in hot water or by exposure to steam.[45] Losses of nutrients during blanching are the result of leaching of water-soluble substances and oxidation of oxidizable nutrients such as ascorbic acid. Steam blanching has the advantage of providing minimum leaching of water-soluble nutrients, but is of no particular advantage from the standpoint of oxidation. Whatever form of blanching is employed, it must achieve the purpose for which the operation is

Table 2

RETENTION OF ASCORBIC ACID, THIAMIN, RIBOFLAVIN, NIACIN, AND CAROTENE IN VEGETABLE CANNING[9]

| Product vitamin | After blanching | | | | After processing | | | |
|---|---|---|---|---|---|---|---|---|
| | Number of observations | Maximum (%) | Minimum (%) | Mean (%) | Number of observations | Maximum (%) | Minimum (%) | Mean (%) |
| Asparagus | | | | | | | | |
| Ascorbic acid | 26 | 100 | 74 | 95 | 32 | 100 | 80 | 82 |
| Thiamin | 12 | 100 | 79 | 92 | 31 | 85 | 60 | 67 |
| Riboflavin | 12 | 100 | 72 | 90 | 26 | 100 | 65 | 88 |
| Niacin | 8 | 100 | 77 | 94 | 22 | 100 | 77 | 96 |
| Green beans | | | | | | | | |
| Ascorbic acid | 38 | 90 | 50 | 74 | 41 | 75 | 40 | 55 |
| Thiamin | 34 | 100 | 82 | 91 | 41 | 90 | 55 | 71 |
| Riboflavin | 29 | 100 | 70 | 95 | 30 | 100 | 85 | 96 |
| Niacin | 29 | 100 | 60 | 93 | 30 | 100 | 80 | 92 |
| Carotene | — | — | — | — | 9 | 96 | 81 | 87 |
| Lima beans | | | | | | | | |
| Ascorbic acid | 12 | 83 | 54 | 72 | 10 | 100 | 60 | 76 |
| Thiamin | 12 | 77 | 36 | 58 | 15 | 67 | 32 | 47 |
| Riboflavin | 8 | 100 | 59 | 76 | 12 | 100 | 50 | 87 |
| Niacin | 8 | 98 | 68 | 81 | 11 | 100 | 77 | 85 |
| Whole kernel corn | | | | | | | | |
| Carotene | — | — | — | — | 4 | 100 | 87 | 97 |
| Thiamin | — | — | — | — | 14 | 48 | 20 | 34 |
| Riboflavin | — | — | — | — | 13 | 100 | 68 | 97 |
| Niacin | — | — | — | — | 13 | 96 | 72 | 86 |
| Peas | | | | | | | | |
| Ascorbic acid | 60 | 90 | 60 | 76 | 43 | 90 | 45 | 72 |
| Carotene | — | — | — | — | 12 | 100 | 88 | 97 |
| Thiamin | 60 | 100 | 73 | 88 | 54 | 70 | 40 | 54 |
| Riboflavin | 37 | 87 | 67 | 75 | 43 | 100 | 70 | 82 |
| Niacin | 39 | 96 | 59 | 73 | 32 | 80 | 50 | 65 |

## Table 2 (continued)
## RETENTION OF ASCORBIC ACID, THIAMIN, RIBOFLAVIN, NIACIN, AND CAROTENE IN VEGETABLE CANNING[a]

| Product vitamin | After blanching | | | | After processing | | | |
|---|---|---|---|---|---|---|---|---|
| | Number of observations | Maximum (%) | Minimum (%) | Mean (%) | Number of observations | Maximum (%) | Minimum (%) | Mean (%) |
| Spinach | | | | | | | | |
| Ascorbic acid | 21 | 78 | 39 | 61 | 21 | 62 | 34 | 52 |
| Carotene | — | — | — | — | 5 | — | — | 100 |
| Thiamin | 4 | — | — | 77 | 5 | — | — | 24 |
| Riboflavin | 4 | — | — | 81 | 5 | — | — | 76 |
| Niacin | 4 | — | — | 89 | 4 | — | — | 78 |
| Tomatoes | | | | | | | | |
| Ascorbic acid | — | — | — | — | 9 | 100 | 87 | 93 |
| Carotene | — | — | — | — | 6 | 89 | 45 | 80 |
| Thiamin | — | — | — | — | 6 | 97 | 92 | 96 |
| Riboflavin | — | — | — | — | 6 | 100 | 91 | 100 |
| Niacin | — | — | — | — | 6 | 100 | 92 | 98 |

designed and it must produce a desirable product. In comparing the effect on nutrient retention of different blanching treatments, the effect on the quality of the finished product must be taken into consideration. Unfortunately, this has not been done in many of the studies on blanching that have been conducted; consequently, the results are difficult to interpret.

Equivalent water blanches may be obtained either by increasing the temperature and decreasing the time or by increasing the time and decreasing the temperature. Wagner et al.,[46] in a study of the effects of blanching on the retention of ascorbic acid, thiamin, and niacin, found that the time of blanching had a much greater effect on the leaching of nutrients than the temperature. For example, blanching peas for 2.5 min at 170 to 180°F and at 200°F gave retentions of ascorbic acid of 86 and 91%, respectively, of 1, 2, and 3 sieve-size peas, whereas blanching for 8 min at 170 to 180°F and at 200°F gave retentions of 65 and 64%, respectively. This same study reported a retention of 100% for 5 and 6 sieve-size peas blanched for 2.5 min at either 170 to 180°F or 200°F, and a retention of 76% for the same type of peas blanched for 8 min at either 170 to 180°F or 200°F. Similar results on peas were obtained by Feaster et al.[47] in the midwestern U.S. and by Lamb et al.[48] in the northwestern U.S.

In an experiment on green beans blanched for 2 and 6 min at 160 and 210°F, Wagner et al.[46] found that the best retentions of ascorbic acid were obtained as a result of blanching for 2 min at 210°F. It would appear that less oxidation of ascorbic acid occurred at the higher temperature because of the elimination of oxygen from the blanch water and/or the inactivation of enzymes.

Most studies have shown steam blanching to be superior to water blanching from the standpoint of retention of water-soluble nutrients. Guerrant et al.[49] found that peas steam-blanched for 6 min at 210°F retained the same amount of their original ascorbic acid (75%), as compared with peas water-blanched for 3 min at 180°F, and 40% when water-blanched 12 min at 200°F. Holmquist et al.[50] showed superior retention in peas steam-blanched 1 to 3 min at 212°F as compared with water blanching for 5 min at 205°F. No superiority of retention of thiamin, riboflavin, or niacin could be demonstrated. Lamb[51] found that spinach steam blanched 2¾ min at 205°F gave an ascorbic acid retention of 97%, as compared to 55% when comparable spinach was blanched in a rotary hot water blancher for 2½ minutes at 206°F. Lamb[51] also reported that asparagus steam-blanched for 2 min at 210 to 212°F retained 96% of its ascorbic acid, whereas comparable asparagus water-blanched for 2½, 5, 10, and 20 min at 190°F retained 95, 91, 83, and 72% of its original ascorbic acid, respectively. Kramer and Smith[52] studied changes in moisture, fat, fiber, ash, carbohydrate, calcium, and phosphorus of peas, lima beans, and spinach during water and steam blanching. Changes found were minor in most instances.

Lamb[51] has shown that with spinach, the type of blanching equipment has a marked effect on nutrient retention, irrespective of the times and temperatures used. Draper blanchers gave markedly better retention of ascorbic acid and other vitamins than rotary blanchers, even though the time of blanching was much longer in the draper blanchers. The reasons given were that in a draper blancher, the spinach moves through the blancher in a thick mass and is held below the surface of the water at all times. Leaching losses are minimized since the blanch water can not freely circulate through the mass of spinach, and oxidation is kept at a minimum since air does not contact the spinach at any time. In a rotary blancher, spinach is tumbled in a revolving cylinder while subjected to hot-water sprays. Conditions for both leaching and oxidation are at a maximum with this type of equipment. In studies of peas blanched commercially in a rotary and tubular blanchers, Lamb et al.[48] found only minor differences in retention.

It might be supposed that blanching successive batches of vegetables in the same blanch water would result in better retention of water-soluble nutrients as the water becomes more nearly saturated with these substances. Guerrant et al.[49] found that five successive lots of peas blanched for 6 min at 190°F in the same blancher water showed only slightly higher retentions of ascorbic acid in the fourth and fifth blanches. These investigators concluded that successive blanching of vegetables in the same water has no practical advantages from the standpoint of nutrient retention.

Conclusions to be drawn from these studies are that nutrient retention during blanching may be improved by utilizing the shortest blanch consistent with the attainment of a high-quality product and by employing conditions permitting minimum contact with air. Temperature of blanching must be high enough (180°F or over) to quickly inactivate enzymes and to dispell air from the blanch water and product. Heberlein et al.[53] found that peas blanched for shorter periods than those commercially employed at that time did not suffer quality degradation as a result of the shorter blanching time. Steam blanching is recommended for those products whose quality is not impaired by this procedure. Asparagus is customarily steamblanched and no quality differences have been found between steam and water blanching. Wagner et al.[46] stated that the canned product prepared from steam-blanched lima beans was of inferior quality to the product prepared from water-blanched beans. The extraction of starchy material from the beans during the blanch appears to be necessary to produce a high-quality product. Steam blanching of spinach is generally considered to produce an inferior color in the final canned product, and many canners are of the opinion that a long, low-temperature blanch produces a greener and more desirable color. These results emphasize that compromise is often necessary in the selection of canning procedures that retain the maximum nutrients without sacrifice of consumer acceptability.

### Effect of Holding Between Blanching and Processing

Studies of step-by-step canning operations show that, with the exception of ascorbic acid, holding for several minutes between blanching and canning is not detrimental to the retention of nutrients. Losses of ascorbic acid were apparent in some products, and Paul et al.[54] conducted a series of studies in which peas, green beans, lima beans, spinach, and asparagus given high- (over 200°F) and low-temperature (170 to 180°F) blanches were either canned immediately or held for 15 to 30 min in air or water. Canning immediately after blanching gave the highest retention of ascorbic acid, and holding either in air or water gave generally lower values; however, the effect of these treatments was minor as compared with the blanch itself. Enzyme inactivation did not appear to be important in these studies; however, Moyer et al.[55] found that whereas adequately blanched peas could be held for as long as 2 hr without appreciable loss of ascorbic acid, peas blanched under conditions in which enzymes were not inactivated (1 to 7 min at 160°F or 1 min at 175°F) underwent "thermal maceration" with the release of enzymes causing rapid destruction of ascorbic acid. Modern canning procedures in which products are blanched sufficiently to inactivate enzymes and processed without delay do not result in significant loss even of ascorbic acid between the time of blanching and heat processing.

### Effect of Heat Processing

With the exception of thiamin and ascorbic acid, nutrients are little affected by heat processing. As originally reported by Kohman and Eddy,[5] ascorbic acid is affected by heat processing only to the extent that oxygen is present in the can. Clifcorn,[34] in a survey of the literature, reported that only ascorbic acid is affected by the type of container. Daniel and Rutherford,[56] Hauck,[57] Leuck and Pilcher,[58] McConnell et al.,[59] and Pederson and Robinson[60] have shown that in low pH products, ascorbic acid is slightly better retained in plain rather than enameled tin-plated cans or glass containers. The reason given is that in plain-bodied cans, a portion of the oxygen trapped in the can is consumed in reactions between the tin plate and fruit acids. In enameled cans and glass containers, reaction with the container is inhibited and most of the oxygen reacts with the ascorbic acid in the product.

After oxygen is consumed, further destruction of ascorbic acid occurs at a very slow rate.[61] Riester et al.[62] point out the advantages of closing the container with a minimum of air. Guerrant and O'Hara[63] and Feaster et al.[64] have shown that in nonacid products such as lima beans and peas, the type of container has no appreciable effect on the retention of ascorbic acid.

The effect of heat processing on thiamin has been the subject of extensive investigation. Bendix et al.[65] have studied factors affecting the stability of thiamin during heat processing of vegetables. Thiamin decreases as the time and temperature of processing increases. Oxygen does not appear to be a factor in thiamin destruction. More mature vegetables are found to retain more thiamin than those less mature. Thiamin is well-retained in acid products such as tomatoes by virtue of the comparatively low heat treatment required for sterilization. The advantage of high-temperature, short-time processes in obtaining the maximum retention of thiamin has been demonstrated by Feaster et al.[64] The retention of thiamin in cream-style corn increased from 40% with a conventional process to 95% with a high-temperature, short-time process using a tubular heat exchanger. Agitating processes were shown to produce better retention of thiamin in whole kernel corn than conventional still processes. More recent studies of green beans[23] and sweet potatoes[25] failed to show any significant difference between still and continuous agitating cooks on ascorbic acid, thiamin, or niacin. Lamb et al.[32] found that can size was a factor in thiamin retention in canned peas when large and small-sized cans were given the same process as a result of the slower rate of heat penetration into the large cans; however, when processes of equivalent sterilizing power were compared, little difference in retention was found. Experiments on green beans showed that slightly less thiamin was retained in No. 10 cans processed for 20 min at 250°F than in No. 303 (303 × 406) cans or 8 oz (211 × 304) cans processed for 11 min at 250°F.[23] The two processes were approximately equivalent in sterilizing value.

## Meat and Fish

Work on the effect of canning on meat and fish products has been concerned primarily with the effect of heat processing on thiamin and amino acids. Other nutrients appear to be well-retained in these products, although certain of the newer B vitamins have not been extensively investigated.

Meat and fish products are heated primarily by conduction rather than by convection as are brine-packed vegetables; hence, more heat is required for sterilization. Arnold and Evehjem,[66] Rice and Beuk,[67] and Greenwood et al.[68] have studied the effect of processing at various times and temperatures on thiamin retention. Greenwood et al.[69] have studied the so-called "core effect" on thiamin retention. Produce near the can wall receives more heat in a conduction-heated product than produce in the center of the can; hence, retention of thiamin is better in the center of the can than it is next ot the can sides. The improvement in retention of thiamin and other heat-labile nutrients depends upon the development of methods that permit rapid and uniform heating of the entire mass of the product. Certain meat products such as canned ham are not heated sufficiently to sterilize the product but depend on refrigeration to prevent spoilage. Newer techniques such as diathermal and electronic heating present a possible means of product sterilization, but commercial application of these methods has not been accomplished.

The presence of an enzyme, thiaminase, in many fish products can contribute to the destruction of thiamin.[70] Fish products packed without the removal of bones such as salmon, sardines, and mackerel may receive a somewhat longer heat treatment to render the bones edible. The nutritional value of the calcium and phosphorus derived from bones is probably greater than that of the heat-labile nutrients that may be destroyed by the extra heating.

Studies on the amino acid content of raw, precooked, and processed meat and fish products were performed by Dunn et al.[71] and Neilands et al.[72] Amino acids were determined by microbiological methods. No differences were found in any of the individual amino acids as a result of precooking and processing. It has been pointed out by several investigators[73,74] that processing can lead to a decrease in the digestability of the protein, probably resulting from cross-linkage of amino acids. These investigators show that there may be a small decrease in the nutritive value of proteins as a result of heat processing meat and fish products, but there is no serious impairment of nutritional value as a result of canning.

## EFFECT OF STORAGE ON NUTRIENT RETENTION

Numerous studies have been performed in which canned foods were stored for various times at different temperatures. Many of these studies have emphasized the effects of storage at abnormal storage temperatures (90°F and above).[75,76,77] These studies were prompted in part by the need of the armed forces to know the effect of outdoor storages in tropical climates on nutritive retention. However, a study of commercial warehouse temperatures performed by Monroe et al.[78] revealed that warehouse temperatures did not average higher than 77°F during year-round storage even in warm climates. The range of average storage temperatures varied from 58°F in New York to 77°F in New Orleans, Louisiana and Tampa, Florida. As a result of this work, storage temperature studies were conducted on canned food at 50, 65, and 80°F by Guerrant et al.,[79] Moschette et al.,[80] and Sheft et al.[81] Warehouse temperatures varied considerably, from 30 to 78°F in New York to 54 to 104°F in Yuba City, California. Retention studies of canned samples stored in these warehouses revealed that in every instance, as good or better retentions were obtained in the products stored in the commercial warehouses as were obtained in the products stored at 80°F. Apparently, large fluctuations in warehouse temperatures do not reflect temperatures in the canned products themselves. Furthermore, Riester et al.[82] demonstrated that insulation of warehouses plus judicious management to take advantage of lower night temperatures can result in a definite saving of ascorbic acid and flavor of canned citrus juices.

The controlled-temperature experiments showed that in almost every instance, storage at 50 or 65°F resulted in better than 80% retention of all nutrients after storage for 24 months. Storage at 80°F had an adverse effect on certain vitamins, particularly ascorbic acid and thiamin. The effect of high-temperature storage varies with the nature of the product and is more pronounced with acid than nonacid products.[83] Ascorbic acid undergoes anaerobic breakdown at a slow rate during storage.[61] The results in Figure 1 show that ascorbic acid in orange juice, a typical acid product, is affected much more seriously by storage at 80°F than ascorbic acid in green beans, a typical nonacid product. Similar results were obtained on the retention of thiamin at 80°F.[34] Riboflavin and carotene are affected by storage to a lesser extent, whereas niacin is largely unaffected by storage.

Riboflavin, niacin, and pantothenic acid of canned pork luncheon meat were not affected to any significant extent by storage at temperatures ranging from 45 to 98°F, whereas thiamin was adversely affected at the higher storage temperatures.[84,85] The need for cool storage of meat products containing important amounts of thiamin is indicated.

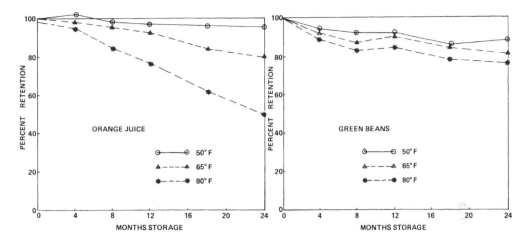

FIGURE 1.    Retention of ascorbic acid during storage of orange juice and green beans.[9]

With the advent of nutrition labeling it became important to know the retention of nutrients during storage for the estimated storage life of the product, since the label statement must represent the nutrient content at the time the product is consumed. Kramer[86] and DeRitter[87] have summarized available information on the stability of nutrients during storage under various conditions.

Retentions of protein, carbohydrate, and fat are largely unaffected by storage. Hydrolyzable carbohydrates, such as sucrose in acid products, undergo hydrolysis during storage — sucrose is converted to glucose and fructose. This has only a minor effect on nutritional value. Minerals are also unaffected by storage with the exception of iron, that increases on storage in products packed in tin-plated steel containers, and minerals such as copper that decrease in concentration as a result of electrochemical reaction with the tin plate.[88] In addition to iron, tin may increase in concentration during storage of products packed in tin-plated cans.

## FACTORS AFFECTING THE RELIABILITY OF RETENTION STUDIES ON COMMERCIALLY CANNED FOODS

As previously stated, many small-scale laboratory experiments, designed to measure retention of nutrients during various canning operations, are not representative of actual commercial conditions and lead to results that are difficult to interpret. Variations can occur in the time of holding products between treatment and analysis, the ratio of product ot blanching water, and the degree of exposure of the product to leaching and oxidation. Commercial canning usually consists of a continuous operation between dumping of the raw product and final processing, in which a steady state is reached with a relatively constant amount of product undergoing treatment at each stage of the operation. Ordinarily, the product is handled with a minimum of delay during those stages of the operation where losses of nutrients may occur. Retention studies should be performed during the period at which a steady state has been achieved and not at a time when operations are abnormal, such as at the beginning or end of a run. By careful timing of each operation, it is possible to select samples representing as nearly as possible the same type of material, but it is not always possible to confine sampling to a given lot of raw product since different lots may be mixed prior to canning. Multiple sampling over a period of time or at different times during which operations are reasonably uniform and averaging of results are generally recommended for obtaining reliable retention values.

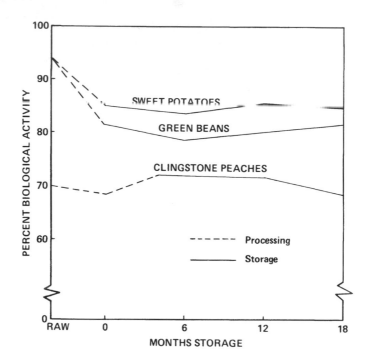

FIGURE 2.    Effect of heat processing and storage on percent biological activity of carotene in canned sweet potatoes, green beans, and clingstone peaches.[90]

Moisture changes in the product brought about by washing, blanching, etc., produce changes in the concentration of nutrients unless a correction is made. This is usually done by calculating results on a dry solids basis; however, when soluble substances are leached from a product, such as may occur during blanching, retention results calculated on a dry basis are too high. It has been pointed out by Lee[89] that retentions of carotene after blanching appear to be in excess of 100% when results are calculated on the dry basis. Lee suggested that alcohol-insoluble solids rather than total solids be used for calculation purposes. Guerrant et al.,[49] Lamb,[51] and Elkins et al.[88] investigated alcohol-insoluble solids, water-insoluble solids, and crude fiber as a basis for eliminating errors caused by leaching. Elkins et al.[88] concluded that errors produced by leaching were negligible except on products with large surface area such as spinach or on products subjected to severe blanching.

Brush et al.,[90] Kramer,[91] and Elkins et al.[88] have studied the distribution of nutrients between solid and liquid portions of canned foods. From these studies it is apparent that a significant portion of the nutrients in canned foods is present in the liquid portion and that these liquids should be utilized to obtain the maximum nutritional benefit from canned foods. Retention studies on canned food customarily include the nutrients present in the packing medium.

Retention values for carotene have been questioned by several investigators because beta carotene is known to undergo isomerization during heating with the production of isomers having less vitamin A activity than the original beta carotene. Sweeney and Marsh[92] reported that as much as 20% of the pro-vitamin A activity of green vegetables and 35% in yellow vegetables may be lost due to stereoisomerism. Weckel et al.[93] reported on stereoisomerism in canned carrots; Lee and Ammerman[94] reported varying amounts of isomerism in sweet potatoes depending upon heat processing conditions. Gebhardt et al.[95] compared the results obtained on carotene in clingstone peaches by the Association of Official Analytical Chemists (AOAC) method[96] and a modification of the Sweeney and Marsh[92] method. Figure 2 shows the effect of heat processing and storage on the percent biological activity of carotene in canned sweet potatoes, green beans, and clingstone peaches. These results show that sweet potatoes and green beans suffer a decrease of about 10% of their biological activity as a result of heat processing, whereas the biological activity of clingstone peaches does not change. None of these products underwent a significant change in vitamin A activity during storage for 18 months at ambient temperature. It would appear that the more severe heat processing required to sterilize sweet potatoes and green beans than that required for clingstone peaches causes a greater degree of isomerization. It has been noted[88] that a large proportion of the biological activity of vitamin A in clingstone peaches is produced by cryptoxanthin, a pigment having 50% of the biological activity of beta carotene; hence the biological activity of the total pigments present in raw clingstone peaches is only 70% that of beta carotene. It may be concluded from these results that previous retention values given for vitamin A in vegetables based upon analysis for carotene by the AOAC method may be slightly high because of partial isomerization of the beta carotene in the vegetable during heat processing. The retention of vitamin A in acid products such as fruits is probably not affected to any significant extent by isomerization during heat processing. Results obtained by the AOAC method may be low by exclusion of cryptoxanthin from the analysis.

An apparent increase in ascorbic acid as determined by reactions with indophenol dye during storage of canned corn and lima beans for periods greater than 9 months was reported by Guerrant et al.[77] Several investigators have reported the interference of reductones and other substances resulting from long storage.[97] Previous studies have made no correction for these substances. In view of these observations some question might be raised concerning the accuracy of retention values obtained after long storage of canned foods when indophenol methods have been used. Methods in which the effect of reductones as well as reduced iron and other interfering substances are reported to have been eliminated include the 2,4 dinitrophenylhydrazine method of Roe et al.[98] an enzymatic method,[99] and the AOAC microfluorimetric method.[97] These methods also measure dehydroascorbic acid, which, if present, would result in low values for vitamin C. Comparisons on a number of products between the indophenol titration and microfluorimetric methods reveal no difference between the methods for several canned fruit and vegetable products.[100] Significant differences were found in samples of tomato puree, tomato paste, and spinach, with the microfluorimetric method giving lower results than the dye titration method. The data presently available would indicate that ascorbic acid retention values determined by indophenol methods for most canned products stored under normal conditions are reasonably accurate. Retention values for vitamin C reported on concentrated products such as tomato puree and paste and certain vegetables, particularly when stored under unfavorable conditions, may be too high when results are obtained by the indophenol titration method. Work reported by Lamb[51] and Elkin et al.[88] indicates that dehydroascorbic acid is not present in significant amounts in canned foods. Future work on retention of vitamin C should be confirmed by a method not affected by reductones and other interfering substances.

## FUTURE STUDIES ON RETENTION OF NUTRIENTS IN CANNED FOODS

Although present studies have established with some certainty the effect of present canning procedures on the retention of nutrients in canned foods, new canning procedures and methods of handling raw products would justify further study. The use of new containers for canned foods, such as the use of pouches and processing with a minimum amount of packing media, would require evaluation of these procedures from the standpoint of nutrient retention. Procedures designed to conserve water and other natural resources could affect nutrient retention. Preliminary studies on hot-gas blanching of vegetables[101] indicate somewhat better retention of vitamin C than was obtained using conventional blanching treatments.

Improvements in methodology, such as procedures for separation and quantitative determination of certain members of the B complex of vitamins, would permit additional studies of these vitamins. Knowledge of the nutritional importance of minerals is creating renewed interest in these substances,[102] and although canning might be expected to have little effect on these minerals, their availability to humans may be affected by the canning procedure. Fiber is being given increased recognition as an essential to nutritional well being.[103] Canning may influence the quality and consequently the biological value of this substance.

Retention studies on canned foods have generally been limited to nonformulated and nonenriched products. With the increasing use of formulated and enriched products the need for additional retention studies is apparent. The application of nutrition labeling to these products requires an accurate knowledge of the effects of canning and storage on their nutrient content.

# REFERENCES

1. **Kohman, E. F.,** *Vitamins in Canned Foods,* National Canners Association, Washington, D.C., 1922, 19-L.
2. **Cameron, E. J.,** The canning industry nutrition program, *Food Technol. (Chicago),* 8, 586-592, 1954.
3. **Kohman, E. F., Eddy, W. H., and Gurin, C. Z.,** Vitamins in canned foods. XI. A canned food diet, *Ind. Eng. Chem.,* 23, 1064, 1931.
4. **Kohman, E. F., Eddy, N. H., White, M. E., and Sanborn, N. H.,** Comparative experiments with canned, home cooked, and raw food diets, *J. Nutr.,* 14, 9, 1937.
5. **Kohman, E. F., Eddy, W. H., and Gurin, C. Z.,** Vitamins in canned foods. XIII. Canning tomato juice without vitamin C loss, *Ind. Eng. Chem.,* 25, 682, 1933.
6. **Kohman, E. F., Eddy, W. H., and Carlsson, V.,** Vitamins in canned foods. II. The vitamin C destruction factor in apples, *Ind. Eng. Chem.,* 16, 1261, 1924.
7. **Anon.,** *Nutritive Aspects of Canned Foods,* American Can Company, Nutrition Laboratory, Maywood, Ill., 1947.
8. **Cameron, E. J. and Esty, J. R.,** Eds., *Canned Foods in Human Nutrition,* National Canners Association, Washington, D.C., 1950.
9. *Retention of Nutrients during Canning,* Research Laboratories, National Canners Association, Washington, D.C., 1955.
10. **Marshall, R. E. and Robertson, W. F.,** Handling and storage procedures for vegetables prior to canning, *Food Technol. (Chicago),* 2, 133, 1948.
11. **Paul, P., Einbecker, B., Kelley, L., Jackson, M., Jackson, L., Marshall, R. E., Robertson, W. F., and Ohlson, M. A.,** The nutritive value of canned foods. XXXII. Changes in ascorbic acid of vegetables during storage prior to canning, *Food Technol. (Chicago),* 3, 228, 1949.
12. **Ingalls, R., Brewer, W. D., Tobey, H. L., Plummer, J., Bennett, B. B., and Paul, P.,** The nutritive value of canned foods. XL. Changes in thiamine content of vegetables during storage prior to canning, *Food Technol. (Chicago),* 4, 264, 1950.
13. **Ingalls, R., Brewer, W. D., Tobey, H. L., Plummer, J., Bennett, B. B., and Ohlson, M. A.,** The nutritive value of canned foods. XXXVIII. Changes in riboflavin content of vegetables during storage prior to canning, *Food Technol. (Chicago),* 4, 258, 1950.
14. **Kelley, L., Bennett, B. B., Rafferty, J. P., and Paul, P.,** The nutritive value of canned foods. XLI. Changes in carotene content of vegetables during storage prior to canning, *Food Technol. (Chicago),* 4, 269, 1950.
15. **U.S. Food and Drug Administration,** Regulations for the enforcement of the federal food, drug and cosmetic act. Nutritional labeling sections 1.17 and 1.18, *Fed. Regist.,* 38, 6959, 1973.

16. Watt, B. K. and Merrill, A. L., Composition of Foods — Raw, Processed, Prepared, Agriculture Handbook No. 8, U.S. Department of Agriculture, Washington, D.C., 1963.

17. Rizek, R. L. and Murphy, E. W., Nutrient Data Bank, Paper delivered at Institute of Food Technologists Short Course, Miami, Fla., 1973.

18. Kinsella, J. E., Lipids and fatty acids in foods: quantitative data needed, *Food Technol. (Chicago),* 29, 22, 1975.

19. Harris, R. S. and Karmas, E., Eds., *Nutritional Evaluation of Food Processing,* 2nd ed., AVI Publishing, Westport, Conn., 1975.

19a. Harris, R. S. and Von Loesecke, H., *Nutritional Evaluation of Food Processing,* John Wiley & Sons, New York, 1960.

20. Lee, C. Y., Effect of cultural practices on chemical composition of processing vegetables, a review, *J. Food Sci.,* 39, 1075—1079, 1974.

21. Farrow, R. P., Lamb, F. C., Elkins, E. R., Jr., Low, N., Humphrey, J., and Kemper, K., Nutritive content of canned tomato juice and whole kernel corn, *J. Food Sci.,* 38, 595—601, 1973.

22. Humphrey, J., Kemper, K., Elkins, E. R., Coryell, P. G., and Chang, B., Nutrient Composition of Green beans, Clingstone Peaches, and Sweet potatoes, in manuscript, 1978.

23. Kemper, K., Lamb, F. C., Elkins, E. R., Humphrey, J., and Coryell, P. G., Effect of Heat Processing and Storage on the Nutrient Content of Green Beans, in manuscript, 1978.

24. Lamb, F. C., Humphrey, J., Kemper, K., Elkins, E. R., Coryell, P. G., Effect of Heat Processing and Storage on the Nutrient Content of Clingstone Peaches, in manuscript, 1978.

25. Elkins, E. R., Humphrey, J., Kemper, K., and Lamb, F. C., Effect of Heat Processing and Storage on the Nutrient Content of Sweet potatoes, in manuscript, 1978.

26. Guidelines for Preparing Nutrient Statements, (Individual Sheets for 24 Products), National Canners Association, Washington, D.C., 1974.

27. Moore, E. L., Wiederhold, E., and Atkins, C. D., Changes occurring in orange and grapefruit juices during commercial processing and subsequent storage in glass and tin-packed products, *Fruit Prod. J.,* 23, 270—275 and 285, 1944.

28. Wagner, J. R., Ives, M., Strong, F. M., and Elvehjem, C. A., Nutritive value of canned foods. IX. Effect of commercial canning and short-time storage on ascorbic acid content of grapefruit juice, *Food Res.,* 10, 469, 1945.

29. Lamb, F. C., Nutritive value of canned foods. XIX. Factors affecting ascorbic acid content of canned grapefruit and orange juices, *Ind. Eng. Chem.,* 38, 860, 1946.

30. Krehel, W. A. and Cowgill, G. R., Vitamin content of citrus products, *Food Res.,* 10, 179, 1950.

31. Strodtz, N. H., Blummer, T. E., and Clifcorn, L. E., The Retention of Carotene During the Canning of Tomato Juice, Proc. Natl. Canners Assoc. Tech. Sessions, Information Letter No. 1371, January 30, 1952, 48—49.

32. Lamb, F. C., Pressley, A., and Zuch, T., Nutritive value of canned foods. XXI. Retention of nutrients during commercial production of various canned fruits and vegetables, *Food Res.,* 12, 273, 1947.

33. Clifcorn, L. E. and Peterson, G. T., The Retention of Vitamin C in Tomato Juice, Suppl. Information Letter No. 1200, National Canners Association, January 31, 1947, 81—85.

34. Clifcorn, L. E., Factors influencing vitamin content of canned foods, in *Advances in Food Technology,* Vol. 1, Academic Press, New York, 1948.

35. Cameron, E. J., Pilcher, R. W., and Clifcorn, L. E., Nutrient retention during canned food production, *Am. J. Public Health,* 39, 756, 1949.

36. Anon., Ascorbic acid destruction factor in tomatoes, *J. Am. Diet. Assoc.,* 29, 152, 1953.

37. Hummel, M. and Okey, R., Relation of composition of canned tomato products to storage losses of ascorbic acid, *Food Res.,* 15, 405, 1950.

38. Lamb, F. C., Lewis, L. D., and White, D. G., The nutritive value of canned foods. XLIII. The effect of storage on the ascorbic acid content of canned tomato juice and tomato paste, *Food Technol. (Chicago),* 5, 269, 1951.

39. U.S. Food and Drug Administration, Tomato juice; amendment of identity standards to permit the optional use of ascorbic acid (Vitamin C), *Fed. Regist.,* 39, 20884, 1974.

40. U.S. Food and Drug Administration, Tomato juice; stay of effective date of order amending identity standards, *Fed. Regist.,* 39, 31898, 1974.

41. Guerrant, N. B., Vavich, M. G., Fardig, O. B., Dutcher, R. A., and Stern, R. M., Changes in the vitamin contents of foods during canning, *J. Nutr.,* 32, 435, 1946.

42. Schroder, G. M., Satterfield, G. H., and Holmes, A. D., Influence of variety, size, and degree of ripeness on the ascorbic acid content of peaches, *J. Nutr.,* 25, 503, 1943.

43. Adam, W. B., Horner, G., and Stanworth, J., Changes occurring during the blanching of vegetables, *J. Soc. Chem. Ind.,* 61, 96, 1942.

44. **Wagner, J. R., Strong, F. M., and Elvehjem, C. A.**, Nutritive value of canned foods. XIV. The effect of commercial canning operations on the ascorbic acid, thiamine, riboflavin, and niacin contents of vegetables, *Ind. Eng. Chem.*, 39, 985, 1947.

45. **Melnick, D., Hockberg, M., and Oser, B. L.**, Steam and hot water blanching, *Food Res.*, 9, 148, 1944.

46. **Wagner, J. R., Strong, F. M., and Elvehiem, C. A.**, Nutritive value of canned foods. XV. Effects of blanching on the retention of ascorbic acid, thiamine, and niacin in vegetables, *Ind. Eng. Chem.*, 39, 990, 1947.

47. **Feaster, J. F., Mudra, A. E., Ives, M. and Tompkins, M. D.**, Nutritive value of canned foods. XXXI. Effect of blanching time on vitamin retention in canned peas, *Canner*, 108(1), 27, 1949.

48. **Lamb, F. C., Lewis, L. D., and Lee, S. K.**, Nutritive value of canned foods. XXXV. Effect of blanching on retention of ascorbic acid and thiamine in peas, *West. Canner Packer*, 40, 6, 1948.

49. **Guerrant, N. B., Vavich, M. G., Fardig, O. B., Ellenberger, H. A., Stern, R. M., and Coonen, H. H.**, Nutritive value of canned foods. XXIII. Effect of duration and temperature of blanching on vitamin retention by certain vegetables, *Ind. Eng. Chem.*, 39, 1000—1007, 1947.

50. **Holmquist, J. W., Clifcorn, L. E., Heberlein, D. G., Schmidt, C. F., and Ritchell, E. C.**, Steam blanching of peas, *Food Technol. (Chicago)*, 8, 437, 1954.

51. **Lamb, F. C.**, Studies of Factors Affecting the Retention of Nutrients during Canning Operations, Western Branch Laboratory, National Canners Association, Berkeley, Calif., 1946.

52. **Kramer, A. and Smith, M. H.**, The nutritive value of canned foods. XXIV. Effect of duration and temperature of blanch on proximate and mineral composition of certain vegetables, *Ind. Eng. Chem.*, 39, 1007, 1947.

53. **Heberlein, D. G., Ptak, L. R., Medoff, S. and Clifcorn, L. E.**, Nutritive value of canned foods. XXIX. Quality and nutritive value of peas as affected by blanching, *Food Technol. (Chicago)*, 4, 104, 1950.

54. **Paul, P. C., Robertson, W. F., Case, W. H., and Marshall, R. E.**, Nutritive value of canned foods. XLIV. Enzyme inactivation and ascorbic acid retention in vegetables blanched and held under different conditions prior to canning, *Food Technol. (Chicago)*, 6, 464, 1952.

55. **Moyer, J. C., Robinson, W. B., Stotz, E. H., and Kertesz, Z. I.**, Effect of blanching and subsequent holding on some chemical constituents and enzyme activities in peas, snap beans and lima beans, *N.Y. Agric. Exp. Stn. Bull.*, No. 754, October 1952.

56. **Daniel, E. R. and Rutherford, M. B.**, Effect of home canning and storage on ascorbic acid content of tomatoes, *Food Res.*, 1, 341, 1936.

57. **Hauck, H. M.**, Vitamin C content of home-canned tomato juice, *J. Home Econ.*, 30, 183, 1938.

58. **Lueck, R. H. and Pilcher, R. W.**, Canning fruit juices, *Ind. Eng. Chem.*, 33, 292, 1941.

59. **McConnell, J. E. W., Esselen, W. B., Jr., and Guggenberg, N.**, Effect of storage conditions and type of container on stability of carotene in canned vegetables, *Fruit Prod. J.*, 24, 133, 1945.

60. **Pederson, C. S. and Robinson, W. B.**, The quality of sauerkraut preserved in tin and glass, *Food Technol. (Chicago)*, 6, 46, 1952.

61. **Huelin, F. E.**, Studies on the anaerobic decomposition of ascorbic acid, *Food Res.*, 15, 633, 1953.

62. **Riester, D. W., Braun, O. G., and Pearce, W. E.**, Why canned citrus juices deteriorate in storage, *Food Ind.*, 17, 742, 1945.

63. **Guerrant, N. B. and O'Hara, M. B.**, Vitamin retention in peas and lima beans after blanching, processing in tin and in glass, after storage and after cooking, *Food Technol. (Chicago)*, 7, 473—477, 1953.

64. **Feaster, J. F., Tompkins, M. D., and Ives, M.**, Retention of vitamins in low acid canned foods, *Food Ind.*, 20, 14, 1949.

65. **Bendix, G. H., Heberlein, D. G., Ptak, L. R., and Clifcorn, L. E.**, Factors influencing the stability of thiamine during heat sterilization, *Food Res.*, 16, 494, 1951.

66. **Arnold, A. and Elvehjem, C. A.**, Processing and thiamine, *Food Res.*, 4, 547, 1939.

67. **Rice, E. E. and Beuk, J. F.**, Decomposition of thiamine in pork, *Food Res.*, 10, 99, 1945.

68. **Greenwood, D. A., Beadle, B. W., and Kraybill, H. R.**, Stability of thiamine to heat. II. Effect of meat-curing ingredients in aqueous solutions in meat, *J. Biol. Chem.*, 149, 349, 1943.

69. **Greenwood, D. A., Kraybill, H. R., Feaster, J. F. and Jackson, J. M.**, Vitamin retention in processed meat. Effect of thermal processing. *Ind. Eng. Chem.*, 36, 922, 1944.

70. **Deutsch, H. F. and Hasler, A. D.**, Distribution of vitamin B$_1$ - destruction enzyme in fish, *Proc. Soc. Exp. Biol. Med.*, 53, 63, 1943.

71. **Dunn, M. S., Camien, M. N., Eiduson, S., and Malin, R. B.**, The nutritive value of canned foods. XXXIII. I. Amino acid content of fish and meat products, *J. Nutr.*, 39, 177, 1949.

72. **Neilands, J. B., Sirny, R. J., Sohljell, I., Strong, F. M., and Elvehjem, C. A.**, The nutritive value of canned foods. XXXIII. II. Amino acid content of fish and meat products, *J. Nutr.*, 39, 187, 1949.

73. **Beuk, J. F., Chornock, F. W., and Rice, E. E.**, Effect of severe heat treatment on the amino acids of fresh and cured pork, *J. Biol. Chem.*, 175, 291, 1948.

74. **Mayfield, H. L. and Hedrich, M. T.**, Effect of canning, roasting, and corning on the biological value of the proteins of western beef, finished on either grass or grain, *J. Nutr.*, 37, 487, 1949.

75. **Brenner, S., Wodicka, V. O., and Dunlap, S. G.**, Effect of high temperature storage on the retention of nutrients in canned foods, *Food Technol. (Chicago)*, 2, 207, 1948.

76. **Feaster, J. F., Tompkins, M. D., and Pearce, W. E.**, Effect of storage on vitamins and quality of canned foods, *Food Res.*, 14, 25, 1949.

77. **Guerrant, N. B., Vavich, M. G., and Dutcher, R. A.**, Nutritive value of canned foods. XIII. Influence of temperature and time of storage on vitamin contents, *Ind. Eng. Chem.*, 37, 1240—1243, 1945.

78. **Monroe, K. H., Brighton, K. W., and Bendix, G. H.**, Nutritive value of canned foods. XXVIII. Some studies of commercial warehouse temperature with reference to the stability of vitamins in canned foods, *Food Technol. (Chicago)*, 3, 292, 1949.

79. **Guerrant, N. B., Fardig, O. B., Vavich, M. G., and Ellenberger, H. E.**, Nutritive value of canned foods. XXVII. Influence of temperature and time of storage on vitamin content, *Ind. Eng. Chem.*, 40, 2258—2263, 1948.

80. **Moschette, D. S., Hinman, W. F., and Halliday, E. G.**, Nutritive value of canned foods. XXII. Effect of time and temperature of storage on vitamin content of commercially canned fruits and fruit juices (stored 12 months), *Ind. Eng. Chem.*, 39, 994, 1947.

81. **Sheft, B. B., Griswold, R. M., Tarlowsky, E., and Halliday, E. G.**, Nutritive value of canned foods. XXVI. Effect of time and temperature of storage on vitamin content of commercially canned fruits and fruit juices (stored 18 and 24 months), *Ind. Eng. Chem.*, 41, 144, 1949.

82. **Riester, D. W., Wiles, G. D., and Coates, J. L.**, Temperature variations in warehousing citrus juice, *Food Ind.*, 20, 372, 1948.

83. **Freed, M., Brenner, S., and Wodick, V. O.**, Prediction of thiamin and ascorbic acid stability in stored canned foods, *Food Technol. (Chicago)*, 3, 148, 1949.

84. **Feaster, J. F., Jackson, J. M., Greenwood, D. A., and Kraybill, H. R.**, Vitamin retention in processed meat—effect of storage, *Ind. Eng. Chem.*, 38, 87, 1946.

85. **Rice, E. E. and Robinson, H. E.**, Nutritive value of canned and dehydrated meat products, *Am. J. Public Health*, 34, 587, 1944.

86. **Kramer, A.**, Storage retention of nutrients, *Food Technol. (Chicago)*, 28, 50, 1974.

87. **DeRitter, E.**, Stability characteristics of vitamins in processed foods, *Food Technol. (Chicago)*, 30, 48, 1976.

88. **Elkins, E. R., Kemper, K., and Lamb, F. C.**, Investigation to Determine the Nutrient Content of Canned Fruits and Vegetables, Final Report Contract USDA-ARS-12-14-11054 (62), National Canners Association Research Foundation, Washington, D.C., 1976.

89. **Lee, F. A.**, Vitamin retention in blanched carrots. Alcohol-insoluble solids as a reference base, *Ind. Eng. Chem. Anal. Ed.*, 17, 719, 1945.

90. **Brush, M. K., Himan, W. F., and Halliday, E. G.**, The nutritive value of canned foods. V. Distribution of water soluble vitamins between solid and liquid portions of canned vegetables and fruits, *J. Nutr.*, 28, 131, 1944.

91. **Kramer, A.**, The nutritive value of canned foods. VIII. Distribution of proximate and mineral nutrients in the drained and liquid portions of canned vegetables, *J. Am. Diet. Assoc.*, 21, 354, 1945.

92. **Sweeney, J. P. and Marsh, A. C.**, Vitamins and other nutrients, *J. Assoc. Off. Anal. Chem.*, 53(5), 937, 1970.

93. **Weckel, K. G., Santons, B., Hernan, E., Laferriere, L., and Gabelman, W. H.**, Carotene components of frozen and processed carrots, *Food Technol. (Chicago)*, 16, 91, 1962.

94. **Lee, W. G. and Ammerman, G. R.**, Carotene sterioisomerism in sweet potatoes as affected by rotating and still retort canning processes, *J. Food Sci.*, 39, 1188—1190, 1974.

95. **Gebhardt, S. E., Elkins, E. R., and Humphrey, J.**, Comparison of two methods for determining the vitamin A value of clingstone peaches, *J. Agric. Food Chem.*, 25, 629-632, 1977.

96. *Official Methods of Analysis*, 12th ed., Horwitz, W., Ed., Association of Official Analytical Chemists, Washington, D.C., 1975.

97. **Freed, H.**, *Method of Vitamin Assay*, 3rd ed., Interscience, New York, 1966, 287.

98. **Roe, J. H., Mills, M. B., Oesterling, M. J. and Damron, C. M.**, The determination of diketo-1-gluonic acid, dehydro-1-ascorbic acid, and L-ascorbic acid in the same tissue extract by the 2-4-dinitrophenylhydrazine method, *J. Biol. Chem.*, 174, 201, 1948.

99. **Marchesini, A., Montuori, F., Muffato, D., and Maestri, D.**, Application and advantages of the enzymatic method for the assay of ascorbic acid, and dehydroascorbic acid, and reductones. Determination in fresh and canned spinach, *J. Food Sci.*, 39, 568, 1974.

100. The NCA Research Laboratories in 1975 Review of Technical Issues and Research Progress, National Canners Association, Berkeley, Calif., 1975, 62.

101. **Ralls, J. W. and Mercer, W. A.**, Continuous In-plant Hot-gas Blanching of Vegetables, EPA-660/ 2-74-091, National Environmental Research Center, Office of Research and Development, U.S. Environmental Protection Agency, Corvallis, Ore., 1974.
102. **Nielsen, F. H.**, "Newer" trace elements in human nutrition, *Food Technol. (Chicago)*, 28, 38, 1974.
103. **Scala, J.**, Fiber, the forgotten nutrient, *Food Technol. (Chicago)*, 28, 34, 1974.

# EFFECT OF PROCESSING ON NUTRITIVE VALUE OF FOOD: FREEZING*

Owen Fennema

## INTRODUCTION

The freezing process consists of prefreezing treatments, freezing, frozen storage, and thawing. This method of long-term food preservation is generally regarded as superior to canning or dehydration when judged on the basis of retention of sensory attributes and nutritive properties. This in no way suggests, however, that the freezing process is perfect, since it is well known that significant amounts of some vitamins are lost during the freezing process. Losses of nutrients during freeze processing can result from physical separation (e.g., peeling and trimming during the prefreezing period or exudate loss during thawing), leaching (especially during blanching), or chemical degradation. The degree of concern given to these losses logically depends on the nutrient, i.e., whether it is abundant or meager in the total average diet and on the importance of the food in the average diet, i.e., whether or not the food is generally relied on as a major source of the nutrient in question.

Attention in this chapter will be limited to fruits, fruit juices, vegetables, and animal tissues, since these categories comprise the majority of foods that are commercially frozen in addition to being the most important frozen foods from a nutritional standpoint. Furthermore, only vitamins and minerals will be considered, since existing evidence indicates that the freezing process, as used commercially, has no significant detrimental effect on nutritive values of lipids, carbohydrates, and proteins.[1]

Changes in the vitamin and mineral contents of major food classes will be considered for each separate stage of the freezing process as well as for the overall freezing process. Although most of the important literature has been reviewed, total coverage is not claimed.

Because of the results available, emphasis will be given to vitamin C in fruits and vegetables and to B vitamins in animal tissues. Values of vitamin C reported in this paper refer to reduced L-ascorbic acid. Vitamin C and thiamin ($B_1$) have been studied extensively since they are water-soluble (cannot be stored in the body and are subject to leaching during processing), are highly susceptible to chemical degradation, are present in many foods, are required in the diet, and are sometimes deficient in the diet. If these vitamins are well retained, it generally can be assumed that other nutrients are also well retained.

When considering the various data that follow, it is important to note that the reference value used for calculating nutrient losses differs depending on the phase of the freezing process that is under consideration. For example, blanching losses are based on the difference in nutrient content between blanched and fresh products, freezing losses in vegetables are based on the difference in nutrient content between blanched-frozen-unstored and blanched-unfrozen products, storage losses are based on the difference in nutrient content between frozen-stored and frozen-unstored products, etc. This is mentioned so that improper conclusions will be avoided. For example, if a given product loses 20% of its vitamin C content during blanching and another 20% of its vitamin C content during frozen storage, the "absolute amounts" of vitamin C lost during these two phases will not be the same, since the calculations are based on different reference values.

* Contribution from the College of Agricultural and Life Sciences, University of Wisconsin-Madison, Madison, Wis.

One final introductory comment is worthy of mention. It is occasionally reported that increases in some vitamins occur during the freezing process. In some instances, this can be attributed to analytical errors or to biological variability; however, there are instances where the increases are too large to be accounted for in this manner. In such instances, it has been suggested that the freezing process releases bound, biologically inactive forms of the vitamin, or converts inactive precursors to the active vitamin. More detailed information on the subject matter covered here is contained in an earlier review.[2]

## LOSSES OF NUTRIENTS DURING PREFREEZING OPERATIONS

Losses of vitamins from fruits and animal tissues during the holding period following harvest or slaughter and prior to freezing are slight, provided the product is maintained at a low nonfreezing temperature and the storage time is limited to no more than a few days.[3-6]

Prior to freezing, most vegetables are blanched to inactivate enzymes that would otherwise result in unacceptable changes in sensory properties and nutritive value during frozen storage. Blanching, particularly when done by immersing the product in hot water, can result in substantial losses of some water-soluble vitamins. Losses of vitamin C during water blanching and cooling of eight common vegetables can range from 1 to 76%, with 20 to 25% losses being typical for green beans, lima beans, Brussels sprouts, cauliflower, and green peas (Table 1). Losses of vitamin C from asparagus are generally less than for other vegetables listed in Table 1, and losses of vitamin C from broccoli and spinach are generally larger than for other vegetables in Table 1.

Losses of vitamin $B_1$ during water blanching and cooling can range from 0 to 80%, with losses of 9 to 11% being typical for green beans and green peas, and considerably larger losses being typical for lima beans and spinach (Table 1).

Water blanching also causes approximately a 30%[14-53] loss of niacin from lima beans,[14,22-23] a 19%[14-24] loss of riboflavin from green peas,[14,16,23,39] a 14%[11-17] loss of riboflavin from green beans,[13,16,19,39] and no significant loss of carotene from broccoli, green peas, green beans, corn, Brussels sprouts, spinach, squash, collards, kale, beet greens, endive, carrots, and sweet potatoes.[14,23,40,42-43]

Losses of water-soluble vitamins during blanching occur primarily by leaching rather than by chemical degradation. This is borne out by the behavior of broccoli and spinach. Both of these products have large surface-to-mass ratios that favor leaching, and both exhibit very large losses of vitamin C during water blanching.

Substantially smaller losses of water-soluble vitamins and most minerals generally occur during steam blanching rather than during water blanching.[8,14,20-21,27,30,33,44-47] This is particularly true when products with large surface-to-mass ratios are being blanched, and when steam blanching is followed by a method of cooling that does not involve liquid water (e.g., air cooling).

## LOSSES OF NUTRIENTS DURING FREEZING

With the possible exception of pork[48,49] and Brussels sprouts,[29] freezing generally has no significant effect on the vitamin contents of vegetables,[7,12,18,22-24,36,40,50-51] fruits,[52-53] and animal tissues.[54-57]

## LOSSES OF NUTRIENTS DURING FROZEN STORAGE

Substantial losses of vitamins can occur during frozen storage of food tissues, and the magnitude of loss depends on the product, prefreezing treatments (especially

Table 1
## LOSS OF VITAMINS C AND B₁ FROM VEGETABLES DURING BLANCHING AND COOLING[a]

| | Loss of vitamins (mean % and range) | | |
|---|---|---|---|
| Product | Vitamin C | Vitamin B₁ | Ref. |
| Asparagus | 10 (6—15) | — | 7—8 |
| Beans, green | 23 (12—42) | 9 (0—14) | 7—21 |
| Beans, lima | 24 (19—40) | 36 (20—67) | 14, 22—26 |
| Broccoli | 36 (12—50) | — | 7—8, 12, 15, 20, 27—28 |
| Brussels sprouts | 21 (9—45) | — | 7—8, 29, 30 |
| Cauliflower | 20 (18—25) | — | 7—8, 21 |
| Peas, green | 22 (1—35) | 11 (1—36) | 9, 14—16, 20, 23—24, 26—27, 31—39 |
| Spinach | 50 (40—76) | 60 (41—80) | 9, 12, 14-15, 20, 38, 40—41 |

[a]  Each value represents the vitamin content after cooling or after freezing, as compared to the vitamin content of the fresh product. The effect of freezing has been shown to be neglibible. Most of the data involve water blanching and cooling.

From Fennema, O., *Nutritional Evaluation of Food Processing*, Harris, R. S. and Karmas, E., Eds., AVI Publishing, Westport, Conn., 1975, 246. With permission.

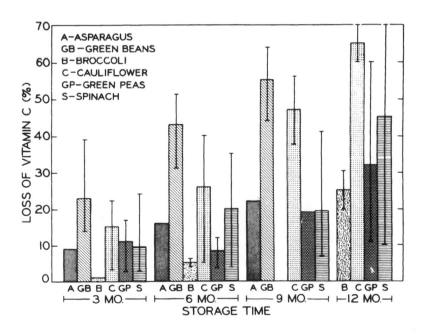

FIGURE 1.  Cumulative losses (after completion of freezing) of vitamin C from vegetables during storage at −18°C (means plus ranges). References: Asparagus (reduced ascorbic acid plus dehydro-ascorbic acid),[7,61-62] broccoli,[7,12,61] cauliflower (reduced ascorbic acid plus dehydro-ascorbic acid),[7,21,61-62] green peas,[9,23-24,63,65-66] and spinach,[9,12,61,65-69] (From Fennema, O., *Nutritional Evaluation of Food Processing*, Harris, R. S. and Karmas, E., Eds., AVI Publishing, Westport, Conn., 1975, 249. With permission.)

## Table 2
## APPROXIMATE LOSSES OF VITAMINS AND MINERALS FROM VEGETABLES DURING FROZEN STORAGE

Loss of nutrients during 12 months at −18°C (%)

| Product | B$_1$ | B$_2$ | Niacin | B$_6$ | Vitamin K | Folic acid | Pantothenic acid | Carotene | Fe | Other[a] minerals | Ref. |
|---|---|---|---|---|---|---|---|---|---|---|---|
| Beans, green | 0—32 | 0 | 0 | 0—21 | 0 | 6 | 53 | 0—23 | 18 | 0 | 10,31,63,69-72 |
| Beans, lima | — | 45 | 26 | 0 | — | — | — | — | — | — | 23,71 |
| Broccoli | — | — | — | 0 | 6 | — | — | 0 | — | — | 72-73 |
| Cabbage | — | — | — | 0 | 0 | — | — | — | — | — | 71-72 |
| Peas, green | 0—16 | 0—8 | 0—8 | 7 | — | 0 | 29 | 0—4 | 20 | 0 | 23,31,39,42,63, 70 |
| Spinach | — | 0 | — | — | 42 | — | — | — | — | — | 39,72 |

[a]  P, Mg, Ca, K, Na.

From Fennema, O., *Nutritional Evaluation of Food Processing*, Harris, R. S. and Karmas, E., Eds., AVI Publishing, Westport, Conn., 1975, 250. With permission.

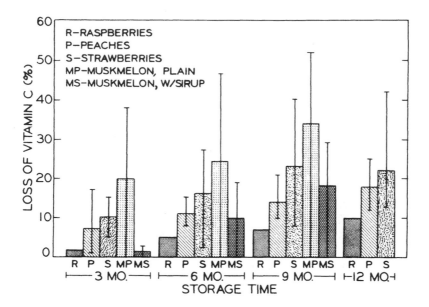

FIGURE 2. Cumulative losses (after completion of freezing) of vitamin C from fruits during storage at −18°C (means plus ranges). References and conditions: Muskmelon — two varieties, sliced, packaged in cellophane-lined pint containers.[60] Peaches — sliced, in syrup, various packages.[61,74,78-79] Raspberries — whole, 3 + 1 part 50% sucrose syrup, retail composite cartons.[80] Strawberries — whole or sliced, sugared or plain, various packages.[61,63-64,74,81-82] (From Fennema, O., *Nutritional Evaluation of Food Processing*, Harris, R. S. and Karmas, E., Eds., AVI Publishing, Westport, Conn., 1975, 263. With permission.

blanching), the type of packaging,[58-59] the type of pack (e.g., with or without syrup),[60] and the storage conditions.

Losses of vitamin C from vegetables stored at −18°C (Fgiure 1) can be substantial, and the extent of loss depends greatly on the product and on storage time. Losses of vitamins other than vitamin C from vegetables stored for 12 months at −18°C range from negligible to large depending on the vitamin and the product (Table 2). Iron is the only mineral for which significant losses have been reported, and this result is probably an analytical inaccuracy rather than a real loss.

Losses of vitamins C, $B_1$, and $B_2$ during frozen storage are usually considerably less in blanched vegetables than in unblanched. For example, some investigators have reported that blanched green beans and spinach stored 9 to 12 months at −19°C lose only 25 to 50% as much vitamin C as comparable unblanched products.[9,11] However, it is not necessarily true that losses incurred by blanching are compensated for by the reduction in losses that would otherwise occur during frozen storage. Such compensation is especially unlikely when products are stored for only a short time at −18°C or lower.

A further point of interest concerns the effect of subfreezing temperatures on the rate of vitamin C degradation in vegetables. The behavior of products for which reasonably good data are available (green beans, cauliflower, green peas, and spinach) indicates that a 10°C rise in temperature, within the range −18 to −7°C, causes the rate of vitamin C degradation to accelerate by a factor of 6 to 20 times ($Q_{10} = 6$ to 20).[2,24,44,62,67-68,74-77] This is an uncommonly large dependence on temperature. Thus, decreases in storage temperature over the range −7 to −18°C will decrease losses of vitamin C in vegetables to a much greater extent than might be predicted based on a normal relationship between reaction rate and temperature.

Table 3

LOSS OF B-VITAMINS FROM ANIMAL TISSUES DURING
FROZEN STORAGE

Loss of vitamins during 6 months storage at −18°C (%)[a]

| Product | B₁ | B₂ | Niacin | Pantothenic acid | Pyridoxine | Ref. |
|---------|----|----|--------|------------------|------------|------|
| Beef steaks[b] | 0 | <1 | + | <10 | 22 | 56 |
| Pork, chops and roasts | + to 18 | 0—37 | + to 5 | 0—8 | 18[b] | 5,48-49 |
| Lamb chops | + | — | + | — | — | 85 |
| Oysters[b] | 33 | 19 | 3 | 17 | 59 | 54 |

[a]    Independent effect of storage except some values include effect of thawing. + indicates an apparent increase in vitamin content.

[b]    Data are of limited value since only one study is involved.

From Fennema, O., *Nutritional Evaluation of Food Processing,* Harris, R. S. and Karmas, E., Eds., AVI Publishing, Westport, Conn., 1975, 272. With permission.

Table 4

LOSS OF VITAMIN C FROM VARIOUS VEGETABLES DURING
THE ENTIRE FREEZING PROCESS[a]

| Product | Typical amount of vitamin C in fresh product[101] (mg/100g) | Loss of vitamin C during 6 to 12 months at −18°C (mean percent and range) | Ref. |
|---------|-----------------------------------------------------------|--------------------------------------------------------------------------|------|
| Asparagus | 33 | 12 (12—13) | 7,27 |
| Beans, green | 19 | 45 (30—68) | 7,9-10,12,21,68 |
| Beans, lima | 29 | 51 (39—64) | 23-24 |
| Broccoli | 113 | 49 (35—68) | 7,12,27 |
| Cauliflower | 78 | 50 (40—60) | 7,21 |
| Peas, green | 27 | 43 (32—67) | 9,23-24, 27 |
| Spinach | 51 | 65 (54—80) | 9,12,91 |

[a]    Simulated commercial conditions.

From Fennema, O., *Nutritional Evaluation of Food Processing,* Harris, R. S. and Karmas, E., Eds., AVI Publishing, Westport, Conn., 1975, 254. With permission.

Losses of vitamin C from fruits stored at −18°C (Figure 2) can be substantial, and the extent of loss depends greatly on the time of storage, the type of product, the type of packaging, and the style of pack (e.g., with or without syrup). Losses of vitamin C from citrus juice concentrates during storage for 9 to 12 months at −18°C usually are less than 5%.[60,63,83-84]

Reminiscent of the situation with frozen vegetables, rates of vitamin C degradation in some frozen fruits are highly temperature dependent. Thus for some peaches, boysenberries, and strawberries, a 10°C rise in temperature in the range of −18 to −7°C causes the rate of vitamin C degradation to increase by a factor of 30 to 70 times ($Q_{10}$ = 30 to 70).[2,59,74,79,82]

Losses of B vitamins from animal tissues stored for 6 months at −18°C are shown in Table 3. With the exception of pyridoxine, losses tend to range from moderate to small. The data are limited, however, and any general conclusion should be accepted with caution.

Table 5
## LOSS OF VITAMIN C FROM FRUITS DURING THE ENTIRE FREEZING PROCESS

| Product | Storage time at −18°C (months) | Loss of vitamin C (%) | Ref. |
|---|---|---|---|
| Strawberries | | | |
| 44 brands "as purchased" | ? | 45 (9—85)[a] | 92 |
| 17 varieties, slices, sugared, in metal cans | 5 | 17 (0—44) | 3 |
| Puree, 5 + 1 or 3 + 1 sugar | 6 | 16 | 60 |
| Whole, no syrup or sugar, in polyethylene bags | 10 | 34 | 81 |
| Partially sliced, 6 + 1 sugar, polyethylene boxes | 10 | 42 | 64 |
| Citrus products | | | |
| Orange juice concentrate 42° Brix | 9 | 1 | 93 |
| Orange juice, unconcentrated | 6 | 32 | 94 |
| Orange segments | 6 | 31 | 94 |
| Grapefruit juice concentrate 42° Brix | 9 | 5 | 93 |
| Grape fruit sections | | | |
| Plain | 9 | 4 | 60 |
| With syrup | 9 | 4 | 60 |
| Apricots in Syrup | 5 | 19 | 95 |
| Apricots in Syrup + Added Vitamin C | 5 | 22 | 95 |
| Cantaloupes | | | |
| In syrup | 5-9 | 9—44 | 60,95 |
| In syrup + added vitamin C | 5 | 23 | 95 |
| Plain | 9 | 65—85 | 60 |
| Cherries | | | |
| Sweet, pitted, in syrup, with or without added vitamin C and citric acid | 10 | 19 (11—28) | 96 |
| Peaches | | | |
| Sliced, in syrup, with added vitamin C, 12 varieties | 8 | 23 (12—40) | 95-96 |
| Sliced, in syrup, 12 varieties, moisture-proof containers | 8 | 69 (38—82) | 96 |
| Sliced, in syrup, in glass jars | 5 | 29 | 95 |

[a]   Based on estimated initial concentration of 60 mg vitamin C per 100 g of product.

From Fennema, O., *Nutritional Evaluation of Food Processing,* Harris, R. S. and Karmas, E., Eds., AVI Publishing, Westport, Conn., 1975, 267. With permission.

## Table 6
## LOSS OF VITAMINS FROM ANIMAL TISSUES DURING THE ENTIRE FREEZING PROCESS

| Product | Storage conditions | Loss of B vitamins (%) | | | | | |
| --- | --- | --- | --- | --- | --- | --- | --- |
| | | $B_1$ | $B_2$ | Niacin | Pantothenic acid | Pyridoxine | Ref. |
| Beef liver, sliced | 60 Days (−20°C) | 32 | 35 | + | — | — | 56 |
| Beef steak, l. dorsi | 6 Month (−18°C) | 8 | 9 | 0 | 8 | 24 | 57 |
| | 10—12 Months (−18°C) | 2 | 43 | 4 | — | — | 57 |
| Beef (l. dorsi and semimembranosus) | 3 Years (−18°C, un-aged) | +34 | +9 | 20 | — | — | 4 |
| | 3 Years (−18°C, aged) | 3 | +8 | +1 | — | — | 4 |
| Pork loins[a] | 1 Year (−18°C) | 11 | +44 | +14 | +6 | — | 97 |
| Poultry, fowls, whole | 8 Months (−18°C) | | | | | | |
| Light meat | | 12 | 3 | +10 | — | — | 98 |
| Dark meat | | 42 | 11 | 0 | — | — | 98 |
| Poultry, less than 84 days old | 8—12 Months (−18°C) | | | | | | |
| Breast | | 16 | 0 | 9 | — | — | 99 |
| Leg | | 5 | 33 | 22 | — | — | 99 |
| Turkeys, 27—36 weeks old | 3 Months (−23°C) | | | | | | |
| Breast | | 0 | 8 | 0 | — | — | 100 |
| Leg | | 18 | 0 | 0 | — | — | 100 |
| Oysters[a] | 6 Months (−18°C) | 22 | 0 | 35 | + | 46 | 54 |

*Note:* Values may or may not include thawing.

[a] Data are highly variable.

From Fennema, O., *Nutritional Evaluation of Food Processing*, Harris, R. S. and Karmas, E., Eds., AVI Publishing, Westport, Conn., 1975, 277. With permission.

A few studies have dealt with nutrient losses during frozen storage of food at fluctuating temperatures as compared to storage at comparable constant temperatures. Results from these studies indicate that losses of vitamins do not differ significantly between the two conditions.[76,86-88]

## LOSSES OF NUTRIENTS DURING THAWING

Only a few studies have been conducted that enable the independent effect of thawing on the nutritive value of food tissues to be determined. The results of these studies tend to indicate that thawing has a small and probably insignificant effect on the vitamin contents of vegetables,[19,34,50,89] fruits,[83,90] and animal tissues.[55,56] Thaw exudate will contain water-soluble vitamins and minerals, however, so losses of these nutrients will be proportional to the amount of thaw exudate, if the thaw exudate is discarded.

## LOSSES OF NUTRIENTS DURING THE ENTIRE FREEZING PROCESS

Shown in Table 4 are losses of vitamin C from seven important vegetables during the entire freezing process (based on differences in the vitamin C contents of fresh products and products that were blanched, frozen, and stored for 6 to 12 months at $-18°C$). Losses differ among products and among different lots and cultivars of the same product. With the exception of the small and large loss values for asparagus and spinach, respectively, losses average about 50%. Losses of vitamin C from vegetables during the entire freezing process are largely attributable to blanching (especially water blanching) and to prolonged frozen storage (6 to 12 months) when this occurs.

Shown in Table 5 are losses of vitamin C from several fruits and fruit juices during the entire freezing process. Losses vary greatly depending on the type of product, the cultivar,[86] whether or not syrup is present, the solids content of juices, and the type of package. Most of the popular fruits, when processed in a recommended manner, lose less than 30% of their original vitamin C contents during the entire freezing process, and concentrated citrus juices lose less than 5%. Most of these losses occur during frozen storage.

Losses of B vitamins from animal tissues during the entire freezing process are shown in Table 6. Changes in thiamin content range from +34% to −42%, changes in riboflavin content range from +44% to −43%, changes in niacin content range from +14% to −35%, and based on limited data, changes in pantothenic acid content range from +6% to −8% and changes in pyridoxine content range from −24% to −46%. Most of the losses listed above occur during frozen storage and thawing (thaw exudate) of the animal tissues.

Additional values for losses of nutrients from foods during the entire freezing process can be computed from data in Agricultural Handbook No. 456.[101] Absolute values for nutrient contents of frozen foods are available in the reference just cited and in reports by Burger et al.[102] and Lowenberg and Wilson.[103]

## REFERENCES

1. **De Groot, A. P.,** The influence of dehydration of foods on the digestibility and the biological value of the proteins. *Food Technol. (Chicago),* 17, 339—343, 1963.
2. **Fennema, O.,** Effects of freeze-preservation on nutrients, in *Nutritional Evaluation of Food Processing,* Harris, R. S. and Karmas, E., Eds., AVI Publishing, Westport, Conn., 1975, 244—288.

3. **Scott, L. E. and Schrader, A. L.**, Ascorbic acid content of strawberry varieties before and after processing by freezing, *Proc. Am. Soc. Hortic. Sci.*, 50, 251—253, 1947.
4. **Meyer, B., Mysinger, M., and Buckley, R.**, The effect of three years of freezer storage on the thiamin, riboflavin, and niacin content of ripened and unripened beef, *J. Agric. Food Chem.*, 11, 525—527, 1963.
5. **Westerman, B. D., Oliver, B., and Mackintosh, D. L.**, Influence of chilling rate and frozen storage on B-complex vitamin content of pork, *J. Agric. Food Chem.*, 3, 603—605, 1955.
6. **Gkinis, A. M.**, Changes in Food Tissues at High Subfreezing Temperatures, Ph.D. dissertation, University of Wisconsin, Madison, 1976.
7. **Gordon, J. and Noble, I.**, Effects of blanching, freezing, freezing-storage, and cooking on ascorbic acid retention in vegetables, *J. Home Econ.*, 51, 867—870, 1959.
8. **Nobel, I. and Gordon J.**, Effect of blanching method on ascorbic acid and color of frozen vegetables, *J. Am. Diet. Assoc.*, 44, 120—123, 1964.
9. **Bedford, C. L. and Hard, M. M.**, The effect of cooling method on the ascorbic acid and carotene content of spinach, peas, and snap beans preserved by freezing, *Proc. Am. Soc. Hortic. Sci.*, 55, 403—409, 1950.
10. **Dawson, E. H., Reynolds, H., and Toepfer, E. W.**, Home-canned versus home-frozen snap beans, *J. Home Econ.*, 41, 572—574, 1949.
11. **Farrell, K. T. and Fellers, C. R.**, Vitamin content of green snap beans. Influence of freezing, canning, and dehydration on the content of thiamin, riboflavin, and ascorbic acid, *Food Res.*, 7, 171—177, 1942.
12. **Fisher, W. B. and Van Duyne, F. O.**, Effect of variations in blanching on quality of frozen broccoli, snap beans, and spinach, *Food Res.*, 17, 315—325, 1952.
13. **Guerrant, N. B. and Dutcher, R. A.**, Further observations concerning the relationship of temperature of blanching to ascorbic acid retention in green beans, *Arch. Biochem.*, 18, 353—359, 1948.
14. **Guerrant, N. B., Vavich, M. G., Fardig, O. B., Ellenberger, H. A., Stern, R. M., and Coonen, N. H.**, Nutritive value of canned foods. Effect of duration and temperature of blanch on vitamin retention by certain vegetables, *Ind. Eng. Chem.*, 39, 1000—1007, 1947.
15. **Hartzler, E. R. and Guerrant, N. B.**, Effect of blanching and of frozen storage of vegetables on ascorbic acid retention and on the concomitant activity of certain enzymes, *Food Res.*, 17, 15—23, 1952.
16. **Lee, F. A. and Whitcombe, J.**, Blanching of vegetables for freezing. Effect of different types of potable water on nutrients of peas and snap beans, *Food Res.*, 10, 465—468, 1945.
17. **Melnick, D. Hochberg, M., and Oser, B. L.**, Comparative study of steam and hot water blanching, *Food Res.*, 9, 148—153, 1944.
18. **Morrison, M. H.**, The vitamin C content of quick frozen green beans, *J. Food Technol.*, 10, 19—28, 1975.
19. **Phillips, M. G. and Fenton, F.**, Effects of home freezing and cooking on snap beans: thiamin, riboflavin, ascorbic acid, *J. Home Econ.*, 37, 164—170, 1945.
20. **Proctor, B. E. and Goldblith, S. A.**, Radar energy for rapid food cooking and blanching, and its effect on vitamin content, *Food Technol. (Chicago)*, 2, 95—104, 1948.
21. **Retzer, J. L., Van Duyne, F. O., Chase, J. T., and Simpson, J. I.**, Effect of steam and hot-water blanching on ascorbic acid content of snap beans and cauliflower, *Food Res.*, 10, 518—524, 1945.
22. **Cook, B.-B., Gunning, B., and Uchimoto, D.**, Variations in nutritive values of frozen green baby lima beans as a result of methods of processing and cooking, *J. Agric. Food Chem.*, 9, 316—321, 1961.
23. **Guerrant, N. B. and O'Hara, M. B.**, Vitamin retention in peas and lima beans after blanching, freezing, processing in tin and in glass, after storage and after cooking, *Food Technol. (Chicago)*, 7, 473—477, 1953.
24. **Guerrant, N. B., Hartzler, E. R., Nicholas, J. E., Perry, J. S., Garey, J. G., Murphy, J. F., Dodds, M. L., and Bennett, G.**, Some factors affecting the quality of frozen foods, *Penn. State Coll. Agric. Exp. Stn. Bull.*, No. 565, 1953.
25. **Gustafson, F. G. and Cooke, A. R.**, Oxidation of ascorbic acid to dehydro-ascorbic acid at low temperatures, *Science*, 116, 234, 1952.
26. **Tressler, D. K., Mack, G. L., and Jenkins, R. R.**, Vitamin C in vegetables. VII. Lima beans, *Food Res.*, 2, 175—181, 1937.
27. **Batchelder, E. L., Kirkpatrick, M. E., Stein, K. E., and Marron, I. M**, Effect of scalding method on the quality of three home-frozen vetebales, *J. Home Econ.*, 39, 282—286, 1947.
28. **Eheart, M. S.**, Effect of microwave vs. water-blanching on nutrients in brocolli, *J. Am. Diet. Assoc.*, 50, 207—211, 1967.
29. **Abrams, C. I.**, The ascorbic acid content of quick frozen Brussels sprouts, *J. Food Technol.*, 10, 203—213, 1975.

30. **Dietrich, W. C. and Neumann, H. J.**, Blanching Brussels sprouts, *Food Technol. (Chicago)*, 19, 1174—1177, 1965.
31. **Barnes, B. and Tressler, D. K.**, Thiamin content of fresh and frozen peas and corn before and after cooking, *Food Res.*, 8, 420—427, 1943.
32. **Feaster, J. F., Mudra, A. E., Ives, M., and Tompkins, M. D.**, Effect of blanching time on vitamin retention in canned peas, *Canner*, 108(1), 27—30, 1949.
33. **Holmquist, J. W., Clifcorn, L. E., Heberlein, D. G., and Schmidt, C. F.**, Steam blanching of peas, *Food Technol. (Chicago)*, 8, 437—445, 1954.
34. **Jenkins, R. R. and Tressler, D. K.**, Vitamin C content of vegetables. VIII. Frozen peas, *Food Res.*, 3, 133—140, 1938.
35. **Lamb, F. C., Lewis, L. D., and Lee, S. K.**, Effect of blanching on retention of ascorbic acid and thiamin in peas, *West. Canner Packer*, 5, 60—62, 1948.
36. **Morrison, M. H.**, The vitamin C and thiamin contents of quick frozen peas, *J. Food Technol.*, 9, 491—500, 1974.
37. **Moyer, J. C. and Tressler, D. K.**, Thiamin content of fresh and frozen vegetables, *Food Res.*, 8, 58—61, 1943.
38. **Tressler, D. K., Mack, G. L., and King, C. G.**, Factors influencing the vitamin C content of vegetables, *Am. J. Public Health*, 26, 905—909, 1936.
39. **Van Duyne, F. O., Wolfe, J. C., and Owen, R. F**, Retention of riboflavin in vegetables preserved by freezing, *Food Res.*, 15, 53—61, 1950.
40. **Sweeney, J. P. and Marsh, A. C.**, Effect of processing on provitamin A in vegetables, *J. Am. Diet. Assoc.*, 59, 238—243, 1971.
41. **Von Kamienski, E. S.**, Retention of vitamin C during the processing of frozen spinach, *Sci. Aliment.*, 18(7), 243—244, 1972.
42. **Stimson, C. R. and Tressler, D. K.**, Carotene (vitamin A) content of fresh and frosted peas, *Food Res.*, 4, 475—483, 1939.
43. **Zimmerman, W. I., Tressler, D. K., and Maynard, L. A.**, Determination of carotene in fresh and frozen vegetables. I. Carotene content of green snap beans and sweet corn, *Food Res.*, 5, 93—101, 1940.
44. **Dietrich, W. C., Nutting, M.-D., Olson, R. L., Lindquist, F. E., Boggs, M. M., Bohart, G. S., Neumann, H. J., and Morris, H. J.**, Time-temperature tolerance of frozen foods. XVI. Quality retention of frozen green snap beans in retail packages, *Food Technol. (Chicago)*, 13, 136—145, 1959.
45. **Moyer, J. C. and Stotz, E.**, Electronic blanching of vegetables, *Science*, 102, 68—69, 1945.
46. **Odland, D. and Eheart, M. S.**, Ascorbic acid, mineral and quality retention in frozen broccoli blanched in water, steam and ammonia-steam, *J. Food Sci.*, 40, 1004—1007, 1975.
47. **Wedler, A.**, Results of experiments on the change in contents of nutritional compounds through processing and preparation of vegetables, *Qual. Plant. Mater. Veg.*, 21 (1—2), 79—95, 1971.
48. **Lee, F. A., Brooks, R. F., Pearson A. M., Miller, J. I., and Wanderstock, J. J.**, Effect of rate of freezing on pork quality. Appearance, palatability, and vitamin content, *J. Am. Diet. Assoc.*, 30, 351—354, 1954.
49. **Lehrer, W. P., Jr., Wiese, A. C., Harvey, W. R., and Moore, P. R.**, Effect of frozen storage and subsequent cooking on the thiamin, riboflavin, and nicotinic acid content of pork chops, *Food Res.*, 16, 485—491, 1951.
50. **Holmes, A. D., McKey, B. V., Esselen, K. O., Crowley, L. V., and Jones, C. P.**, Vitamin content of field-frozen kale, *Am. J. Dis. Child.*, 70, 298—300, 1945.
51. **Secomska, B., Iwanska, W., and Nadolna, I.**, Retention of some vitamins in cooked potatoes stored in the frozen state, *13th Int. Congr. Refrig.*, 3, 311—316, 1973.
52. **Loeffler, H. J.**, Retention of ascorbic acid in raspberries during freezing, frozen storage, pureeing, and manufacture into velva fruit, *Food Res.*, 11, 507—515, 1946.
53. **Sulc, S.**, The influence of different freezing methods, temperature, and time, on the preservation of important factors, *13th Int. Congr. Refrig.*, 3, 447—454, 1973.
54. **Fieger, E. A.**, Vitamin content of fresh, frozen oysters, *Quick Frozen Foods*, 19(4), 152 and 155, 1956.
55. **Kahn, L. N. and Livington, G. E.**, Effect of heating methods on thiamin retention in fresh or frozen prepared food, *J. Food Sci.*, 35, 349—351, 1970.
56. **Kotschevar, L. H.**, B-vitamin retention in frozen meat, *J. Am. Diet. Assoc.*, 31, 589—596, 1955.
57. **Lee, F. A., Brooks, R. F., Pearson, A. M., Miller, J. I., and Volz, F.**, Effect of freezing rate on meat. Appearance, palatability, and vitamin content of beef, *Food Res.*, 15, 8—15, 1950.
58. **Guadagni, D. G. and Nimmo, C. C.**, The time-temperature tolerance of frozen foods. III. Effectiveness of vacuum oxygen removal, and mild heat in controlling browning in frozen peaches, *Food Technol. (Chicago)*, 11, 43—47, 1957.

59. Guadagni, D. G., Nimmo, C. C., and Jansen, E. F., Time-temperature tolerance of frozen foods. VI. Retail packages of frozen strawberries, *Food Technol. (Chicago),* 11, 389—397, 1957.

60. Wolfe, J. C., Owen, R. F., Charles, V. R., and Van Duyne, F. O., Effect of freezing and freezer storage on the ascorbic acid content of muskmelon, grapefruit sections, and strawberry puree, *Food Res.,* 14, 243—252, 1949.

61. Guerrant, N. B., Changes in light reflectance and ascorbic acid content of foods during frozen storage, *J. Agric. Food Chem.,* 5, 207—212, 1957.

62. Jenkins, R. R., Tressler, D. K., Moyer, J., and McIntosh, J., Storage of frozen vegetables. Vitamin C experiments, *Refrig. Eng.,* 39, 381—382, 1940.

63. Derse, P. H. and Teply, L. J., Effect of storage conditions on nutrients in frozen green beans, peas, orange juice, and strawberries, *J. Agric. Food Chem.,* 6, 309—312, 1958.

64. Pierce, R. T., Shaw, M. D., Heck, J. G., and Bennett, G., Small storage temperature differences can affect the quality of frozen strawberries and green beans, *Refrig. Eng.,* 63 (11), 52—57, 1955.

65. Volz, F. E., Gortner, W. A., and Delwiche, C. V., The effect of desiccation on frozen vegetables, *Food Technol., (Chicago),* 3, 307—313, 1949.

66. Weits, J., Van Der Meer, M. A., and Lassche, J. B., Nutritive value and organoleptic properties of three vegetables fresh and preserved in six different ways, *Int. Z. Vitaminforsch.,* 40, 648—658, 1970.

67. Dietrich, W. C., Boggs, M. M., Nutting, M.-D., and Weinstein, N. E., Time-temperature tolerance of frozen foods. XXIII. Quality changes in frozen spinach, *Food Technol. (Chicago),* 14, 522—527, 1960.

68. Jurics, E. W., Comparative investigations of the vitamin C contents of frozen and fresh vegetables in the raw and cooked states, *Nahrung,* 14, 107—114, 1970 (in German).

69. Tinklin, G. L. and Filinger, G. A., Effects of different methods of blanching on the quality of home frozen spinch, *Food Technol., (Chicago),* 10, 198—201, 1956.

70. Lee, F. A., Gortner, W. A., and Whitcombe, J., Effect of freezing rate on vegetables, *Ind. Eng. Chem.,* 38, 341—346, 1946.

71. Richardson, L. R., Wilkes, S., and Ritchey, S. J., Comparative vitamin $B_6$ activity of frozen, irradiated and heat-processed foods, *J. Nutr.,* 73, 363—368, 1961.

72. Richardson, L. R., Wilkes, S., and Ritchey, S. J., Comparative vitamin K activity of frozen, irradiated and heat-processed foods, *J. Nutr.,* 73, 369—373, 1961.

73. Martin, M. E., Sweeney, J. P., Gilpin, G. L., and Chapman, V. J., Factors affecting the ascorbic acid and carotene content of broccoli, *J. Agric. Food Chem.,* 8, 387—390, 1960.

74. Bennett, G., Cone, J. F., Dodds, M. L., Garey, J. C., Guerrant, N. B., Heck, J. G., Murphy, J. F., Nicholas, J. E., Perry, J. S., Pierce, R. T., and Shaw, M. D., Some factors affecting the quality of frozen foods. II., *Penn. State Coll. Agric. Exp. Stn. Bull.,* No. 580, 1954.

75. Dietrich, W. C., Lindquist, F. E., Miers, J. C., Bohart, G. S., Neumann, H. J., and Talburt, W. F., The time-temperature tolerance of foods. IV. Objective tests to measure adverse changes in frozen vegetables, *Food Technol. (Chicago),* 11, 109—113, 1957.

76. Dietrich, W. C., Nutting, M.-D., Boggs, M. M., and Weinstein, N. E., Time-temperature tolerance of frozen foods. XXIV. Quality changes in cauliflower, *Food Technol., (Chicago),* 16, 123—128, 1962.

77. Lindquist, F. E., Dietrich, W. C., and Boggs, M. M., Effect of storage temperature on quality of frozen peas, *Food Technol. (Chicago),* 4, 5—9, 1950.

78. DuBois, C. W. and Colvin, D. L., Loss of added vitamin C in the storage of peaches, *Fruit Prod. J. Am. Food Manuf.,* 25, 101—103, 1945.

79. Guadagni, D. G., Nimmo, C. C., and Jansen, E. F., The time-temperature tolerance of frozen foods. II. Retail packages of frozen peaches, *Food Technol. (Chicago),* 11, 33—42, 1957.

80. Guadagni, D. G., Nimmo, C. C., and Jansen, E. F., Time-temperature tolerance of frozen foods, X. Retail packages of frozen red raspberries, *Food Technol. (Chicago),* 11, 633—637, 1957.

81. Crivelli, G., Rosati, P., and Monzini, A., Chemical stability of frozen strawberries during storage, in *Frozen Foods,* International Institute of Refrigeration, Paris, 1969, 67—71.

82. Guadagni, D. G., Downes, N. J., Sanshuck, D. W., and Shinoda, S., Effect of temperature on stability of commercially frozen bulk pack fruits — strawberries, raspberries, and blackberries, *Food Technol. (Chicago),* 15, 207—209, 1961.

83. Huggart, R. L., Harman, D. A., and Moore, E. L., Ascorbic acid retention in frozen concentrated citrus juices, *J. Am. Diet. Assoc.,* 30, 682—684, 1954.

84. McColloch, R. J., Rice, R. G., Bandurski, M. B., and Gentili, B., The time-temperature tolerance of frozen foods. VII. Frozen concentrated orange juice, *Food Technol. (Chicago),* 11, 444—449, 1957.

85. Lehrer, W. P., Jr., Wiese, A. C., Harvey, W. R., and Moore, P. R., The stability of thiamin, riboflavin, and nicotinic acid of lamb chops during frozen storage and subsequent cooking, *Food Res.,* 17, 24—30, 1952.

86. **Boggs, M. M., Dietrich, W. C., Nutting, M.-D., Olson, R. L., Lindquist, F. E., Bohart, G. S., Neumann, H. J., and Morris, H. J.,** Time-temperature tolerance of frozen foods. XXI. Frozen peas., *Food Technol. (Chicago),* 14, 181—185, 1960.

87. **Gortner, W. A., Fenton, F., Volz, F. E., and Gleim, E.,** Effect of fluctuating storage temperatures on quality of frozen foods, *Ind. Eng. Chem.,* 40, 1423—1426, 1948.

88. **Guadagni, D. G. and Nimmo, C. C.,** Time-temperature tolerance of frozen foods. XIII. Effect of regularly fluctuating temperatures in retail packages of frozen strawberries and raspberries, *Food Technol. (Chicago),* 12, 306—310, 1958.

89. **Fenton, F. and Tressler, D. K.,** Losses of vitamin C during commercial freezing, defrosting, and cooking of frosted peas., *Food Res.,* 3, 409—416, 1938.

90. **Bauernfeind, J. C., Jahns, F. W., Smith, E. G., and Siemers, G. F.,** Vitamin C stability in frozen fruit processed with crystalline L-ascorbic acid, *Fruit Prod. J.,* 25, 324—330, 347, 1946.

91. **Von Kamienski, E. S.,** Retention of vitamin C during the processing of frozen spinach, in *Frozen Foods,* International Institute of Refrigeration, Paris, 1969, 53—55.

92. **Fagerson, I. S., Anderson, E. E., Hayes, K. M., and Fellers, C. R.,** Vitamin C and frozen strawberries, *Quick Frozen Foods,* 16(9), 84—85, 1954.

93. **Marshall, J. R., Hayes, K. M., Fellers, C. R., an DuBois, C. W.,** Stability of ascorbic acid in citrus concentrates during storage, *Quick Frozen Foods,* 17(12), 50—52, 129, 1955.

94. **Tingleff, A. J. and Miller, E. V.,** Studies on ascorbic acid retention in frozen juice, segments, and whole oranges, *Food Res.,* 25, 145—147, 1960.

95. **Crow, L. S. and Scoular, F. I.,** Effects of antioxidant ascorbic acid upon the ascorbic acid content of frozen fruits, *J. Home Econ.,* 47, 259—260, 1955.

96. **Strachan, C. C. and Moyls, A. W.,** Ascorbic, citric, and dihydroxymaleic acids as antioxidants in frozen pack fruits, *Food Technol. (Chicago),* 3, 327—332, 1949.

97. **Westerman, B. D., Vail, G. E., Kalen, J., Stone, M., and Mackintosh, D. L.,** B-complex vitamins in meat. III. Influence of storage temperature and time on the vitamins in pork muscle, *J. Am. Diet. Assoc.,* 28, 49—52, 1952.

98. **Millares, R. and Fellers, C. R.,** Vitamin and amino acid content of processed chicken meat products, *Food Res.,* 14, 131—143, 1949.

99. **Morgan, A. F., Kidder, L. E., Hunner, M., Sharokh, B. K., and Chesbro, R. M.,** Thiamine, riboflavin, and niacin content of chicken tissues, as affected by cooking and frozen storage, *Food Res.,* 14, 439—448, 1949.

100. **Cook, B. B., Morgan, A. F., and Smith, M. B.,** Thiamin, riboflavin, and niacin content of turkey tissues as affected by storage and cooking, *Food Res.,* 14, 449—458, 1949.

101. **Adams, C. F.,** *Nutritive Value of American Foods in Common Units,* Agric. Handb. No. 456, U.S. Department of Agriculture, Washington, D.C., 1975.

102. **Burger, M., Hein, L. W., Teply, L. J., Derse, P. H., and Krieger, C. H.,** Vitamin, mineral, and proximate composition of frozen fruits, juices and vegetables, *J. Agric. Food Chem.,* 4, 418—425, 1956.

103. **Lowenberg, M. E. and Wilson, E. D.,** *Nutrients in Frozen Foods,* National Association of Frozen Food Packers, Washington, D.C., 1959.

# EFFECT OF PROCESSING ON NUTRITIVE VALUE OF FOOD: FREEZE-DRYING*,**

## James M. Flink

## INTRODUCTION

Of the various dehydration processes, freeze-drying has generally been conceded to be the most "gentle," since it can take place while the sample is at a low temperature. On the basis of this understanding, freeze-drying has often been used as a method for converting wet samples into a dry material, suitable for subsequent analysis.

For example, Ang et al.[4] have freeze-dried samples of food products for protein quality analysis. They stated that the samples are freeze-dried for 2 to 3 days; on the second day a moderate heating to 38°C was applied to accelerate the drying. Posati et al.[49] imply that no changes occur during freeze-drying since they lyophilized their wet samples to prepare dry powders for tryptophane analysis. No freeze-drying conditions were specified. Wing and Alexander[64] have freeze-dried ground samples prior to analysis for vitamin $B_6$. They noted that the heating(?) plate temperature is not allowed to go above 0°C in order to minimize possible destruction of vitamin $B_6$. They did not cite any references or indicate the use of an internal control.

In most cases there are no control experiments conducted to determine the loss of the component during the freeze-drying process. Instead, the methods section of a research paper will merely note that the material was freeze-dried (or lyophilized) and then subjected to some particular analysis. Thus, it can be said that the field has accepted (right or wrong) the concept of low losses during freeze-drying.

In the course of preparing this section, it was somewhat surprising to note how few articles in the literature completely report the freeze-drying conditions, probably indicating that many of the freeze-dryers in use are poorly instrumented. This makes it quite difficult to report really meaningful data on nutrient retention in freeze-drying. It must be recognized, however, that nutrient degradation is, at a minimum, time, temperature, and moisture-content dependent, and thus the observed nutrient loss will be intimately related to the process conditions used. The importance of this will become increasingly apparent below during the discussion of freeze-drying.

It has been noted that the scientific literature on freeze-drying and product quality generally presents data from either of two approaches — organoleptic evaluation or nutrient content determination. In many cases these two are closely related, such as in nonenzymatic browning (organoleptic) and the loss of available lysine or ascorbic acid content (nutrient). In this case, either could be considered as a measure of nutrient value, though one would be an indicator while the other would be a direct measure. Goldblith and Tannenbaum[25] discuss the results of Tuomy and Felder[61] in this respect.

It must be noted that the method of evaluation for nutrient value will also have some influence. For example, it has been noted in the literature that an evaluation of protein value by loss of available lysine is valid only when lysine is the limiting amino acid in the diet.[8,14,30] Thus, when animal feeding studies are used to evaluate protein quality, often there is no reduction in nutritive value as a result of the freeze-drying process, even though the conditions used would register changes in the food product when evaluated according to other criteria.

The freeze-drying process is, at a minimum, two processes — freezing and sublimation drying. While this is undoubtedly a simplification it does point to an additional

* Manuscript submitted 27 October 1976.
** Tables appear at end of text.

problem in evaluating nutrient retention in freeze-drying; namely, how much of the overall production process to consider. In some studies it has been shown that the largest loss of certain nutrients occurs in the processing steps prior to the freezing step, as with the washing and blanching of vegetables.[8,29,37,38] The reported nutrient loss can therefore vary greatly, depending on how much of the total process is included. As an aside, it has been noted in reviewing the literature that many authors refer to the large losses in cooking which greatly overshadow the losses in freeze-drying.

The storage stability of freeze-dried products has been a subject of much study. Information regarding the retention of nutrients during freeze-drying can sometimes be obtained from these studies if and when the authors have thought to report the nutrient content of their original raw material. In most cases examined, however, this was not found to be reported.

In the discussion that follows, the freeze-drying process will be briefly described and the process factors that can be expected to influence the nutritive value of freeze-dried foods will be discussed. Following that will be tabulated data for nutrient retention (or loss) during the freeze-drying process; this will generally refer to changes occurring in the period in which the product is in the freeze-dryer. Changes in preliminary steps (such as blanching, washing, etc.) or in storage in the dry state will generally not be included. However, the limitations noted above must always be considered. When original sources were not available, the sources from which the data were obtained are noted in the References. In addition, a survey of *Chemical Abstracts* and *Food Science and Technology Abstracts* indicates a number of references in the area of nutrient value. While the information in the abstracts was often of limited value, it was decided that rather than discard the potentially useful references, they would be included, but referenced only by their abstract number.

## THE FREEZE-DRYING PROCESS AND NUTRIENT RETENTION

When describing the freeze-drying process itself, the steps include freezing of the product water to ice, sublimation of the ice crystals so produced, and desorption (or evaporation) of the unfrozen water. This results in a dry porous product, though there will always be some small amount of residual water remaining. The rate at which dry product is produced depends on a number of physical factors that influence the relative rates of heat and mass transfer.

When describing nutrient retention, what is being considered are the positive aspects of nutrient loss. Nutrient loss mechanisms can be quite variable, but in general, those of importance in the freeze-drying process depend primarily on a number of physical factors that affect the rate at which the nutrients undergo chemical degradation.

For the most part, the physical factors that influence the rate of drying are the same as those that affect the rate of nutrient loss — namely, temperature, moisture, and time. Other factors that are often of importance relative to nutrient loss, such as oxygen content and light, are not of significance in the freeze-drying process proper.

### Factors Affecting Kinetics of Nutrient Loss

As noted above, sample temperature, moisture content, and exposure time are the important parameters in determining the extent of nutrient loss in the freeze-drying process. The influence of these factors has been shown on a number of occasions, mostly with respect to the storage stability of dried food products.[34,38,39,62] Labuza[39] and Bluestein and Labuza[8] have presented extensive reviews of the information presently available that can be used for kinetic analyses of nutrient loss. They note a definite shortage of kinetic data on nutrient loss, thus making predictive-type evaluations of the effects of freeze-drying process parameters on nutrient loss difficult or impossible.

Storage stability studies are generally conducted at conditions of temperature, moisture, and time that are quite different from freeze-drying conditions. This means that determining the freeze-drying nutrient loss from storage stability kinetics will require a significant extrapolation of exposure conditions. However, in studies on the nonenzymatic browning of dry systems at high temperatures that model extreme conditions found in the dry layer during freeze-drying,[19] there are indications that the extrapolations are valid if the mechanism of degradation and the systems physical properties do not change.

The study by Flink et al.[19] shows that the influence of temperature, moisture, and time on the chemical degradation behavior during conditions modelling extreme freeze-drying are not unexpected. Since there is an interaction between the three factors, equal extents of degradation could be achieved by an almost infinite variety of combinations of these process variables. Individually, increasing temperature, moisture, or time results in increased chemical degradation. Thus, with respect to nutrient loss alone, the kinetic aspects of degradation are relatively simple. As will be noted below, however, incorporating freeze-drying kinetics will complicate the stiuation somewhat.

**Factors Affecting Kinetics of Freeze-Drying**

As noted above, freeze-drying involves freezing the water in the sample, subliming the ice formed, and then desorbing the unfrozen water. It is a process that requires the input of energy (heat transfer) and the removal of moisture (mass transfer). The heat and mass transfer relationships for freeze-drying have been extensively discussed by King[36] and Karel.[33] Technically, the first dehydration occurs during the freezing step, since the formation of ice results in the removal of water from the remainder of the solutes. This dehydration occurs at a low temperature with the product input temperature generally being the highest temperature encountered at this stage of the process; since heat is being removed in this step, the environment will be at a lower temperature. While acceleration of chemical reactions can occur at sub-zero temperatures due to changes in the concentrations of reactants in the unfrozen phase, this will be of no significance with respect to freeze-drying itself.

In contrast to the freezing step, sublimation of ice and desorption of unfrozen water requires the input of heat. It is generally accepted[36] that the heat and mass transfer behavior can be expressed in terms of the so-called "uniformly retreating ice front" model (URIF) in which the partially dry product is considered to consist of a frozen layer and a dry layer (Figure 1). In most practical freeze drying cases, heat is supplied to the sample surface by radiation or a combination of radiation and conduction. This heat is transferred by conduction across the dry layer to the ice-dry layer interface, where it is used to sublime some ice, causing the ice layer to retreat slightly further. The sublimed ice is transported to the product surface and eventually to the freeze-dryer condenser. Desorption of water occurs continually and simultaneously at all locations in the dry layer. The two transport phenomena occur because gradients of temperature and moisture exist in the dry layer. Thus there are different values of temperature and moisture at every location in the dry layer.

Results of studies[1,23,46] indicate that the moisture content for a given material, at any point in the dry layer, is dependent only on the ice-front temperature and the temperature at that point. The length of time that a point in the dry layer is at a particular temperature and moisture content depends on the drying rate and, therefore, on the temperature and moisture gradients. Therein lies a part of the complexity associated with freeze-drying because the temperature and moisture gradients are opposed to each other; the warmest point is also the driest and the wettest point is also the coldest. Thus, as drying proceeds, the tendency for an increase in the rate of nutrient degradation associated with increasing temperature will be balanced to some extent by

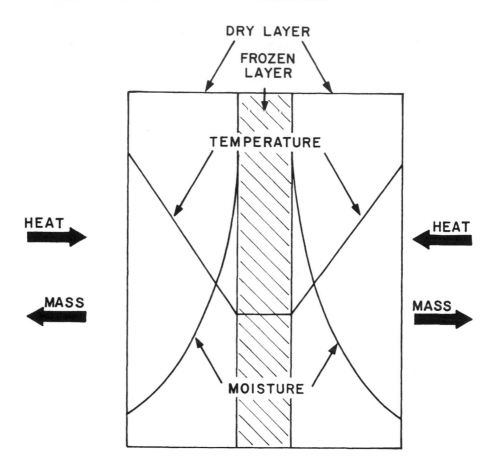

FIGURE 1.   Schematic of heat and mass transfer during freeze-drying showing the temperature and moisture profiles.

the tendency for a decrease in the rate of nutrient degradation associated with decreasing moisture.

The entire freeze-drying process can be conducted at or below room temperature. In this case, heat is supplied from shelves at ambient temperature and the product temperature never rises above ambience. This is often done in the laboratory where drying time is not critical. However, economic operation requires more rapid rates of drying, generally achieved by increasing the heat transfer rate until one of a number of limiting conditions generally related to structural changes of the sample are reached. The heat transfer rate is increased by raising the heat supply temperature, resulting in higher temperatures in the dry layer. This leads to the second complexity associated with freeze-drying; though an increased temperature gradient results in higher local temperatures, they are present for shorter periods of time.

## Summary

The freeze-drying process can be conducted over a very wide range of process variables that are for the most part interrelated, but in such a way that to change one in a direction giving a higher nutrient loss will cause the values of the others to show lower nutrient loss. Thus, the rate of freeze-drying can be increased significantly compared to ambient operation and still give a product with high nutrient retention levels. This generalization breaks down when an acceleration of the drying rate through increases in the dry-layer temperature gradient results in excessively high surface temperatures for the required exposure times.

The interaction and opposition of the gradients also means that nutrient loss will probably not be uniformly distributed throughout the product. Thus, excessive loss at the surface need not be the sole criterion of product quality; rather, average nutrient level might be more valuable.

In the foregoing discussion it was assumed that radiation and/or conduction was the mode of heat transport and that sample dimensions remain unchanged. However, drying rates can be increased without increases in temperature gradients by using microwave energy to supply the heat of sublimation to the ice interface. The drying rate can be increased with smaller increases in the surface temperature by decreasing the sample dimensions when possible. In each of these cases, nutrient levels can be expected to be higher.

## SURVEY OF NUTRIENT RETENTION DATA

Examination of information on the stability of nutrients[5,16,31] yields little indication of their stability under freeze-drying conditions, for where temperatures and moistures vary widely, pH can change in the unfrozen regions, and oxygen, light, and UV light are absent. Thus, what follows are tables on the experimental determinations of nutrient retention levels in freeze-drying. Goldblith and Tannenbaum[25] reviewed some of these examples earlier, but for completeness they are included here. Table 10 gives information on some additional sources of nutrient retention data. This table gives the *Chemical Abstract* reference number, and thus these items are not repeated in the reference list. In addition, three recent reviews (Eboli,[18] Larousse,[40] and Ammu and Sharma,[3]) listed in *Food Science and Technology Abstracts* are given in the reference list with their FSTA reference number. Also, Speiss[56] has been referenced by King[36] as having presented information on nutrient loss in freeze-drying.

### Amino Acids and Proteins

Experimental determinations of the retention of nutritive value for amino acids and proteins following freeze-drying are given in Table 1. For the conditions tested, nutrient retention is essentially complete. Some additional information that does not fit into a tabular format is given below.

Bender[7] reviews the mechanisms of protein damage associated with processing and describes methods for evaluation of this damage. De Groot[14] discusses the problem of limiting amino acids in the diet vs. amino acid lost discussed earlier. Hackler[28] has heated soy milk to inactivate trypsin inhibitor and then freeze-dried the product. The results are difficult to interpret, since he does not give the initial trypsin inhibitor activity (TIA) after heating and prior to freeze-drying. Also, two separate experiments do not give the same TIA after "identical" process conditions (probably due to product variations). Karandaeva[32] has noted that nitrogen balances observed in feeding studies indicate some slight damage when freeze-drying protein foods. Speckman et al.[55] compared a diet of dehydrated products (mainly freeze dried; some compressed) with an equivalent but not identical diet of fresh, frozen, and thermally processed materials. They showed that the coefficients of average digestibility with respect to energy and crude protein were the same for the two diets, and that the average daily nitrogen balance was the same, with the subjects being in balance. Sauvegeot[52] has indicated that freeze-drying causes deterioration of protein quality in meat as a result of protein or amino acid aggregation or through the Maillard reaction.

Ford[22] evaluated the availability of selected amino acids after freeze-drying cod for 24 hr with a maximum temperature of 24°C. While he does not compare availability before and after freeze drying, presumably the high levels of availability observed after freeze-drying (Table 2) indicate no occurrence of damage during the freeze-drying process for the specified conditions.

### Vitamins

**Ascorbic Acid** — Experimental determinations on the retention of nutritive value for ascorbic acid (vitamin C) following freeze-drying are given in Table 3. It can be seen that the retentions are either in the range of 50 to 70% or 90 to 100%. This probably reflects the difficulty of determining which data refers to raw material and which to blanched material. It seems that ascorbic acid will be well-retained in the freeze-drying process itself.

**Carotenoids and vitamin A** — Experimental determinations on the retention of nutritive value for carotenoids and vitamin A following freeze-drying are given in Table 4. It can be seen that retention is quite high, generally above 95%. Sweeney and Marsh[57] conducted an extensive survey into the stability of the various carotene isomers. They noted that since they do not all exhibit equal vitamin A activity, the change in distribution is more significant than just total decrease in carotene content. In Table 5 it can be seen that, for the most part, the distribution remained unchanged following freeze-drying, even though the total content was reduced.

**Thiamin** — Experimental determinations on the retention of thiamin (vitamin $B_1$) following freeze-drying are given in Table 6. The results reported for thiamin are fewer and they are more variable. In general, the retention levels associated with freeze-drying alone can be considered to be above 75%. Again the failure to specify drying conditions and complete process schemes limits the interpretation of the available data.

**Riboflavin** — Experimental determinations on the retention of riboflavin (vitamin $B_2$) following freeze-drying are shown in Table 7. The retention is essentially complete, being above 90% in almost all the cases in which freeze-drying alone was considered.

**Other vitamins** — Experimental determinations on the retention of a number of other vitamins following freeze-drying are shown in Table 8. With the exception of the low values for pyridoxine retention given by Thomas and Calloway,[58] the retentions are generally high and in the 80 to 100% range. Labuza[38] attributed some data given by Schroeder[54] as being data of retention following freeze-drying. Examination of Schroeder's tables, however, indicates that these values were for dried products, but not necessarily freeze-dried. The confusion probably arose from Schroeder placing his data for dried products in the table column headed frozen products and denoted "dried" by a superscript.

### Other Nutrients

Some studies have investigated the retention of fats during freeze-drying. Pol and Groot[48] noted that spray-dried milk had a 30 to 40% larger loss of essential fatty acids than lyophilized milk. Calloway[11-12] measured the retention of polyunsaturated fatty acids (Table 9). Watts et al.[63] measured the retention of total fat (Table 9).

Richter and Handle[50] noted that there was no additional loss of available calcium in freeze-dried spinach due to the formation of insoluble calcium oxalate from soluble oxalic acid. Karandaeva[32] noted that calcium and phosphorous balances in human subjects were unchanged when they switched from a diet of fresh foods to one of freeze-dried products. Speckmann et al.[55] showed that the coefficient of average digestibility for fat was the same for a dehydrated (mainly freeze-dried) diet as it was for its equivalent fresh, frozen, and thermally processed counterpart.

### Other Data Sources

As noted earlier, in the course of preparing this review an examination of the *8th Collective Index of Chemical Abstracts,* covering the years 1967 to 1971, showed a number of potentially useful references located in journals of limited worldwide circulation. Rather than discard the information found in the abstracts consulted, they have been listed in Table 10 by the first author and by the respective *Chemical Abstract* number. Since it was apparent that limited numerical data were given in the abstracts, earlier indexes were not examined. It should be recognized, however, that these sources could be expected to supply additional information.

## Summary

On the basis of the foregoing tables, it can be said that freeze-drying of foods can give dehydrated products with little loss of nutritional value beyond that occurring in the predrying steps. The extent to which the process can be accelerated without significant nutrient degradation is not known, and would seem to be an important area for scientific investigation. It was also noted that in many studies the freeze-drying conditions and especially product temperatures are not specified. The value of nutrient retention data will be greatly enhanced if future studies include explicit descriptions of the freeze-drying conditions.

While it is not in the scope of this chapter to present data on nutrient loss during storage of freeze-dried foods, a few general comments would seem in order. Freeze-drying generally results in a highly porous product, which means that oxygen and moisture can "penetrate" easily to the product interior, giving a high potential for degradation reactions, especially those involving oxidative deterioration. These facts put a premium on careful packaging, preferably with vacuum or inert gas headspaces. The recently developed technique of compression of freeze-dried foods eliminates much of this void volume and should result in improved stability in storage.

## Table 1
## RETENTION OF NUTRITIVE VALUE OF AMINO ACIDS AND PROTEINS FOLLOWING FREEZE-DRYING

| Food material | Content | | | Percentage retention | Notes | Ref. |
|---|---|---|---|---|---|---|
| | Initial | Final | Units | | | |
| Beef | 586 | 604 | mg/g N | 103 | 3,2[a,b] | 12 |
| | 148 | 143 | mg/g N | 97 | 24,23[a,c] | 12 |
| | 234 | 245 | mg/g N | 105 | 30,27[a,d] | 12 |
| | 74.2 | 74.5 | see note G | 100 | [e,f,g] | 14 |
| | 101.4 | 101.5 | see note H | 100 | [e,f,h] | 14 |
| | 75.5 | 75.7 | see note I | 100 | [e,f,i] | 14 |
| Beef, ground | 21.54 | 25.91 | % of fresh | 110 | — | 63 |
| | 45.4 | 46.6 | g/100g dry | 103 | [j] | 59 |
| Chicken | 586 | 608 | mg/g N | 104 | 7,4[a,b] | 12 |
| | 178 | 170 | mg/g N | 96 | 24,24[a,c] | 12 |
| | 234 | 248 | mg/g N | 106 | 31,27[a,d] | 12 |
| | 72.4 | 73.5 | see note G | 102 | [e,g,k] | 14 |
| | 100.4 | 100.9 | see note H | 100 | [e,h,k] | 14 |
| | 72.9 | 74.4 | see note I | 102 | [e,i,k] | 14 |
| | 3.36 | 3.29 | see note L | 98 | [l] | 24 |
| | 102.4 | 100.3 | see note M | 98 | [m] | 24 |
| | 81.7 | 85.3 | g/100 g dry | 104 | [j] | 59 |
| Crabmeat | 3.11 | 3.51 | see note L | 113 | [l] | 24 |
| | 94.8 | 107.0 | see note M | 113 | [m] | 24 |
| Egg, whole | 12.07 | 12.37 | % of fresh | 102.5 | — | 63 |
| | 68.5 | 68.7 | see note N | 100 | [n,o] | 44 |
| Egg, white | 96.5 | 96.5 | see note N | 100 | [n,o] | 44 |
| Egg, yolk | 35.4 | 35.1 | see note N | 99 | [n,o] | 44 |
| Fish patty (fried) | 83.2 | 83.7 | see note G | 101 | [e,g,p] | 14 |
| | 97.8 | 98.7 | see note H | 101 | [e,h,p] | 14 |
| | 81.3 | 82.4 | see note I | 101 | [e,i,p] | 14 |

## Table 1 (continued)
## RETENTION OF NUTRITIVE VALUE OF AMINO ACIDS AND PROTEINS FOLLOWING FREEZE-DRYING

| Food material | Content Initial | Final | Units | Percentage retention | Notes | Ref. |
|---|---|---|---|---|---|---|
| Green beans (sulfited) | 56.8 | 55.4 | see note G | 98 | e.g.q | 14 |
|  | 81.6 | 80.8 | see note H | 99 | e.h.q | 14 |
|  | 46.4 | 45.0 | see note I | 97 | e.i.q | 14 |
| Haddock | 83.0 | 84.3 | see note G | 102 | e.g.r | 14 |
|  | 100.0 | 101.0 | see note H | 101 | e.h.r | 14 |
|  | 83.1 | 85.3 | see note I | 103 | e.i.r | 14 |
| Meat, fish | — | — | — | ≈100 | — | 29 |
| Milk, homogenized | 3.71 | 4.07 | % of fresh | 106.7 | — | 63 |
| Pork loin | 631 | 639 | mg/g N | 101 | 3,2a.b | 12 |
|  | 158 | 151 | mg/g N | 96 | 24,21a.c | 12 |
|  | 258 | 242 | mg/g N | 94 | 30,28a.d | 12 |
|  | 38.3 | 46.6 | g/100 g dry | 121 | j | 59 |
| Shrimp | 599 | 633 | mg/g N | 106 | 6,3a.b | 12 |
|  | 182 | 188 | mg/g N | 103 | 26,20a.c | 12 |
|  | 256 | 262 | mg/g N | 102 | 30,22a.d | 12 |
|  | 3.02 | 3.24 | see note L | 107 | l | 24 |
|  | 92.1 | 98.8 | see note M | 107 | m | 24 |
|  | 92.8 | 92.3 | g/100 g dry | 99 | j | 59 |
| Sweet corn (sulfited) | 76.0 | 75.3 | see note G | 99 | e.g.s | 14 |
|  | 97.0 | 97.5 | see note H | 101 | e.h.s | 14 |
|  | 73.7 | 73.5 | see note I | 100 | e.i.s | 14 |

a    Numbers in "Notes" refer to % of amino acid in raw and freeze dried material freed by pepsin, which is presumed to be a measure of digestibility and protein quality.

b    Lysine.

c    Methionine.

d    Phenylalanine.

e    All products were cooked before freeze-drying; initial content is for cooked product; standard deviations are given in original paper.

f    Freeze drying conditions = 66°C, 23 hr.

g    Biological value.

h    Digestibility.

i    Net protein utilization = (biological value) (digestibility) ÷ 100.

j    Total protein content.

k    Freeze drying conditions = 41°C/0.75 torr/24 hr.

l    Protein efficiency ratio (PER) = gram gain in weight ÷ gram food intake; casein PER = 3.28.

m    Protein quality value (PQV) = $PER_{sample} \div PER_{casein} \times 100$; casein PQV = 100.

n    Digestible protein as percent of dry matter; unclear if electrophoretic technique.

o    Freeze drying conditions = 40°C/0.4 torr/20 hr.

p    Freeze drying conditions = 43°C/0.6 torr/18 hr.

q    Freeze drying conditions = 60°C/0.5 torr/18 hr.

r    Freeze drying conditions = 46°C/0.6 torr/18 hr.

s    Freeze drying conditions = 43°C/0.75 torr/18 hr.

## Table 2
## AVAILABILITY OF AMINO ACIDS
## IN FREEZE-DRIED COD

| Amino acid | Amino acid concentration (g/16 g of nitrogen) | | Available (%) |
|---|---|---|---|
| | Total | Available | |
| Valine | 5.7 | 5.8 | 102 |
| Histidine | 2.0 | 1.9 | 95 |
| Arginine | 6.1 | 5.5 | 90 |
| Methio-nine | 3.3 | 3.2 | 97 |
| Leucine | 8.0 | 7.5 | 94 |
| Lysine | 9.1 | 8.4 | 92 |

From Ford, J. E., A microbiological method for assaying the nutritional value of proteins. IV. Analysis of enzymatically digested foods by sephadex gel-filtration, *Br. J. Nutr.*, 19, 277, 1965, Cambridge University Press. With permission.

## Table 3
## RETENTION OF NUTRITIVE VALUE OF ASCORBIC ACID FOLLOWING FREEZE-DRYING

| Food material | Content | | | Percentage retention | Notes | Ref. |
|---|---|---|---|---|---|---|
| | Initial | Final | Units | | | |
| Asparagus | 112.2 | 114.2 | mg/100 g dry | 102 | — | 41 |
| Bananas | 46.0 | 48.2 | mg/100 g dry | 105 | a | 17 |
| | 46.0 | 48.2 | mg/100 g dry | — | a.b | 17 |
| Fruit | — | — | — | ≈100 | c.d | 37 |
| Green beans Seminole | 206.8 | — | mg/100 g | 58 | e | 20 |
| | 206.8 | — | mg/100 g | 63 | f | 20 |
| | 206.8 | — | mg/100 g | 56 | g | 20 |
| Ideal | 188.7 | — | mg/100 g | 52 | e | 20 |
| | 188.7 | — | mg/100 g | 74 | f | 20 |
| | 188.7 | — | mg/100 g | 50 | g | 20 |
| Contender | 213.1 | — | mg/100 g | 42 | e | 20 |
| | 213.1 | — | mg/100 g | 77 | f | 20 |
| | 213.1 | — | mg/200 g | 40 | g | 20 |
| Mont-Calme | 241.4 | — | mg/100 g | 53 | e | 20 |
| | 241.4 | — | mg/100 g | 77 | f | 20 |
| | 241.4 | — | mg/100 g | 40 | g | 20 |
| Guava juice | 587 | 578 | mg/100 g dry | 98 | h.i | 21 |
| | 567 | 560 | mg/100 g dry | 99 | h.j | 21 |
| Mangoes | 268 | 276 | mg/100 g dry | 103 | k.l | 2 |
| | 268 | 284 | mg/100 g dry | 106 | k.m | 2 |
| Onions | 54.2 | 51.9 | mg/100 g dry | 96 | — | 41 |
| Orange juice | 452 | 440 | mg/100 g dry | 97 | n.q | 21 |
| | 451 | 437 | mg/100 g dry | 97 | o.q | 21 |
| | 441 | 434 | mg/100 g dry | 98 | p.q | 21 |
| Parsley | 187.4 | 165.4 | mg/100 g dry | 88 | — | 41 |
| Peach juice | 310 | 305 | mg/kg fresh | 98 | r | 53 |
| Peas | 67.8 | 52.2 | mg/100 g dry | 77 | — | 41 |
| | | | | 70 | — | 45 |

## Table 3 (continued)
## RETENTION OF NUTRITIVE VALUE OF ASCORBIC ACID FOLLOWING FREEZE-DRYING

| Food material | Content: Initial | Content: Final | Content: Units | Percentage retention | Notes | Ref. |
|---|---|---|---|---|---|---|
| Variety 1 | 116 | 107 | mg/100 g dry | 92 | s | 29 |
| | 71 | 75 | mg/100 g dry | 106 | t | 29 |
| | 50 | 45 | mg/100 g dry | 90 | u | 29 |
| Variety 2 | 136 | 115 | mg/100 g dry | 85 | s | 29 |
| | 116 | 90 | mg/100 g dry | 78 | t | 29 |
| | 84 | 77 | mg/100 g dry | 92 | u | 29 |
| | 31.00 | 23.25 | mg/100 g | 75 | v | 13 |
| Raspberries | 75 | 70 | % of fresh | 93 | w | 43 |
| Whole | 290 | 280 | mg/kg fresh | 97 | r | 53 |
| Juice | 525 | 515 | mg/kg fresh | 98 | r | 53 |
| Red cabbage | 891.1 | 755.1 | mg/kg dry | 85 | — | 41 |
| Spinach | 34.00 | 19.30 | mg/100 g | 57 | x | 13 |
| Strawberries | 575 | 550 | mg/kg fresh | 96 | r | 53 |
| Yogurt | — | — | — | 65—80 | — | 47 |

[a] Freeze dried 24 hr at 50 to 80 mtorr; no heating temperature given.
[b] $SO_2$ treated.
[c] Fruits: strawberry, black currant, rose hips.
[d] Freeze drying conditions: 7 hr with heating plates — 85°C (period 1), 60°C (period 2), 38°C (period 3); residual moisture about 4%; average sublimation rate of 1.1 to 1.3 kg $H_2O/m^2/hr$.
[e] Water blanch — retention value includes blanching.
[f] Steam blanch — retention value includes blanching.
[g] $NaHCO_3$ blanch — retention value includes blanching.
[h] Maximum sample surface temperature during freeze drying = 50°C; vacuum = 50 — 100 mtorr; drying time for 12 mm thick slab = 11 hr.
[i] Pasteurized.
[j] Nonpasteurized.
[k] Dipped into 0.5% ascorbic acid solution; heating plates at 20°C; 0.12 torr; 60 hr drying time; original data given on product weight basis.
[l] Fast freezing in Freon-12®.
[m] Slow freezing.
[n] 13% total solids.
[o] 20% total solids.
[p] 36% total solids.
[q] Maximum sample surface temperature during freeze drying = 60°C; vacuum = 50 — 100 mtorr; drying time for 12 mm thick slab = 16 hr for 13% total solids (approximately 0.65 kg $H_2O/m^2/hr$). 18.5 hr for 20% total solids (0.5), 26 hr, for 36% total solids (0.3).
[r] Includes 8 day storage in dry state before analysis.
[s] Small.
[t] Medium.
[u] Large.
[v] Freezing alone gave 50% retention; based on 100 g initial weight.
[w] Initial content is for blanched; freezing alone showed no loss from blanched state.
[x] Freezing alone gave 41% retention; based on 100 g initial weight.

Table 4
RETENTION OF NUTRITIVE VALUE OF CAROTENOIDS FOLLOWING
FREEZE-DRYING

| Food material | Content | | | Percentage retention | Notes | Ref. |
|---|---|---|---|---|---|---|
| | Initial | Final | Units | | | |
| Apricot juice | 10.7 | 8.7 | mg/kg fresh | 81 | a | 53 |
| Carrots | 91.4 | 80.2 | mg/100 g fresh | 88 | b | 57 |
| | n— | — | — | 100 | — | 29 |
| | 77.5-105 | 52.6-89 | mg/100 g dry | 85 | c,d,e | 15 |
| Green beans | | | | | | |
| Seminole | 3.1 | — | mg/100 g | 96 | f | 20 |
| | 3.1 | — | mg/100 g | 100 | g | 20 |
| | 3.1 | — | mg/100 g | 90 | h | 20 |
| Ideal | 3.4 | — | mg/100 g | 83 | f | 20 |
| | 3.4 | — | mg/100 g | 91 | g | 20 |
| | 3.4 | — | mg/100 g | 76 | h | 20 |
| Contender | 3.1 | — | mg/100 g | 99 | f | 20 |
| | 3.1 | — | mg/100 g | 99 | g | 20 |
| | 3.1 | — | mg/100 g | 92 | h | 20 |
| Mont-Calme | 3.7 | — | mg/100 g | 96 | f | 20 |
| | 3.7 | — | mg/100 g | 98 | g | 20 |
| | 3.7 | — | mg/100 g | 91 | h | 20 |
| Juices | — | — | — | 90—98 | — | 11 |
| Orange juice | 1.69 | 1.63 | mg/100 g dry | 96 | i,l | 21 |
| | 1.60 | 1.56 | mg/100 g dry | 98 | j,l | 21 |
| | 1.58 | 1.50 | mg/100 g dry | 95 | k,l | 21 |
| Rose hips | — | — | — | ≈100 | m | 37 |
| Tomato juice | 9.1 | 9.15 | mg/kg fresh | 101 | n | 53 |
| | 7.6 | 7.6 | mg/kg fresh | 100 | o | 53 |
| | 8.5 | 7.4 | mg/kg fresh | 87 | p | 53 |
| Vegetables | — | — | — | ≈100 | — | 11 |
| Yogurt | — | — | — | 85—90 | — | 47 |

[a]  No sulfite.
[b]  Values for total carotene; see Table 5 for retention data for individual carotene isomers.
[c]  Percent retention based on blanched; initial content of fresh = 62.2 to 100 mg/100 g dry.
[d]  Isomerization occurs during drying; only trans $\beta$-carotene has 100% vitamin A activity; if fresh, 100% trans; freeze-dried has 89% of carotene as trans and thus only 80% of original trans.
[e]  Freeze-drying conditions: 71°C/1 torr/4 to 5 hr.
[f]  Water blanch — retention value includes blanching.
[g]  Steam blanch — retention value includes blanching.
[h]  $NaHCO_3$ blanch — retention value includes blanching.
[i]  13% total solids.
[j]  20% total solids.
[k]  36% total solids.
[l]  Maximum sample surface temperature during freeze drying = 60°C; vacuum of 50 to 100 mtorr; drying time for 12 mm thick slab = 16 hr for 13% total solids (approximately 0.65 kg $H_2O/m^2/$ hr), 18.5 hr for 20% total solids (0.5), 26 hr for 36% total solids (0.3).
[m]  Freeze-drying conditions: 7 hr with heating plates — 85°C (period 1), 60°C (period 2), 38°C (period 3); residual moisture about 4%; average sublimation rate of 1.1 to 1.3 kg $H_2O/m^2/$hr.
[n]  Natural.
[o]  Pasturized.
[p]  Concentrated.

Table 5
## RETENTION OF CAROTENE ISOMERS FOLLOWING FREEZE-DRYING

| Carotene type | Biopotency | Fresh | (%)[a] | Freeze-Dried | (%)[b] | Retention[c] (%) |
|---|---|---|---|---|---|---|
| Neo-α-carotene B | 38 | 1,645 | 1.8 | 1,524 | 1.9 | 93 |
| All-trans-α-carotene | 100 | 39,211 | 42.9 | 33,764 | 42.1 | 86 |
| Neo-α-carotene U | 53 | 731 | 0.8 | 561 | 0.7 | 77 |
| Neo-β-carotene B | 13 | 4,661 | 5.1 | 4,010 | 5.0 | 86 |
| All-trans-β-carotene | 53 | 44,055 | 48.2 | 39,458 | 49.2 | 90 |
| Neo-β-carotene U | 16 | 1,097 | 1.2 | 802 | 1.0 | 73 |
| Total | | 91,400 | 100.0 | 80,200 | 99.9 | 88 |

[a]  Percent of total carotene in fresh carrots.
[b]  Percent of total carotene in freeze-dried carrots.
[c]  Percent of isomer retained following freeze-drying.

From Sweeney, J. P. and Marsh, A. C., *J. Am. Diet. Assoc.*, 59(3), 243, 1971. With permission.

Table 6
## RETENTION OF NUTRITIVE VALUE OF THIAMINE FOLLOWING FREEZE-DRYING

| Food material | Content Initial | Final | Units | Percentage retention | Notes | Ref. |
|---|---|---|---|---|---|---|
| Beef | — | — | — | 98 | — | 60 |
| | 0.133 | 0.146 | mg/100 g dry | 100 | [a] | 59 |
| Chicken | 0.109 | 0.102 | mg/100 g | 94 | [b,d,f] | 51 |
| | 0.058 | 0.054 | mg/100 g | 93 | [c,d,f] | 51 |
| | 0.176 | 0.162 | mg/100 g | 92 | [b,e,f] | 51 |
| | 0.100 | 0.069 | mg/100 g | 69 | [c,e,f] | 51 |
| | 0.250 | 0.202 | mg/100 g dry | 81 | [a] | 58-59 |
| | 0.250 | 0.122 | mg/100 g dry | 49 | [c,g] | 58 |
| Meat, shrimp | — | — | — | 100 | [h] | 12 |
| Mutton | — | — | — | 70 | — | 29 |
| Peas | — | — | — | ≈100 | — | 12 |
| Pork | — | — | — | >90 | — | 12 |
| | 3.08 | 1.98 | mg/100 g dry | 64 | [i] | 35 |
| | 2.06 | 2.15 | mg/100 g dry | 100 | [a] | 59 |
| Shrimp | 0.113 | 0.049 | mg/100 g dry | 43 | [a,c,g] | 58-59 |
| Yogurt | — | — | — | 52—80 to 60—72 | [j] | 47 |

[a]  Data in Reference 59 appears to be too high by a factor of 10; accounted for in the data here.
[b]  Raw.
[c]  Cooked.
[d]  Light meat.
[e]  Dark meat.
[f]  Maximum product temperature is 29°F; desorbed to dryness in desiccator.
[g]  Initial content apparently is for raw items; therefore, retention value is for combined cooking and freeze-drying processes.
[h]  Meat = beef, chicken, and pork.
[i]  Original data is on a wet basis.
[j]  Two sets of results since two sources of information (see References).

Table 7
RETENTION OF NUTRITIVE VALUE OF RIBOFLAVIN
FOLLOWING FREEZE-DRYING

| Food material | Content | | | Percentage retention | Notes | Ref. |
|---|---|---|---|---|---|---|
| | Initial | Final | Units | | | |
| Beef | — | — | — | 100 | — | 60 |
| | 0.436 | 0.473 | mg/100 g dry | 109 | — | 59 |
| Chicken | 0.104 | 0.108 | mg/100 g | 104 | a,b,d | 51 |
| | 0.106 | 0.101 | mg/100 g | 95 | a,b,d | 51 |
| | 0.241 | 0.212 | mg/100 g | 88 | a,b,e | 51 |
| | 0.247 | 0.229 | mg/100 g | 93 | a,c,e | 51 |
| | 0.760 | 0.522 | mg/100 g dry | 69 | c,f | 58—59 |
| | 0.760 | 0.680 | mg/100 g dry | 89 | — | 58—59 |
| Fruits | — | — | — | ≈100 | — | 41 |
| Meat, fish | — | — | — | 100 | — | 29 |
| Mutton | — | — | — | 70 | — | 29 |
| Pork | — | — | — | ≈100 | — | 11 |
| Pork | 0.502 | 0.403 | mg/100 g dry | 80 | — | 59 |
| Shrimp | 0.125 | 0.125 | mg/100 g dry | 100 | — | 58 |
| | 0.125 | 0.109 | mg/100 g dry | 87 | — | 59 |
| Vegetables | — | — | — | ≈100 | — | 11 |
| Yogurt | — | — | — | 100 | — | 47 |

[a] Maximum sample temperature is 29°F; desorbed to dryness in desiccator.
[b] Raw.
[c] Cooked.
[d] Light meat.
[e] Dark meat.
[f] Initial content apparently is for raw items; therefore, retention value is for combined cooking and freeze drying processes.

Table 8
RETENTION OF NUTRITIVE VALUE OF MISCELLANEOUS VITAMINS
FOLLOWING FREEZE-DRYING

| Nutrient | Food material | Content | | | Percentage retention | Notes | Ref. |
|---|---|---|---|---|---|---|---|
| | | Initial | Final | Units | | | |
| Folic acid | Beef | 77 | 111 | µg/100 g dry | 144 | — | 59 |
| | Chicken | 174 | 264 | µg/100 g dry | 152 | — | 59 |
| | Shrimp | 197 | 244 | µg/100 g dry | 124 | — | 59 |
| Niacin | Beef | — | — | — | 100 | — | 60 |
| | | 10.51 | 9.81 | mg/100 g dry | 93 | — | 59 |
| | Chicken | 10.50 | 9.32 | mg/100 g | 89 | a,c | 51 |
| | | 10.76 | 11.06 | mg/100 g | 103 | b,c | 51 |
| | | 5.30 | 5.31 | mg/100 g | 100 | a,d | 51 |
| | | 5.37 | 5.37 | mg/100 g | 100 | b,d | 51 |
| | | 30.00 | 31.27 | mg/100 g dry | 104 | — | 59 |
| | Meat, fish | — | — | — | 70—100 | — | 29 |
| | Pork | — | — | — | ≈100 | — | 11 |
| | | 11.48 | 12.42 | mg/100 g dry | 108 | — | 59 |
| | | 11.48 | 12.42 | mg/100 g dry | 108 | — | 59 |
| | Shrimp | 5.99 | 2.39 | mg/100 g dry | 40 | — | 59 |
| | Vegetable | — | — | — | ≈90 | — | 11 |

## Table 8 (continued)
## RETENTION OF NUTRITIVE VALUE OF MISCELLANEOUS VITAMINS FOLLOWING FREEZE-DRYING

| Nutrient | Food material | Initial | Final | Units | Percentage retention | Notes | Ref. |
|---|---|---|---|---|---|---|---|
| Pantothenic acid | Beef | 1.18 | 1.02 | mg/100 g dry | 87 | — | 59 |
| | Chicken | 4.17 | 4.02 | mg/100 g dry | 96 | — | 59 |
| | Meat, fish | — | — | — | 70—100 | — | 29 |
| | Pork | 1.67 | 0.74 | mg/100 g dry | 44 | — | 59 |
| | Shrimp | 1.32 | 0.18 | mg/100 g dry | 14 | — | 59 |
| | Vegetables | — | — | — | ≈90 | — | 11 |
| Pyridoxine | Beef | 0.77 | 0.91 | mg/100 g dry | 118 | — | 59 |
| | Chicken | 2.17 | 0.26 | mg/100 g dry | 12 | — | 59 |
| | | 2.16 | 0.14 | mg/100 g dry | 6 | b,c | 58 |
| | Meat | — | — | — | 100 | f | 11—12 |
| | Milk, raw | — | — | — | 91 | g | 26 |
| | | — | — | — | 69 | h | 26 |
| | Pork | 1.05 | 1.37 | mg/100 g dry | 131 | — | 59 |
| | Shrimp | 0.53 | 0.62 | mg/100 g dry | 118 | — | 59 |
| | | | 0.41 | mg/100 g dry | 77 | b,c | 58—59 |
| Tocopherol | Beef | 2.03 | 1.19 | mg/100 g dry | 59 | — | 59 |
| | Chicken | 1.83 | 1.17 | mg/100 g dry | 64 | — | 59 |
| | Pork | 0.95 | 0.94 | mg/100 g dry | 99 | — | 59 |
| Vitamin $B_{12}$ | Meat, fish | — | — | — | 70—100 | — | 29 |
| | Yogurt | — | — | — | 80 | — | 47 |

a   Raw.
b   Cooked.
c   Light meat.
d   Dark meat.
e   Loss includes cooking and freeze-drying.
f   Meat = beef, pork, and chicken.
g   Drying temperature of 20°C.
h   Drying temperature of 50°C.

## Table 9
## RETENTION OF FATS AND POLYUNSATURATED FATTY ACIDS FOLLOWING FREEZE-DRYING

| Food material | Initial | Final | Units | Percent retention | Ref. |
|---|---|---|---|---|---|
| **Beef** | | | | | |
| Δ2a | 0.69 | 0.74 | g/100 g crude fat | 107 | 59 |
| Δ3 | 0.45 | 0.50 | g/100 g crude fat | 111 | 59 |
| Δ4 | 0.10 | 0.09 | g/100 g crude fat | 90 | 59 |
| Δ5 | 0.07 | 0.08 | g/100 crude fat | 114 | 59 |
| Δ6 | 0.03 | 0 | g/100 g crude fat | 0 | 59 |
| Total | 1.34 | 1.41 | g/100 g crude fat | 105 | 59 |
| **Chicken** | | | | | |
| Δ2 | 21.77 | 18.35 | g/100 g crude fat | 84 | 59 |
| Δ3 | 1.47 | 1.46 | g/100 g crude fat | 99 | 59 |
| Δ4 | 2.06 | 1.17 | g/100 g crude fat | 57 | 59 |
| Δ5 | 0.36 | 0.27 | g/100 g crude fat | 75 | 59 |
| Δ6 | 0.34 | 0.26 | g/100 g crude fat | 76 | 59 |
| Total | 26.00 | 21.51 | g/100 g crude fat | 83 | 59 |

### Table 9 (continued)
## RETENTION OF FATS AND POLYUNSATURATED FATTY ACIDS FOLLOWING FREEZE-DRYING

| | Content | | | Percent | |
| Food material | Initial | Final | Units | retention | Ref. |
| --- | --- | --- | --- | --- | --- |
| Pork | | | | | |
| Δ2 | 7.01 | 6.02 | g/100 g crude fat | 86 | 59 |
| Δ3 | 0.52 | 0.50 | g/100 g crude fat | 96 | 59 |
| Δ4 | 0.21 | 0.21 | g/100 g crude fat | 100 | 59 |
| Δ5 | 0.06 | 0.04 | g/100 g crude fat | 67 | 59 |
| Δ6 | 0.05 | 0.06 | g/100 g crude fat | 120 | 59 |
| Total | 7.85 | 6.83 | g/100 g crude fat | 87 | 59 |
| Shrimp | | | | | |
| Δ2 | 1.07 | 1.34 | g/100 g crude fat | 125 | 59 |
| Δ3 | 2.30 | 1.63 | g/100 g crude fat | 71 | 59 |
| Δ4 | 5.23 | 3.50 | g/100 g crude fat | 67 | 59 |
| Δ5 | 10.76 | 7.01 | g/100 g crude fat | 65 | 59 |
| Δ6 | 7.07 | 5.84 | g/100 g crude fat | 83 | 59 |
| Total | 26.43 | 19.32 | g/100 g crude fat | 73 | 59 |
| Beef, ground | 11.54 | 11.50 | % of fresh | 99.7 | 63 |
| Egg, whole | 10.43 | 11.20 | % of fresh | 107 | 63 |
| Milk, homogenized | 3.76 | 4.07 | % of fresh | 108 | 63 |

[a] Δ indicates number of double bonds.

### Table 10 (continued)
## *CHEMICAL ABSTRACTS'* LISTING OF SOURCES OF ADDITIONAL INFORMATION ON RETENTION OF NUTRITIVE VALUE FOLLOWING FREEZE-DRYING[a]

| Chemical Abstract number | First author | Food material | Nutrition | Losses during lyophilization (%) |
| --- | --- | --- | --- | --- |
| 66:18074z | Hamed | Green beans | Vitamin C | 24 |
| | | | Carotene | 5 |
| 66:18123q | Hamed | Tomato juice | Vitamin C, carotene | N.G.[b] |
| 66:45578 | Lempka | Cauliflower | Vitamin C | 13—86[c] |
| 66:45592y | Lempka | Black currants | Vitamin C | 16—33 |
| | | Raspberries | Vitamin C | <44 |
| | | Strawberries | Vitamin C | 15—43 |
| 70:105282s | Popovskii | Apricots, peaches, plums, strawberries | Vitamin C, carotene | Some |
| 71:2230q | Popovskii | Apricots, peaches, fruit berry puree, strawberries | Vitamin C, carotene | Small or none |
| 72:99352n | Kyzlink | Strawberries | Vitamin C | 4—10 |
| 73:38517u | Kassam | Pharmaceutical | Vitamin B complex | N.G. |
| 74:52259p | Weits | Green beans, peas, spinach | Ascorbic acid, carotene, riboflavin, thiamine, K. P, Ca | N.G. |
| 75:139542v | Lempka | Green peas | Vitamin C, carotene, riboflavin | [d] |

**Table 10 (continued)**
**CHEMICAL ABSTRACTS' LISTING OF SOURCES OF**
**ADDITIONAL INFORMATION ON RETENTION OF NUTRITIVE**
**VALUE FOLLOWING FREEZE-DRYING[a]**

[a] From *Chemical Abstracts 8th Collective Index*.
[b] N.G. = not given.
[c] Depends on time of harvest.
[d] Nutrient retention in green peas:

| | Fresh | Frozen | Freeze-dried | Percentage retention (based on fresh) |
|---|---|---|---|---|
| | | (mg% dry basis) | | |
| Vitamin C | 111 | 99 | 132 | 119 |
| Carotene | 0.32 | 0.40 | 0.50 | 156 |
| Riboflavin | 0.30 | 0.42 | 0.58 | 149 |

# REFERENCES

1. **Aguilera, J. M. and Flink, J. M.,** Technical note: determination of moisture profiles from tempera-ture measurements during freeze drying, *J. Food Technol.,* 9, 391—396, 1974.
2. **Aliaga, T. J. and Luh, B. S.,** Quality and storage stability of freeze dried mangoes, in *Proceedings XIIIth Int. Cong. Refrigeration,* Vol. 3, AVI Publishing, Westport, Conn., 1973, 757—763.
3. **Ammu, K. and Sharma, T. R.,** Changes in the nutritional value of the AFD (accelerated freeze-dried) foodstuffs during processing and storage, *Indian Food Packer,* 29(2), 5—10, 1975; *Food Sci. Tech-nol. Abst.,* 8, 2681, 1976.
4. **Ang, C. Y. W., Chang, C. M., Frey, A. E., and Livingston, G. E.,** Effects of heating methods on vitamin retention in six fresh or frozen prepared food products, *J. Food, Sci.,* 40, 997—1003, 1975.
5. **Barratt, R.,** Nutrition. II. Effects of processing, *Food Can.,* 1973(2), 28—31, 1973.
6. **Bender, A. E.,** Nutritional effects of food processing, *J. Food Technol.,* 1, 261—289, 1966.
7. **Bender, A. E.,** Processing damage to protein food, *J. Food Technol.,* 7, 239—250, 1972.
8. **Bluestein, P. B. and Labuza, T. P.,** Effects of moisture removal on nutrients, in *Nutritional Evalu-ation of Food Processing,* Harris, R. S. and Karmas, E., Eds., AVI Publishing, Westport, Conn., 1975, 289—323.
9. **Burger, I. H. and Walters, C. L.,** The effect of processing on the nutritive value of flesh foods, *Proc. Nutr. Soc.,* 32, 1—8, 1973.
10. **Cain, R. F.,** Water soluble vitamins: changes during processing and storage of fruit and vegetables, *Food Technol. (Chicago),* 21, 998—1007, 1967.
11. **Calloway, D.,** Dehydrated foods, *Nutr. Rev.,* 20, 257—260, 1962.
12. **Calloway, D. H.,** Nutritonal properties of unrefrigerated animal products, *Food Technol. (Chicago),* 102—106, 1962.
13. **Cook, D. J.,** Nutritional loss in food processing — vitamin C, Process Biochem., 9(5), 21—24, 1974.
14. **DeGroot, A. P.,** The influence of dehydration of foods on the digestibility and the biological value of the protein, *Food Technol. (Chicago),* 17, 339—343, 1963.
15. **DellaMonica, E. S. and McDowell, P. E.,** Comparison of beta-carotene content of dried carrots prepared by three dehydration processes, *Food Technol. (Chicago),* 19, 1597—1599, 1965.
16. **De Ritter, E.,** Stability characteristics of vitamins in processed foods, *Food Technol. (Chicago),* 30, 48—51, 54, 1976.
17. **Draudt, H. N. and Haung, I-Yih,** Effect of moisture control of freeze dried peaches and bananas on changes during storage related to oxidative and carbonyl-amine browning, *J. Agric. Food. Chem.,* 14(2), 170—176.
18. **Eboli, V.,** Freeze Dried Foods (in Italian), *Ind. Aliment.* (Pinerolo, Italy), 11(7/8), 89—99, 1972; *Food Sci. Technol. Abstr.,* 4, 12E493, 197 1972.

19. **Flink, J. M., Hawkes, J., Chen, H., and Wong, E.,** Properties of the freeze drying "scorch" temperature, *J. Food Sci.,* 39, 1244—1246, 1974.
20. **Foda, Y. H., El-Waraki, A., and Zaid, M. A.,** Effect of dehydration, freeze drying and packaging on the quality of green beans, *Food Technol. (Chicago),* 21(7), 1021—1024, 1967.
21. **Foda, Y. H., Hamed, M. G. E., and Abd-Allah, M. A.,** Preservation of orange and guava juices by freeze-drying, *Food Technol. (Chicago),* 24, 1392—1398, 1970.
22. **Ford, J. E.,** A microbiological method for assaying the nutritional value of proteins. IV. Analysis of enzymatically digested foods by sephadex gel-filtration, *Br. J. Nutr.,* 19, 277—293, 1965; Reference 25.
23. **Gentzler, G. L. and Schmidt, F. W.,** Thermodynamic properties of various water phases relative to freeze-drying, *Trans. Am. Soc. Agric. Eng.,* 16(1), 179—182, 1973.
24. **Goldblith, S. A.,** Freeze dehydration of foods, in, *Aspects Theoriques et Industriels de la Lyophilisation,* Rey, L., Ed., Hermann, Paris, 1964, 555—572.
25. **Goldblith, S. A. and Tannenbaum, S. R.,** The nutritional aspects of the freeze-drying of foods, in *Proc. Seventh Int. Congr. Nutrition,* Vol. 4, Hamburg, 1966, 1—16.
26. **Görner, F. and Oravcova, V.,** *Dairy Sci. Abstr.,* 33, 867, 1970; Reference 27.
27. **Gregory, M. E.,** Reviews of progress in dairy science: water-soluble vitamins in milk and milk products, *J. Dairy Res.,* 42, 197—216, 1975.
28. **Hackler, L. R.,** Effect of heat treatment on nutritive value of soy milk protein fed to weanling rats, *J. Food, Sci.,* 30, 723—728, 1965.
29. **Hanson, S. W. F., Ed.,** *The Accelerated Freeze Drying of Foods,* Her Majesty's Stationery Office, London, 1961.
30. **Harris, R. S. and Karmas, E., Eds.,** *Nutritional Evaluation of Food Processing,* AVI Publishing, Westport, Conn., 1975.
31. **Harris, R. S. and Von Loesecke, H., Eds.,** *Nutritional Evaluation of Food Processing,* John Wiley & Sons, New York, 1960.
32. **Karandaeva, V. P.,** Comparative nutritive values of meat dehydrated in a hot-air drier and by freeze drying, *Nutr. Abstr. Rev.,* 34, 433, 1964.
33. **Karel, M.,** Heat and mass transfer in freeze drying, in, *Freeze Drying and Advanced Food Technology,* Goldblith, S. A., Rey, L., and Rothmayr, W. W., Eds., Academic Press, London, 1975, 177—202.
34. **Karel, M. and Nickerson, J. T. R.,** Effects of relative humidity, air and vacuum on browning of dehydrated orange juice, *Food Technol. (Chicago),* 18, 1214—1218, 1964.
35. **Karmas, E., Thompson, J. E., and Peryman, D. B.,** Thiamine retention in freeze-dried irradiated pork, *Food Technol. (Chicago),* 16(3), 107—108, 1962.
36. **King, C. J.,** *Freeze-Drying of Foods,* CRC Press, Boca Raton, Fla., 1971.
37. **Krebes, T. and Behun, M.,** Quality and manufacture of freeze-dried fruit nectars, in *Proc. XIth Int. Congr. Refrigeration,* Vol. 2, 1963, 1597—1600.
38. **Labuza, T. P.,** Nutrient losses during drying and storage of dehydrated foods, *CRC Crit. Rev. Food Technol.,* 3(2), 217—240, 1972.
39. **Labuza, T. P.,** Effects of dehydration and storage, *Food Technol. (Chicago),* 27, 20—26, 1973.
40. **Larousse, J.,** Manufacture, value and utilization of freeze-dried foods, *Rev. Fr. Diet.,* 19(72), 7—13, 1975 (in French); *Food Sci. Technol. Abstr.,* 7, 11G699.
41. **Lempka, A. and Prominski, W.,** Changes in the vitamin contents of lyophilized fruits and vegetables, *Nahrung,* 11(3), 267—276, 1967; Reference 53.
42. **Mann, E. J.,** Freeze-dried dairy products, *Dairy Ind.,* 39(4), 123—124, 1974.
43. **Mapson, L. W.,** *Br. Med. Bull.,* 12, 73, 1956; Reference 6.
44. **Mitkov, S., Bakalivanov, St., Nikolova, T., and Vitanov, T.,** Determination of optimal parameters in lyophilization of egg white, egg yolk, and mixture of both, in *Proc. XIIIth Int. Congr. Refrigeration,* Vol. 3, AVI Publishing, Westport, Conn., 1973; 379—748.
45. **Mrak, E. M. and Pfaff, H. J.,** *Food Technol. (Chicago),* Recent advances in the handling of dehydrated fruits, 1, 147, 1947; Reference 38.
46. **Oetjen, G. W.,** Continuous freeze-drying of granulates with drying times in the 5 - 10 minutes range, in *Proc. XIIIth Int. Congr. Refrigeration,* Vol. 3, AVI Publishing, Westport, Conn., 1973, 697—706.
47. **Petrova, Z. Y.,** *Dairy Sci. Abstr.,* 34, 414, 1972; Refernces 27 and 42.
48. **Pol, G. and Groot, E. H.,** *Med. Melk - en Zuiveltijdechr,* 14, 158, 1960; Reference 6.
49. **Posati, L. P., Holsinger, V. H., DeVilbiss, E. D., and Pallansch, M. J.,** Effect of instantizing on amino acid content of nonfat dry milk, *J. Dairy Sci.,* 57, 258—260, 1974.
50. **Richter, E. and Handle, S.,** Influence of blanching and conservation by air drying at different temperatures, deep freezing and freeze drying on oxalic acid of spinach, *Z. Lebensm. Unters. Forsch.,* 153, 31—36, 1973 (in German).
51. **Rowe, D. M., Mountney, G. J., and Prudent, I.,** effect of freeze drying on the thiamine, riboflavin and niacin content of chicken muscle, *Food Technol. (Chicago),* 17, 1449—1450, 1963.

52. Sauvegeot, F., *Ind. Aliment,* (Pinerolo, Italy), 7, 122, 1968; Reference 9.

53. Sauvegeot, F., La lyophilisation et les just de fruits, *Ind. Aliment. Agric.,* 1969, 529—537, 1969.

54. Schroeder, H. A., Losses of vitamins and trace minerals resulting from processing and preservation of foods, *Am. J. Clin. Nutr.,* 24, 562—573, 1971.

55. Speckmann, E. W., Smith, K. J., Vanderveen, J. E., Homer, G. M., and Wiltsic Dunco, D., Nutritional acceptability of a dehydrated diet, *Aerosp. Med.,* 36(3), 256—260, 1965.

56. Speiss, W. E. L., *Kaltetechnik,* 16, 349, 1964; Reference 36.

57. Sweeney, J. P. and Marsh, A. C., Effect of processing on provitamin A in vegetables, *J. Am. Diet. Assoc.,* 59(3), 238—243, 1971.

58. Thomas, M. H. and Calloway, D. H., Nutritional Evaluation of Dehydrated Foods and Comparison with Foods Processed by Thermal and Radiation Methods, Q.M.F.C.I.A.F. Report 2—61, 1961, Reference 25.

59. Thomas, M. and Calloway, D., Nutritional value of dehydrated food, *J. Am. Diet. Assoc.,* 39, 105—116, 1961.

60. Tischer, R. C., Meat, quick-serve meals and the future army, *Food and Nutrition News,* 29(9), 1958; Reference 10.

61. Tuomy, J. M. and Felder, J., Effect of processing temperatures and cooking methods on the quality of freeze-dried cooked pork, *Food Technol. (Chicago),* 18(12), 1959—1960, 1964.

62. Wanninger, L. A., Jr., Mathematical model predicts stability of ascorbic acid in food products, *Food Technol. (Chicago),* 26, 42—45, 1972.

63. Watts, J. H., Booker, L. K., Wright, W. G., and Williams, E. G., The effects of various drying methods on the nitrogen and fat contents of biological materials, *Food Res.,* 21(5), 528—533, 1956.

64. Wing, R. W. and Alexander, J. C., Effect of microwave heating on vitamin B$_6$ retention in chicken, *J. Am. Diet. Assoc.,* 61(6), 661—664, 1972.

# EFFECT OF PROCESSING ON NUTRITIVE VALUE OF FOOD: FERMENTATION

## E. Dworschák

In the narrow sense of the term "fermentation" refers to alcoholic and lactic acid fermentation, which includes the process of Embden-Meyerhof-Parnas. The multistage process begins with glucose and then branches off at pyruvate; as a result of alcoholic fermentation, pyruvate develops first into acetaldehyde and then into ethanol. By way of lactic acid fermentation, lactic acid is produced from pyruvate.

In a broader sense fermentation is considered to be the process during which microorganisms (bacteria, yeast, and mold) multiply in the alimentary substance regarded as a culture medium, consume a certain amount, mostly of the carbohydrate component, transform the composition of the culture medium itself in the process and enrich it with the products of their metabolism. Hence, not only alcohols and acids but also vitamins are developed; moreover, the protein structure may undergo basic changes. Because of fermentation, changes may also occur in the nutritive value of foodstuffs. In the ensuing chapter the effect of fermentation on the biological value of major foodstuffs will be demonstrated.

## YOGURT FERMENTATION

Rasic and Stojsavljevic[11,13] produced yogurts on a culture medium with a 1:1 ratio of 2% *Streptococcus thermophilus* and *Lactobacillus bulgarious*. Using the standard procedure, the inoculated yogurt culture was incubated at 41 to 42°C for 2 to 3 hr. It was kept in the refrigerator at 4 to 7°C for 18 to 20 hr. The modified procedure is as follows: the inoculated culture is incubated at 42°C for an hour, then the incubation is continued at 30 to 32°C for 5 to 6 hr until coagulation. After the incubation the product is kept in the refrigerator at 4 to 7°C for 18 to 20 hr. Yogurt can be produced from both spray-dried and sheep's milk.

Fermentation caused no changes in the composition of amino acids. At the same time the authors examined the in vitro digestibility of the pepsin-pancreatin enzyme system. In Figure 1 the results of the in vitro digestibility of various milk species are presented, which were termed by the authors as the biological activity of amino acids. In Figure 2 the biological activity of amino acids of the yogurts produced from these milk species is presented, following the incubation. A comparison of the two figures indicates clearly that, at the effect of fermentation in the yogurt produced from milk, the activity of arginine, alanine, isoleucine, leucine, and tyrosine increased.

In the yogurt produced from powdered milk, only the relative quantity of alanine and leucine increased, whereas the level of aspartic acid, serine, glycine, and tyrosine decreased. In the yogurt produced from sheep's milk the biological activity of threonine and valine increased, while that of aspartic acid, serine, glutamic acid, and isoleucine decreased.

The biological values marked by the pepsin-pancreatin digest index (Tables 1 and 2) indicate that in the course of yogurt fermentation the in vitro digestibility of proteins, and especially the release of amino acids, increases, resulting in an improvement of the nutritive value. A comparison of the biological evaluation of proteins in yogurt species produced from different native substances is given in Figure 2.

Apart from amino acids the fermentation of yogurt has an effect on some parts of vitamin B complex.[5] The loss of vitamins $B_1$ and $B_2$ under the influence of pasteurization, vacuum condensation, and fermentation is summed up in Table 3.

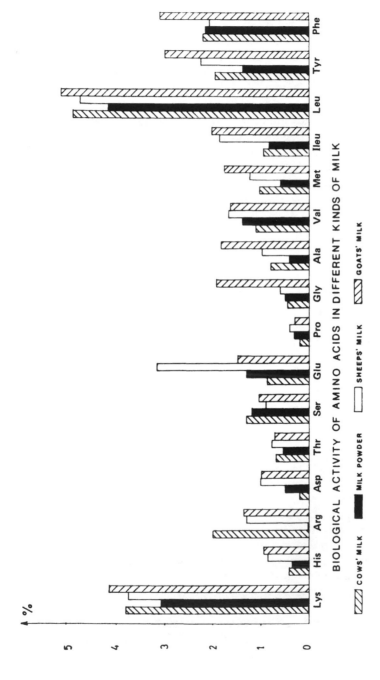

FIGURE 1. Biological activity of amino acids in different kinds of milk. (From Stojslavljevic, T., Rasic, J., and Curcic, R., *Milchwissenschaft*, 26, 147, 1971. With permission.)

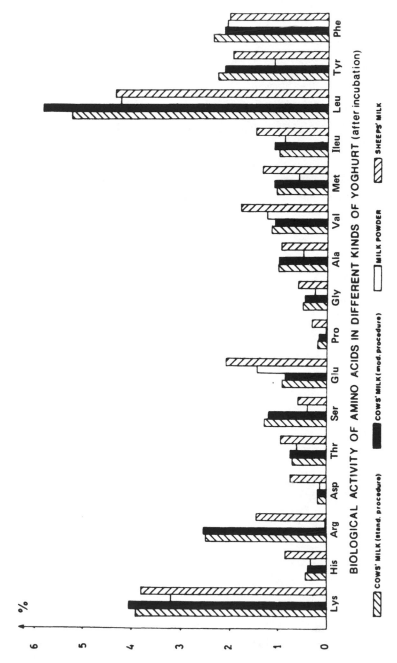

FIGURE 2.  Biological activity of amino acids in different kinds of yogurt (after incubation). (From Rasic, J., Stojslavljevic, T., and Curcic R., *Milchwissenschaft*, 26, 219, 1971. With permission.)

Table 1

## BIOLOGICAL VALUES OF MILK PROTEINS

|  | Cow's milk | Spray-dried milk | Goat's milk | Sheep's milk |
|---|---|---|---|---|
| Estimated biological values of the proteins[a] | 81.4 | 77.5 | 85.4 | 83.5 |

[a]     As compared to whole egg.

From Stojslavljevic, T., Rasic, J., and Curcic, R., *Milchwissenschaft*, 26, 147, 1971. With permission.

Table 2

## BIOLOGICAL VALUES OF YOGURT PROTEINS

| Estimated biological values of the proteins[a] | Yogurt | | | |
|---|---|---|---|---|
|  | Cow's milk (standard method) | Cow's milk (modified method) | Spray-dried milk | Sheep's milk |
| After incubation | 85.2 | 84.1 | 78.6 | 88.9 |
| After incubation and refrigeration | 87.3 | 85.6 | 79.8 | 89.3 |

[a]     As compared to whole egg.

From Rasic, J., Stojslavljevic, T., and Curcic, R., *Milchwissenschaft*, 26, 219, 1971. With permission.

Table 3

## VITAMIN B LOSS IN THE PROCESS OF YOGURT PRODUCTION

|  | $B_1$ vitamin loss | $B_2$ vitamin loss |
|---|---|---|
| Pasteurization at 85°C | 13.5% | 6% |
| Vacuum condensation | 14% | 6% |
| Fermentation at 42 to 45°C for 2.5 to 3 hr then storage at 6—10°C for 15 to 17 hr | 12% | 10% |

From Görner, F. and Oravcova, V., *Polnohospodarstvo*, 15, 825, 1969. With permission.

## THE EFFECT OF FERMENTATION ON THE COMPOSITION OF CHEESE

In the process of cheese production a significant loss of vitamins occurs because of the wearing out of whey. For example, Nilson et al.[10] pointed to the fact that in cheese curds, a basic material of cheese, the following percentage of vitamins in relation to whey is retained: nicotinic acid, 22%; vitamin $B_6$, 10%; biotin, 28%; folic acid, 40%; panthotenic acid, 28%; and vitamin $B_{12}$, 11%.

During cheese ripening the deterioration of some vitamins in the B group may continue, while the synthesis of others may begin, depending on the type of bacteria used. Many authors have studied the behavior of vitamin B complex under the influence of

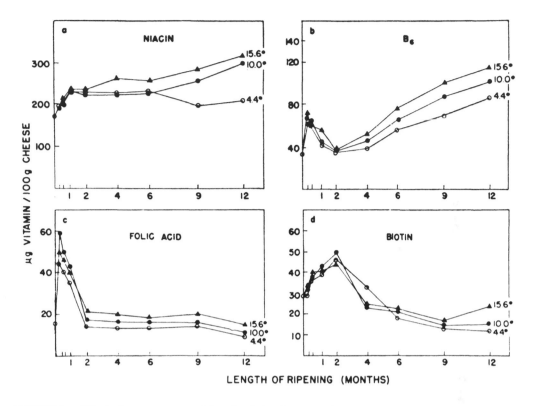

FIGURE 3. Effect of temperature and length of ripening upon the niacin, vitamin B₆, folic acid, and biotin content of Cheddar cheese (average of five lots). (From Nilson, K. M., Vakil, J. R., and Shahani, K. M., *J. Nutr.*, 86, 362, 1965. With permission.)

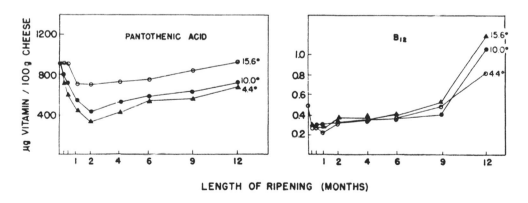

FIGURE 4. Effect of temperature and length of ripening upon the pantothenic acid and vitamin B₁₂ content of Cheddar cheese (average of five lots). (From Nilson, K. M., Vakil, J. R., and Shahani, K. M., *J. Nutr.*, 86, 362, 1965. With permission.)

fermentation or, more precisely, cheese ripening. According to Nilson et al.[10] the increase of ripening temperature in the case of Cheddar cheese caused an increase of the vitamin content (Figures 3 and 4). The following curves were made for the levels of some types of vitamins as a function of ripening time:

1.  The vitamin content increases proportionally with the ripening time (niacin; Figure 3).

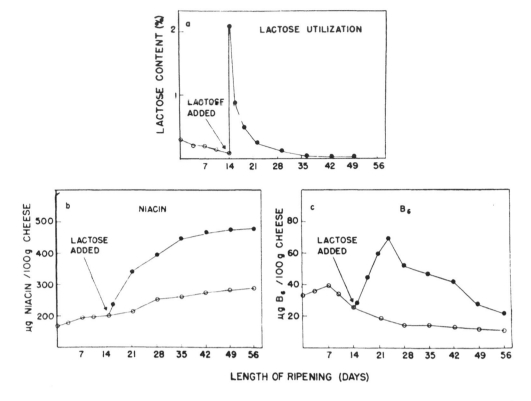

FIGURE 5.   Relationship between lactose metabolism and the biosynthesis of niacin and vitamin $B_6$ in Cheddar cheese (average of five lots). (From Nilson, K. M., Vakil, J. R., and Shahani, K. M., *J. Nutr.*, 86, 362, 1965. With permission.)

2.   At the early stages of ripening the vitamin level decreases; later it increases (pantothenic acid, vitamin $B_{12}$, Figure 4).

3.   At the early stages of ripening the vitamin level shows an increase, then it decreases (folic acid, biotin; Figure 3).

4.   The vitamin concentration exhibits several breaks in the function of ripening time (vitamin $B_6$; Figure 3).

Nilson et al.[10] also pointed out that if the fermentation promoting lactose is added to the Cheddar cheese, lactose transforms in a short period of time, whereas the quantity of certain vitamins (niacin, vitamin, and $B_6$) increases abruptly (Figure 5).

The analysis of the quantity of vitamins belonging to the B group as a function of ripening time usually resulted in an increase. Kisza[8] observed in Roequefort-type cheese a 15% increase of vitamin $B_{12}$/6 mg/100 g salt-free dry matter during 3 months.

According to Görner and Oravcova,[5] in ripened Gouda cheese the vitamin $B_1$ was 96 µg, and vitamin $B_2$ was 312 µg in relation to 100 g of dry matter, which when compared to the young cheese showed a 313 to 322% increase, respectively.

Some literary data indicate that in the process of cheese ripening, vitamin $B_2$ and niacin production are performed mainly on the surface.[1] The mold breeding on the surface of cheese increases the niacin synthesis. For example, on the surface of Camembert cheese 2.3 mg% niacin was present, while inside there was only 0.35 mg%. In the rind of Gruyere cheese 50% more niacin was found than in the inner parts.

According to the studies of Berger-Grüner[1] in the process of Sortsalute cheese ripening the production of vitamin $B_2$ caused by bacteria and their deterioration was almost in an equilibrium, whereas the niacin content during the ripening of the cheese was increasing (Table 4).

Table 4
THE NIACIN CONTENT
OF SORTSALUTE
CHEESE AS A
FUNCTION OF
RIPENING TIME

Niacin mg% Counted on
DM

| Day | Charge | Day | Charge |
|-----|--------|-----|--------|
| 3   | 0.234  | 3   | 0.264  |
| 12  | 0.346  | 14  | 0.349  |
| 20  | 0.349  | 21  | 0.351  |

From Berger-Grüner, M., *Milchwissenschaft*, 21, 222, 1966. With permission.

Table 5
INFLUENCE OF BACTERIAL STRAINS ON
VITAMIN $B_{12}$ CONTENT IN EDAM CHEESE IN
THE PROCESS OF THE RIPENING

| Bacterial strains | Increase in percent of vitamin $B_{12}$ |
|-------------------|------------------------------------------|
| *Propioni bacterium shermanii* | 134 |
| *P. pentosaceum* | 83 |
| *P. raffinosaceum* | 78 |
| *P. freuden-reichii* | 69 |

From Janicki, J. and Obrusiewicz, T., *Rocz. Technol. Chem. Zywn.*, 19, 59, 1970. With permission.

The increase of vitamin B in cheese depends also upon the bacteria strain used. Janicki and Obrusiewicz[7] analyzed the change of vitamin $B_{12}$ concentration in Edam cheese. Unripened young cheese contained 1.4 µg/100 g vitamin $B_{12}$. The increase of vitamin content in the selected four best strains is summarized by percentage in Table 5.

## EFFECT OF FERMENTATION ON THE NUTRITIVE VALUE OF SOYBEANS AND OTHER CEREALS

Fermented soybean foods are very popular in the Far East, and the most familiar among them is the tempeh of Indonesian origin. Practically, tempeh is prepared as follows: partly smashed soybeans are cooked with water, cooled, and dried, and are then inoculated with *Rhizopus oligosporus*. After fermentation for various lengths of time the mold is killed by steaming. Some authors[14] tried fermentation similar to tempeh with other food products, e.g., wheat, also with *R. oligosporus* strains.

Weight gain and food consumption by rats receiving a diet containing fermented wheat were significantly increased over the wheat control group. However, the weight gain of rats fed diets containing fermented soybeans was not significantly different from the weight gain by rats on the control diet, although food consumption was less than for the control group (Table 6).

## Table 6
## WEIGHT GAIN, FOOD CONSUMPTION, AND PROTEIN EFFICIENCY RATIO OF RATS FED FERMENTED OR UNFERMENTED GRAINS AS PROTEIN SOURCE

| Protein source | Weight gain (g) | Food consumption (g) | PER (gram weight gain per gram protein consumed) |
|---|---|---|---|
| Casein | 98.0 ± 6.6[a] | 347 ± 13[a] | 2.81 ± 0.10[a] |
| Wheat, control | 37.6 ± 2.7 | 295 ± 13 | 1.28 ± 0.05 |
| Wheat, fermented | 55.0 ± 1.6[b] | 322 ± 7[b] | 1.71 ± 0.05[b] |
| Soybeans, control | 76.5 ± 2.3 | 353 ± 10 | 2.17 ± 0.03 |
| Soybeans, fermented | 72.9 ± 3.3 | 321 ± 12[b] | 2.27 ± 0.05 |
| Soybeans and wheat, control | 97.1 ± 3.2 | 389 ± 8 | 2.49 ± 0.04 |
| Soybeans and wheat, fermented | 94.2 ± 2.2 | 338 ± 12[b] | 2.79 ± 0.04[b] |

[a]   Standard error of mean.
[b]   Significantly ($p < 0.05$) different from corresponding unfermented grain.

From Wang, H. L., Ruttle, D. I., and Hesseltine, C. W., *J. Nutr.*, 96, 109, 1968. With permission.

## Table 7
## INFLUENCE OF FERMENTATION TIME ON PROTEIN QUALITY OF WHEAT

| Time (hr) | Weight gain (g) | Food consumption (g) | PER (gram weight gain per gram protein consumed) |
|---|---|---|---|
| 0 (Control) | 29.3 ± 1.7[a] | 235 ± 13[a] | 1.25 ± 0.07[a] |
| 12 | 28.9 ± 2.3 | 225 ± 9 | 1.28 ± 0.05 |
| 24 | 40.7 ± 2.1[b] | 228 ± 9 | 1.78 ± 0.07[b] |
| 48 | 49.5 ± 2.2[b] | 269 ± 11[b] | 1.84 ± 0.04[b] |
| 72 | 39.4 ± 3.0[b] | 226 ± 11 | 1.73 ± 0.06[b] |

[a]   Standard error of mean.
[b]   Significantly ($p < 0.05$) different from control.

From Wang, H. L., Ruttle, D. I., and Hesseltine, C. W., *J. Nutr.*, 96, 109, 1968. With permission.

Thus, fermentation unanimously improved the biological value of proteins in the above mentioned process. The PER (protein efficiency ratio) of fermented soybean-wheat mixture was near that of the caseine.

Wang et al.[14] also studied the effect of fermentation time on PER value (Table 7). Rats receiving wheat diets fermented for 24 hr increased in body weight and PER value. The increase in body weight and PER value of rats consuming diets after 48 hr fermentation was the highest. The consumption of diets after 72 hr fermentation was reduced because of the flavor change; this caused a reduction in weight gain.

The nutritive value of proteins in the tempeh itself changed with the function of fermentation time.[12] The PER and Essential Amino Acid Index (EAAI) increased after 12 to 36 hr fermentation. The correlation coefficient between PER and EAAI in the case of 12 to 72 hr fermentation was 0.97 (Figure 6). The increase of EAAI and PER value corresponded to a 30% increase of tryptophan during fermentation.[12] Murata et al.[9] noticed an increase of tryptophan and phenylalanine in some samples of fermented tempeh.

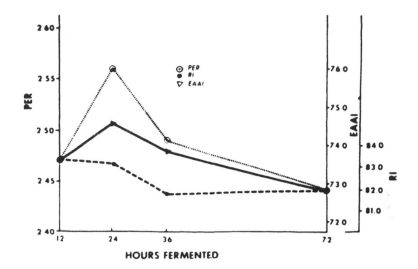

FIGURE 6. Effect of tempeh fermentation-time on the protein efficiency ratio (PER), essential amino acid index (EAAI), and requirement index (RI). (From Wang, H. L., Ruttle, D. I., and Hesseltine, C. W., *J. Nutr.*, 96, 109, 1968. With permission.)

In conformity with the analysis of Wang et al.,[14] the ratio of essential amino acids in fermented soybean and wheat preparations did not change when compared to one another. The glutamic acid decreased by 30%, while the alanine increased by 50%. The authors stated that the change of amino acids was in relation to the increased glutamic-pyruvic transaminase activity of mold. The result was a decrease of the quantity of nonessential amino acids compared to that of essential amino acids.

The pepsin-pancreatin digestibility of wheat preparations fermented by *R. oligosporus* increased, and many essential amino acids became free on the effect of enzymes (Table 8). According to Wang et al.[14] the enzymes produced by mold probably attack the proteins, simplifying the further activity of proteolytic enzymes.

Murata et al.[9] examined changes of vitamin B complex on the effect of fermentation in tempeh. As a result of fermentation thiamin decreased; at the same time vitamin $B_2$, $B_6$, and nicotic acid increased four to eight times over the amount in the unfermented soybeans. The vitamin levels in a slightly overfermented sample marked B were much higher than that of the others (Table 9).

As to the effect of fermentation time, the vitamin $B_1$ level during 24 hr showed an increase then decreased (Figure 7). The 48 hr fermentation, from the point of palatability, seemed optimal; the vitamin $B_1$ level was equal to that of unfermented soybeans.

## EFFECT OF FERMENTATION PROMOTING ADDITIVES ON THE NUTRITIVE VALUE OF BAKERY PRODUCTS[3]

The good quality of bakery products cannot always be ensured by direct dough production. For this reason fermentation is increased by food additives (e.g., amylolitic enzymes) in order to obtain a proper dough porosity. Thus, the effect of fermentation-promoting technological processes (e.g., bread production with sponge technology and food additives) on the nutritional value of bakery products was investigated.

Sample breads of 360 g were baked. Three flours (ash content 0.55) of low, average, and high amylase activity were used, since fermentation is largely influenced by amylase activity. Fermentation-promoting additives were used, including the mold amylase

Table 8
## EFFECT OF FERMENTATION ON ESSENTIAL AMINO ACIDS RELEASED BY PEPSIN AND PANCREATIN DIGESTION OF WHEAT

| Amino acids[a] | Control (mg/g N) | Fermented (mg/g N) | Total essential amino acids | |
|---|---|---|---|---|
| | | | Control (mg/g) | Fermented (mg/g) |
| Lysine | 94 | 118 | 119 | 137 |
| Histidine | 17 | 25 | 22 | 29 |
| Threonine | 136 | 134 | 173 | 156 |
| Valine | 57 | 55 | 72 | 64 |
| Total sulfur-containing amino acids | 62 | 71 | 80 | 83 |
| Isoleucine | 54 | 62 | 69 | 72 |
| Leucine | 179 | 199 | 229 | 231 |
| Total aromatic amino acids | 186 | 197 | 237 | 228 |
| Total essential amino acids | 785 | 862 | — | — |

[a]    Tryptophan was destroyed during the picric acid procedure and not determined in the enzyme hydrolysates.

From Wang, H. L., Ruttle, D. I., and Hesseltine, C. W., *J. Nutr.,* 96, 109, 1968. With permission.

Table 9
## VITAMIN CONTENT OF INDONESIAN TEMPEH AND UNFERMENTED SOYBEANS

In Dry Matter

| | Tempeh made in Indonesia (sun dried) | | | |
|---|---|---|---|---|
| | Unfermented control, sample number A-1 | Tempeh, sample number A-2 | Unfermented control, sample number B-1 | Tempeh, sample number B-2 |
| Thiamin (mg%) | 0.22 | 0.13 | 0.26 | 0.16 |
| | (1)[a] | (0.6) | (1) | (0.6) |
| Riboflavin (mg%) | 0.06 | 0.49 | 0.03 | 1.41 |
| | (1) | (8.1) | (1) | (47) |
| Vitamin B$_6$ (mg%) | 0.08 | 0.35 | 0.04 | 0.58 |
| | (1) | (4.4) | (1) | (14) |
| Nicotinic acid (mg%) | 0.90 | 4.39 | 0.21 | 4.31 |
| | (1) | (4.9) | (1) | (20) |

[a]    Rate of value in tempeh to value in unfermented soybeans.

Reprinted from Murata, K., Ikehata, H., and Miyamoto, T., *Food Technology/Journal of Food Science,* Vol. 32, p. 580, 1967. Copyright © by Institute of Food Technologists. With permission.

preparation Cereáz® manufactured by the Hungarian Biogal Pharmaceutical Works. The breads contained 3% yeast to the amount of flour and the duration of baking was uniformly 25 min at 260°C.

Apart from tryptophan, with regard to the components examined, the various fermentation-increasing methods (included the bread production with sponge technology) did not show significant differences. Therefore, the data obtained are contracted in the figures.

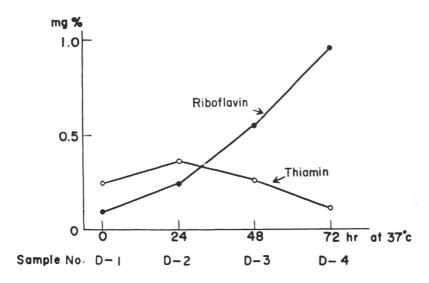

FIGURE 7. Changes in thiamin and riboflavin content of tempeh (D) during fermentation. (Reprinted from Murata, K., Ikehata, H., and Miyamoto, T., *Food Technology/Journal of Food Science,* Vol. 32, p. 580, 1967. Copyright © by Institute of Food Technologists, With permission.)

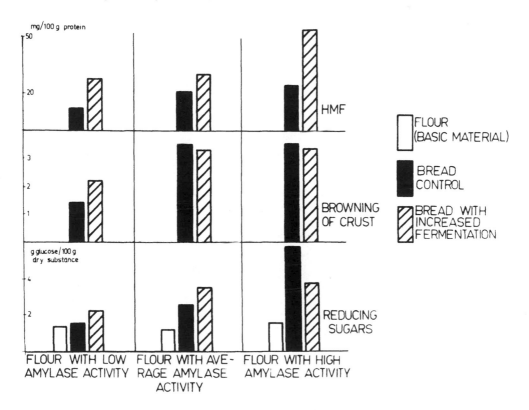

FIGURE 8. The HMF, reducing sugar, and crust browning values of sample breads produced from flours of various amylase activity in the function of fermentation. (From Dworschák, E., Molnár, E. B., and Szilli, M., *Lebensm. Wiss. Technol.,* 6, 14, 1973. With permission of Forster-Verlag AG, Ottikerstrasse 59, CH-8033, Zurich, Switzerland.)

Figure 8 reflects the results of HMF (5-hydroxymethylfurfural) crust browning and

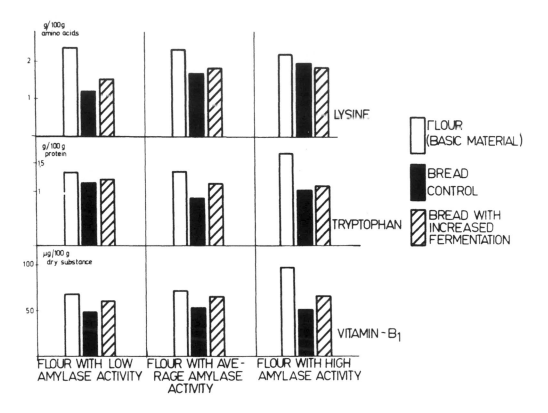

FIGURE 9.   The vitamin $B_1$, lysine, and tryptophan contents of flours with various amylase activity and that of sample breads produced from the former materials in the function of fermentation. (From Dworschåk, E., Molnår, E. B., and Szilli, M., *Lebensm. Wiss. Technol.*, 6, 14, 1973. With permission of Forster-Verlag AG, Ottikerstrasse 59, CH-8033, Zurich, Switzerland.)

sugar. It can be seen that the increase of the examined components was proportional to that of the enzyme activity in flour. The HMF and sugar content of the samples exposed to an increased fermentation was higher than in the controls, except for breads produced from flour of high enzyme activity. In the consecutive reactions of sugar production and fermentation, the latter's speed was probably higher. The crust browning after a certain degree of sugar concentration did not increase.

Data of lysine, tryptophan, and vitamin $B_1$ are presented in Figure 9. All three components significantly decreased in breads in comparison to the flour. The decrease of lysine in controls resulting from the flour of low enzyme activity was 50%. In increasingly fermented breads the average lysine, tryptophan, and vitamin $B_1$ values were higher than in the controls, even if this difference was not considerable in each case. Only the lysine content in breads baked from flour of high enzyme activity was an exception. In this context the difference between the lysine content of the flour and the bread produced from it decreased with the increase of amylase activity in flours. Data about tryptophan can be found in Table 10. The table demonstrates the different technological modifications, in an approximately increasing order, with the intensity of fermentation. The tryptophan content of bread correlates with the increase of fermentation; its decomposition gradually diminishes in relation to the flour. This trend does not apply to flours of high enzyme activity.

The decrease of amino acid and vitamin $B_1$ content of breads compared to the flour can be due to the Maillard reaction and the heat lability of vitamin $B_1$. In the highly fermented dough the amount of sugar is increased by the enzyme activity, which could result in a more intensive Maillard reaction during baking. This assumption seems to

Table 10
## EFFECT OF VARIOUS DOUGH FERMENTATION METHODS ON THE TRYPTOPHAN CONTENTS OF BREADS

Grams per 100 g Protein

| Means of treatment, basic material | Flour | Bread control | Sucrose | Cereâz® | Cereâz® + sucrose | Sponge + sucrose | Sponge + Cereâz® | Sponge + Cereâz® + sucrose | Sponge + Cereâz® increased |
|---|---|---|---|---|---|---|---|---|---|
| Flour of low enzyme activity | 1.33 | 1.13 | 1.03 | 1.12 | — | 1.20 | 1.20 | — | 1.25 |
| Flour of average enzyme activity (0.03 SKB units) | 1.31 | 0.86 | 1.02 | 0.91 | 1.19 | 1.15 | 1.25 | 1.24 | 1.34 |
| Flour of high enzyme activity (0.7 SKB units) | 1.60 | 1.04 | 1.09 | 0.80 | — | 1.01 | 1.37 | — | 1.14 |

From Dworschák, E., Molnár, E. B., and Szilli, M., *Lebensm. Wiss. Technol.*, 6, 14, 1973. With permission of Forster-Verlag AG, Ottikerstrasse 59, CH-8033, Zurich, Switzerland.

be supported by data of crust browning and HMF content, which have so far been considered the sensitive indicators of Maillard reaction. It is to be expected that the amount of sensitive amino acids decreases in breads produced from dough of higher amylase activity and sugar content, in comparison to the controls; namely, it is in inverse ratio the HMF content. As can be seen in previous figures, amino acid levels in heat-treated samples did not diminish; even the tryptophan and lysine content increased. Consequently, the reducing activity of sugar concentration to the amino acids seems to be counteracted by some other effect appearing during the processing.

It was observed that the pH decreases during fermentation. According to literary data on the Maillard reaction, the amino acid decomposition in the presence of sugars is promoted by the pH increase.[2] On the other hand, the acid medium decreases the thermal decomposition of vitamin $B_1$.[4] If formation of acids was higher in breads produced with increased fermentation than in the controls, the protecting effect of this technology on essential amino acids and vitamin $B_1$ would be explained. During dough making some organic acids (lactic acid, acetic acid, etc.) are produced because of fermentation and other parallel reactions. The increase in fermentation by additives is followed by the increase in quantity of organic acids.[6]

In order to prove the mechanism connected with pH changes, breads were prepared from flour of average enzyme activity: (1) adjusted to a 0.4% level by lactic acid, (2) soured by fermentation with sugar and Cereâz®, and (3) control. The lysine content of the doughs and the final products were determined. Figure 10 shows that lactic acid resulted in higher pH changes than increased fermentation and prevented the lysine decomposition to a greater extent than did the acid medium in the two other samples. There is only a slight difference between the lysine content of fermented and control samples in favor of the former, due presumably to the slight pH change.

The increased fermentation promoted the HMF formation and crust browning and at the same time exerted a protecting effect on the decomposition of amino acids. The rise of the acidity in the medium was followed by the increase of HMF, caramel, and dextrine formation, whereas the intensity of the Maillard reaction decreased.

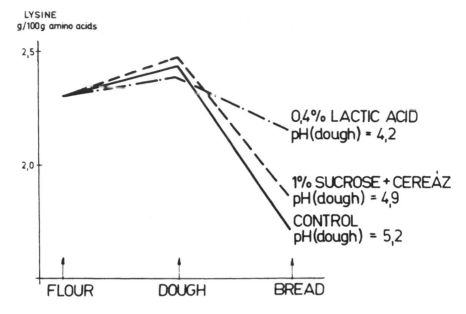

FIGURE 10.   Lysine content of dough: (1) control, (2) soured with lactic acid, (3) soured with fermentation; and that of breads made from the former materials. (From Dworschák, E., Molnár, E. B., and Szilli, M., *Lebensm. Wiss. Technol.*, 6, 14, 1973. With permission of Forster-Verlag AG, Ottikerstrasse 59, CH-8033, Zurich, Switzerland.)

# REFERENCES

1. Berger-Grüner, M., *Milchwissenschaft,* 21, 222—225, 1966.
2. Burton, H. S. and McWeeny, D. J., *Nature (London),* 197, 226-268, 1963.
3. Dworschák, E., Molnár, E. B., and Szilli, M., *Lebensm. Wiss. Technol.*, 6, 14-18, 1973.
4. Farrer, K. T. H., *Adv. Food Res.*, 6, 257-306, 1955.
5. Görner, F. and Oravcova, V., *Polnohospodarstvo,* 15, 825-831, 1969.
6. Hunter, I. R. and Pence, J. W., *J. Food Sci.*, 26, 578-580, 1961.
7. Janicki, J. and Obrusiewicz, T., *Rocz. Technol. Chem. Zywn.*, 19, 59-74, 1970.
8. Kisza, J., *Zesz. Nauk. Wyzsz. Szk. Roln. Olsztynic,* 23, 523-544, 1967.
9. Murata, K., Ikehata, H., and Miyamoto, T., *J. Food Sci.*, 32, 580-586, 1967.
10. Nilson, K. M., Vakil, J. R., and Shahani, K. M., B vitamin content of Cheddar cheese, *J. Nutr.,* 86, 362—368, 1965.
11. Rasic, J., Stojslavljevic, T., and Curcic, R., A study on the amino acids of yoghurt. I, *Milchwissenschaft,* 26, 219-224, 1971.
12. Stillings, B. R. and Hackler, L. R., Amino acid studies on the effect of fermentation time and heat processing of tempeh, *J. Food Sci.*, 30, 1043-1048, 1965.
13. Stojslavljevic, T., Rasic, J., and Curcic, R., A study on the amino acids of yoghurt. 2, *Milchwissenschaft,* 26, 147-151, 1971.
14. Wang, H. L., Ruttle, D. I., and Hesseltine, C. W., Protein quality of wheat and soybeans after Rhisopus oligosporus fermentation, *J. Nutr.*, 96, 109-114, 1968.

# ENZYMES AND FOOD QUALITY

P. F. Fox and P. A. Morrissey

## INTRODUCTION

Enzymes are specialized proteins possessing catalytic activity on which all living organisms depend to promote the various vital reactions necessary to maintain life. Some 2000 enzymes have been isolated and classified into six principal subgroups:

1. Oxidoreductases: catalyzing oxidation — reduction reactions
2. Transferases: catalyzing group transfer reactions
3. Hydrolyzases: catalyzing hydrolytic reactions
4. Lyases: catalyzing the addition of groups to double bonds and vice-versa
5. Isomerases: catalyzing isomerizations
6. Ligases (Synthetases): catalyzing the condensation of two molecules coupled with the cleavage of a P-P bond of ATP or similar triphosphate

In addition to relevant chapters in general biochemistry textbooks, specialized texts on general enzymology include Dixon and Webb,[164] Whitaker,[752] Barman[34,35] Nielands and Stumpf,[514] Commission on Biochemical Nomenclature,[124] Boyer,[73] and Colwich and Kaplan.[123]

With a few minor exceptions, our food was once living tissue, plant, animal, microbial, or secretions of living tissue and was, therefore, synthesized through the action of enzymes. During life our future food depended on enzymes to maintain life. Following death these various enzymes remain active for periods dependent on such environmental factors as temperature, pH, oxygen supply, availability of substrate, cofactors, etc. Conversion of living tissue to food depends on the continued activity of indigenous enzyme systems post-mortem or post-harvest; indeed *de novo* synthesis post-harvest is an important feature of many fruits and vegetables. However not all enzymic changes are desirable and much food spoilage occurs through the continued action of indigenous enzymes and of enzymes produced by contaminating living microorganisms or released by them on lysis.

Since essentially all food constituents are enzyme substrates they may be modified by adding exogenous enzymes to improve food quality or to convert a food commodity from one form to another. With the increasing tendency toward processed convenience foods, the use of exogenous enzymes is assuming a major significance made possible by advances in enzyme technology. The growing interest in the use of novel, unconventional food sources for human food has opened up additional avenues for enzyme applications in food processing; indeed some of these developments have been made possible only through the application of enzymes.

General references on food enzymology include Underkofler et al.,[707] Reed,[588] Underkofler,[706] Schultz,[613] de Becze,[44] Schwimmer,[618] Anon.,[403a] Eskin et al.,[185] Wieland,[760] Whitaker,[753] Monsan and Durand,[481] Dewdney,[158] Beck and Scott,[42], Fox,[208] Skinner,[644] Desmazeaud et al.,[152] Drapron and Ribadeau-Dumas,[000] Jones,[347] Shahani et al.,[626] Kretovich et al.,[396] Richardson,[593] Gams,[227] and Villadsen.[717]

Food enzymology can be divided into three well-defined areas:

1. Indigenous enzymes
2. Exogenous, added enzymes
3. Enzymes produced by microorganisms presented either as contaminants or added as cultures

Although the third category is very important in food technology, it will not be considered in the present discussion. Suffice it to say that fermentation has been a classical method of food preservation throughout history. Among the more important food products which owe their identity to the activity of microbial enzyme systems are cheeses and other fermented dairy products, fermented meat products, pickled fruits and vegetables, beers, wines, and spirits. However the consequences of microbial activity are not always beneficial and on the debit side are food spoilage and food poisoning. Among the many important texts and major reviews on changes in food produced by microbial enzymes produced *in situ* are Foster et al.,[205] Frazier,[215] Schormuller,[635] Jay,[337] Kyoto,[403a] Dwivedi,[172] and Kinsella and Hwang.[378]

### Indigenous Enzymes

In a recent paper, Schwimmer[619] wrote "It is not too great an exaggeration to maintain that food processing and technology may be considered as the art and science of the promotion, control and/or prevention of cellular disruption and its metabolic consequences at the right time and at the right place in the food processing chain. In this context cellular disruption with respect to food can (1) create identity; (2) improve quality; (3) be deleterious." Although Schwimmer was writing principally of the influence of cellular disruption in food processing, the quotation is an equally eloquent description of modern food enzymology.

Indigenous food enzymes can be considered from at least two aspects: (1) changes, desirable and undesirable, induced in food quality by enzymic activity and (2) as indexes of the history of a food product. Although this latter aspect is of considerable importance to the food processor, it is not directly relevant to the present discussion and will not be discussed further.

### *Changes Induced by Indigenous Enzymes*

Indigenous enzymes catalyze numerous desirable changes in most food groups but the importance of these changes depends on the particular product; a desirable change in one product may be deleterious in another and this may apply even between different products of the same group. However, in many cases desirable changes are overshadowed by deleterious effects. Consequently, early efforts in food enzymology were principally concerned with inactivating undesirable enzymes, usually by thermal processing and less frequently by chemical agents or by reducing their activity by low-temperature storage. Increased knowledge of enzyme characteristics, their compartmentalization within cells, and genetic selection of plants and animals has made it possible in many cases to improve food quality and methods of food conservation by exploiting beneficial enzymes or selectively suppressing undesirable ones.

### Added Enzymes

Crude enzyme preparations have been unwittingly used in food processing since prehistoric times, e.g., calf vells in cheese manufacture, bruised papaya leaves to tenderize meat, and malt in brewing and distilling. Increased availability of commercially pure enzymes has markedly expanded and diversified the range of applications which fall into three general categories:

1.  Those in which enzyme treatments form an essential part of the process, e.g., the production of cheeses, beers, and spirits.
2.  Those in which enzymes are used to improve product quality where alternative procedures may or may not be available, such as meat tenderization, loaf volume and quality, and functional properties of food constituents, e.g., dextrins and other starch derivatives, proteins, and lipids.

3.  Those in which enzymes are used to improve the economic or technological aspects of a process, e.g., extraction of fruit juices and essential oils, manufacture of liquid center candies, and continuous bread manufacture.

Enzymes possess many unique properties which make them very attractive agents in food processing: (1) they are specific and hence can be used to modify an individual food constituent without significantly affecting other constituents; (2) enzymes are required only in catalytic rather than stoichiometric amounts and hence do not per se alter the physico-chemical properties of the food; (3) they generally require moderate conditions of pH, temperature, ionic strength, etc., and hence induce specific changes without concomitant secondary changes which might result from more severe processing conditions; and (4) when enzymes have catalyzed the desired change they may be inactivated by relatively mild changes of temperature or pH and so induce no further change in the product.

However, these same characteristics may be disadvantageous under certain circumstances, e.g., narrow pH-activity range, inactivation by various inorganic ions, or excessively narrow specificity. Hence, careful selection of enzymes for particular applications is required.

Because of their specificity, enzymes are ideal reagents for many analytical applications. However, this aspect will not be considered in this review and the interested reader is referred to Bergemeyer,[52] Guildbault,[266] and Boehringer-Mannheim.[64] The review by de Becze[44] also contains useful information on enzyme units and methods of analysis.

According to Marshall[459] 2100 patents on the use of enzymes in food processing were issued in the U.S. alone in the period of 1950 to 1970, in addition to countless scientific publications. Of the 2100 patents, 500 dealt with the use of enzymes to increase food production or to increase the acceptability of food products; approximately 300; the majority using microbial enzymes, pertained to the flavor of foods. Beck and Scott[42] claim that of the approximately 2000 enzymes which have been identified and classified to date, less than 20 are commercially used on a scale that has significant impact on either the food industry or the enzyme industry. The considerations necessary for the successful commercialization of enzymes in food technology are extensively discussed by Beck and Scott,[42] who estimated that the value of the enzyme industry in 1973 was $100 million per annum worldwide of which $45 million worth were used in food applications. These values are similar to those cited by Skinner[644] from a survey by Bernard Wolnak and associates (Table 1).

The production of enzymes for food and industrial applications has developed into a high-technology industry of considerable economic importance. The numerous texts and reviews on commercial enzyme production include Spencer,[656] Wiseman,[764] and Skinner.[644]

Perhaps the most significant recent development in the industrial application of enzymes has been the immobilization of enzymes on solid supports. A variety of approaches and techniques have been developed for the immobilization of enzymes which will not be reviewed here. The principal advantage of immobilized enzymes over their soluble counterparts is the very considerable reduction in enzyme costs offered by the possibility of re-using enzymes, sometimes over a very considerable period; with soluble enzyme systems, the enzyme was denatured or discarded once one batch of substrate had been transformed. Other advantages such as greater enzyme stability, somewhat altered characteristics (not always an advantage), continuous-flow operation, and the possibility of performing sequential transformations by linked enzyme reactors also accrue from the immobilization of enzymes. In addition to the specific applications of immobilized enzymes in food processing cited later, the following are some general

Table 1
VALUE OF ENZYMES USED IN FOOD
PROCESSING (MILLIONS OF DOLLARS)

| Enzyme | 1971 | 1975 | 1980 |
|---|---|---|---|
| Amylases | 8.31 | 12.50 | 14.20 |
| Amyloglucosidases | 1.70 | 2.10 | 2.60 |
| Fungal amylases | 2.01 | 2.40 | 3.10 |
| Bacterial amylases | 4.60 | 8.00 | 8.50 |
| Proteases | 17.34 | 23.36 | 28.11 |
| Fungal | 0.76 | 0.82 | 0.91 |
| Bacterial | 0.83 | 1.00 | 1.30 |
| Pancreatin | 0.80 | 0.80 | 0.80 |
| Rennets (animal and microbial) | 7.50 | 12.00 | 15.00 |
| Pepsin | 2.75 | 3.64 | 5.00 |
| Papain | 4.70 | 5.10 | 5.10 |
| Other Enzymes | 9.61 | 14.25 | 20.80 |
| Glucose oxidase | 0.35 | 0.50 | 0.90 |
| Cellulase | 0.10 | 0.25 | 0.40 |
| Invertase | 0.10 | 0.20 | 0.20 |
| Glucose isomerase | 1.00 | 3.00 | 6.00 |
| Pectinases | 2.56 | 3.00 | 3.50 |

Reprinted with permission of the copyright owner, The American Chemical Society, from the 53(33), 25, 1975 issue of *Chem. Eng. News.*

Table 2
APPLICATIONS OF ENZYMES IN FOOD TECHNOLOGY

| Food | Enzyme | Food | Enzyme |
|---|---|---|---|
| Beer | Proteinases | Meat | Proteinase |
| | Amylases | | |
| | β-Glucanase | | |
| | Glucose oxidase | Fruit and veg. | Cellulase |
| | Catalase | | Pectinases |
| | Diacetyl reductase | | Glucose oxidase |
| Bread | Proteinases | | Catalase |
| | Amylases | | Alliinase |
| | Lipoxidase | | Naringinase |
| | β-Galactosidase | | Proteinases |
| | Pentosanases | | Tannase |
| Egg products | Glucose oxidase | | α-Galactosidase |
| | Catalase | Starches/sugars | Amylases |
| Dairy products | Rennets | | Invertase |
| | Other proteinases | | Sucrose phosphorylase |
| | Lipases | | Glucose isomerase |
| | Catalase | | Pullanase |
| | β-Galactosidase | | α-Galactosidase |

references on immobilized enzymes with particular reference to food technology: Olson and Cooney,[528] Greenfield and Laurence,[256] Weetall,[743-745] and Skinner.[644]

Some of the very numerous applications of enzymes in food processing are tabulated in Table 2. Many of these are probably of minor significance and the more important ones are considered in some detail below; the numerous references cited should be consulted if greater detail is desired.

It was decided to approach the review from a commodity viewpoint; the significance and application of indigenous and added enzymes in each of the major sectors of the food industry are considered separately. We have however excluded consideration of the enzymology of enology and brewing and have thus restricted the discussion to food in the narrow sense.

## DAIRY PRODUCTS

### Indigenous Enzymes

Milk contains about 20 enzymes (Table 3) many of which have been isolated in homogeneous form and well characterized. This research has been reviewed by Shahani,[625] Groves,[264] Shahani et al.,[627] Dwivedi,[172] and Johnson.[340] The distribution of the principal enzymes between the fat and aqueous phases was reviewed and studied by Kitchen et al.[381] Although milk enzymes are regarded by some authors as serving a definite positive role in milk, it is generally presumed that enzymes occur in milk simply as spill-over from the secretory cells. Most of the enzymes are present at low levels, have no natural substrates in milk, and are of no consequence technologically.

However, a few enzymes cause serious defects in milk and its products and dairy processes are designed to curtail or eliminate their activity. Significantly none of the indigenous milk enzymes with the possible exception of sulphydryl oxidase, is responsible for desirable changes and consequently their preservation during processing is not a consideration. Destruction of pathogenic bacteria is the prime objective of thermal processing of milk but many enzymes are coincidently inactivated. Some milk enzymes are very thermo-stable and survive normal HTST pasteurization conditions; higher processing temperatures produce injurious changes in the physicochemical properties of milk proteins.

Technologically the most important milk enzymes are: lipase, xanthine, oxidase, proteinase, and possibly acid phosphatase and sulphydryl oxidase.

Milk contains at least one lipase and possibly a lipoprotein lipase as well as a number of esterases; the subject has been extensively reviewed.[101,102,166,207,538] Milk lipase is not normally active in milk because the enzyme and its substrate are separated (compartmentalized) by the fat globule membrane. However when this membrane is ruptured by homogenization, agitation, or temperature fluctuations lipolysis occurs.[294,329,339] Free fatty acids released on lipolysis cause a defect, hydrolytic rancidity, due principally to the highly flavored short-chain acids; long chain acids cause a soapy taste. The milks of some cows become rancid simply on cooling (without further activation treatments); this phenomenon occurs in 3 to 35% of cows according to Roadhouse and Henderson[597] and Tarassuk[688] or in <20% according to Hunter et al.[324] The cause(s) of difference in susceptibility of milks to lipolysis is uncertain; Tarassuk and Frankel[689] suggest that "spontaneous" milks contain a higher level of membrane-bound lipase than normal milks but this has been questioned by many authors. Drissen and Stadhouders[169] suggest that spontaneous lipolysis may be due to a lipoprotein lipase but Downey[166] says that such a hypothesis is unnecessary and suggests that susceptible milks have weak membranes or possibly contain a "colipase" (i.e., a stimulatory factor). Hydrolytic rancidity is a serious defect in milk but may be avoided if due precautions are observed.[329] Lipolysis is desirable in Blue cheeses, milk for which is normally homogenized to activate the milk lipase system. Milk lipase is quite heat labile and is readily inactivated by HTST pasteurization; there are reports that milk lipase may become reactivated.

Milk is rich in xanthine oxidase, an enzyme capable of oxidizing a range of aldehydes and purines. The enzyme, which is associated with the fat globule membrane, has been isolated by a number of workers, e.g., Mangino and Brunner;[441] it requires FAD, Fe, Mo, and Cu as cofactors. In milk it is activated by a number of treatments which dissociate it from the FGM.[255,265,326] The significance of xanthine oxidase in milk lies

Table 3

INDIGENOUS MILK
ENZYMES

| Enzyme | Classification Number |
|---|---|
| Aldolase | 4.1.2.7. |
| α-Amylase | 3.2.1.1. |
| β-Amylase | 3.2.1.2. |
| Arylesterase | 3.1.1.2. |
| Carbonic anhydrase | 4.2.1.1. |
| Catalase | 1.11.1.6. |
| Cytochrome reductase | 1.9.3.1. |
| Diaphorase | 1.6.4.3. |
| Esterase | 3.1.1.1. |
| β-Galactosidase | 3.2.1.23. |
| Lipase | 3.1.1.3. |
| Lysozyme | 3.2.1.17. |
| Peroxidase | 1.11.1.7. |
| Phosphatase (acid) | 3.1.3.2. |
| Phosphatase (alkaline) | 3.1.3.1. |
| Phospholipase | 3.1.3— |
| Proteinase | 3.4.— |
| Rhodanase | 2.8.1.1. |
| Ribonuclease | 2.7.7.16. |
| Sulphydryl oxidase | |
| Superoxide dismutase | 1.15.1.1. |
| Xanthine oxidase | 1.2.3.2. |

in its possible involvement in spontaneous lipid oxidation,[24] and its oxidative capability is doubled on heat treatment.[5] It has also been proposed that xanthine oxidase may be a predisposing factor in the development of atherosclerosis through oxidation of aldehydes,[781] however little, if any, direct correlation between xanthine oxidase activity and atherosclerosis has been established experimentally.

It has been recognized for many years that milk contains an indigenous proteinase at very low concentration[741] which has been highly purified by a number of workers.[170,356,771] There are suggestions that milk contains two proteinases — one with trypsin-like properties, the other chymotrypsin-like.[359] The enzyme is relatively heat stable[170] and its activity is reported to be increased by HTST pasteurization.[515] It is capable of hydrolyzing both $α_s$- and β-caseins with a preference for the latter.[515] Its significance in milk has not been definitely established but because of its heat stability it may cause proteolysis in milk and milk products even though its activity in milk is low and the pH of milk is quite far removed from its optimum (pH 8.0). It has been proposed that the γ-caseins which appear to correspond to the C-terminal segments of β-caseins are derived from the latter by proteolysis possibly by milk proteinase.[243,355,358,768] The concentration of γ-casein in milk is inversely related to that of β-casein and increases with advancing lactation, advancing age of cow, and mastitic infection.[141] There are suggestions that milk proteinase is identical with blood plasmin which increases in milk on increased cell membrane permeability. Isolated plasmin rapidly hydrolyzes β-casein to γ-casein;[177] it hydrolyzes $α_{s1}$-casein more slowly but does not appear to be capable of hydrolyzing K-casein,[178] which is fortituous in view of the importance of K-casein to the physicochemical stability of casein micelles. Indigenous milk proteinase may play a minor role in proteolysis in cheese during ripening.[524]

Milk contains a number of phosphatases of which alkaline phosphomonesterase (pH 10.0) and acid phosphomonoesterase (pH 4.0) are best characterized. While the alkaline enzyme is of very considerable significance in dairy technology as an index of pasteurization efficiency, it appears to have no further significance. The acid enzyme, although present at a much lower concentration than alkaline phosphatase, may be of greater technological significance because it is more heat stable (survives HTST pasteurization), is much more active on casein phosphate esters and its pH optimum (4.0) is closer to the pH of many dairy products.[57,58] It may, therefore, cause dephosphorylation of casein in dairy products thereby altering its properties. Direct experimental evidence on this point is lacking but the report of Davies and Law[141] of a phosphorous-deficient β-casein in milk is of interest.

Apart from its usefulness as a test-enzyme for the efficiency of flash pasteurization, lactoperoxidase may have some involvement in lipid oxidation, probably due to the heme group since the heat denatured enzyme is more active than the native enzyme.[180]

The milks of most species contain a lysozyme but human milk is particularly rich, containing 3000 times the level of lysozyme normally present in bovine milk.[104] Procedures for the isolation of lysozyme from human milk have been published by Jolles[344] and Parry et al.,[537] and for bovine lysozyme by Chandan et al..[103] Lysozyme may play an antibacterial role in milk and in the digestive tract; if so the very high level of lysozyme in human milk may assume nutritional significance. Indeed a number of claims have been made for the benefits accruing from the addition of egg white lysozyme to baby food formulations, especially for premature babies.[483]

The only other indigenous milk enzyme which may influence milk quality is sulphydryl oxidase. This enzyme has been isolated and characterized by Kiermeier and Petz[375-377] and Janolino and Swaisgood.[336] The enzyme is capable of catalyzing the oxidation of sulphydryl groups using molecular oxygen; since these groups are responsible for the cooked flavor of heated dairy products, sulphydryl oxidase may have an ameliorating effect on the side-effects of high heat treatments.

### Added Enzymes

Enzymes are used in relatively few dairy processes but some of these are major and traditional applications.

### Rennets

Cheese, a traditional dairy product of major economic importance in Western countries, is manufactured essentially as follows:

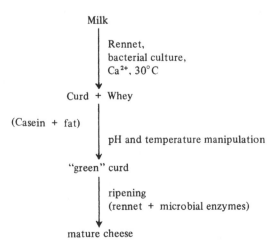

The primary reaction in cheese manufacture involves destabilization of casein micelles via a limited proteolytic reaction. Casein, which represents ≈80% of total milk protein, is a heterogeneous protein system containing four principal groups of proteins: $\alpha_{s1}(\alpha_{s0},\alpha_{s1})$, $\alpha_{s2}(\alpha_{s2},\alpha_{s3},\alpha_{s4},\alpha_{s6})$, $\beta$, and K in the approximate ratio 4:1:4:1.[141] $\alpha_{s0}$- and $\alpha_{s1}$- caseins have a common polypeptide chain but contain nine and eight phosphate residues, respectively.[444] $\alpha_{s2}$-, $\alpha_{s3}$-, $\alpha_{s4}$-, and $\alpha_{s6}$-caseins have a common polypeptide chain but 13, 12, 11, and 10 phosphate residues, respectively.[77] Some $\beta$-casein is degraded to $\gamma_1$, $\gamma_2$, and $\gamma_3$, possibly by milk protease (see milk protease above) and to an uncharacterized $\beta$-casein containing four rather than five phosphate residues.[141] The K-casein fraction contains five proteins with a common polypeptide chain but with different levels of carbohydrate.[430] In addition to the level of heterogeneity described, all the caseins, except $\alpha_{s2}$, exhibit genetic polymorphism. The chemistry of the caseins has been reviewed by, among others, Gordon and Kalan,[244] Farrell and Thompson,[190] McKenzie,[468] Swaisgood,[679] Lyster,[429] and Whitney et al.[758]

Most ($\approx 95\%$) of the casein occurs in large aggregates, micelles (avg. dia. = 100 nm), the detailed structure of which is not agreed.[190,468,646] The micelles are stabilized by hydration and zeta potential and it is generally agreed that K-casein is the principal stabilizing factor with a major contribution from colloidal calcium phosphate.

The first step in cheese manufacture is the specific hydrolysis of the phenylalanine-methionine bond (residues 105-106) of K-casein by chymosin and similar proteinases.[135] The hydrophilic C-terminal third of K-casein is split off from the micelle, thus reducing the zeta potential[251,545] and pre-disposing the micelle system to coagulation by $Ca^{2+}$ at temperatures >20°C. The process of rennet coagulation generally has been reviewed by Mackinlay and Wake[431] and Ernstrom and Wong.[184]

Most of the added rennet is lost in the whey at draining; the actual amount retained in the curd is strongly influenced by the pH of the curd at draining.[309] The rennet retained by the curd is however essential for cheese ripening as it is primarily responsible for the proteolysis which occurs during ripening as indicated by gel electrophoresis and protein solubility at pH 4.6.[383,523,524,723,723a] Proteolysis of this type is essential for the development of the proper texture of cheese and it may also contribute to flavor development. However excessive proteolysis or proteolysis of the wrong type may lead to off flavor development, especially bitterness.[425]

Chymosin (3.4.4.3) from the stomachs of young suckled calves is the traditional enzyme used in cheese manufacture. Chymosins are characterized by a high ratio of milk clotting to proteolytic activity.[201,525] However, for various reasons (supply and demand, religious taboos, good business opportunities) there has been an active search for suitable "rennet substitutes", especially during the past 10 years.[149,497] Most proteinases will coagulate milk under suitable conditions but most are too proteolytic, yield cheese with very soft body and bitter off flavor, and are unsuitable as rennet substitutes. Of the very numerous proteinases that are available and have been tested only four have been found to be at least acceptable in hard and semi-hard long-ripened cheeses, viz., pig pepsin, bovine pepsin, and the proteinases from *Mucor miehei* and *M. pusillus*. A protease from *Endothia parasitica* has been considered acceptable by some authors and sheep pepsin has been suggested as suitable on the basis of preliminary screening trials only.[525] Comprhensive reviews on milk coagulants include Nelson,[506] Martens and Naudts,[458] and Green.[252]

The possibility of using immobilized coagulants has been receiving attention from three different viewpoints: (1) separation of the first and second stages of milk coagulation; (2) as a technique for identifying the location of K-casein on the micelle; and (3) cheese manufacture. To date the latter has received only theoretical attention; the technique may have industrial application but it would appear necessary to incorporate some coagulant in the curd to cause proteolysis in the ripening cheese. References on immobilized coagulants include Green and Crutchfield,[253] Ashoor et al.,[20] Ferrier et al.,[195] Arima et al.,[16] Cooke and Caygill,[127] Cheryan et al.,[109,110] Hicks et al.,[301] Brown and Swaisgood,[84] Olson and Richardson,[531] and Taylor et al..[692]

Obviously cheese manufacture alters the nutritive value of milk very significantly; all cheese varieties are free or nearly so of lactose which may be of significance in the nutrition of lactase-deficient patients. While cheese is a protein-rich product its proteint ratio is lower than that in milk and the 20% of total milk protein lost in the whey is superior nutritionally to casein which is somewhat deficient in methionine. The protein of all ripened cheese varieties undergoes at least some proteolysis and very extensive proteolysis occurs in surface ripened varieties. The nutritional significance of a high level of medium-sized peptides in the diet has not been investigated. Many extensively ripened cheese contain a high level of amines; the possibility exists that these may become involved in nitrosamine formation. Many of these amines are vasodilators and may be fatal if taken in combination with certain drugs.

*Lipases*

Lipases have a number of relatively low-volume applications in dairy processing which have been reviewed by Anti,[10] Seitz,[623] Arnold,[17] Shahani et al.,[626] and Huang and Dooley.[315] A considerable amount of information has been accumulated on the characteristics of lipolytic systems from different sources which makes it possible to select a lipase best suited for a specific purpose.

Perhaps the major applications of lipases in dairy processing at present are in the production of various cheese varieties. The Italian cheeses, Romano and Provolone owe their characteristic sharp flavors to a high content of short-chain fatty acids, especially butyric acid.[501] Early attempts in the U.S. to manufacture these cheeses using rennet extracts were unsuccessful and led to the isolation of a lipase, pregastric esterase, from the rennet paste preparations normally used in Italy.[188,189,279-281] Preparations of pregastric esterases from calf, kid, and lamb are now commercially available for use in the manufacture of Italian cheeses. The three enzymes differ slightly in specificity, but all show high specificity for short chain fatty acids. Lipases produced by *Mucor miehei* are reported to give Italian cheese of satisfactory quality,[315,548] and this enzyme has been characterized by Moskowitz et al.[485]

The fat in Blue cheese also undergoes extensive lipolysis during ripening.[142] The free fatty acids in Blue cheese contribute directly to its flavor but possibly more importantly, they serve as substrates for fungal enzymes which produce methyl ketones which are major contributors to the typical flavor of Blue cheese.[378] The predominant lipolytic system in Blue cheese is that of *Penicillium roqueforti* but indigenous milk lipase also makes a significant contribution and it is common practice to homogenize raw milk or its cream phase to activate the milk lipase system prior to Blue cheese manufacture. Blue cheese is a popular ingredient for salad dressings and cheese dips. For such purposes high quality natural cheese is not normally required and considerable interest has developed in the production of Blue cheese flavor in milk fat by culturing with *P. roqueforti* or perhaps by treatment with the isolated lipolytic system of *P. roqueforti*.[174,503,504] Jolly and Kosikowski[345] have reported a method by which the natural ripening agents in blue cheese can be supplemented by fungal (Aspergillus) lipases added to the curd at salting; ripening time was reduced from the normal period of 6 to 9 months at 10°C to 30 to 45 days at 5°C. Not all lipases gave satisfactory results: only two of ten fungal lipases investigated were suitable and these also gave results superior to goat or calf gastric lipases. The lipase preparations probably contained a proteinase also and presumably the increased free fatty acid content caused by added lipase stimulated the oxidative system of *P. roqueforti*[406,407] to produce higher levels of methyl ketones and secondary alcohols. Addition of exogenous lipase was found to have no beneficial effect in the quick-ripening method for Blue cheese described by Harte and Stein.[282]

A more radical approach was adopted by Jolly and Kosikowski[346] in the development of a "Blue Cheese Food". Skim milk was concentrated to 45 to 50% solids by ultrafiltration. Pasteurized heavy cream (40% fat), plastic cream (80% fat), or pure coconut oil were separately incubated with food-grade microbial lipase (*Aspergillus oryzae*), *P. roqueforti* spores and 0.1% lactic acid culture at 20° C for 48 hr with vigorous shaking. Typical Blue cheese flavor developed in the cream which was then mixed with freeze- or spray-dried protein retentate to give a product with approximately 46% water, 16% protein, 18% fat, 2% (added) NaCl and pH 5.7 to 5.8. The mix was heated at 77°C for 3 min, packaged, and chilled. The product had a texture similar to Neufchatel cheese, was free of visible mold mycelia, and had a flavor reminiscent of good quality Blue cheese. The product contained levels of free fatty acid and methyl ketones comparable to those in normal Blue cheese and appears to be well-suited for use in dips, sauces, and dressings.

Compared with Blue and Italian cheeses, Cheddar and Dutch cheeses undergo only a low level of lipolysis.[591,661,662] It has been reported that addition of pre-gastric esterase, especially to pasteurized milk, increases flavor intensity of Cheddar cheese.[27,521,595] Several patents have been awarded to the Kraftco corporation and to Dairyland Food laboratories for methods of improving the flavor of cheese and processed cheese.[17] The ripening of Cheddar cheese may also be accelerated by addition of lipases.[389-391] Lipases are used to hydrolyze milk fat for a variety of uses in the confectionary, candy, chocolate, sauce, and snack food industries; the partially hydrolyzed fat imparts a greater intensity of butter-like flavor to the products and delays staling presumably through the emulsifying influence of the di- and monoglycerides present.[17,626] Rancid flavor in liquid milk, which is carefully avoided in most countries, appears to be favored in Japan where selected microbial lipases are added to produce controlled lipolysis.[522] Lipase is also used in the preparation of yogurt in Japan to eliminate unclean and fishy odors and to accelerate the rate of fermentation.[623] A number of other minor applications of lipase in diary products are cited by Seitz.[623]

*Catalase*

Hydrogen peroxide is used as a milk preservative in warm countries lacking refrigeration and possibly pasteurization facilities; the addition of 0.05% $H_2O_2$ to milk intended for Swiss and Cheddar cheeses is permitted in the U.S. While $H_2O_2$ is a very effective sterilant, it does produce certain defects in cheese even when used properly.[206,427] Treatment with $H_2O_2$ oxidizes a number of amino acids particularly methionine,[134,445,446,647] and reduces the biological value of proteins.[496] Oxidation does however improve the function properties of milk proteins in bread-baking presumably through modification of the whey proteins,[88,268,539] and improves the foamability of whey protein/CMC complexes.[277]

Added $H_2O_2$ is generally reduced by catalase prior to consumption or further processing of the treated milk. Milk contains an indigenous catalase, but the low concentration of enzyme usually present is denatured by the added $H_2O_2$ prior to complete reduction of the latter. Therefore, extraneous catalase (beef liver, *A. niger* or *Micrococcus lysodeikticus*) is normally added. The possibility of using catalase immobilized on cellulose or cheesecloth has been investigated but has not been successful to date due to the rapid denaturation of catalase by $H_2O_2$.[596] An immobilized catalase reactor (catalase immobilized on collagen) is described by Chu et al.[113]

*β-Galactosidase (Lactase)*

Lactase hydrolyses lactose to glucose and galactose and shows a high specificity for galactose in β-glycosidic linkage. Bovine milk contains ≈5% lactose, and concentrated and dehydrated dairy products contain pro rata concentrations. Among sugars, lactose shows many fairly unique characteristics: it has low solubility (≈20 g/100 ml $H_2O$ at

20°C); has a marked tendency to form supersaturated solutions; crystallizes as small, hard, sharp crystals which impart a sandy mouth-feel to foods; its crystallization behavior is complicated by its mutarotation characteristics as the two forms, $\alpha$ and $\beta$, have considerably different solubilities and degree of hydration; it has a low sweetness value ($\approx$16% that of sucrose at 1% concentration); and it has a marked tendency to adsorb flavors, odors, and pigments. The chemistry and properties of lactose have been comprehensively reviewed by Nickerson[512] and some of the unique properties of lactose as a food ingredient have been discussed by Fox.[210]

Most animals secrete $\beta$-galactosidase on the brush border of the small intestine. The level of lactase secretion reaches a maximum shortly after birth and declines to a relatively low level in normal adults. However a very high proportion of Asian and African adults secrete a very low or zero level of lactase,[601] and show total or partial lactose intolerance, i.e., they are unable to metabolize lactose in the small intestine; some lactose is absorbed through the intestine wall and is excreted in the urine, but some passes into the large intestine where it is metabolized by enteric bacteria with gas formation resulting in flatulence and diarrhea. The consensus among earlier workers was that patients suffering from lactase deficiency would be unable to consume lactose-containing dairy products but the problem does not appear to be quite as serious as was initially indicated and lactase-deficient patients apparently adjust to diets containing lactose.[466,575] Dosage levels and other dietary constituents also modify the response to lactose of lactase-deficient patients who may not exhibit the normal symptoms of lactose intolerances at all.[584] However a small proportion of babies of all races are deficient in lactase from birth and must be fed on lactose-free diets.

The dairy industry has developed methods of controlling the physico-chemical problems posed by lactose[512] and it is possible to produce lactose-reduced dairy products by various techniques, e.g., ultrafiltration or "synthetic" milks based on casein or soya protein. However, the various problems posed by lactose, technological and nutritional, may be solved by prehydrolysis of lactose with added lactase, soluble, or immobilized. The voluminous literature on lactase and its applications in dairy processing accumulated over the past 10 years or so, has been reviewed by, among others, Wallenfels and Malhota,[738] Pomeranz,[556] Weetal et al.,[746] Reed,[587] and very comprehensively by Shukla.[636]

Perhaps of more interest to dairy technologists than solving the above lactose-associated problems is finding suitable and profitable uses for the huge amounts of lactose available in whey from cheese or casein manufacture and which in many cases poses a major effluent disposal problem. Lactase is seen as one viable approach to this problem by converting a sugar of low solubility and low sweetness to sugars (glucose and galactose) which are considerably more soluble and sweeter. The production of sugar syrups from acid whey with 90% lactose hydrolysis is described by Wierzbicki and Kosikowski[762] using a soluble lactase. A basically similar process using immobilized lactase is described by Weetal et al.[746] These syrups have been satisfactorily incorporated into a number of food products, e.g., sweetened yogurts, maple syrups, and puddings.

The syrups prepared by these workers are about 70% as sweet as sucrose syrups on an equal weight basis. Glucose and galactose are less sweet than sucrose (sucrose = 100; lactose = 16; glucose = 70; galactose = 70; fructose = 173). Thus, the isomerization of glucose and/or galactose to fructose would permit the production of sweeter syrups better suited for certain applications. The technology already exists for the conversion of glucose (produced by enzymatic hydrolysis of starch) to fructose using immobilized glucose isomerase.[18,33,414] Thus, using two linked immobilized enzyme reactors it is possible to produce a sweet glucose-fructose-galactose syrup from lactose:

$$\text{lactose} \xrightarrow{\text{lactase}} \text{glucose + galactose}$$
$$\text{glucose} \downarrow \text{isomerase}$$
$$\text{glucose + fructose + galactose}$$

To the authors' knowledge a process of this type is not in commercial operation, but it should be technically feasible. The obvious next step might be to seek an enzyme which would convert galactose to glucose and then to fructose.

Some other benefits accruing from the prehydrolysis of lactose include: (1) improved baking quality of milk powder, i.e., better gas production from glucose fermentation by baker's yeast and better crust resulting from Maillard Browning reactions of galactose and protein amino groups;[556] (2) accelerated acid production in yogurt;[526] and (3) accelerated acidification and ripening of cheese,[622] although the latter claim appears open to question.[549a]

*Miscellaneous*

Direct acidification of dairy products is becoming fairly common.[211] Acidification is normally performed by an acidogen (generally gluconic acid-δ-lactone) or by an acidogen plus acid. Instead of using preformed GDL it is suggested[579,580] that the formation of GDL *in situ* from glucose using glucose oxidase would afford better control of acid production. The following scheme might be envisaged:

$$\text{lactose} \xrightarrow{\text{lactase}} \text{glucose + galactose}$$
$$\downarrow \text{glucose oxidase}$$
$$\text{gluconic acid}$$

Lactose may be converted directly to lactobionic acid by lactase dehydrogenase and this reaction may have application in the acidification of dairy products and other foods.[767]

Treatments of milk with phospholipase C or D or trypsin improves the stability of milk to oxidative rancidity.[633] The effect is probably due to a modification of the fat globule membrane; trypsin may also owe its effectiveness to improved copper binding by trypsin-modified milk proteins, thereby removing copper from the fat phase.

A number of studies have implicated peroxidases in combination with $H_2O_2$ and thiocyanate ions as antibacterial agents. The possibility of using immobilized peroxidase as a pasteurizing agent is discussed by Richardson and Olson[596] and Olson and Richardson.[531]

Production of protein hydrolyzates for use in dietetic foods or to modify functional properties is potentially an important avenue of protein utilization. The production of tryptic digests of whey protein is described by Jost and Monti.[353] The possibility of improving the functional properties of undenatured whey proteins (prepared by gel filtration) by limited proteolysis was investigated by Kuehler and Stine;[398] emulsification capacity was decreased by proteolysis and while foamability was increased, foam stability decreased. The low heat stability of whey proteins restricts their usefulness as food supplements because of restrictions imposed on heat processing; limited tryptic hydrolysis renders whey protein stable at 134°C for 5 min.[302]

## MEAT

### Introduction

Meat is defined as the flesh of animals which has undergone certain biochemical changes after death thereby rendering it suitable for use as food. Although some 3000 mammalian species exist, only a few dozen domesticated animals and aquatic organ-

## Table 4
### COMPOSITION OF LEAN MUSCLE TISSUE (%)[323]

| Species | Water | Protein | Lipid | Ash |
|---------|-------|---------|-------|-----|
| Beef | 70—73 | 20—22 | 4—8 | 1 |
| Pork | 68—70 | 19—20 | 9—11 | 1.4 |
| Chicken | 73.7 | 20—23 | 4—7 | 1 |
| Lamb | 73 | 20 | 5—6 | 1.6 |
| Cod | 81.2 | 17.6 | 0.3 | 1.2 |
| Salmon | 64 | 20—22 | 13—15 | 1.3 |

isms form the bulk of muscle tissue consumed by man. The food scientist interchanges the term "muscle" and "meat"; the former is essentially the functional locomotive tissue and the latter refers to the post-mortem tissue and also includes some adipose tissue and bone. Meat can be subdivided into the categories of "red" meat from cattle, sheep and pigs; and "white" meat which comes essentially from poultry; sea foods are the flesh of all aquatic organisms including clams, oysters, lobster, etc.

Meat is an excellent source of high quality protein and of the B-complex vitamins and for these reasons contributes significantly to the dietary balance of meals. Meat composition varies mostly in lipid content but the species, specific cuts used, the extent of trimming, processing, and mode of storage must also be considered. However, for general consideration an overall composition is suitable.[323]

As shown in Table 4, protein makes up about 20% of the lean portion of meat and is popularly regarded as being nutritionally superior to plant proteins. The importance of meat in the diet has been summarized by Bender.[51] The data show that in 1971 meats of all kinds contributed 17% of the intake of energy; 20% of the protein, and 30% of the fat of the average United Kingdom diet. Meat also contributed 20% of vitamin $B_1$ and $B_2$, and 37% of the niacin. Meat is an important source of iron, which not only is readily absorbed itself, but appears to assist the absorption of iron from other sources.[409]

According to the first law of nutrition "Meat must be consumed in order to be of nutritional value"; therefore the acceptability of meat by the consumer is a matter of concern to the physiologist, biochemist, meat scientist, butcher, and processor. The acceptability of meat to the consumer depends upon color, water holding capacity, juiciness, and odor. Considerable variability in these attributes have been apparent as long as man has consumed meat. Intra-species differences do not, in general, reflect differences in composition, but are due to the influence of pre- and post-mortem glycolytic rates on protein denaturation and water retention. Fresh meat color is frequently determined by the rate and extent of enzymic action, as is texture. Pale, soft, exudative pork is an example of abnormal enzymic activity occurring both immediately prior to slaughter and post slaughter. Consequently, meat quality can be discussed primarily in terms of enzyme functionality and activity.

## Muscle Structure

The number of studies contributing to an understanding of striated muscle, contractile protein biochemistry, and the molecular basis of contraction is enormous. The reader should consult a number of excellent books and reviews for more detailed information and specific literature references. Special mention should be made of Needham's[500] monumental treatise on the historical development of muscle physiology and biochemistry, and the four volumes on *The Structure and Function of Muscle* edited by Bourne.[70] Other important studies include: Bendall,[45,47] Cold Spring Harbor Symposium,[122] Cassens,[98] Wilkie,[763] Briskey et al.,[82,83] Price and Schweigert,[573] Smith,[649]

Lawrie,[408] Forrest et al.[202] Other important books, reviews, and articles, particularly on contractile protein biochemistry, the molecular basis of contraction, and post-mortem muscle changes will be discussed where relevant.

Skeletal muscles are usually attached to the bone of the skeleton via inelastic tendon and each muscle is surrounded by a layer of connective tissue which in turn branches out to divide the muscle into bundles. The muscle bundles are composed of a large number of approximately longitudinal muscle fibers which constitute 75 to 92% of the total muscle volume. Each muscle fiber extends for a considerable distance along the length of the muscle and some may even extend along the whole length.[47] The diameter of the muscle fiber usually lies in the range 10 to 100 nm and each fiber is surrounded by the sarcolemma, which is a trilaminar membrane approximately 100 Å thick.[361] Nerve fibers end in the sarcolemma in specialized regions called the "motor end plate". From the "motor end plate" the electrical stimulus is carried to the contractile elements in the fiber via the transverse tubules or T-system. For more detailed discussion on the "motor end plate" the reader should consult Couteaux.[129] The T-system arises from invaginations of the sarcolemma surrounding the fibers.[736] The ends of the T-system meet in the interior of the cell close to two terminal sacs of the sarcoplasmic reticulum (SR). The SR membrane is somewhat analagous to the endoplasmic reticulum of other cells. Details of the T-tubule and SR system are discussed by Porter and Franzini-Armstrong[560] and Franzini-Armstrong[212]

The function of the T-tubule and SR system is twofold: (1) to transmit electrical stimuli to the interior of the fiber and (2) to control the level of calcium ions in the sarcoplasmic fluid, to release it during muscle contraction, and to sequester calcium ions during relaxation. The SR membranes contain an ATP-dependent $Ca^{2+}$ pump which maintains the sarcoplasmic $Ca^{2+}$ concentration in resting muscle at a level ($<10^{-7}M$) below that needed for activation of cross-bridge interaction between the thick myosin and the thin actin filaments. Upon stimulation, an electrical signal is transmitted along the T-tubules to the terminal cisternae of the SR, causing a rapid release of $Ca^{2+}$ into the sarcoplasmic fluid thereby increasing the concentration of $Ca^{2+}$ to a level ($10^{-5}M$) necessary to promote cross-linking between myosin and actin and resulting in muscle tension.

### The Contractile Elements

The contractile force is produced by cylindrical organelles called myofibrils which fill over 80% of the volume of the muscle. The myofibrils are surrounded by the sarcoplasm, the T-tubule system, sarcoplasmic reticulum, and mitochondria. A schematic diagram of the organization of skeletal muscle is shown in Figure 1.

The myofibrils are usually 1 to 2 $\mu$m in diameter, and an average fiber contains at least 1000 units. The alternating light and dark zones arise from the arrangement of thick and thin filaments.[492]

The thick filaments of muscle consist almost entirely of the protein myosin. Reviews of various aspects of the chemical and physicochemical properties of myosin have been given by Perry,[549] Lowey et al.,[424] Young,[778] Briskey and Fukazawa,[80] and Ebashi and Nonomura.[176] The thick filaments also contain two other proteins called C-protein and M-protein. Bands of C-protein encircle the myosin filament at regular intervals and appear to play a role in binding the myosin molecules together into bundles. The M-protein, which has an aggregation-promoting action on myosin, is located at the center of the A-band.

Actin constitutes about 20 to 25% of the myofibrils and is the main protein present in the thin filaments. Its elemental unit is a globular protein of molecular weight less than 50,000 called G-actin. These basic monomeric units have a tendency to form long actin filaments called F-actin in the presence of ATP and $Mg^{2+}$. Two other proteins,

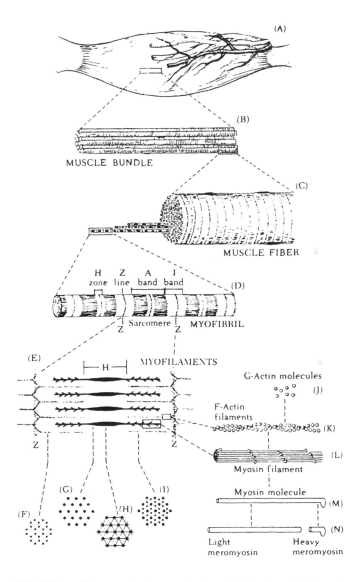

FIGURE 1. Diagram of the organization of skeletal muscle from the gross structure to the molecular level. (A) Skeletal muscle; (B) a bundle of muscle fibers; (C) a muscle fiber; (D) a myofibril; (E) a sarcomere; (F-I) cross-sections at various locations in the sarcomere; (J) G-actin molecule; (K) an actin filament; (M) a myosin filament; showing the head and tail region; (N) The light meromyosin (LMM) and heavy meromyosin (HHM) portions of the myosin molecule. (From *Principles of Meat Science*, by John C. Forrest, Elton D. Aberle, Harold B. Hedrick, Max D. Judge, and Robert A. Merkel, W. H. Freeman and Company. Copyright © 1975. With permission.

namely tropomyosin and troponin, are present at a concentration of 8 to 10% each in the myofibrils. These proteins, plus $Ca^{2+}$, are concerned with the regulation of the fundamental process of contraction carried out by myosin, actin, ATP, and $Mg^{2+}$. Tropomyosin is a rod-like molecule about 40 nm long and 2 nm wide and is located in the grooves of F-actin. Troponin, a globular protein, is bound to tropomyosin and is located at 38.5 nm intervals along the thin filaments. Troponin is composed of three polypeptide chains: TN-I (mol wt = 23,000) the tropomyosin binding subunit; TN-T(mol wt = 37,000), the subunit which inhibits actomyosin ATP-ase activity; and TN-

**Table 5**
**THE COMPONENTS OF THE MYOFIBRIL[519]**

| Protein | Location | Approximate % of total myofibrillar protein | Molecular weight | Number of polypeptide chains and chain wt. |
|---|---|---|---|---|
| Myosin | Thick filaments | 55 | 460,000 | 2 × 190,000 (heavy chain) <br> 1.2 × 21,000 (A-1 light chain) <br> 2 × 18,000 (DTNB light chain) <br> 0.8 × 17,000 (A-2 light chain) |
| C-protein | Thick filaments (located at nine sites spaced about 43 nm apart in each half of the A band) | 2 | 140,000 | 1 × 140,000 |
| M-line protein | M-line[a] | | 88,000 | 2 × 44,000 |
| Actin | Thin filaments | 23 | 41,700 | 1 × 41,700 |
| Tropomyosin | Thin filaments | 6 | 70,000 | 2 × 35,000 |
| Troponin | Thin filaments (located at sites spaced 38.5 nm apart throughout the thin filament) | 6 | 80,000 | 1 × 37,000 (TN-T) <br> 1 × 23,000 (TN-I) <br> 1 × 18,000 (TN-C) |
| α-Actinin | Z disc[a] | 1 | 180,000 | 2 × 90,000 |

[a]    Probably other proteins are also present in the M-line and Z-disc.

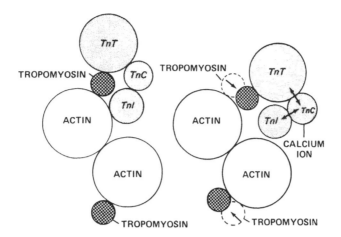

FIGURE 2. The thin filament is seen schematically, end on. In the resting state (left) the Tn-T subunit binds to tropomyosin and the inhibitory subunit TnI binds to actin. In the active state (right) when Ca²⁺ is high, the link between TnI and actin is weakened and tropomyosin moves deeper into the actin groove, exposing the site at which myosin can bind. (From Cohen, C., *Sci. Am.*, 233, 45, 1975. With permission.)

| | |
|---|---|
| 1. **Muscle at Rest** | (a) Uncharged ATP cross-bridges extended |
| | (b) Ca²⁺ stored in sarcoplasmic reticulum |
| | (c) Actin and myosin uncomplexed |
| 2. **Excitation** | (a) Nerve release of acetyl choline |
| | (b) Plasmalemma and T-tubule depolarization |
| | (c) Ca²⁺ released from the sarcoplasmic reticulum |
| | (d) Calcium saturates troponin |
| | (e) Troponin moves tropomyosin from blocking position |
| | (f) Cross bridge attachment |
| 3. **Contraction** | (a) ATP $\xrightarrow{\text{ATPase}}$ ADP + Pi + Energy |
| | (b) Energy used to swivel cross-bridges |
| | (c) Actin slides over myosin and muscle shortens |
| 4. **Recharging** | (a) CP + ADP $\longrightarrow$ ATP + C |
| | (b) Actomyosin $\longrightarrow$ Actin + Myosin |
| 5. **Relaxation** | (a) Nerve impulse ceases |
| | (b) Sarcoplasmic reticulum sequesters Ca²⁺ |
| | (c) Tropomyosin moves to blocking position |
| | (d) Cross bridges detach and muscle returns to resting state |

FIGURE 3. Summary of events occurring during muscle contraction cycle.

C (mol wt = 18,000), the calcium binding subunit. The main characteristics of the myofibrillar units are summarized in Table 5. For more detail on the regulatory proteins the reader should consult Bourne,[70] Weber and Murray,[735] Fuchs,[219] and Cohen.[120]

*Muscle Contraction*

When the central nervous system decrees that a muscle contract, an action potential begins at the myoneural junction and progresses longitudinally along the sarcolemma and stimulates the entire length of the fiber. The arrival of an action potential causes the release of acetylcholine at the "motor end plate" of the muscle fiber. The acetylcholine diffuses across the tiny space to the sarcolemma receptor sites and causes alteration in the cell membrane's permeability, allowing $Na^+$ to diffuse rapidly across the membrane. The membrane's polarity is reversed. The depolarization wave passes down the T-tubule to the terminal cisternae of the SR system, thereby causing a rapid release of $Ca^{2+}$ and an elevation of the sarcoplasmic $Ca^{2+}$ to approximately $10^{-5} M$. The released $Ca^{2+}$ in promoting cross-linking between actin and myosin is shown in Figure 2.

At low $Ca^{2+}$, TN-I binds stongly to actin; tropomyosin is in the blocking position and prevents the attachment of the myosin head to actin. The release of $Ca^{2+}$ from the sarcoplasmic reticulum strengthens the linkage of TN-C to the troponin subunits and weakens the TN-I-actin linkage. TN-I may then move away from the actin and tropomyosin is free to move to a deeper position in the thin filament grooves. The myosin binding-site on the actin is now exposed and in the "on position" and cross-bridges result. The myosin heads go through their power stroke which causes the two sets of filaments to slide past each other.[492] When the contraction signal ceases, the sarcoplasmic reticulum pumps calcium out of the sarcoplasm and reestablishes a concentration of $10^{-7}$ mol/$l$ of intracellular calcium. Troponin now changes its conformation and tropomyosin moves to the blocking position. The cross-bridges can no longer attach to the thin filaments and consequently actin and myosin slide passively over one another. The whole process may then be repeated in response to another nerve signal. The sequence of events in the contraction-relaxation cycle is summarized in Figure 3. For more detail on the mechanism of muscle contraction the reader should consult the main reference above.

## Muscle Metabolism

Muscle requires a large outlay of energy to rapidly operate the contractile apparatus. This energy for contraction is provided by the hydrolysis of ATP. The chemical reactions resulting in the hydrolysis of ATP take place on the head regions of the myosin molecule, and myosin ATP-ase, which requires the presence of $Mg^{2+}$ and $Ca^{2+}$, catalyzes the breakdown.

Mammalian muscle would require the hydrolysis of about 1 mmol of ATP per gram muscle per minute during activity. However the amount actually present is about 5 $\mu$mol/g which is sufficient for only 0.3 sec of activity. It is well-known that ATP content of muscle before and after a single contraction shows essentially no decrease, nor is there an increase in ADP content. Therefore, the most immediate problem in the cell is the resynthesis of ATP. The primary source of ATP is the so-called Lohmann reaction, catalyzed by creatine kinase:

$$ADP + \text{Creatine Phosphate (CP)} \xrightarrow{\text{Creatine Kinase}} ATP + \text{Creatine (C)}$$

The content of CP is about 20 $\mu$mol/g, which is adequate for short term activity.[192]

In vivo, the major source of ATP is its resynthesis from ADP by respiration, whereby muscle glycogen is oxidized to carbon dioxide and water. Lipid metabolism may also be an important source of utilizable energy where the work load is not high.[290] Resting muscle mainly uses fatty acids and acetoacetate as fuel; very little glucose is removed from the blood under these conditions. However, during maximum activity glucose becomes the major fuel.

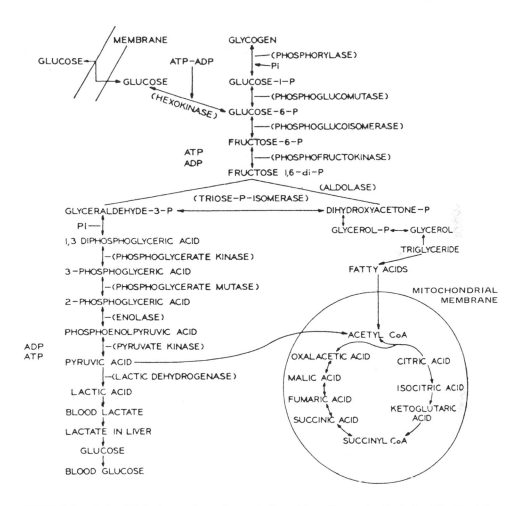

FIGURE 4. A simplified scheme of muscle metabolism. (From Kastenschmidt, L. L., *The Physiology and Biochemistry of Muscle as a Food*, Part 2, Briskey, E. J., Cassens, R. G., and Marsh, B. B., Eds., © University of Wisconsin Press, Madison, 1970, 736. With permission.)

## Aerobic Metabolism

Muscle metabolism has been reviewed extensively and only some of the recent pertinent reviews will be referred to here.[31,70,363,405,712] The most efficient mechanism for ATP synthesis and one which occurs in red muscle and in muscles which are not working at maximum output is aerobic glycolysis. Most of the energy is supplied via the Krebs cycle and the mitochondrial electron transport system, and nutrients such as carbohydrates, proteins, and lipids are degraded to carbon dioxide and water. The conversion of glycogen to glucose and to two molecules of pyruvate occurs in the sarcoplasm and does not require oxygen. The overall scheme of muscle metabolism is shown in Figure 4.

Pyruvate, formed from glucose in the sarcoplasm, then enters the mitochondria for aerobic oxidation via the Krebs cycle and the cytochrome system. Most of the rephosphorylation occurs in the cytochrome chain. When a single glucose molecule, derived from glycogen, is degraded to carbon dioxide and water, 37 ADP molecules are converted to 37 ATP molecules (Figure 5).

## Anaerobic Metabolism

When the muscle is under heavy stress, i.e., exposed to severe activity, abnormal

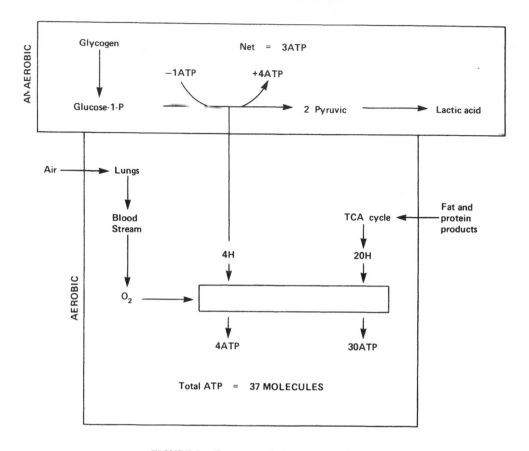

FIGURE 5.    Energy supply for muscle activity.[202]

temperature, humidity, and atmospheric pressure, or exposed to low oxygen tension, electric shock, or injury,[408] mitochondrial function is not maintained and anaerobic metabolism may then become dominant. Essentially, glycolysis produces more NADH than can be oxidized by the aerobic glycerol phosphate shuttle. In this case the aerobic glycolysis is supplemented by the anaerobic system whereby glycolytic NADH is reoxidized via the anaerobic pathway (Figure 6) involving reduction of pyruvate to lactate.[712] In this case ATP production is much less efficient than it is in aerobic respiration and only 2 or 3 moles of ATP per mole of glucose are produced. The production of lactic acid during anaerobic contraction, particularly in the white skeletal muscle, may lead to temporary reduction of pH in the living muscle cell.[471] However, this lactate rapidly diffuses out of muscle into the blood stream, which carries it to the liver where it is converted back to glycogen by a process called gluconeogenesis (Cori cycle). The extra oxygen consumed in the post-exercise phase (oxygen debt) is used to convert some of the lactate to $CO_2$ and $H_2O$. The Cori Cycle is shown in Figure 7.

### Post-Mortem Glycolysis

Post-mortem muscle glycolysis has been the subject of a number of reviews.[48,97,148,363,509] The principal changes following death are summarized in Figure 8. Following death, circulation of the blood ceases, resulting in a complex series of changes within the muscle. The most immediate effect of the cessation of blood circulation is the depletion of the oxygen supply to the tissue. This results in an inability to resynthesize ATP via the electron transport chain and oxidative phosphorylation mechanisms. We are, therefore, principally interested in anaerobic metabolism because it

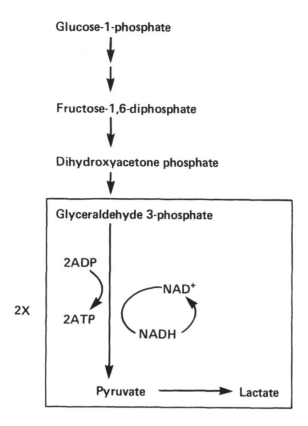

FIGURE 6.  Anaerobic breakdown of glucose in a muscle cell.

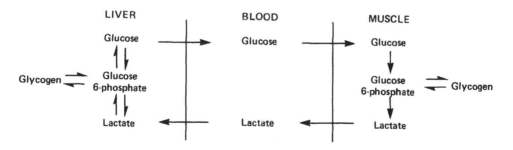

FIGURE 7.  The Cori Cycle.

has an important bearing on the food quality of the muscle. The pathways which provide for ATP synthesis by rephosphorylation in the living muscle also attempt to maintain ATP level after death. However, metabolism of some substrates, such as lipid, ceases at the time of death. The rate of post-mortem metabolism is a variable quantity and has important implications in the ultimate usefulness of muscle as a food.[79,363,364,415] Regulation of the glycolytic system has been discussed by Lardy[405] and Hers et al.;[295] and according to Hessel-de-Heer et al.,[296] the control mechanism for glycolysis seems to be phospho-fructokinase activity, while the relationship between ADP and ATP is an alternate control mechanism. Newbold and Lee[510] showed that the phosphorylase step, i.e., the conversion of glycogen to glucose-*1*-phosphate to be the controlling step. The rate of post-mortem glycolysis has been classified as follows:[363]

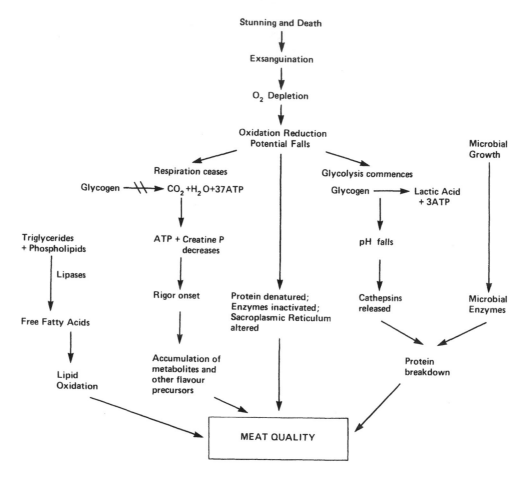

FIGURE 8.    Principle changes in muscle following death.

1.  "Fast-glycolyzing" muscles are those having a pH of 5.5 or less at 30 min post-mortem.
2.  "Slow-glycolyzing" muscles have a pH of 6.0 or higher at 60 min post-mortem.
3.  "Stress-resistant" animals are those which can withstand ante-mortem stress and whose muscles after death are usually slow glycolyzing.
4.  "Stress-susceptible" animals are those which cannot tolerate ante-mortem stress. They usually have fast-glycolyzing muscles or expire before they can be exsanguinated.

The sequence of chemical steps by which ATP is produced is essentially the same post-mortem as in vivo when the oxygen supply may become temporarily inadequate for the provision of energy. However, the extent of change and the concomitant production of lactic acid is much more extensive in post-mortem glycolysis. These changes are discussed in detail by Bendall[48] and are shown in Figure 9.

Very simply there is a disappearance of CP and glycogen and later of ATP, and the concomitant formation of lactate which is accompanied by a fall of pH. Glycolytic activity may cease because of exhaustion of substrate or, more likely, because of the decrease in pH caused by glycolysis. As glycolytic activity slows down, ATP concentration decreases; this usually takes about 24 hr. In all cases the patterns of change are similar, but differences in time scale can be enormous according to temperature, stress, etc. (these will be discussed more fully later).

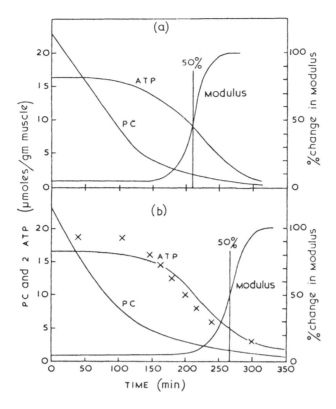

FIGURE 9. Decline of PC and ATP levels and increase of modules in rabbit psoas muscle at 38°C. Initial pH = 7.10; (a) animal depleted in glycogen before death; ultimate pH = 6.58; (b) high initial glycogen level; ultimate pH = 5.7. (From Bendall, J. R. *The Structure and Function of Muscle,* Vol. 2, 2nd ed., Bourne, C. H., Ed., Academic Press, New York, 1973, 259. With permission.)

The rate of glycolysis in post-mortem muscle can be easily estimated by following pH decline. Both the rate of pH decline and the ultimate pH are important in controlling meat quality. A too-rapid pH drop has been associated with the pale-soft-exudative (PSE) condition that is especially common in pork. If a substantial decline in pH occurs before the muscle has been cooled to a sufficiently low temperature, denaturation is excessive and pale, soft, and exudative (PSE) symptoms are likely to be observed. Lister[415] observed that the amount of drip released from a sample of muscle can be predicted with some accuracy if the temperature is known at which a pH of about 6.0 is reached. On the other hand, lack of substrate yields high pH meat which tends to be very dark in color, firm, and dry.

The rate at which the pH decline proceeds after the animal has been exsanguinated and to the extent of total drop in pH are both highly variable. In fact, Briskey[78] outlined six distinct types of pH pattern, which are shown in Figure 10.

The classifications are as follows:

1. A pH drop of only a few tenths of a unit during the first hour or so post-slaughter and an ultimate pH of 6.5 to 6.8 (dark muscle).
2. A slow gradual decrease to an ultimate pH of 5.7 to 6.0 (slightly dark).
3. A gradual decrease from approximately pH 7.0 to a pH of about 5.6 to 5.7 within 8 hr post-mortem, and then to an ultimate pH of 5.3 to 5.7 after 24 hr (normal muscle).

4.    A relatively rapid decrease to about 5.5 in 3 hr, with an ultimate pH of 5.3 to 5.6 (slightly PSE).

5.    A very rapid decrease to around 5.4 to 5.6 during the first hour post-slaughter and ultimate pH of 5.3 to 5.6 (extremely PSE).

6    A gradual but extensive decrease to a final pH of approximately 5.0 (extremely exudative, slightly pale).

The implications of these changes and other abnormal glycolytic patterns are discussed below.

### Rigor Mortis

One of the most dramatic changes which takes place in the muscle after death is the stiffening of the muscle. These changes are discussed extensively by Bendall.[48] Loss of elasticity and extensibility, and shortening accompany the development of rigor mortis. Bendall distinguishes the following types of rigor: acid rigor, alkaline rigor, and an intermediate type. The type of rigor which occurs at any temperature is strictly determined by the magnitude of the initial CP, ATP, and glycogen contents. We have already seen that the initial and final pH values are indirect measures of these constituents.

### Abnormal Types of Glycolysis

The time course of the changes in post-mortem glycolysis and rigor onset have been well documented.[48] Of particular interest are abnormal types of glycolysis and rigor encountered when tissue is cooled rapidly after slaughter and the extremely rapid glycolysis in pigs which leads to the pale, soft, and exudative conditions in pork.

The sarcoplasmic reticulum and its role in muscle contractions has been previously described. The fact that the SR system plays such an important role in muscle contraction and relaxation and in controlling myofibrillar ATP-ase activity suggests that the maintenance or loss of its functional integrity may be related to post-mortem changes in muscle. Calcium activates myofibrillar ATP-ase activity by tenfold or greater.[248] Thus, any changes in the SR sequestering properties would lead to a more rapid ATP breakdown, an accelerated rigor mortis development, and a stimulation of the glycolytic process.

The function and stability of the SR postmortem have been carefully considered by a number of researchers in the cause-effect relationship. Nauss and Davies[498] have suggested that the sarcoplasmic reticulum gradually loses its ability to bind $Ca^{2+}$ postmortem and that the effect initiates glycolysis. The loss of calcium-accumulating ability was demonstrated by Greaser et al.[249] The ability to accumulate $Ca^{2+}$ decreased by approximately 40% during the first 3 hr post-mortem and by 80% at 24 hr. The rate of loss of binding capacity was much greater (50% loss in 30 min and 80% in 3 hr) in muscles which had a rapid pH decline.

Thus, the sarcoplasmic reticulum appeared to be relatively labile after death. However, it was not clear whether the loss of sarcoplasmic reticulum function was causing the pH to drop more rapidly or whether the pH decline was causing a disruption in the sarcoplasmic reticulum. Greaser et al.[250] have shown that pH values of below 6.0, a condition that occurs in most post-mortem muscle, reduce the ability of SR membranes to bind $Ca^{2+}$. The inactivation was also found to be greater at higher temperatures. Thus, low muscle pH and high temperatures may be responsible for the inactivation of the $Ca^{2+}$-accumulating ability. The obvious conclusion is that the membrane was being denatured or structurally altered. Goll et al.[239] proposed on the basis of exogenous enzyme action, that limited proteolysis disrupted the sarcoplasmic reticulum function and produced the same effect on SR fragments as post-mortem aging. Similar results were obtained after treatment with cathepsins.[748]

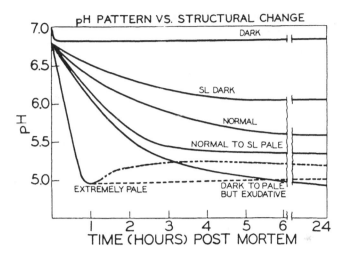

FIGURE 10. pH pattern types. (From Briskey, E. J., *Adv. Food Res.*, 13, 98, 1969. With permission.)

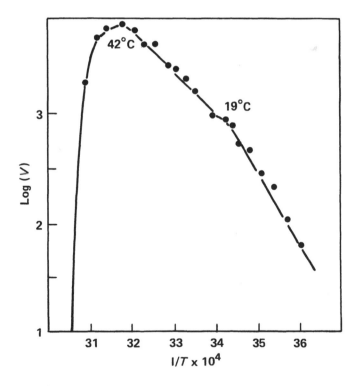

FIGURE 11. Semi-logarithmic plot of initial rates of $Ca^{2+}$ accumulation by the sarcoplasmic reticulum of rabbit muscle as a function of reciprocal temperature. (With permission from Inesi, G., Millman, M., and Eletr, S., *J. Mol. Biol.*, 81, 483, 1973. Copyright by Academic Press, Inc. (London) Ltd.

Temperature has also been suggested as a significant factor and in this context the work of Inesi et al.[330] is most interesting. They observed a transition in the tempera-ture-dependence of $Ca^{2+}$ accumulation and ATP-ase activity at 20°C in SR membranes. The transition is characterized by an abrupt change in the activation energies for the

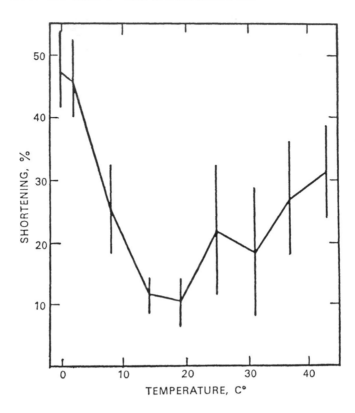

FIGURE 12.     Ultimate shortening of muscles at various storage temperatures. (From Locker, R. H. and Hagward, C. J., *J. Sci. Food
Agric.*, 14, 788, 1963. With permission.)

cation transport process and the associated enzyme activity. When the $Ca^{2+}$-accumu-
lating ability of the SR was plotted as a function of reciprocal temperature (Figure
11), it was shown that a change in the apparent activation energy for the process occurs
about 20°C and another at 40°C. The rates between 5° and 20°C fit a process with an
apparent activation energy of 28 kcal $mol^{-1}$. Above 20°C activation energy is lower,
17 kcal $mol^{-1}$, until the temperature reaches 40°C. If the temperature is increased above
40°C, the rate of $Ca^{2+}$-accumulation drops sharply. The 20°C transition was shown to
involve primarily the lipid component and the effect observed in the 40°C region is
primarily associated with changes in protein conformation. Thus, at temperatures in
the 37°-40°C range a large effluence of $Ca^{2+}$ occurs and at temperatures below 10°C
similar effluxes occur. The increase in free calcium is undoubtedly associated with
contraction during the rigor mortis process.

*Cold Shortening*

    The most important change taking place during rigor onset is the extent of shorten-
ing which is of major importance to meat tenderness. Increase in $Ca^{2+}$ in the sarcoplasm, which is associated with high ADP levels,[287] undoubtedly causes the contraction
during development of rigor mortis. The spectacular excessive shortening that occurs
in muscle during glycolysis at 0 to 5°C, shown in Figure 12 from Locker and  Hagyard,[419] has been termed cold shortening and has been studied extensively because of
the pronounced increase in toughness.[453,509] The history of the affect of temperature
on meat tenderness have been recently reviewed by Locker et al.[420] The great bulk of
the changes occur very rapidly, before the onset of the rapid phase of ATP breakdown.
The time-course of events has been reviewed by Bendall.[48] Figure 13 shows that short-

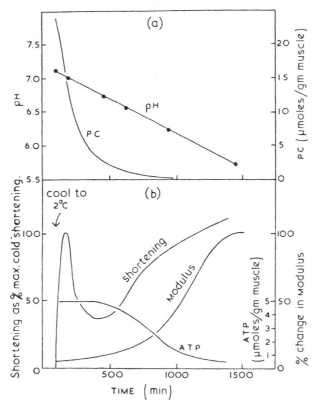

FIGURE 13. Cold-shortening of beef muscle placed at 2°C, 100 min after death. a) Changes in PC and pH; (b) Changes in modulus shortening and ATP. (From Bendall, J. R., *The Structure and Function of Muscle*, Vol. 2, 2nd ed., Bourne, C. H., Ed., Academic Press, New York, 1973, 291. With permission.)

ening begins almost as soon as the muscle is placed at 2°C and reaches a maximum after about 60 min, while both PC and ATP levels are still high. The shortening is superseded by lengthening which is rapid at first and then slows down, to be finally superseded by a new shortening which coincides in time with the disappearance of ATP from the muscle.

Since the release of calcium from the calcium pump is the process necessary for activating the contractile system, the temperature dependence of the shortening process can be explained by the temperature dependent calcium accumulative ability observed by Inesi et al.[330] The practical aspects of cold shortening were recently reviewed by Marsh,[454] who outlined various means whereby the extreme development of contraction may be avoided when chilling lamb. The problem is of particular interest to the New Zealand lamb processors because customers had begun to complain of the toughness of their chilled lamb. One of the more interesting methods used to overcome the problem was the process of rigor acceleration. Carse[96] found that pH decline normally taking 16 hr would occupy only 3 hr when a post-mortem electrical stimulation of 250 V was applied. More recently, Crystall and Hagyard[133] reported a total conditioning immediately after slaughter with a 3000 V capacitive discharge.

### Thaw Rigor

This phenomenon has also been extensively studied and is reviewed by Bendall[48] and by Locker et al.[420] The importance of thaw rigor in muscle quality was recognized by Sharp and Marsh.[631] The phenomena of drastic shortening accompanied by copious drip, observed when muscle is frozen prerigor and rapidly thawed, is known as thaw rigor. Marsh and Thompson[452] found that lamb muscle frozen immediately and thawed

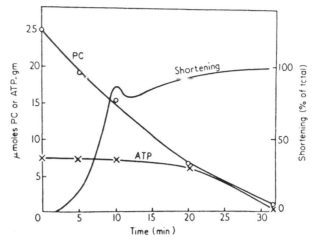

FIGURE 14. Pattern of chemical and physical changes in rabbit psoas strip, frozen pre-rigor at −20°C, and then allowed to thaw in air at 17°C. (From Bendall, J. R., *The Structure and Function of Muscle*, Vol. 2, 2nd ed., Bourne, C. H., Ed., Academic Press, New York, 1973, 288. With permission.)

at 16 to 20°C gave an average shortening of 72% with a 27% loss in weight as drip. Muscle frozen in rigor and thawed shortened by only 5% with 3% drip. Bendall[48] showed that rigor sets in at about 25 min, when only half the ATP has been destroyed. Figure 14 shows that the time for half change of ATP is only 25 min compared to 540 min for normal rigor. The rapid shortening sets in soon after thawing begins and is completed in about 10 min, while ATP is still high. We see an accelerated metabolic run-down with the pH fall and ATP loss completed in almost an hour. Rupture of the sarcoplasmic membrane resulting in high serum levels of $Ca^{2+}$ has been proposed by Kushmerick and Davies[403] as the reason for thaw rigor. Thus, cold shortening and thaw rigor are related in their dependence on calcium release. The resulting abnormal enzymatic activity and extreme shortening is a major cause of meat toughness.

### Pale and Dark Cutting Meat

The onset of rigor mortis in skeletal muscle is associated with a fall in the concentrations of ATP and CP in the tissue, breakdown of glycogen, and accumulation of lactic acid. It is generally accepted, as already pointed out, that the rate of post-mortem metabolism in muscle is a variable quantity and it is equally well-accepted that this variable rate of post-mortem metabolism has important implications in the ultimate use and quality of muscle as a food. High rates of anaerobic glycolysis occur frequently in pig muscle post-mortem. The combination of low pH and high temperature which results from such glycolysis brings about changes in the properties of the muscle proteins which cause tissue to become pale, soft, and exudative.[49,50,236,472,604] Pale, soft, and exudative (PSE) tissue is a problem of great practical concern to the meat industry and the monetary implications of this problem and its allied phenomenon of porcine stress syndrome (PSS) is highlighted by the recent estimates by Hall[274] that the problems result in a 230 to 320 million dollars loss per annum to the pig industry in the U.S.

The subject of PSE has been reviewed by Briskey[79] and Bray,[76] and more recently Cassens et al.[100] have reviewed the subject of PSE and animal physiology in relation to meat quality. In addition, a number of important symposia have dealt extensively with the problem.[99,296,672,696] The above references provide an excellent and comprehensive coverage of the subject and consequently we intend to be selective in our treatment of the subject.

*Incidence of PSE*

The incidence of PSE muscle varies between breeds of pigs, and is particularly high in stress-susceptible breeds such as the Poland China and the Pietrain.[296] In general, Forrest et al.[203] showed that 18% of all hams examined were pale, soft, and exudative. Van Logtestijn et al.[714] calculated that the incidence in most European countries was between 10 and 20%. The incidence of PSE is greater in pigs that have been subjected to temperature fluctuations during hauling and holding prior to slaughter.[136]

*Stress Susceptible and Stress Resistant Pigs*

It is well recognized that animals, in particular pigs, can be classified as having stress susceptibility or stress resistance. The nature of the stressors which are capable of causing disturbance is varied. According to Lawrie[408] be associated with activity, temperature, humidity, atmospheric pressure, oxygen tension, nutrition, pathology, drugs, toxins, and psychology (fear, light, sound). Irrespective of stressor, the stress-susceptible animal exhibits extensive anaerobic glycolysis and accumulation of lactate in muscle during life. High body temperatures, high venous blood $pCO_2$, and low $pO_2$ are also evident. It has been suggested that the muscles of stress-susceptible pigs are in a highly anaerobic state prior to or simultaneous to death.[81] This anaerobic state would then stimulate glycolysis. It has been observed[204,354,611] that the muscles of stress-susceptible pigs have a fast rate of glycolysis, a short-time course of rigor mortis, and become pale, soft, and exudative. On the other hand, stress-resistant pigs, i.e., animals able to maintain normal temperatures, blood pH, high $pO_2$, and low $pCO_2$, have a slow rate of glycolysis, a long-time course of rigor mortis, and retain a normal color and gross morphology post-mortem.

The effect of stimulation on meat quality has been examined by a number of workers. Bendall[46] curarized large white pigs which produced an extremely high pH in the longissimus dorsi after bleeding and a slow rate of pH decline. Curare is a neuromuscular blocking agent and would be expected to reduce the rate of post-mortem glycolysis. Although it does so in stress-resistant pigs,[470,471] it does not reduce the rate of post-mortem glycolysis in stress-susceptible pigs such as the Poland China[606] or the Pietrain. The effect of injecting relaxing doses of magnesium has been shown by Lister and Ratcliff[417] to be influenced by the breed of animal (Figure 15).

A marked retardation of the pH changes in muscle post-mortem was observed in all cases. However the changes were more rapid in the Pietrain pigs. The change in pH of the muscle closely followed the disappearance of ATP and CP. Lister and Ratcliff[417] conclude that it is the mechanisms regulating the turnover and degradation of ATP in muscle, which control the rate of change in its pH post-mortem. The inhibition of ATP-ase activity accounts for the beneficial effects of magnesium sulfate.

Bendall in his review[48] points to the indirect evidence of the role of $Ca^{2+}$ and membrane permeability in the PSE phenomenon:

1. According to Lister[416] the plasma $K^+$ levels rise sharply post-slaughter and can only be accounted for by substantial release of internal $K^+$ from the musculature.
2. The failure of curare to prevent rapid P turnover in anaerobic Pietrain muscle shows that the trouble lies on the membrane side of the neuromuscular junction. Since curare specifically inhibits the depolarizing effect of acetylcholine release on the post-synaptic membrane.

The higher the metabolic turnover in Poland, China, and Pietrain pigs post-mortem, the more rapid the change in pH, and the higher the muscle temperature will be at the lower pH values. The combined effect of temperature and pH leads to loss of the calcium-accumulating ability of the sarcoplasmic reticulum post-mortem[249] and dena-

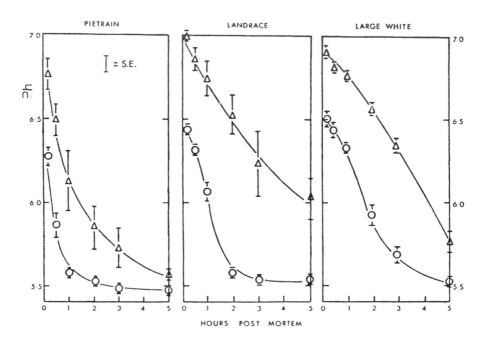

FIGURE 15. Changes in pH of porcine muscle post-mortem. Δ = magnesium injected, O = control. (From Lister, D. and Ratcliff, P. W., in *Proc. 2nd Int. Symp. Cond. Meat Qual. Pigs*, Hessel-de-Heer, J. C. M., et al., Eds., Wageningen, Netherlands, 1971, 144. With permission.)

turation and precipitation of sarcoplasmic proteins on the myofibrils.[469,612] The precipitation of the sarcoplasmic protein is responsible for the production of pale, soft, and exudative pork, the practical and commercial consequences of which have been previously outlined.

Dark-cutting, firm, and dry muscle condition can be produced in meat from animals that are stress-resistant or where the animal has survived a stress of sufficient duration to deplete the glycogen reserves. Dark-cutting meat occurs frequently in beef (3%) pork and lamb. A chemicophysical manifestation or preslaughter glycogen depletion is an ultimate pH above 6.5.

The deeper color of high pH meat is due to the muscle pigment remaining in the reduced state. At high pH the surviving activity of the cytochrome system is greater and this results in depletion of oxygen[408] and myoglobin oxygenation does not occur. Ashmore et al.[19] concluded that the failure of bright red color to develop in meat results from high mitochondria activity at the high pH of dark-cutting beef. Dark-cutting meat is generally considered not to be completely acceptable commercially. However it is recognized that there is some reduction in shrink on curing and curing losses are also reduced.

The presence of brown pigment metmyoglobin in meat is also highly undesirable. Fortunately this pigment can be reduced back to purplish myoglobin by enzymes present in meat. Dean and Ball[146] were perhaps the first to recognize the existence of natural metmyoglobin reducing systems in fresh meat. Walters and Taylor[737] demonstrated a slow enzymatic reduction of purified ferrimyoglobin under anaerobic incubation of same with pork muscle at pH 6. Although the enzymatic reduction of metmyoglobin has been demonstrated in meat, the enzyme systems responsible for reduction have not been fully isolated and studied. A cytoplasmic flavoenzyme, DT diaphorase was detected histochemically in meat by Bodwell et al.[62] This enzyme has been shown to be capable of reducing metmyoglobin. Matsui et al.[460] recently reported on the purification of two metmyoglobin reducing systems from dolphin skeletal muscle. One system, termed a diaphorase, contained two FAD per molecule and uses $NADH_2$, but not $NADPH_2$, as a source of reducing equivalents. The second reducing system, called ferrimyoglobin reductase, was much more effective in the presence of $NADH_2$ and $NADPH_2$, as a source of reducing equivalents. For a detailed discussion on the reduction of metmyoglobin, the enzyme systems, role of electron transport, and concentration of various substrates the reader should consult the following recent reviews: Govindarajan[245] and Giddings.[234,235]

Enzyme systems also play a role in the formation of cured meat pigment. Mitochondrial and cytochrome C involvement in cured-meat color development has been extensively studied by Walters et al.[739] They indicate that mitochondria appear to survive the bacon curing process and may function in the transfer of NO from nitrosylferricytochrome C to ferrimyoglobin to form MbNO in cured meat. Metmyoglobin (MetMb) is formed when nitrite is added into the muscle (anaerobic conditions prevail). In addition, ferrocytochrome C is oxidized by nitrite to ferricytochrome C and the NO is bound to cytochrome C. The nitrosylferricytochrome C is now reduced by NADH and a dehydrogenase system to ferroytochrome C. The NO is liberated and is transferred to MetMb (Figure 16), yielding nitrosomyoglobin (MbNO).

### Action of Proteolytic Enzymes on Meat

Over the years considerable research has been done in establishing the effect of pre-slaughter factors such as species, breed, age, sex, and nutrition, and of post-slaughter treatments such as aging and the use of artificial tenderizers. As already outlined shortening occurs during the onset of rigor mortis. Rate and extent of shortening depends on the rate and extent of pH decline, storage temperature, and species. This shortening causes increased toughness.[372]

The traditional butcher's method of hanging or conditioning meat is known to improve tenderness, flavor, and aroma of meat. It is now generally recognized that these changes are due to autolysis; however the mechanism whereby these changes occur has been shrouded in controversy and confusion.

The tenderizing of meat has been the subject of two comprehensive reviews.[41,751] More recently, Goll et al.[238] have discussed specific biochemical change in myofibrillar proteins during post-mortem storage. A number of research papers have also appeared on this topic.[137,140,371,747] However, much research in recent years has centered on the mechanism of protein-enzyme systems in post-mortem proteolysis.[65,93,143-145]

### Resolution of Rigor

Shortening occurs during the onset of rigor mortis. The rate and extent of shortening depends upon the species of animal from which the muscle is obtained and on storage temperature.[291] When ATP levels fall almost to zero in post-mortem muscle all crossbridges stop in that part of their cycle in which they are attached because ATP is necessary for detachment of cross-bridges from thin filaments.[241] Secondly, the sarcoplasmic reticular membranes lose the ability to retain bound $Ca^{2+}$ during post-mortem storage[239] and since $Ca^{2+}$ causes sarcomere shortening in living muscle it would appear that loss of $Ca^{2+}$ accumulating ability of the sarcoplasmic reticular membranes causes post-mortem sarcomere shortening.

However several groups of workers[671,681] have reported that, after 24 hr post-mortem, shortened sarcomeres gradually lengthen to some extent. It has been shown that the characteristically low elastic modulus of prerigor muscle and the equally characteristic reversibility of its stretch deformation — recovery curves, are slowly reestablished in the post-rigor period. Bendall[48] showed that resolution can be seen very clearly during rigor at 38°C and that the process is highly pH-dependent, occurring very rarely in exhausted muscle (ultimate pH 7.1) or muscle from starved animals (ultimate pH

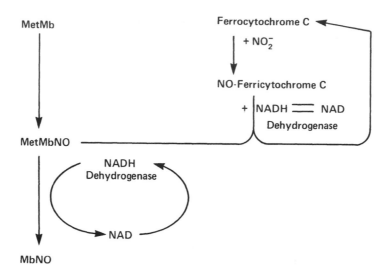

FIGURE 16.    Enzymatic formation of nitrosomyoglobin.

6.4 to 6.8). The sarcomere lengthening occurs during the same period that resolution of rigor is observed[237,239] and, according to Fukazawa and Briskey,[220] is associated with post-mortem tenderization of muscle. This finding is not unexpected since sarcomere shortening markedly decreases meat tenderness;[418] sarcomere lengthening through weakening of the actin-myosin interaction would be expected to increase tenderness.

On the basis of accepted muscle biochemistry, lengthening of post-mortem muscle must originate from transverse breaks or cracks in the myofibrils. An interesting theory proposed by Bendall[48] is that resolution is basically a denaturation process, probably of the $\alpha$-actinin and tropomyosin which are the linking proteins between the ends of the actin filaments in the Z-band.

Post-mortem Z-disk disintegration was observed by a number of groups[140,221,671,681] and occurs most quickly and most extensively at storage temperatures above 25°C. Degradation of Z-bonds weakens attachments between sarcomeres and therefore predisposes the muscle to rupture into pieces from one Z-band to the adjacent Z-bands.

A third structural change that is observed is the gradual degradation of M-lines which occurs after 24 hr of post-mortem storage.[240] The rate and extent of degradation is greater at high storage temperatures and in porcine or rabbit muscle than in bovine muscle.

Some workers[48,238] are of the opinion that agents other than proteolytic enzymes may be involved. However, the weight of evidence suggests that limited proteolysis occurs in post-mortem muscle. The fact that resolution of rigor is highly pH-dependent[48] further implicates proteolytic enzymes in meat aging.

*Proteolysis in Meat*

Proteolysis of collagen and elastin of connective tissue might appear to be the most likely change causing increased tenderness. However, Sharp[629] has conclusively shown that no increase in water-soluble hydroxyproline-containing derivatives occurred during conditioning of muscle. Goll et al.[238] identified a number of sites in the myofibril that are known to be vulnerable to added proteolytic enzymes. Myosin is readily degraded to heavy meromyosin and light meromyosin by the action of trypsin, chymotrypsin, or subtilisin. The second site of proteolysis is at or near the Z-band[671] and Ebashi and Kodama[175] have shown that the tropomyosin-troponin complex is also readily degraded by trypsin. Goll et al.[240] have shown that very brief treatment with trypsin of supercontracted myofibrils increases sarcomere length of these myofibrils from 1.3 $\mu$m to 1.8 $\mu$m. This change can occur in the complete absence of ATP and must indicate that trypsin treatment has weakened the actin-myosin complex.

*Lysosomal Enzymes in Meat Tenderness*

Studies based on histochemical and biochemical methods have indicated that intracellular proteolytic enzymes (cathepsins) are present in skeletal muscle,[267,350,392,393,428,652,742] but their role in tenderizing is not well-documented. The tissue proteinases are located in cells either in the lysosomes proper or in granules such as those of the neutrophil granulocytes. The identity of lysosomes was established almost simultaneously by two groups of investigators, Walker and Levy,[734] working with mouse liver $\beta$-glucuronidase and de Duve and co-workers.[53,54] In fact de Duve is most frequently associated with their discovery.

Most of the functional characteristics of lysosomes have been well documented[37-39,147,163,664] and they are now considered to be a heterogeneous group of cytoplasmic organelles forming part of a complex dynamic membraneous system. The pH optima are in the acid range.

Novikoff[516] and Novikoff et al.[517] have described in detail the involvement of lysosomes in cellular physiology and pathology and formed the opinion that "pure lysosomes" are present in all cells including muscle and blood. Dreyfus et al.[168] observed that healthy muscles may be poor in lysosomes even though there is a well-defined turnover in muscle protein in mature animals. Following tissue injury or in diseased muscle there is a pronounced infiltration by macrophages and other phagocytic leukocytes. Hamdy et al.[276] showed that increases in proteolytic activity occurred during the course of healing in bruised chicken muscle, while Tappel et al.[685,686] reported high correlation between increased acid hydrolase activities and histological evidence of infiltration by macrophages into muscles of vitamin E deficient rabbits.

Studies on the role of cathepsins during aging of meat has been hampered by observations which suggest that proteolytic activity in bovine skeletal muscle is low in comparison with the activity of similar enzymes in organ tissues such as liver, spleen, lungs, and kidney. Zender et al.[780] gave comparative characteristics of the proteolytic activities of various organs and tissues extracted with a 2% KCl solution:

|  | Units of activity |
|---|---|
| Kidneys | 1.900 |
| Liver | 1.500 |
| Lungs | 1.000 |
| Heart | 0.330 |
| Psoas major muscle | 0.025 |

Another comparison of activities is found in the measurements of cathepsins in rat tissues by Bouma and Gruber.[71] Comparing the activity of cathepsins, with spleen arbitrarily set at 100, they recorded activities of 20, 204, and 30 for liver and the low activities of <5, 8, and 11 for heart and <5, <5, and <5 for skeletal muscle for cathepsins B, C, and D, respectively. Limited studies by Fruton et al.[218] indicated that proteinases of relatively low activity are present in bovine skeletal muscle and are active in the pH ranges 4.0 to 6.5 and 8.5 to 9.5. Landmann[404] concluded that the general proteolytic activity in beef muscle is due to two enzyme systems, one with a pH optimum at 5 which is strongly activated by $Fe^{2+}$ and one with an optimum of pH 2 and activated by EDTA. The acid proteinase system was found to contain cathepsins B and C. Landmann noted that the optimal pH of these isolated fractions is in the pH range of meat which is favorable for enzymic action during aging. However, Bodwell and Pearson[61] were unable to attribute the proteolytic activity in extracts of bovine skeletal muscle to either cathepsin B or C and in agreement with the work of Sharp[630] concluded that the sarcoplasmic proteins were the major substrates for the natural proteolytic enzymes. Randall and MacRae[583] examined the proteolytic activity of the water-soluble proteins of bovine skeletal muscle separated by starch gel electrophoresis and presumed the presence of proteolytic activity resembling that of cathepsin B and C. More recently, Lutalo-Bosa and MacRae[428] determined the proteolytic activity of cathepsins B, C, and D in skeletal muscle and concluded that the activities of cathepsins B and D are higher in bovine skeletal muscle than previously indicated. Huang and Tappel[316] showed that cathepsin D is the most important of the cathepsins since it initiates protein hydrolysis and produces peptides that are further broken down by other cathepsins such as cathepsin C. In view of the increased lysosomal proteolytic activity in diseased and injured muscle, it is conceivable that lysosomal activity increases in post-mortem muscle and that these lysosomal hydrolyzases play a part in modification of meat quality. However, the relationships are difficult to demonstrate.

Fish muscle cathepsins have not been studied in the same detail as those from mammals. Siebert[639] found that the cathepsin activity of fish muscle was ten times greater than that of mammalian tissue; cathepsins have been observed to play a role in the spoilage of fish prior to processing.[640] Sinnhuber and Landers[643] reported that heat treatment was required prior to irradiation to inactivate the enzymes that cause release of amino nitrogen in cod muscle. Purification studies on fish muscle cathepsin have been carried out by Groninger,[259] Ting et al.,[695] and Reddi et al.[585] The significance of fish cathepsins in muscle tenderness is not known and is probably not very important due to the extremely perishable nature of fish. In certain fish, particularly fish that have been feeding actively, autolytic spoilage occurs readily.[687] Pacific Northwest herring and feeding salmon must be carefully treated by rapid chilling or evisceration. Visceral proteolysis, called "torn bellies", arise from penetration by the natural proteolytic digestive enzymes of the visceral tract into the flesh. Enzymes from the feed itself, or from bacteria in the digestive tract cannot be ruled out.

Shestakov[634] suggested that some proteolytic activity in muscle may be due to residual blood in the muscle since badly bled muscles undergo the tenderizing changes of conditioning to a greater extent than do those which are bled. It is well recognized that even with effective bleeding, only about 50% of the total blood is removed. We have already discussed the infiltration of injured or diseased tissue by macrophages. The main source of macrophages are blood monocytes and tissue histocytes. Maturation of blood monocytes into macrophages is believed to be induced by blood polymorphonuclear leukocytes or their degradation products. That polymorphonuclear leukocytes themselves contain numerous hydrolytic enzymes was demonstrated by Cohn et al.,[121] working on the degradation of bacteria by phagocytic cells. Bradley[74] implicated blood as a source of proteolytic enzymes when he pointed out that the active red muscles of the chicken's leg carry out autolysis much more intensely than the inactive pectoral muscles. The red muscles of cattle, rabbits, and dogs possess greater proteolytic activity than the white muscles of birds. Similar trends were noted for fish. More recently, the role of blood lysosomal hydrolyzases in muscle proteolysis has been actively studied at the University of Missouri.[28,715] Porcine leukocytes were isolated from blood after sedimenting erythrocytes with dextrin. The lysosomes were suspended in cold 0.25 $M$ sucrose and the lysosomes were separated by sonication followed by differential sedimentation. Degradation of various myofibrillar proteins by reaction with leukocyte lysosomal proteases was demonstrated by a variety of techniques. Reductions in muscle fiber extensibility were observed in muscle treated with the proteinase fraction. Degradation of actomyosin, actin, troponin, and tropomyosin was also observed.

*Ca²⁺-Activated Enzyme*

One of the most interesting findings in recent years was the presence in skeletal muscle cells of a $Ca^{2+}$-activated factor capable of removing Z-disks from intact myofibrils of rabbit psoas strips that had been incubated in $Ca^{2+}$-containing saline solutions for 9 hr at pH 7.2 and 37°C.[93,238] Z-disks in muscle strips from the same animal suspended under identical conditions in the same solution but containing 1 mM EGTA, a $Ca^{2+}$ chelator instead of 1 mM $Ca^{2+}$, were structurally intact after 9 hr of incubation. Incubation in 1 mM $Ca^{2+}$-containing solutions of purified myofibrils that had no membrane, and which had been washed free from sarcoplasmic proteins, had no effect on Z-disk structure, even after long incubation times. Thus, the above authors concluded that some factor in the muscle cell sarcoplasm was being activated by $Ca^{2+}$ and that this factor was removing Z-disks. This $Ca^{2+}$-activated "proteolytic" factor was termed CAF. The importance of $Ca^{2+}$ was previously noted by Haga et al.[271] and by Davey and Gilbert.[139] The former found that $Ca^{2+}$ promoted the separation of actin from Z-lines, while the latter showed that both the weakening of lateral attachments and the disappearance of Z-lines during ageing were inhibited by EDTA.

*Purification and Properties of CAF*

A crude enzyme system with similar properties was previously isolated by Kohn[385] and it is very likely that CAF is identical with the kinase activating factor that was purified to 60% homogeneity by Huston and Krebs.[325] The active fraction was isolated from a pH 4.9 to 6.2 precipitate of sarcoplasmic proteins.[93] The isoelectrically precipitated protein was dissolved in 30 mM Tris-acetate pH 7.0, 1 mM EDTA and then salted out between 0 and 40% ammonium sulfate saturation. The enzyme was further purified by using five column chromatographic procedures in succession:[144] (1) 6% agarose, (2) DEAE-cellulose, (3) Sephadex® G200, (4) DEAE-cellulose with a very shallow KCl gradient, and (5) Sephadex® G100. Based on yield of purified CAF they concluded that porcine skeletal muscle contained 3.4 μg CAF per gram fresh muscle weight. The purified enzyme had a molecular weight of 110,000 daltons and contains one 80,000-dalton subunit and one 30,000-dalton subunit per molecule. The pH optimum on either myofibril or casein substrates is 7.5 and it is considered to be an extremely active proteinase. The enzyme also requires sulphydryl reducing agents and 1 mM $Ca^{2+}$ for optimum activity.

Purified CAF partly degrades M-lines, troponin and tropomyosin, and C-protein, but has no effect on myosin, actin, or α-actinin. Dayton et al.[145] on the basis of molecular weight, amino acid composition, and other properties ruled out the possibility that CAF actually originated from blood or connective tissue present in the minced muscle and on the basis of their analyses conclude that CAF is not one of the known catheptic enzymes found in muscle cells. On the basis of differential centrifugation of porcine muscle homogenates, the above authors conclude that CAF is an intracellular proteolytic enzyme located in the sarcoplasm of muscle cells and is not confined to membrane-enclosed particles such as lysosomes.

*Role of CAF in Meat Tenderness*

According to Dayton et al.,[143] CAF is the first proteolytic enzyme with the ability to degrade intact myofibrils that has been purified from skeletal muscle and because purified CAF is maximally active near the in vivo pH in living muscle cells, they suggest that CAF has a physiological role in metabolic turnover in myofibrils and myofibrillar proteins. Studies in the same laboratory[529,530] have shown that the effects of CAF on myofibrils are remarkably similar to the effect of post-mortem aging on myofibrils. These studies later showed that post-mortem Z-disk degradation is also caused by a $Ca^{2+}$-activated enzyme found in the sarcoplasm of muscle cells. The amount of $Ca^{2+}$-

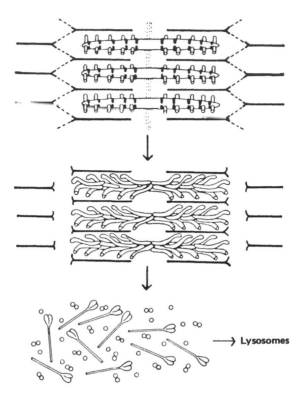

FIGURE 17.  A schematic diagram showing how CAF
could act to initiate myofibrillar breakdown. (From Day-
ton, W. R., Goll, D. E., Stromer, M. H., Reville, W. J.,
Zeece, M. G., and Robson, R. M., in *Cold Spring Harbor
Conference on Cell Proliferation, Vol. II, Proteases and
Biological Control,* Cold Spring Harbor, New York, 1975.
With permission.)

activated enzyme in muscle can be correlated directly with the amount of post-mortem
Z-disk degradation that occurs in the muscle. The semitendinosus muscle has approximately three times more CAF activity than psoas muscle immediately after death and
after 6 days of post-mortem storage, the CAF activity remaining in bovine semitendinosus muscle may be 20 to 30 times greater than the CAF activity remaining in bovine
psoas muscle.[529] Fragmentation of myofibrils as measured by an absorbance technique
increased significantly in semitendinosus muscle during post-mortem storage, but remained relatively unchanged in psoas muscle during the same period.[530] The degree of
myofibrillar fragmentation that occurred was correlated directly with the amount of
post-mortem tenderization in the particular muscle. They therefore, concluded that
CAF is a major factor causing post-mortem changes in meat quality.

The mode of action of CAF in increasing tenderness may in fact, be similar to that
schematically outlined by Dayton et al.[143] for myofibrillar turnover. The mode of action proposed by these authors is shown in Figure 17 and described below.

CAF degredation of Z-disks and C-protein (Figure 17 top) should cause disordering of the three dimen-
sional array of thick and thin filaments (Figure 17 middle). Moreover, degradation of tropomyosin and
troposin by CAF should initiate disassembly of thin filaments of actin monomers or dimers (Figure 17
bottom), and degradation of the M-line possibly by some agent other than CAF, could initiate disassembly
of the thick filaments (Figure 17 bottom). The actin and myosin monomers released by this disassembly
might then be degraded by lysosomes.

Table 6
RELATIVE POTENCIES OF TWELVE ENZYME
PREPARATIONS ON THE MUSCLE TISSUE
COMPONENTS BASED ON STRUCTURAL
MANIFESTATION

| Enzyme preparations | pH | Muscle fibers | Connective tissue fibers | |
|---|---|---|---|---|
| | | Actomyosin | Collagen | Elastin |
| Protease 15 | 6.4 | + + + | – | – |
| Rhozyme P-11 | 6.8 | + + | – | – |
| Rhozyme A-4 | 7.3 | + + | – | – |
| HT Proteolytic | 6.9 | + + + + | trace | – |
| Fungal amylase | 7.1 | + + + | trace | – |
| Hydralase D | 7.4 | + + + | trace | – |
| Hydralase TP | 6.9 | + + | trace | – |
| Ficin | 5.2 | + + + | + + + | + + + + |
| Papain | 5.1 | + + | + | + + |
| Bromelin | 6.3 | trace | + + + | + |
| Trypsin | 5.7 | + + | + | + |
| Viokase | 5.8 | + + +[a] | + | + |

[a]  Sarcolemma not affected.

From Landmann, W. A., *Proc. Meat Tenderness Symp.*, Campbell Soup Co., Camden N.J., 1963, 95. With permission.

However, the model does propose a role for lysosomes and it is possible that the catheptic enzymes and in particular, leukocyte lysosomes, may be the causative agent in M-line destruction and in the weakening of actin-myosin cross-links. Lysosomes have a pH optimum of 5.0 or less and in this respect it is significant to note that resolution of rigor is highly pH dependent, occurring most rapidly in muscles with an ultimate pH between 5.3 and 5.8.[48]

### Added Enzymes

The use of added enzymes to accelerate ripening of meat and upgrade poor quality cuts was introduced in 1949 and a variety of enzymes are now widely used.[654,751] Commercially used enzymes fall into three groups: those of bacterial or fungal origin, such as Protease 15, Rhozyme, subtilisin, pronase, and hydrolase D; those of plant origin such as papain, bromelain and ficin; and those of animal origin, such as trypsin. It is now claimed that 30 to 40% of the worlds meat supply is artifically tenderized and that such treatment increases the percentage of salable prime cuts from 30 to 70%. The chemistry and histological aspects of added enzyme action on meat proteins have been studied by Miyada and Tappel,[479] Wang et al.,[740] and Kang and Rice.[360] According to Miyada and Tappel,[479] the greatest change among the various protein fractions occurred in the transformation of soluble protein nitrogen to nonprotein nitrogen due to hydrolysis, mainly of actomyosin. The activity of the various enzymes toward meat decreased in the order: ficin, bromelain, trypsin, papain, and rhozyme. Both the plant and microbial enzymes tested degraded collagen to some extent.

Wang et al.,[740] using histological techniques were able to identify the sites of enzyme action and show that enzymes of different origins preferentially attack different muscle components. Table 6 summarizes the findings.

Somewhat similar results were obtained by Kang and Rice.[360] Collagenase, bromelain, and trypsin degraded the stroma fraction more strongly than the myofibrillar fraction.

Table 7

PRE-RIGOR ENZYME INJECTION

| Meat | Tenderness of meat, points | | Increase in tenderness as a result of treatment points |
|---|---|---|---|
| | Control | Treated with enzyme | |
| Freshly killed | 2.7 | 4.2 | + 1.5 |
| Chilled | 3.0 | 3.8 | + 0.8 |
| Defrosted | 3.0 | 3.6 | + 0.6 |

The enzymes are usually applied in three ways:

1.  Sprinkling a powdered preparation on the surface of the meat or immersing the meat in an enzyme solution. These methods are applicable only to small cuts and even then tenderization may be uneven.
2.  Preslaughter intraveneous injection of oxidized papain. This is a patent of Swift & Co., Chicago[710] and is termed the Proten® process. Oxidized papain at a level of 1.5 mg/lb live weight is injected about 30 min before slaughter. The animals are slaughtered, dressed, and chilled conventionally. The papain is reduced to the active forms by the reducing atomosphere in the muscles post-mortem. There is an increase in tenderness in all carcass cuts but organs with a good blood supply (heart, liver, tongue) tend to disintegrate on cooking.[574] The plant enzymes are inactive on undenatured protein at chill temperatures. All papain proteolytic action takes place during cooking in the range 50° to 82°C.
3.  Post-mortem pre-rigor pumping of dressed carcasses is practiced in the U.S.S.R.[654] This may be done either by intravenous injection or by intramuscular injection using a series of needles. This method allows more rigorous control of enzyme localization between tough and tender joints. The desirability of pre-rigor injection is seen from the following data.[654]

*Use of Other Enzymes*

Denton et al.[151] proposed that proteolytic enzymes of plant or animal origin and proteolytic enzymes derived from fungal or bacterial sources may be used, singly or in combination, to assist the mechanical removal of meat from bone. Hyaluronidase is used to assist the distribution of seasoning throughout poultry carcasses.[488]

**Enzymes in Meat Flavor**

The flavor of meat and fish is an important property, but it is also extraordinarily complex as is evident from a number of recent reviews. Most of the reviews relate to meat flavor, however, it is probable that nitrogenous, carbohydrate, and lipid substances are the flavor sources in both systems. For a more detailed discussion on the role of enzymes, particularly in tissue flavor, the reader should refer to Herz and Chang,[300] Dwivedi,[173] and Patterson.[543]

The ultimate flavor of cooked meat depends upon a number of preslaughter and post-mortem factors. For instance, species, breed, sex, age, fattiness, and feed have been listed as preslaughter factors influencing the flavor of meat.[543] Stress at time of slaughter, post-mortem aging, and storage temperature are also important. The concentration of meat flavor precursors depends very much on metabolic activity in the animal body. Consequently, the concentration of suitable substrates, the nature and concentration of enzymes, time-course of temperature and pH post-slaughter, the ultimate pH, and storage temperature must be considered.

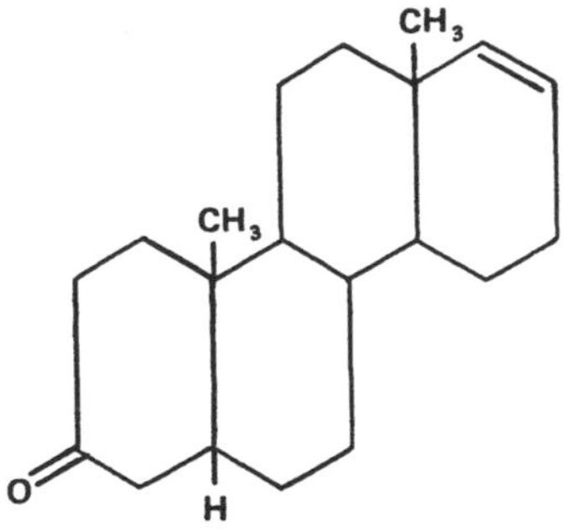

FIGURE 18. 5 α-androst-16-en-3-one.

Table 8
NUCLEOTIDE CONTENT OF RAW
AND ROASTED BEEF (mg/100 g
DRY, FAT-FREE TISSUE)

| Nucleotide | Raw | Heated to 77°C |
|---|---|---|
| Cytidylic acid | 13.1 ± 2.0 | 13.0 ± 3.2 |
| Adenylic acid | 12.1 ± 3.5 | 41.3 ± 4.1 |
| Uridylic acid | 7.1 ± 1.2 | 5.3 ± 2.5 |
| Inosinic acid | 278.4 ± 24 | 170.3 ± 38.0 |
| Guanylic acid | 2.2 ± 4.9 | 3.1 ± 4.6 |

The flavor quality of lean tissue was found to be related to breed. European-type cattle give a better flavored meat than do Brahmin cattle.[317] Similar results were reported by Branaman et al.,[75] where beef-type Hereford meat had a more desirable flavor than the dairy-type Holstein. Change in the composition of muscle with age is also an important factor,[132] and more recently Tuma et al.[704] and Tuma[703] observed that flavor of cooked meat generally increased with age of the animal and once maturity was reached and metabolic turnover stabilized, the flavor remained largely unchanged.

The sex of animals also influences the flavor of meat. Male pigs at maturity are frequently associated with an unpleasant "boar taint" on cooking. The compound contributing to the sex odor is 5 α-androst-16-en-3-one (Figure 18), which occurs mainly in the adipose tissue at low concentration.[542] This compound is similar to the steroidal hormones and is associated with normal male metabolism.

Post-mortem muscle metabolism is also important in meat flavor. A relationship between the ultimate pH of muscle and its flavor has been reported.[72] A relatively high pH of meat post-mortem produced a definite loss of flavor,[343] which was probably associated with the evolution of hydrogen sulfide during cooking of high pH meat.[547]

The nucleotides as a group of substances possess flavor enhancing properties and have been implicated in the modification of meat flavor.[349] It has been shown that the only isomer of IMP which is flavorous is 5'IMP and 5'GMP is even more flavorous. The 2' or 3' nucleotides are not effective. Nucleotides occur in raw muscle; Macy et al.[434] reported on the changes in individual 5'-nucleotides during cooking to an internal temperature of 77°C. The major change is in the level of inosinic acid which decreases from 278 to 170 mg per 100 g dry tissue (Table 8).

We have already discussed the decrease in ATP during post-mortem rigor. The formation of adenosine-5'-monophosphate (AMP) results from the autolytic removal of

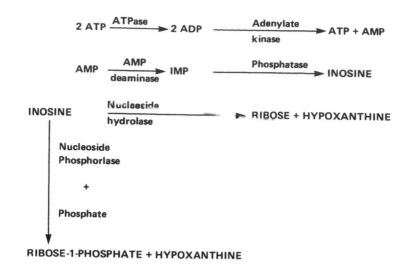

FIGURE 19.    Conversion of ATP to hypoxanthine in post-mortem muscle.

two terminal phosphate groups of ATP by the combined catalytic action of ATP-ase and myokinase (Figure 19). AMP is then deaminated to IMP by the action of AMP deaminase. Further degradation of IMP into inosine and hypoxanthine occurs during storage. Hypoxanthine has a bitter flavor and has been implicated as the cause of off-flavor in fish[348] and may also cause off flavors in irradiated beef since some enzymatic activity remains. Hashimoto[286] established the importance of IMP to the flavor of good quality fresh fish. In species in which IMP is rapidly degraded, flavor losses have been related. More recently Groninger and Spinelli[260] showed that, if nucleotide activity was blocked in fish by treatment with EDTA, the treated fish were preferred to untreated fish. While IMP degradation may be correlated with flavor in fish no such relationship has been reported for meat from warm-blooded animals. Nucleic acids are substantially degraded during aging[138] and it is well recognized that this change occurs during a period where flavor is markedly enhanced by cooking. Hence, it may be deduced that nucleic acid breakdown is not directly responsible for desirable meat flavor.

Examination of nucleotide degradation in fish muscle as a means for assessing fish freshness and quality has received considerable attention.[55,304] Measurement of the accumulation of hypoxanthine in particular has shown potential as an index of freshness, especially in marine fish.[91,92,213,214,362,657] Some work has been done on fresh water fish[55] and hypoxanthine measurement has shown potential value. Recently Jahns et al.[334] introduced a simple visual enzyme test paper for hypoxanthine determination in fish which is suitable for use at wholesale and retail outlets.

Hydrolytic and oxidative rancidity both occur in frozen muscle; the former is catalyzed by lipases and the latter by heme compounds. Both changes are temperature-dependent. Fatty acids are mainly formed from lecithin[423] first by a phospholipase enzyme to yield lysolecithin and this is further degraded to glycerophosphorylcholine by a lysolecithinase enzyme. Awad et al.[25] showed that when fresh water fish were stored at −10°C for 16 weeks the free fatty acid content rose to about 21.4% of the total lipid. It is generally accepted that lecithinase activity and fatty acid oxidation are greater in the red muscle of fish.

It appears doubtful that free fatty acids as such contribute significantly to undesirable flavors in muscle. However, they are more readily oxidized than the parent glyceride esters and may thus tend to accelerate oxidative rancidity development in the stored muscle and contribute to off-flavor development and loss of nutritive value.

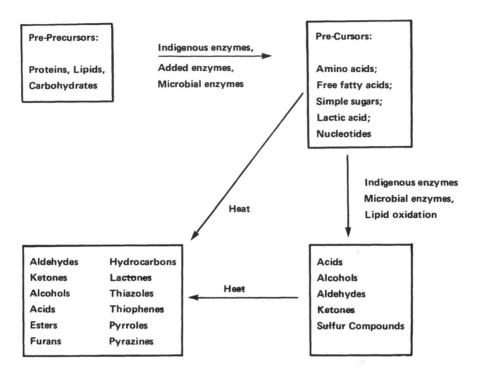

FIGURE 20.    Scheme of flavor production in meat and fish.

Early workers[410,590] suggested that lipoxygenase may be responsible for lipid oxidation in animal tissues. However, in more recent studies,[478] lipoxygenase activity has been ruled out and Whitaker[752] reports that efforts to isolate an enzyme which has a specificity similar to that of lipoxygenase have been unsuccessful. It is generally concluded that oxidation of unsaturated fatty acids in animal tissues is due mainly to heman catalysis.

Lipid hydrolysis is also of major interest to the protein chemist because a correlation has been shown to exist between the hydrolysis of tissue lipid and denaturation and loss of extractability of muscle proteins. Insolubilization occurred as a result of free fatty acid-protein interaction[527] which leads to loss of texture, flavor, and nutritional value. The nature of the association has been discussed by Anderson and Ravesi[9] who suggest that loss in protein extractability is due to the solvent environment becoming increasingly nonpolar.

Autolytic enzymes are considered relatively unimportant organoleptically in spoiling of fish held around freezing temperatures. Evidence from studies with other protein foods suggests that spoilage microorganisms of the *Pseudomonas* group produce considerable proteolysis and off-flavor in muscle.[89] Similarly Herbert and Shewan[292] could find no evidence to show that autolytic enzymes are directly involved in the production of volatile sulfides in chill-stored cod. *Pseudomonas* spp. were responsible for the production of hydrogen sulfide and methylmercaptan as a result of degradation of cysteine and methionine.

The role of enzymes in the development of food flavors has been discussed for dairy products by Dwivedi[172] and by the same author for meat and meat products.[173] In his 1975 review he discusses the important role of bacterial proteinases, lipases, and other enzymes in the development of flavor compounds and flavor precursors in fermented sausages. The metabolic pathways for the production of meat precursors are also discussed in detail.

Figure 20 summarizes the main mechanisms involved in the production of flavorants and their precursors.

## Thiaminase Activity

Most of the enzyme systems discussed influence the nutritional value of food in an indirect manner. Some improve the color, flavor, texture, and water-holding capacity of the tissue while others induce color and flavor changes which make the food unacceptable. A number of reactions have a direct influence on the nutritional status of the food. For example, the production of hydroperoxides by lipoxygenase activity and the destruction of carotene by various enzyme systems. Perhaps the most intriguing enzyme system is that of thiaminase which hydrolyses thiamin to 2-methyl-6-amino-5-hydroxymethyl pyrimidine and 4-methyl-5-hydroxymethyl thiazole, thus destroying this vitamin. The presence of antithiamin substances in fish has been known since Chastekparalysis was induced by inclusion of raw carp in fox diets.[254] Thiaminase occurs in many species of fish and shellfish. In general, the enzyme seems to be confined to certain types of freshwater fish. However, a number of salt water fish, particularly herring, also contain the antivitamin factor. The enzymes are either an intrinsic part of the flesh or occur indirectly through microorganisms in the intestines or on the surface.

The following fish have been reported as active in the antithiamin factor:[67]

| Freshwater species | Marine species |
|---|---|
| Carp | Capelin |
| Chub | Herring |
| Smelts | Menhaden |
| Minnow | Garfish |
| | Whiting |

Fortunately boiling or cooking the fish in most cases inactivates the enzyme. However, Kundig and Somogyi[399] found a thermostable antithiamin factor in carp viscera. Thus, it appears that different antithiamin enzymes exist and studies by Tang and Hilker[682] indicated that more than one factor was present in Skipjack tuna.

The presence of thiaminase in waste material which may ultimately be converted in feed for poultry, fur animals, trout in hatcheries, and pets may lead to deficiency signs. Yudkin[779] was of the opinion that consumption of raw fish or unheated fermented fish products by certain Asian peoples may contribute to the incidence of beri-beri. The consumption of mollusks and salted or cured herring may raise the requirement for thiamin. In fact salted herring has been shown to destroy 50 to 60% of added thiamin within 6 hr.[779]

Endemic thiamin deficiency has been shown to persist in certain parts of Japan despite administration of thiamin. It is generally accepted that this form of beri-beri is caused by thiaminase-producing microorganisms that inhabit the intestinal tract.[67]

Certain plants also contain thiaminase activity. The enzyme has been observed in rice polishings, beans, and mustard seed. Thus, in regions where people consume an exclusive unpolished rice diet, the thiamin requirements may not be met.

## CEREALS

Cereal products form a major item in the human diet throughout the world. While many species of cereal are used for human consumption, by far the dominant ones are wheat in Europe, America, and Oceania and rice in Asia. The discussion will concern itself only with the indigenous enzymes in wheat flour and the use of exogenous enzymes in the baking of wheat flour.

## Indigenous Enzymes

Good quality wheat flour contains a number of enzymes of which $\alpha$ and $\beta$-amylases, proteinase, lipase, lipoxidase, and phytase are the most important from the viewpoint of the food technologist. Most of these enzymes are present at a low level in flour from ungerminated wheat, but nevertheless play a significant role in the functional and nutritive attributes of flour and bread. On germination the concentration of most enzymes increases and their activity so alters the functional properties of flour as to make it unsuitable for baking.

Attempts to permit the baking of bread from sprouted wheat have included the manufacture of small loafs and the use of high salt levels and low pH (4.5) which increase the rate of denaturation of $\alpha$-amylase, the use of lower flour extraction rates since $\alpha$-amylase is concentrated in the outer endosperm layers, and heating grain with superheated steam in an attempt to denature the enzymes in the grain. In addition to the six enzymes listed above, wheat contains a battery of enzymes necessary to initiate germination and which increase in concentration at germination; the synthesis of many additional enzymes is initiated at germination. The enzymes involved in the germination process, located principally in the wheat germ, will not be discussed as it is assumed that under modern farming and milling practices flour is produced only from ungerminated wheat.

The chemistry and technology of wheat and bread-making are discussed in numerous texts and review articles including Geddes,[231] Kent,[368] Kent-Jones and Amos,[369] Matz,[461,462] and Pomeranz.[555]

Early work on the importance of indigenous enzymes in baking technology is reviewed in a monograph edited by Anderson[8] and by Kent-Jones and Amos;[369] and in later work by Pomeranz,[555] Reed and Thorn,[589] and Pratt.[562]

*Amylases*

Amylases are the most important indigenous enzymes in flour. Flour contains a low level of fermentable sugar (normally $\approx 0.5\%$) which is insufficient to support sufficient yeast growth to produce adequate $CO_2$ to give good-sized, well-aerated bread. During dough fermentation further fermentable sugars are produced from damaged starch granules by indigenous amylases (granular starch is not susceptible to hydrolysis by amylase but flour normally contains $\approx 9\%$ (7 to 12%) of starch damaged during milling, hard wheats being more susceptible to damage, or present in abnormal granules, susceptible to hydrolysis; $\alpha$-amylases are more effective on damaged granules). It was recognized early that ungerminated cereals contained an abundance of $\beta$-amylase which hydrolyzes alternate $\alpha$-1-4 glycosidic bonds in amylose and amylopectin to yield maltose (it is frequently referred to as a saccharifying enzyme). It is capable of hydrolyzing amylose essentially completely to maltose, but being unable to hydrolyze $\alpha$-1-6 glycodic linkages it leaves a large limit dextrin unhydrolyzed in amylopectin. After some early controversy, there is now agreement that ungerminated wheat contains only a low and variable level of $\alpha$-amylase, but the concentration of this enzyme increases at least 1000-fold on germination. $\beta$-Amylase is able to convert only $\approx 60\%$ of the available starch to maltose and if the concentration of damaged starch is low, the level of maltose produced may be insufficient to support optimum yeast growth. Prior to the widespread use of the combined harvester some spouting normally occurred during harvesting and the resulting $\alpha$-amylase ensured an adequate level of fermentable sugar. It is now common practice to add an exogenous $\alpha$-amylase to flour to ensure adequate sugar levels.

Amylases are concentrated in the outer starchy layers of the endosperm with relatively little activity in the inner portions: the aleurone cells and bran contain no $\beta$-amylase but are relatively rich in $\alpha$-amylase; the amylytic activity of the germ is concentrated in the scutellum. The level of amylases changes during the course of maturation and there are some intervaretial differences.[589]

Both $\alpha$- and $\beta$-amylases from wheat have been isolated and crystallized; multiple forms of both enzymes occur. The pH optima of both enzymes is in the range pH 4 to 5 but the exact value is subject to the usual experimental variables (assay temperature, ionic strength, ionic composition). The temperature optimum for $\beta$-amylase is $\approx$ 50°C and that for $\alpha$-amylase 60 to 66°C; denaturation of both enzymes is pH-dependent, being most stable at pH 4 to 5. This difference is technologically significant because $\alpha$-amylase retains significant activity at temperatures sufficiently high to induce gelatinization of starch (normally 3 to 4 min is required for the internal temperature of a 500 g loaf to pass through the temperature range 60 to 75°C, the gelatinization range of starch) and thus while present only at low concentration they may produce more hydrolysis of starch during baking than does the more thermo-labile $\beta$-amylase. Malt or indigenous wheat $\alpha$-amylases are more stable than fungal $\alpha$-amylases but considerably less stable than bacterial $\alpha$-amylases (50% inactivation at 73, 71, and 78°C, respectively).

Excessive $\alpha$-amylase activity causes undesirably extensive hydrolysis of starch leading to loss of water-binding capacity and to stickiness and gumminess in bread crumb; hence the undesirability of sprouting which results in excessive levels of $\alpha$-amylase and renders wheat unmillable. As discussed earlier a low level of $\alpha$-amylase activity is desirable to produce an adequate level of fermentable sugars but this is best done by adding an exogenous source of $\alpha$-amylase (malt).

*Protease*

It has been recognized since 1884 that flour contains a proteinase, now thought to be a sulfydryl proteinase (papain type).[589] The enzyme appears to be normally inactive but is activated by reducing agents. The early extensive literature on the nature of flour proteinase was reviewed in detail by Hildebrand.[303]

More recent work using starch gel electrophoresis and gel permeation chromatography indicates the presence of numerous proteolytically active components some of which probably arise from self-association of the enzyme or association with non-enzymatic proteins, but there appears to be at least two distinct proteinases one of which is extractable with 10% NaCl, the other being strongly associated with gluten. One of the proteinases appears to be a sulfydryl enzyme.[645] Wheat also contains a number of peptidases and the levels of both proteinases and peptidases increase markedly on germination.[589] Both proteinase and peptidase activity are concentrated in the germ and outer layers with relatively little in the endosperm; consequently patent or 72% extraction flours contain relatively little proteolytic activity.[311]

The significance of the indigenous proteinases in dough, which have wide proteolytic specificity, remained controversial for many years but it appears to play only a minor role, with physicochemical changes in the flour proteins due to pH and salt being of greater significance. The proteinase content of wheat increases about 20-fold on germination with detrimental effects on baking quality of flour.

The improving effect of oxidizing agents on flour quality was previously held to be due to the inhibiting influence of these agents on flour proteinases but this viewpoint does not now appear to be tenable; rather they appear to act directly by crosslinking the gluten.[675]

*Phosphatases*

Wheat and other cereals contains phytic acid (a hexaphosphate of the hexahydric alcohol, inositol) which sequesters calcium, iron, and other polyvalent cations rendering them unmetabolizable; children fed on high-bread diets may suffer from rickets (which is the basis of calcium fortification of flours in the U.K.),[85,463,464] although there is some disagreement on this point.[513,732] Phytase is a phosphatase which hydrolyses the phosphate ester bonds of phytic acid which is concentrated in the bran layers and germ of the wheat kernel with relatively little in the endosperm. Thus, the degree of extraction influences the level of phytic acid in flour and hence its nutritive value; and this may be significant in diets low in calcium and iron. The latter is also influenced by the extent to which the indigenous phytase of flour hydrolyzes phytic acid; more extensive hydrolysis occurs during long fermentation times; 60% of the phytic acid in flour is hydrolyzed during a 3 hr fermentation. Phytase is relatively heat-stable and probably remains active during the early stages of baking. It is a nonspecific phosphomonoesterase which is activated by $Mg^{2+}$ and inhibited by $Zn^{2+}$ and $Mn^{2+}$; it has a pH optimum at $\approx 5.2$ and a temperature optimum of $\approx 55°C$.

Phytase, which increases approximately six-fold on germination, has been highly purified from wheat bran.[495] Maize flour is very rich in phytic acid and diets containing high proportions of maize flour, as in Africa and South America, may be deficient in available calcium; Amoa and Muller[7] recommend that maize flour be supplemented with 1% fermented wheat flour (rich in phytase) which would hydrolyze phytic acid during dough fermentation; fermented maize was less effective. Many animal species secrete an active intestinal phytase and consequently the interference of ingested phytate with mineral metabolism is less serious than in man which apparently does not secrete a phytase although some hydrolysis of phytate occurs in the intestine probably due to microbial phytase and nonenzymic catalysis.[582] These authors investigated the survival and activity of ingested wheat phytase in the human gastro-intestinal tract and concluded that wheat phytase did contribute to phytate hydrolysis in man, particularly in the stomach. It would appear therefore that flour and bread with high phytase activity are nutritionally beneficial, especially in high-cereal diets; the addition of phytase preparations to flour might warrant consideration. Wheat contains many other phosphatases[589] which have not been highly purified and which are of no apparent commercial consequence.

### Lipase

The wheat kernel contains a considerable amount of lipase but much of the earlier work did not differentiate between true esterases (which act on esters in solution) and lipase-type esterases (which hydrolyse emulsified esters only). The early work has been reviewed by Sullivan.[674] It appears to be generally agreed that lipolytic activity is concentrated in the scutellum and aleurone layer with relatively little in the germ and endosperm,[674] but the actual ratio of lipolytic activity of the different fractions depends on the substrate used for assay, presumably indicative of a number of esterases with different substrate specificities. Lipolytic activity increases three- to four-fold on malting, much less than the change in $\alpha$-amylase.

Earlier investigators were of the view that wheat contained only one lipase but later studies using improved fractionation techniques indicate the presence of three esterases/lipases.[196,663] The pH optimum has usually been reported to be between pH 7 and 8, varying somewhat with substrate, and the temperature optimum to be between 35 and 40°C. The enzyme is inhibited by sulfydryl blocking agents but the effect is considered to be due to stearic hindrance rather than to interaction at the active site.[230]

Storage of wheat under adverse conditions of temperature and humidity usually results in an increase in free fatty acid levels probably due to a combination of wheat and microbial lipases. However, while relatively low levels of free fatty acids lower consumer acceptability of bread, the functional properties of flour are not affected greatly even though long-chain unsaturated fatty acids cause a very "short" gluten; these unsaturated fatty acids significantly effect baking quality only if they become oxidized when the resultant dough is "dead" and the bread is of poor volume. Yeast has a much higher level of lipolytic activity than flour and at a 2% level would contribute about ten times as much lipase as flour.[589] All the lipases in bread are inactivated during baking and hence do not contribute to the deterioration of bread.

Storage under adverse conditions results in an increase in free fatty acids, amino nitrogen, and inorganic phosphate. The former precedes the other changes and is, therefore, a good indicator of grain deterioration during storage.

### Lipoxidase

The tissues of many plant species contain an enzyme; lipoxidase, which catalyses the peroxidation of unsaturated fatty acids. The enzymes do not contain a heam prostetic group and show a high specificity for *cis-cis* methylene-interrupted dienoic fatty acids. They are inactive on monoenoic fatty acids or *cis-trans* isomers, some of which may be competitive inhibitors. Soya bean is the richest source of lipoxidase and contains about 40 times as much as wheat. Although standard 72% extraction flour contains only ≈ 2% lipid, this is relatively rich in polyenoic acids which are very susceptible to peroxidation. The significance of lipid oxidiation is mostly nutritional: (1) destruction of essential polyunsaturated fatty acids and (2) oxidation and destruction of carotenoids and ascorbic acid by coupled oxidation with the lipoperoxides. Since bakery products are normally only minor sources of carotenoids and essential fatty acids such losses are probably not of major consequence. The breakdown products of hydroperoxides (aldehydes, ketones, and alcohols) give rise to off-flavors termed oxidative rancidity.

### Other Enzymes

Wheat and flour contain numerous other enzymes which have been purified and characterized in some detail[589] and which may have some technological and/or nutritional significance.

Polyphenoloxidase is present at fairly high concentration; the enzyme may cause discoloration and loss in nutritive value due to interaction of quinones with protein amino groups but oxidation is unlikely to progress that far.

A catalase has been isolated from flour. This enzyme could couple the oxidation of carotenoids resulting in bleaching and loss in vitamin A activity. A perioxidase has also been identified and characterized.

Flour contains an ascorbic acid oxidase. Ascorbic acid is known to improve the functionality of flour probably due to the oxidation of sulfydryl groups by dehydroascorbate. Ascorbic acid oxidase of course reduces the biological value of flour. With increasing opposition to the use of chemical oxidizers in flour ascorbic acid is considered to have potential as an oxidizing agent, exploiting the indigenous ascorbic acid oxidase of flour.[702]

### Exogenous Enzymes

There are a few large-volume applications of exogenous enzymes in cereal technology, principal of which are amylases, proteinases, and lipoxidase. Reviews include Gams,[228,229] Pyler,[576,577] Pomeranz,[557] and Waldt.[731]

### Amylases

The influence of added amylase on the quality of bread was recognized by the end of the 19th century and citing earlier workers Kneen and Sandstadt[394] listed five reasons underlying the use of amylase supplementation of flour: (1) to increase gas production, (2) to improve crust color; (3) to improve the moistness and keeping quality; (4) to impart additional flavor; and (5) to increase the gas-retaining ability of the dough. Although probably included in three, the use of amylases as antistaling agents has now become a major application. The effectiveness of amylases in modifying most of these characteristics has already been discussed under indigenous flour enzymes viz., the production of yeast-fermentable sugars and the availability of higher sugar concentrations for Maillard browning reactions (color and flavor); antistaling aspects will be discussed later.

Barley malt was originally the principal source of exogenous amylase, principally α-amylase, but this was gradually replaced by malted wheat (cf. Reed[586] for properties, specifications, etc.). Only very small amounts of malt are required (0.2% of flour weight). Early work showed that other α-amylases, pancreatic or mold amylases (which are more thermo-labile than cereal α-amylase), were also effective but contamination with proteinases and higher costs delayed their commercialization. Bacterial α-amylases are more thermo-stable than the malt enzymes and unless careful selection and use is made of these enzymes they cause excessive starch hydrolysis. Malt α-amylase is about seven times as effective in producing maltose in dough as fungal α-amylase when added on an equal activity basis as predetermined by in vitro test, possibly due to differences in the inhibitory effect of salt, or enzyme adsorption on damaged starch granules.

The problem of inadequate fermentable sugars in flour can be readily solved by the addition of 6 to 8% sucrose or glucose directly to the flour as is fairly widely practiced in the sponge dough process, but this practice is not satisfactory with the straight dough process where the use of amylase is essential. However, amylases perform functions in addition to sugar production; in particular they reduce the viscosity of dough through modification of the water holding capacity of damaged starch, independent of any effect due to contaminating proteinases on gluten; and the formation of dextrins improve crumb texture and compressibility, although excessive dextrinization leads to a gummy, sticky crumb. The effectiveness of an amylase in this regard is very much dependent on its thermo-stability (bacterial > cereal > fungal). The temperature at the center of a 500 g loaf increases 4 to 6°C/min during normal baking.

The first successful introduction of enzymes other than those of malted wheat or barley into the baking industry resulted from research conducted by the Rohm & Hass Company in 1936.[632] Trials in various laboratories showed that malted wheat flour and fungal α-amylase preparations (Rohm & Hass) were entirely acceptable for bread production; bacterial α-amylase, though undesirable, was usable, while pancreatic α-amylases were found to be unsatisfactory. It is important in the production of fungal α-amylases for baking that the proteinase content of the preparation be rigorously controlled; failure to do this led to failure during the early days of fungal enzyme application.[232,557,632] In the U.S., only malt may be added to flour at the mill (according to Pyler,[576,577] 56 to 60 million lbs of malt are used annually); fungal amylases, usually from *A. oryzae*, may be added at the bakery only and are commercially available in tablet form. Some of the potential enzyme preparations contain solubilizing agents, yeast food (salts), and sometimes proteinases, lipoxidases, and oxidizing agents also. In Europe most countries permit the addition of fungal amylases to flour at the mill. Since malt, fungal, and bacterial amylases show different amylytic and stability characteristics, careful standardization of enzyme preparations is required; a number of alternative procedures are available as discussed by Pyler[576,579] and Geddes.[232]

The use of fungal enzymes in continuous bread-making processes is advocated[261,729] particularly when a high level (45%) flour is used in the brew or when a high-protein (strong) flour is used. These preparations contained amylases and proteinases, the activity of both being required for the desired effect.

The advantages of fungal enzyme preparations over malt were summarized by Wichser[759] as follows: (1) the ratio of amylolytic to proteolytic activity can be conveniently varied to meet the changing requirements of the flour proteins; (2) flours with excessively strong proteins can be mellowed by increased levels of fungal proteinases;

(3) baking schedules can be more readily maintained because fungal proteinases reduce mixing times and optimum fermentation times; and (4) the lower inactivation temperature of fungal α-amylases prevents the occurrence of gumminess in bread crumb.

The organoleptic quality of bread deteriorates following baking; the changes leading to this deterioration are collectively referred to as staling which is a very complex process including changes in flavor, texture, and redistribution of moisture in the crumb; the topic has been extensively reviewed, among others, by Maga.[435] The molecular changes responsible for the textural changes appear to involve association of the outer branches of amylopectin to form quasicrystalline structures, a process referred to as retrogradation; aggregation of amylose molecules to form an insoluble network also occurs but this does not appear to contribute to subsequent firming of bread crumb. It was felt early that hydrolysis of amylopectin would reduce the tendency to retrogradation but fungal and cereal amylases were not effective since they are denatured during baking. Careful use of heat-stable bacterial α-amylases were reported by Waldt[730,731] to be quite effective in delaying staling without concomitant ill-effects on other desirable quality attributes; however very careful control of the use of bacterial α-amylase is required to avoid excessive starch hydrolysis which would lead to sticky crumb texture.

*Proteinases*

Since proteolytic as well as amylytic activity increases significantly on malting, the addition of malt to flour increases its protinase content. The view was held that proteolysis may have been responsible for the stickiness which developed in dough to which too much malt was added. However Hildebrand[303] argues that the amount of proteinase normally added in malt is small compared with that of the flour itself and concludes that the proteinase contributed by malt is entirely without significance. In addition, yeast supplies a considerable amount of proteolytic activity which is generally not quantified accurately, and contaminating microorganisms may supply some proteinases. The use of exogenous proteinases in baking, while dating back to the 1920s, did not assume major significance until the 1950s when fungal amylases began to replace malt. As discussed above, the proteinases in fungal amylase preparations initially caused production problems by excessively softening dough. With flours of medium strength or adequate dough-mixing times, fungal proteinases are unnecessary and perhaps undesirable but their advantages for strong (high protein) flours on tight mixing schedules (e.g., continuous processes) quickly became apparent and it is now normal practice to standardize fungal enzyme preparations with respect to both amylytic and proteolytic activity. Fungal enzyme preparations are much more proteolytically active than malt and are normally diluted with flour before addition to the dough mix. Fungal proteinases are normally added to the sponge rather than to the dough to avoid the inhibitory effect of salt and to allow them sufficient time to act on the protein. Higher levels of proteinases are normally required in continuous mixing or liquid ferment processes because of the shorter mellowing times.[576,577]

The effect of proteolytic enzymes in baking is to mellow the dough by modifying the effect of oxidizing agents; the effect is described schematically by Silberstein.[641] Sulfydryl and disulfide groups play key roles in the functionality of gluten in bread production. Reducing agents break intermolecular S-S linkages, allowing gluten molecules to slide easily, resulting in a slack dough in which a gluten network is not formed and gas retention is impaired. Oxidizing agents have the opposite effect: -SH groups are oxidized to S-S bonds, thereby increasing intermolecular bonding; when this occurs in excess, a bucky dough with reduced extensibility is produced. By controlled cleavage of peptide bonds, proteinases reduce buckyness but the -S-S bonds are still intact and promote network formation.

The addition of proteinases to flour intended for cracker production is particularly beneficial as a slack, extensible dough is required for this type of product to permit control of both texture and product volume.

*A. oryzae* is the normal source of proteinases for baking; bacterial proteinases and trypsin depress loaf volume very markedly, but preparations from *A. niger* are fairly satisfactory.[558]

## Lipoxidase

Lipoxidase added to flour in crude form as soy bean meal (0.5 to 1% of flour) is commonly used as a bleaching agent. The bleaching effect is due to the coupled oxidation of carotene and unsaturated fatty acids, peroxides of the latter acting as oxidizing agents. Lipid peroxides also oxidize -SH groups and so improve the functionality of gluten. Peroxidized fat is also reported to contribute a nutty flavor to bread.[382]

## Lactase

The addition of skim milk powder to flour mixes is common practice in many countries. The lactose of the milk powder is not fermentable by bakers yeast, but following hydrolysis by lactase to glucose and galactose, the glucose moiety is fermentable thereby improving loaf volume while the nonfermentable galactose is available for Maillard browning reactions and so contributes to bread flavor and crust color (for references on lactase cf. dairy section, in particular Pomeranz[556]).

## Invertase

Addition of invertase to chemically leavened bread is fairly common; for such products it is frequently more convenient and cheaper to use sucrose rather than monosaccharides as a sugar source, but, being a nonreducing sugar, sucrose is unable to participate in Maillard browning reactions. Hence the addition of invertase increases the availability of reducing sugars which enhance flavor and crust color.

## Pentosanases

Wheat flour contains ≈ 2.5% pentosans which have a detrimental effect on loaf volume and quality.[540] Limited research has been conducted on the use of pentosanases to eliminate this problem.[698,766]

## Glycosidase

Patients with celiac disease are allergic to the gliadin fraction of wheat or rye flour which cause atrophy of the villi of the brush border of the small intestine resulting in diminished secretion of various hydrolyzases and reduced metabolic activity. Treatment requires total exclusion of wheat and rye flour from the diet. The specific allergic protein has not been isolated and attempts to eliminate the toxicity factor by proteolysis were unsuccessful.[476] Phelan et al.[550] suggest that the toxic factor may be a glycopeptide and present evidence that treatment of wheat flour with a glycosidase (as yet not characterized) from *A. niger* reduces its toxic effect in celiac patients.

## STARCH

Starchy foods have formed a major item of the human diet since prehistoric times, principally because they are cheap sources of energy. Industrial applications of starch in the sizing of paper and textiles and in adhesives were also recognized early. Today, starch and its derivatives (produced mainly from maize and potato) are major items of commerce for both industrial and food applications. The latter uses represent a relatively small proportion of total starch output; however a major proportion of prod-

Table 9

SHIPMENTS BY THE U.S. CORN WET MILLING
INDUSTRY OF CORN STARCH BY TYPE OF END USE,
AND OF PRODUCTS MADE FROM STARCH, 1958

| Shipments of corn starch for: | Million pounds | % of shipments |
|---|---|---|
| Paper products | 835.7 | 44.44 |
| Grocers, brewers, bakers, and other food uses[a] | 460.3 | 24.48 |
| Textiles manufacturers | 286.9 | 15.26 |
| Building materials, laundries, miscellaneous uses | 186.4 | 9.91 |
| Export | 111.2 | 5.91 |
| | | |
| Shipments of products from corn starch[b] | | |
| Corn syrup | 1798.88 | 58.91 |
| Corn sugar | 834.4 | 27.33 |
| Dextrin | 159.2 | 5.21 |
| Miscellaneous | 261.1 | 8.55 |

[a]   Includes confections, chewing gum, ice cream and dairy products, jellies, jams, preserves, meat, sugar, salad dressing and mayonnaise, pickles, etc.
[b]   Mostly for food applications.

From Farris, P. L., *Starch: Chemistry and Technology*, Part 1, Whistler, R. C. and Paschall, E. P., Eds., Academic Press, New York, 1965, 27. With permission.

ucts derived from starch are used in the food industry. The data in Table 9 give some idea of the relative importance of the various applications of starch. The utilization of isolated starch and starch products by the food industry represents only a small proportion of total starch actually consumed with cereals and potatoes representing huge quantities.

The chemistry and general properties of starch are discussed in all biochemistry texts; a very comprehensive text on the chemistry and technology of starch is edited by Whistler and Paschall.[750]

The principal use of isolated starch in the food industry is as a thickening and bodying agent in a myriad of products. Varying properties of starch are required for different products and different applications are discussed in detail by Osman[532] and to some extent also by other authors in Whistler and Paschall.[750] The functionality of starch for both food and industrial applications may be improved by various modifications, e.g., crosslinking, oxidation, esterification, addition of charged groups, etc. The production, properties, and uses of modified starches is discussed by various authors in Whistler and Paschall[750] and by Kennedy.[366] Aspects of carbohydrates of interest to the food technologist are considered in the text edited by Birch and Green.[59]

As shown in Table 9, starch hydrolyzates represent a greater proportion of the starch used in foods than starch or chemically modified starches. Hydrolyzed starches fall into three catagories depending on the degree of hydrolysis: dextrins, syrups, and glucose. Hydrolysis may be performed by acid or by amylases, a wide range of which, with differing specificities and physicochemical characteristics, is now available.[455,456] By using the various amylases which are now available it is possible to degrade starch in a specific manner to give all possible products from glucose to maltohexose.

## Dextrins

Dextrins are rather ill-defined polymers of glucose; in the broadest sense they include all polymers greater than disaccharides,[187] but as used in the food industry they represent larger oligosaccharides with DE values of 10 to 20. Dextrins are water-soluble, have lower viscosity than starch for similar concentrations, give very clear pastes, and are free of the "cereal" off-flavor characteristic of unmodified starches. The functional properties and applications of dextrins in foods are discussed by Murray.[489,490]

Acid hydrolysis has been the standard method of producing dextrins. This process, which is discussed by Evans and Wurzburg,[187] has a number of limitations, including rather fixed composition of hydrolyzate for a given DE value, reversion (resynthesis of polysaccharide), and branch formation. A more flexible range of products may be obtained by using a combination of acid/enzyme ($\alpha$-amylase) or enzyme hydrolysis alone. A heat stable $\alpha$-amylase is required to survive the temperature required for gelatinization (ungelatinized starch is not susceptible to enzyme hydrolysis). The stable enzyme quickly reduces the high viscosity of gelatinized starch, permitting the use of high solids content.

## Syrups

Syrups represent a more extensively hydrolyzed starch with DE values in the range 25 to 95. They have numerous applications in the confectionary, candy, ice cream, preserves, and soft drinks industries. They contain varying levels of glucose, maltose, and higher saccharides depending on the extent of hydrolysis. Syrups were traditionally produced by acid hydrolysis, but the range of such products was quite restricted because (1) for a given DE value acid hydrolysis always produces a fixed ratio of mono-, di-, tri- and higher saccharides; (2) bitterness increases with extended hydrolysis, restricting the DE of acid-hydrolyzed syrups to 58 to 60; and (3) crystallization of glucose also occurs in high DE acid syrups. To overcome these problems and to produce syrups with a greater range of composition, a combination of acid and enzymatic hydrolysis was introduced about 1940. Gelatinized starch may be converted to syrups solely by enzymatic means using a combination of amylytic enzymes to give the desired mix of sugars; e.g., a heat stable $\alpha$-amylase to reduce viscosity; a high level of amyloglucosidase if a high glucose syrup is desired; or a high level of $\alpha$-amylase if a high dextrin syrup is desired. Syrups with a very wide range of compositions may be obtained by such combinations.[150,310,708] The latter parts of this reaction may be performed by immobilized amylases and amyloglucosidase.

## Glucose

Starch may be hydrolyzed completely to glucose by acid and until recently this was the sole commercial method. However, acid hydrolysis has a number of serious disadvantages for glucose production: (1) because of reversion, yields are very much below theoretical (<80% compared with a theoretical yield of 111%); (2), the mother liquor left after glucose crystallization is bitter, which largely restricts its application even as an animal feed; (3), the source of starch must be pure and free from protein; otherwise considerable Maillard browing occurs, resulting in reduced yields; (4), enzymatic hyrolysis of starch to glucose requires a lower investment than acid hydrolysis for which corrosion-resistant materials are required; and (5), twice the starting level of starch may be used than with acid hydrolysis.

Amyloglucosidase which hydrolyzes starch completely to glucose has been available for some time but commercial preparations were contaminated with a transglucosylase which considerably reduced the yield of glucose. Preparations of amyloglucosidase essentially free of transglucosylase have been available since the mid-1960s either by using selected microbial strains or by using chemical purification methods. With the currently available amyloglucosidase preparations, almost theoretical yields of glucose may be produced with very high (>90%) recovery rates.

The production of glucose may be completely enzymatic using a heat-stable $\alpha$-amylase to prehydrolyze gelatinized starch to reduce viscosity followed by amyloglucosidase, or prehydrolysis may be performed by acid. Syrups produced by enzyme-enzyme reactions have very high DE values (98) and contain 97% glucose with only trace amounts of maltose and high saccharides.

The ready commercial availability of the debranching enzymes, pullanase and iso-amylases (which hydrolyze, α1,6 glucosidic linkages only with varying degrees of specificity) may have commercial applications in the starch industry:

1.    Combined with bacterial α-amylase and amylo-glucosidase, to produce very high DE (98 to 99) syrups for glucose or glucose-fructose manufacture
2.    Combined with bacterial α-amylase and malt enzymes for the production of high maltose syrups for certain food applications (exhibit less tendency to crystallize and are nonhygroscopic)[87]
3.    The production of high-amylose starches which yield quick-setting, stable gels, act as good binders, form strong transparent films and act as excellent barriers to oxygen and fats

The technology and use of debranching enzymes has been reviewed by, among others, Allen and Dawson.[6]

**High Fructose Syrups**

The most exciting recent development in the application of enzymes in the starch industry, indeed in the entire food industry, has been the commercial development of glucose isomerase; it is also the outstanding commercial success of immobilized enzymes. Although an enzyme capable of isomerizing glucose-6-phosphate to fructose-6-phosphate was identified by Lohmann in 1933 it was not until 1957 that an enzyme capable of isomerizing glucose to fructose was identified and patented.[457] Since then progress has been very rapid through extensive research, principally in the U.S. and Japan, which has been reviewed by Linko, Pohjola and Linko.[414] The enzyme has been used commercially in both soluble and immobilized form,[18,33,387,388,744] and a technique for the entrappment of whole cells *(Actinoplanes missouriensis)* which eliminates the cost of enzyme purification and gives a higher recovery of enzyme, has been described.[414] Microorganisms capable of producing higher enzyme activity are constantly being produced by selection and mutation.[711] The physicochemical characteristics of soluble and immobilized glucose isomerase are reviewed by Gams.[228-229]

Corn starch is the normal starting material (potato and wheat starch have also been used) and this is normally hydrolyzed to glucose by immobilized α-amylase and amyloglucosidase. Thus, three linked enzyme reactors are necessary to convert starch to synthetic invert sugar:

$$\text{Starch} \xrightarrow[\text{α-amylase}]{\text{acid or}} \text{dextrins} \xrightarrow{\text{Amyloglucosidase}} \text{glucose}$$

$$\text{glucose} \downarrow \text{isomerase}$$

$$\text{glucose + fructose}$$

The theoretical equilibrium is ≈ 55% fructose, but in commercial practice the economic rate of conversion is 41 to 45% fructose. Higher conversion rates (up to 90%) may be obtained by complexing fructose with borate or calcium which complex preferentially with fructose; further research may make the production of pure fructose commercially feasible.

The rate of growth in output of high-fructose syrups has been quite remarkable: in the U.S. production has increased from 185,000 tons of sugar equivalent in 1972 to ≈ 1.9 million tons in 1977 and to a projected output of 4.5 million tons in 1980; already ≈ 30% of the total industrial sweetener market in the U.S. is filled by high-fructose syrups. Growth in Europe has been slower: 70,000 tons in 1976 and probably 400,000 tons in 1977.[414] The potential of high fructose syrups world wide is discussed by Fullbrook.[222]

From a nutritional viewpoint the principal attraction of high fructose syrups is their higher sweetness compared with sucrose (sucrose = 100, glucose = 70; fructose = 170; lactose = 16), and hence the caloric value may be reduced for equal sweetness. From a technological viewpoint fructose syrups have application in synthetic honey and in preserves where they are twice as effective in influencing osmotic pressure as sucrose on an equiweight basis. High fructose syrups may be produced considerably cheaper from corn starch than can sucrose from beet and probably from cane. Assuming that legal and political barriers are not imposed, it appears that high-fructose syrups have a very bright future. The design and operation of a new plant for the production of high fructose syrups in the U.S. is described by Russo.[603] The plant, with a capacity of $4 \times 10^6$ lb of product per day, uses soluble bacterial $\alpha$-amylase to liquify starch to 10 DE, followed by soluble amyloglucosidase to produce a 96 DE syrup which is then isomerized using immoiblized glucose isomerase to a syrup containing 42% fructose and 52% glucose.

## Sucrose

Invertase, which hydrolyzes sucrose to glucose and fructose, has been commercially available for many years for the production of invert sugar which is used, among other applications, in the preparation of artificial honey (other applications of invertase are discussed under miscellaneous applications of enzymes). Invertase has been successfully immobilized.

Invertases from some sources, e.g., Aspergillus, catalyze the synthesis of sucrose under certain conditions, especially at low water concentration. This reaction is considered by Butler, Squires, and Kelly[94] as a possible means of producing sucrose synthetically from glucose-fructose syrups (produced from starch). However, these authors consider the synthesis of sucrose from glucose-*1*-phosphate and fructose, catalyzed by sucrose phosphorylase, to be more feasible; fructose could be obtained by crystallization from glucose-fructose syrups (from starch), while glucose-*1*-phosphate could be obtained by hydrolyzing starch with phosphorylase in the presence of inorganic phosphate. The phosphorylase reaction appears to be energetically more favorable than the invertase reaction, and research is focused on optimizing the growth of *L. mesenteroides* for phosphorylase production and immobilizing the enzyme.

## FRUIT AND VEGETABLES

By far the greatest part of our food is of vegetable origin and if we consider that plant tissues are consumed by animals, then all of man's food comes from plants. Fresh fruits and vegetables supply us with carbohydrates, some protein and little fat, and a variety of minerals and vitamins. While fruits and vegetables are important sources of energy, their main characteristic is succulence, i.e., they have a high water content, ranging from 70 to 90% and they also add color and variety to the diet. The composition of fruits and vegetables is highly variable, being influenced by such factors as genetics, cultural practices, regions and rate of growth, variety, and climatic conditions. For instance, the amount of water in the tissue depends on the amount of water absorbed through the roots and the amount lost by transpiration. A detailed discussion on plant composition and chemical components may be obtained from texts edited by Harris and Karmas,[278] Hulme,[318,319] Fennema.[194]

In general, during the maturation of fruit there is a significant increase in sugars and total solids and a decrease in starch, acidity, and astringency. Marked changes in composition of vegetables also occur during maturation. The most significant change and one which will be discussed later, is the increase in starch content of most vegetables, e.g., potato tubers and peas, and a decrease in sugars and water. Ripening and maturation continue during storage and the extent of change depends primarily upon the temperature and length of storage. During this phase each plant or fruit behaves as an independent unit and respiratory processes play a major role. In this section, certain aspects of the metabolism of maturing and stored fruit and vegetables will be discussed. The food technologist and processor is constantly looking for ways to control the maturation of tissue and ideally would like to be able to inhibit or accelerate the ripening process at will to ensure optimum quality at the retail outlet. The storage and handling of fresh fruit and vegetables have therefore received considerable attention over the years. Salunke and Wu[609] discuss various agents that accelerate or delay ripening and senescence. The application of hormones to control physiological changes was reviewed earlier by Haard,[269] and the post-harvest physiology, handling, and utilization of fruits and vegetables are discussed at length in a recent text edited by Pantastico.[536]

Ripening of fruit and vegetables involves a series of changes in color, flavor and texture, and despite the diversity in composition and morphological origin, most fruits and vegetables are markedly similar in metabolic behavior. All the changes which occur are elaborated by the native enzymes. The glycolytic-tricarboxylic acid cycle and the pentose pathway assume a dominant role in most plant respiration. A number of fruits exhibit a characteristic sharp rise in respiratory activity following harvest and visible changes in ripening occur shortly after the maximum rate of respiration has been achieved. Kidd and West[373] considered that the relatively sudden change in the level of respiration marked the transition from the growth to the senescence phase of life. They called the increase in respiration "the climacteric" and since they were specifically referring to a pattern of respiratory changes, most recent workers call it the "respiration climacteric". Thomas[694] defined "climacteric" as a "state of autostimulation in which yellowing and enhanced respiration are two of the attendant effects". Kidd and West[374] recognized the importance of enzyme activity in ripening and discussed two types of changes which might account for the climacteric respiration: (1) an increase in effective enzyme concentrations; and (2) an increase in substrate concentration. However, it is important to recognize that the biochemical processes of ripening are not exclusively catabolic in nature. For instance, a number of anabolic processes have been observed during ripening such as the synthesis of pigments, lipids, nucleic acids, and in the case of some vegetables, starch synthesis occurs.

Control of enzymic activity may be expected to play a very important role in the ripening phase. Increased enzymic activity could occur in response to a number of factors which may regulate enzyme content and/or activity at specific stages of ripening. Tager and Biale[680] observed a marked increase in carboxylase and aldolase activity during the ripening of bananas. An increase in apple malic enzyme activity during ripening was reported by Dilley[160] and Hulme and Wooltorton,[321] and the activity of pyruvic carboxylase increased sharply during ripening of the same fruit.[320] The increased activity is due either to (1) *de novo* synthesis of enzymes;[162,217,592] (2) destruction of enzyme inhibitors;[567] or (3) breakdown of the compartmentalization of living systems.[619] Ethylene acts as a ripening hormone in triggering these changes; however its mode of action is still a subject of speculation.[467]

Although enzyme inhibitors will not be discussed in this section their role in regula-

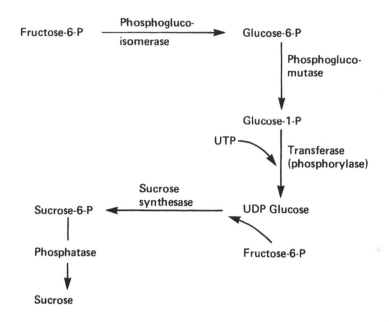

FIGURE 21.   Synthesis of sucrose.

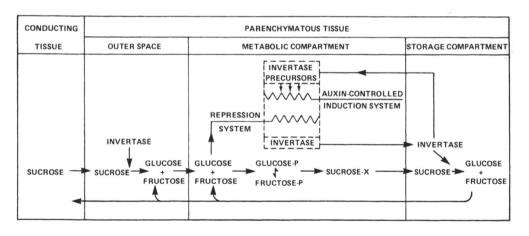

FIGURE 22.   Schematic representation of the sugar accumulation cycle. (From Sacher, J. A., Hatch, M. D., and Glasziou, K. T., *Plant Physiol.*, 38 (3), 352, 1963. With permission.)

tory mechanisms must be borne in mind. Pressey[567] outlines the possible application of enzyme inhibitors in food processing to control deterioration of certain fresh products.

In this section we do not intend to discuss in detail the various enzyme systems of fruit and vegetables. Instead, the focus will be on particular enzymatic reactions which affect color, texture, and flavor and for a recent comprehensive review of enzymes, particularly in fruit, the reader is referred to the chapter by Dilley[161] and other sections in *The Biochemistry of Fruit and their Products.*[318,319]

### Metabolism of Starch and Sugars

It is not possible to discuss in specific detail the metabolism and biochemical pathways accounting for starch-sugar interconversion in fruit and vegetables. The subject has been extensively reviewed by Whiting.[757] We shall discuss changes in sugar and starch occurring in specific circumstances in fruits and particularly in vegetables. The synthesis of starch or its degradation post-harvest is of extreme economic importance in the potato processing industry and harvesting of peas, corn, and beans. In the first case formation of simple sugars is undesirable while starch production in the latter leads to undesirable textural conditions.

Sucrose is the principal sugar synthesized by photosynthesis in the leaves and transported to the growing storage cells where it is converted to starch. The mechanism by which sucrose is accumulated has been reviewed and discussed by Sacher et al.[605] They discuss and elaborate the concept of a circulatory system in the sugar cane plant. The outlined process may be similar for fruit and vegetables. Carbon dioxide is fixed photosynthetically in the leaves and then moves to the stalk. In photosynthesis, $CO_2$ is converted to fructose-6-P via pathways which involve the pentose system. The fructose-6-P is converted to sucrose as seen in Figure 21.

There are three distinct cell compartments through which sucrose moves when accumulated from the medium into storage cells. The compartments are termed the outer space, the metabolic area, and the storage compartment. The various zones are characterized on the basis of metabolic activity and on the permeability of the membrane to sugars and anions. A cyclic scheme by which sugars are moved into the storage compartment or returned from storage for local utilization was outlined by Sacher et al.[605] and is shown in Figure 22.

In fruit the carbohydrate present is usually a mixture of low molecular weight sugars, e.g., monosaccharides, disaccharides, and short chain oligosaccharides. However, many young fruits, e.g., apple, tomato, mango, and banana, contain starch. In some fruits an initial increase in concentrations of starch is followed by a decrease while in others the concentration may increase up to maturity. For example, the starch content of bananas increases to 20% at maturity.[56] In the case of the plum very little starch is present in either the immature or ripened fruit.

The metabolic pathway by which sucrose may be converted to starch is reviewed by Eskin et al.[185] and is shown in Figure 23. Starch, having been formed in the storage cells and tissues, may become transformed into sugars, particularly sucrose, glucose, and fructose during the post-harvest period. The rate and extent of change depends on conditions of storage, temperature, and time, and on the physiological state of the cell. It is not known precisely which enzymes are involved, although increases in the activity of amylases, phosphorylases, and invertase have been reported. Eskin et al.[185] proposed the scheme outlined in Figure 24 for starch degradation during ripening and storage. The decreasing starch content and increase in reducing sugars of ripening bananas have been reported by von Loesecke[713] and are shown in Table 10.

In some foods, particularly peas, corn, beans, and underground tubers (sweet potato, potato, carrot), synthesis of starch rather than degradation predominates both pre- and post-harvest. Premium quality peas with a high sugar content can only be obtained when the peas are harvested in the "immature" state and cooled rapidly. As maturation progresses, the sugar concentration decreases in the pea seed and this is accompanied by a concomitant increase in starch content. Starch synthesis predominates at temperatures above ambient, consequently rapid cooling immediately post-harvest is essential to good quality. The enzymes involved in starch synthesis are principally those associated with photosynthetic tissue, namely fructose *trans*-glycosidase, adenosine diphosphate, glucose, starch glucosyl transferase, UDPG pyrophosphorylase, and ADPG pyrophosphorylase.[270]

### Reactions Occurring In Specific Foods

Nonenzymatic browning in potato processing is of immense interest to the food scientist and enzymologist. Potatoes are known to respond to stresses such as temperature extremes and ionizing radiation by converting some of their starch to sugar. The

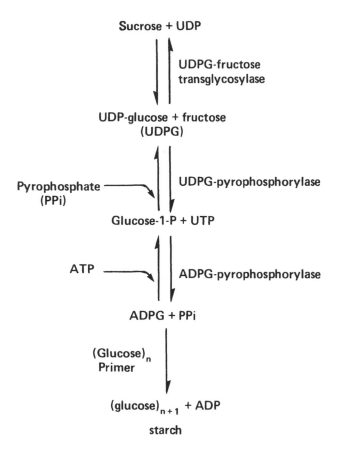

FIGURE 23.    Scheme for starch formation. (From Eskin, N. A. M.,
Henderson, H. M., and Townsend, R. J., *Biochemistry of Foods*,
Academic Press, New York, 1971, 54. With permission.)

extent of change depends upon the temperature and length of storage (Figure 25).[713]
The sugars, especially reducing sugars, are responsible for poor texture after boiling
and an undesirable sweet taste and darkening after frying. Storage of potato tubers at
4°C causes degradation of starch and accumulation of free sugars (sucrose, glucose,
and fructose). The build-up of sugars at low temperatures has been extensively documented and the early literature has been reviewed by James.[335] Because of the economic
importance of the phenomenon, much attention was paid to its possible causes and
Schwimmer[617] proposed a metabolic cycle for starch/sugar interconversion. In general,
it was assumed that activation of degradative enzymes might play the main role in the
degradation process and much work concerning the activities of enzymes involved in
the pathways of starch synthesis and degradation has accumulated.[442,648] The major
question to be answered relates to the trigger mechanism for starch degradation. Most
of the enzymes involved maintain normal activity. Paez and Hultin[534] showed that
potato mitochondria display a temperature response typical of that of enzyme reactions. It has been suggested that phosphorylase is important in causing sugar accumulation at low temperatures. Phosphorylase as already shown is believed to play a focal
role in the metabolism of starch.[749] More recently Hyde and Morrisson[327] reported that
phosphorylase activity was generally greater in tubers stored at 4°C than those conditioned at 21°C. However, Ioannou et al.[331] observed that low temperature induction
of starch degradation is not related to the appearance of additional total phosphorylase
or to the formation of unique isozyme or molecular species. This work has since been

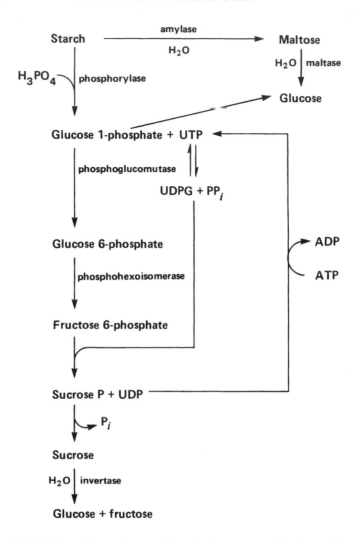

FIGURE 24.    Scheme for starch degradation. (From Eskin, N. A. M., Henderson, H. M., and Townsend, R. J., *Biochemistry of Foods,* Academic Press, New York, 1971, 55. With permission.)

confirmed by Kennedy and Isherwood[367] who found that changes in phosphorylase activity was small and the increase in sucrose concentration at 2°C could not be related to components of the phosphorylase system. The activity of a number of enzymes in the starch/sugar interconversion system were examined by Polock and Rees[554] and it was observed that the rate of sugar accumulation at 2°C exceeded the activity of sucrose synthetase, glucose-6-phosphate dehydrogenase, and aldolase. They suggest that sucrose accumulation at low temperatures is catalyzed by sucrose phosphate synthetase, but is not due to changes in maximum catalytic activities of any of the enzymes studied. The trigger mechanism may, however, be related to the susceptibility of key glycolytic enzymes to cold.

Invertase activity in potatoes has received considerable attention. All the studies have indicated low and sporadic levels of activity in tubers. Among the factors which have been reported to influence invertase activity in tubers are the occurrence of sprouting, elemental nutrition of the plant, and the temperature of storage.[600] They also obtained evidence that potato tubers contain a nondialyzable inhibitor. According to Pressey and Shaw[571] the accumulation of reducing sugars in potato tubers ex-

Table 10
CHANGES IN SUGAR AND STARCH DURING RIPENING OF
BANANAS

| Constituent | Number of days in ripening room | | | | | |
|---|---|---|---|---|---|---|
| | 0 | 3 | 5 | 7 | 9 | 11 |
| Reducing sugars | 0.24 | 2.81 | 7.24 | 10.73 | 12.98 | 15.31 |
| Nonreducing sugars (as sucrose) | 0.62 | 4.85 | 6.52 | 6.12 | 3.89 | 2.60 |
| Starch | 20.65 | 12.85 | 5.00 | 2.93 | 1.73 | 1.21 |

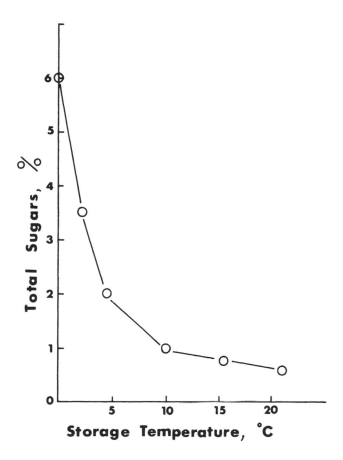

FIGURE 25. Total sugar content of Irish Cobbler potatoes stored for 3 months at different temperatures.[713]

posed to low temperatures occurs with concomitant increase in invertase activity. During the initial period of cold storage when reducing sugars increase rapidly, invertase formation occurs and the level of enzyme exceeds that of the invertase inhibitor. On transfer of cold-stored tubers to warmer temperatures, sugars and invertase decrease sharply and a large excess of inhibitor develops. The increased invertase activity during low temperature storage may in fact be related to a protective action against frost damage.[564] The potato inhibitor has been purified and characterized by Pressey.[565] It is a thermolabile protein with a molecular weight of about 17,000. Inhibition is maximal at about pH 4.5 and is independent of substrate concentration. Protein inhibitors of potato invertase have also been isolated from red beets, sugar beets, and sweet potatoes,[566] and from maize endosperm.[338] The actual trigger mechanism for invertase inhibitor formation, enzyme synthesis, and enzyme turnover has been the subject of considerable research. Recently, Ohad et al.[520] discussed the possibility that increases in enzymatic activity are related to changes in the distribution of enzymes or substrates within the subcellular compartments of the potato tuber. They observed a correlation between reduction of starch content, elevation of sugar level, changes in the composition of the amyloplast membranes, and morphological changes of these membranes. If membrane damage and changes in its permeability to degradative enzymes were the key mechanisms, then one would expect increased degradation when cold-stored tubers are subsequently stored at 25°C. However, sugar production falls off at the high temperature and the reaction is reversible when the tubers are again subjected to cold storage. Ohad et al.[520] do not rule out the possibility of membrane repair at 25°C.

### Structural Changes During Ripening of Fruit and Vegetables

It is generally accepted that softening of fruit and vegetables during ripening is related to alterations in the pectic substances through the action of pectic enzymes. It has been suggested also that cellulase, in addition to pectic enzymes, might contribute to softening of fruit.[159,275] The activities of cellulase and hemicellulases in cell walls during ripening have been discussed by Isherwood[332] but their role in tissue softening is not quite clear according to Hobson.[307] More recently, Coggins and Knapp[119] and Hasegawa and Smolensky[285] discussed the active role of cellulase in the production of high quality dates. Toughening of vegetative tissue, such as peas and asparagus, is associated with the synthesis of cell wall material during maturation and harvesting.[728]

*Pectic Enzymes*

The substrates for pectic enzymes are polymers of galacturonic acid called pectin and pectic acid. The chemistry, classification, occurrence, properties, manufacture, and industrial application of pectic substances have been reviewed extensively.[165,199,200,352,370,508,551,697,765] Research on pectic substances and pectic enzymes during the sixties were reviewed by Voragen and Pilnik.[724]

Pectic enzymes may be divided conveniently into two main groups: the saponifying enzymes or pectic-esterases, and the depolymerizing pectic enzymes. The saponifying enzyme simply removes methoxyl residues from pectin and is commonly called pectinesterase or pectin-methyl-esterase and abbreviated PE. The International Enzyme Commission classified PE as a pectin-pectylhydrolase (E.C. 3.1.1.11).

Prior to 1960 the depolymerizing enzymes were classified as hydrolases with specific activities pertaining to the degree of esterification of the substrate and to random or terminal cleavage.[157] However, Albershein et al.[4] discovered transeliminative cleavage of the $\alpha$-1-4 glycosidic bond by an enzyme present in a commercial pectinase preparation. Both endo- and exo-transeliminative enzymes were identified in the following years and a new classification for pectic enzymes became necessary. The new classification was made by Neukom[507] who subdivided the enzymes which split the $\alpha$-1-4-glycosidic bonds between galacturonic monomers in pectic substances. The enzymes were classified according to their specific activities pertaining to the degree of esterification, into endo- or exo-mechanism of action and to breakdown mechanism. Based on these criteria Neukom[507] arrived at eight groups of depolymerizing enzymes. Each of these eight groups comprises enzymes which can be further subdivided according to pH optima, inhibition, or activation with cations, stability and, in the case of exoenzymes, attacks on reducing or nonreducing ends, and degree of polymerization of end product. Koller[386] assigned numbers based on the recommendations on enzyme nomenclature of the International Union of Biochemistry. The Neukom and Koller classification is shown in Table 11.

## Table 11
## CLASSIFICATION OF DEPOLYMERIZING PECTIC ENZYMES: GLYCOSIDASES AND LYASES

### Pectic Enzymes Acting on Pectin

Polymethylgalacturonases (PMG)
   Endo-PMG (EC 3.2.1.41) causes random cleavage of $\alpha$-1 → 4-glycosidic links of pectin, preferentially degrades highly esterified pectin
   Exo-PMG, causes sequential cleavage of $\alpha$-1 → 4-glycosidic linkages from the non-reducing end of the chain
Pectin lyases[a] (PL)
   Endo-PL (E.C. 4.2.2.3), causes random cleavage of $\alpha$-1 → 4 glycosidic links of pectin by transelimination process; the type of degradation results in galacturonide esters with unsaturated bonds between $C_4$ and $C_5$ at the nonreducing end of the fragment
   Exo-PL, results in sequential breakdown of pectin by transeliminative cleavage

### Pectic Enzymes Acting on Pectic Acid

Polygalacturonase (PG)
   Endo-PG (EC 3.2.1.15) causes random hydrolysis of $\alpha$-1,4-glycosidic linkages of pectic acid
   Exo-PG (EC 3.2.1.40) causes sequential breakdown of $\alpha$-1-4-glycosidic linkages
Pectate Lyase (PAL)
   Endo-PAL (EC 4.2.2.1), hydrolyzes in a random manner $\alpha$-1-4-glycosidic bonds by transelimination
   Exo-PAL (EC 4.2.2.2), causes sequential cleavage of $\alpha$-1-4 linkages by transelimination

[a]   The term "lyase" is preferred to "trans-eliminases" by the International Union of Biochemistry.

The parent pectic substance present in unripe fruit is known by the generic name protopectin and it is accepted that this water-insoluble protopectin is enzymatically decomposed into soluble form during the course of ripening, but no evidence has so far been presented for such an enzyme to exist. According to Pilnik and Voragen[551] the softening of tissue and solubilization of protopectin could be achieved by nonpectinolytic degradation of polysaccharides by cellulases and hemicellulases which break down the cell wall and middle lamella, resulting in solubilization of pectin, as well as a macerating effect. Another group of enzymes, the oligouronidases, which split oligouronides in preference to long chain substrates have been isolated from microorganisms.[284,484]

Since pectic enzymes have been reviewed extensively in recent years,[106,157,199,433,551,587,598,724,725] further discussion will be limited to their occurrence in foods, role in ripening of fruit, in textural changes, and as added enzymes in food processing.

### Occurrence

The occurrence of pectic enzymes in plants and microorganisms has been extensively reviewed by Pilnik and Voragen[551] and by Rombouts and Pilnik.[598] The occurrence of these enzymes are summarized in Table 12. Lyases have been isolated from only one higher plant, the pea seedling. However, many microorganisms produce lyases.[598] Pectate lyases (PAL) are generally produced by bacteria and pectin lyases (PL) only by fungi. These transaliminases may, therefore, be important to fruit technology and fruit preservation.[655]

### Pectic And Other Enzymes In Fruit Textural Changes

The softening of fruit during ripening and senescence is frequently attributed to the enzymatic degradation of cell wall material. Dilley[161] reports that a close association had been established between textural changes and the activity of pectinesterase and

Table 12
PECTINOLYTIC ENZYMES
OCCURRING IN SOME
PLANTS

| Plant | P.E. | P.G. | PL |
|---|---|---|---|
| Bananas | + | | |
| Cherries | + | + ? | |
| Cucumber | + | | |
| Currants | + | | |
| Papaya | + | | |
| Pears | + | | |
| Apples | + | | |
| Tomatoes | + | + | |
| Strawberries | + | + | |
| Grapes | + | | |
| Citrus | + | | |
| Pineapple | | + | |
| Avocado | | + | |
| Carrots | | + | |
| Peaches | | + | |
| Mispel | | + | |
| Pea seedling | | | + |
| Apricots | + | + | |

polygalacturonase during maturation and ripening of tomatoes. A fivefold increase in pectinesterase activity from the mature green to the ripe stages of development was observed. Polygalacturonase activity was not found in green tomatoes,[306] but a 200-fold increase took place as they passed from the green-orange to the red stage. The activity of this enzyme-system has also been shown to correlate well with the loss of firmness in peaches.[572] Most of the polygalacturonases isolated and implicated in the ripening of fruit[283,306,572] are of the endo-type. Their action on a relatively few bonds could markedly alter the pectin molecule and consequently the cell wall. However, some polygalacturonases are exo-splitting enzymes; notably the enzyme in carrots,[288] peaches,[569] and cucumber,[570] and since random cleavage is not probable, the physiological role of an exo-polygalacturonase is not clear. Pressey and Avants[570] suggest that certain linkages susceptible to exo-polygalacturonase action might be critical bonds in the cell wall. The probable role of other enzymes, particularly cellulolytic enzymes, in softening of fruit during ripening has been discussed by a number of workers. Hobson[307] found increases in cellulase activity during the ripening of tomatoes but found no correlation between cellulase activity and firmness among several tomato varieties and concluded that flesh softening during ripening of tomatoes is primarily controlled by the pectic enzyme system. More recently Hasegawa and Smolensky[285] attributed cell disruption and production of a high quality textured date to the action of cellulase. The same enzyme may have some significance in peaches[305] and strawberries.[36]

A recently published abstract[568] suggests that while pectic enzymes may be important in fruit softening, the major mechanism probably involves degradation of all cell wall components leading to loosening of walls and separation of cells. In this respect the structural polysaccharides are as important as the pectic components.

The study and conclusions of Barnes and Patchett[36] in relation to cell wall disruption and softening of strawberries are perhaps the most interesting. They found that polygalacturonase and polymethylgalacturonase are not present at any stage of the fruit's development. Secondly, pectin methylesterase showed minimum activity at the senescent "over-ripe" stage. This latter finding was significant in the light of the earlier studies by Neal[499] who suggested that a key factor in the maintenance of fruit firmness in strawberries is the chelation of calcium ions as cross-links between carboxyl groups of adjacent polyuronide chains. He attributes separation of cell wall at the middle lamella to methylation of polyuronides, thereby destroying $Ca^{2+}$ cross-links. The reduction in demethylating activity observed by Barnes and Patchett[36] in over-ripe strawberries would therefore add support to the above theory. The increase in cellulase activity in "over-ripe" fruit would complement the reduced pectin methylesterase activity. Increased activity of pectin methylesterase has been associated with hardening of fruits in canned tomatoes[312] and with firming of potatoes heated at moderate temperatures (50 to 80°C) and subsequently boiled.[40] This effect is attributed to a loss of plasmalemma integrity at temperatures above 50°C and release of potassium which activates pectin methylesterase.[40] The enzyme increases the amount of free carboxyl groups of the cell wall pectin and $Ca^{2+}$ and $Mg^{2+}$ from the cell interior increase the number of metal bridges.

## Pigment Changes

In senescing plant tissues one of the more obvious changes that occurs is the change in color, particularly with green plants. This involves the degradation of cholorophyll, resulting in the exposure of the yellow carotenoid pigments or red color due to the formation of anthocyanins. The chemistry of plant pigments has been reviewed extensively.[112,194,242,318,319,449,637,716] The biochemical pathway by which chlorophyll disappears in green plants is by no means fully understood. The enzyme chlorophyllase has not been studied extensively and the main question is whether chlorophyllase is involved in chlorophyll biosynthesis or degradation.

The enzyme chlorophyllose could catalyze the degradation as follows:

$$\text{Chlorophyll} + H_2O \xrightarrow{\text{Chlorophyllase}} \text{Phytol} + \text{chlorophyllide}$$

However, the available evidence[465,733] suggests that chlorophyllase does not catalyze the initial step of chlorophyll degradation. However, it may catalyze the removal of phytol at a later step in the degradative pathway. There is a rise of chlorophyllase activity during the climacteric phase and Looney and Patterson[421] observed that chlorophyll degradation can be promoted by treatment with ethylene. Since chlorophyllase is localized within the chloroplasts, which are altered structurally during ripening, the increased activity during the climacteric phase may be due to enhanced enzyme-substrate interaction. The importance of the compartmentalization of enzyme and substrate has been previously discussed.[322,619]

Lipoxygenase is known to contribute to loss of chlorophyll in frozen vegetables and is, in fact, the most common catalytic agent for carotenoid destruction in cereals and vegetables. Lipoxygenase (as 0.5 to 1.0% soyabean flour) is used to oxidize unsaturated fatty acids and the resultant peroxides bleach $\beta$-carotene yielding, for example, a bread with a white crumb. Anthocyanases have been shown to exist in fruit and can catalyze destruction of anthocyanins.[727] Beside anthocyanase, polyphenoloxidases have been implicated in anthocyanin destruction in a number of fruit and vegetables.[607] Pang and Markakis[535] suggested that the loss of anthocyanin was a nonenzymatic oxidation reaction in which quinone, formed by enzymatic oxidation of catechol, functioned as the oxidizing agent (Figure 26). Removal or partial removal of anthocyanin from blackberries, strawberries, raspberries, grapes, bilberries, and cranberries may be desirable when discoloration is a problem during storage. Huang[314] proposed the use of a fungal enzyme for this purpose. This enzyme could be used to remove excess

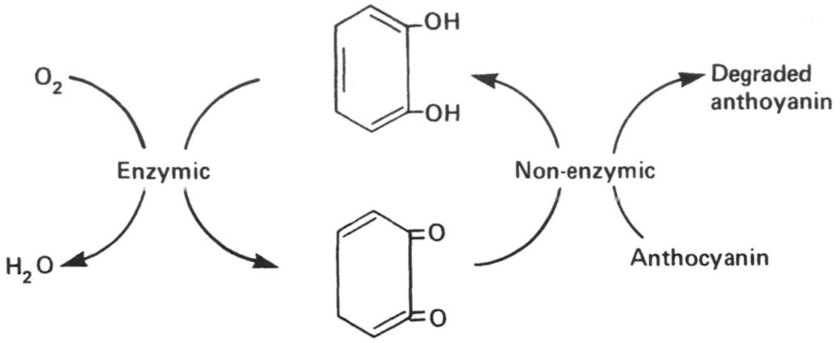

FIGURE 26.    Mechanism of anthocyanin degradation by phenolase.

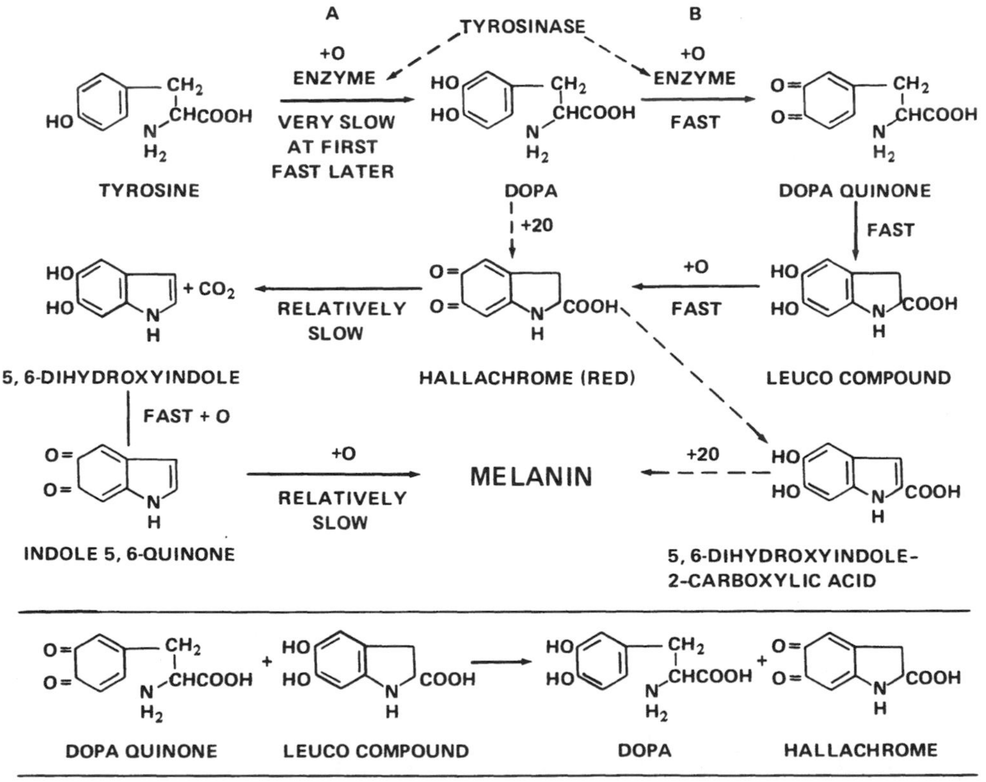

FIGURE 27.    The formation of melanin pigments resulting from the oxidation of tyrosine by phenolase. (From Lerner, A. B. and Fitzpatrick, T. B., *Physiol. Rev.*, 30, 95, 1950. With permission of the American Physiological Society.)

anthocyanins from fruit juices and for the production of white wines from red grapes.[313.776]

*Enzymatic Browning*

Enzymatic browning occurs in fruit and vegetables when the cellular integrity is destroyed and the enzymes and substrates are no longer compartmentalized. This type of browning occurs in mushrooms, avocados, peaches, melons, olives, squash, plums, pears, grapes, bananas, potatoes, shrimp, and many other foods, when the tissue is cut, bruised, peeled, or diseased. In the above cases discoloration results in a loss of consumer acceptability. However, in the case of the date, a high quality product depends on cellular disruption and activation of pectinases, cellulases,[285] and polyphenol oxidases.

Enzymatic browning has been reviewed by Ponting,[559] Eskin et al.,[185] Lerner and Fitzpatrick,[411] Adams and Blundstone,[1] Reed,[587] and Richardson.[593] The enzyme system responsible for browning in foods has been designated as o-diphenol: oxygen oxidoreductase (E.C.1.10.3.1) by the Enzyme Commission. However the enzymes are commonly known as phenoloxidase, cresolase, dopaoxidase, catecholase, tyrosinase, polyphenoloxidase, potato oxidase, and sweet potato oxidase. The major substrate is tyrosine, but other phenolic compounds such as caffeic acid, protocatechuic acid, and chlorogenic acid serve as substrates and the reaction takes place in the presence of oxygen.

The phenolase reaction can be divided into two events: the phenol hydroxylase or cresolase activity, and the oxidation reaction referred to as polyphenol oxidase or catecholase activity. Both reactions are illustrated in Figure 27. Enzymatic browning is a serious problem in food processing, particularly in fruits and vegetables, and during the dehydration processing of these commodities. It is also a problem in fruit juices and is of particular concern to the potato processor. The prevention of enzymatic browning is important to potato processing in general and in particular in the processing of prepeeled raw potatoes.[447,620] The most important phenolic substrate in potato is tyrosine, the level of which and consequently, the propensity to browning after peeling, varies with variety, growing conditions, and the level of potassic fertilizers.[448,486]

*Control Of Enzymatic Browning*

All three reactants (enzyme, phenolic substrate, and oxygen) are required for browning to take place so control is based on rendering at least one of these inactive. This is generally done by avoiding cellular damage due to bruising, peeling, and cutting, or by partially or totally inactivating the enzyme either by heat (blanching) or chemical inhibition (sulfur dioxide, ethylene-diaminetetracetic acid (EDTA), acidulants). Re-reduction of phenoloxidase-produced quinone delays the appearance of undesirable discoloration. Cysteine,[487] ascorbic acid,[559] as well as reversal of oxidative phosphorylation by ATP,[451] have been used to effect the reduction. It appears that these agents function without affecting the intrinsic activity of the polyphenoloxidase enzyme. One of the more interesting methods of inhibition is substrate modification by antiphenolase enzymes.[197] This involves enzymatic methylation of hydroxyl groups and ring cleavage (Figure 28) resulting in the formation of substances which are no longer substrates for enzymatic browning and may even act as competitive inhibitors. In the first example, caffeic acid in the presence of a methyl donor is enzymatically methylated by the action of O-methyl transferase. A second enzyme system which can modify substrate is protocatechuate oxygenase. This reaction involves ring cleavage and the formation of dibasic acids from O-diphenols. The main disadvantage of these enzyme systems is the high pH optima for enzyme action which consequently limits their use in fruit processing.

**Flavor Enzyme Systems in Fruit and Vegetables**

The development of flavor compounds in fruit and vegetables is very important in relation to quality as well as their identity. The aroma of various fruits and vegetables has been the subject of investigation by many workers and many excellent reviews have been published.[90,107,365,518,608,628,754] Reviews on some sulfur-containing compounds associated with foods have been written by Maga.[436-438] Flavor enzymes have been reviewed by Richardson[593] and the flavor compounds of bananas[699] and tea[610] have been discussed in great detail. For a critical review on lipoxygenase see Axelrod[26] and Eskin et al.[186] The aroma of fruits and vegetables and aroma precursors are conceived to

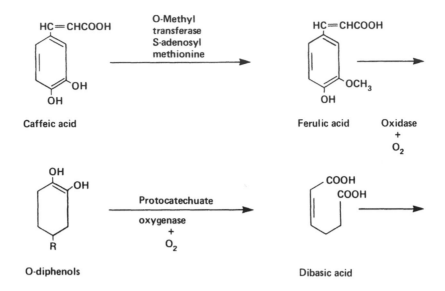

FIGURE 28.    Substrate modification as a means of inhibiting phenolase activity.

### Table 13
### CLASSES OF FLAVOR-FORMING MECHANISMS IN FOOD SYSTEMS

| Class | Description | Examples |
|---|---|---|
| Biosynthetic | Flavor constituents formed directly by biosynthetic processes | Flavors based on terpenoid and ester compounds such as mint, citrus, muskmelon, pepper, banana, etc. |
| Direct enzymic | Flavor constituents formed by enzymes acting on specific flavor precursors | Formation of onion flavor by action of alliinase sulfoxides, cabbage |
| Oxidative (indirect enzymic) | Flavor constituents formed by oxidation of flavor precursors by enzymically-formed oxidizing agents | Flavors characterized by presence of carbonyl and acid compounds such as tea |
| Pyrolytic | Flavor constituents formed from precursors by a heating or baking treatment | Flavors characterized by presence of pyrazines (coffee, chocolate, etc.), furans (bread), etc. |

originate from the basic constituents present in the plant.[614] In this sense flavor production in fruits and vegetables is similar to that reported for meat by Dwivedi,[173] i.e., the flavor component or its precursor is a metabolite produced in animal or vegetable organisms by intracellular biogenic pathways. The flavor-forming mechanisms with characteristic examples have been summarized in Table 13 by Sanderson and Graham[610] and the representative compounds formed have been presented by Salunkhe and Do.[609]

Compounds which may have a role in the development of fruit and vegetable flavors and some precursors are given in Figures 29 to 31. A comprehensive list of vegetable volatiles has been compiled by Johnson et al.[341,342] and Nursten,[518] and the sulfur-containing flavor compounds have been listed by Schutte[614] and Shankaranarayana et al.[628] As outlined in Figures 29 to 31, flavor compounds may be formed directly by

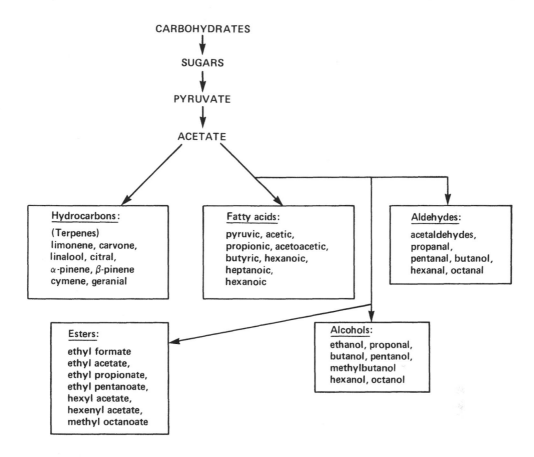

FIGURE 29. Formation of volatiles from carbohydrates.

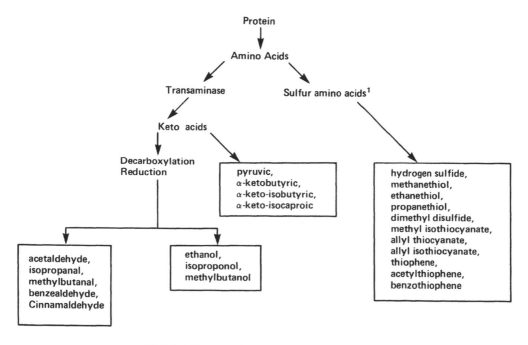

FIGURE 30. Protein and aroma compounds.[614,628]

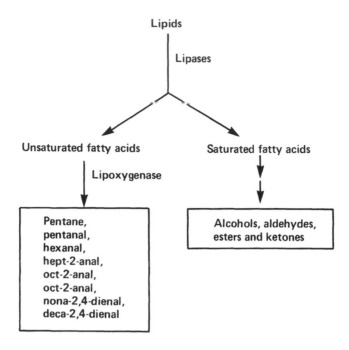

FIGURE 31.     Formation of volatiles from lipids.[263]

biosynthetic processes. The typical flavors of most climacteric fruits are not produced during the growth phase, but are produced during the climacteric rise in respiration that follows the rise in ethylene production. The development of flavor in bananas is a typical biosynthetic process which has been studied extensively by Tressl and Drawert.[699] Labeling experiments are described by these authors and the volatiles produced from some amino acids are listed in Table 14. These authors discuss in particular and show a possible pathway for the production of volatiles from phenylalanine during ripening (Figure 32). Unripe fruits also produce a variety of fatty acids which are converted, during the ripening stage, into a variety of esters, ketones, and alcohols. Tressl and Drawert[699] outline a scheme for the conversion of octanoic acid into esters and alcohols (Figure 33) and a similar pathway for the conversion of $C_{14}$ to $C_{18}$ acids into wax esters has been described by Kolattukudy.[384]

In Class 2,[610] direct enzymic action on a precursor takes place in order to form the flavor compound. This phenomenon is of practical as well as theoretical interest to those concerned with the flavor and other organoleptic properties of fruit and vegetables since the reaction usually takes place when the tissue is physically damaged. A classic example is the formation of garlic and onion flavor when the bulbs are crushed. The onion flavor literature up to 1966 has been reviewed by Carson[95] and a comprehensive review on the same subject was recently published by Whitaker.[754] These plants possess flavors that are characterized by disulfides, trisulfides, and related compounds. The key compounds in the intact onion and garlic bulbs which serve as precursors of antibacterial and flavor and odor compounds are the alkyl- and alkenylcysteine sulfoxides. In garlic, the major compound is S-allyl-L-cysteine sulfoxide.[666] Onions were shown to contain similar compounds, S-methyl- and S-propyl-L-cysteine sulfoxide.[720] The principal flavor precursor in the onion is *trans-S*(+)-1-propenyl-L-cysteine sulfoxide. All these compounds are cleaved by an indigenous S-alkyl-L-cysteine sulfoxide lyase (called alliinase or lyase). The enzymes prepared from garlic and onion have similar specificity and require the L-cysteine sulfoxide portion of the substrate molecule. The enzymes from the two sources differ primarily in their response to pH; the

## Table 14
### VOLATILES PRODUCED FROM SOME AMINO ACIDS[699]

Volatile Components

| L-Leucine | L-Valine | L-Phenylalanine |
|---|---|---|
| Ethyl acetate | 2-Methyl-1-propanal | β-Phenylethanol |
| 3-Methylbutanal | 2-Methylpropyl acetate | Eugenol |
| 2-Methylbutyl acetate | 2-Methylpropionic acid | Eugenol methyl ether |
| *n*-Butyl acetate | 2-Ketoisovaleric acid | β-Phenylethyl acetate |
| Ethyl 3-methylbutyrate | | β-Phenylethyl butyrate |
| 3-Methylbutyl acetate | | Elimicin |
| 3-Methyl-1-butanol | | 5-Methoxyeugenol |
| *n*-Butyl butyrate | | |
| 3-Methylbutyl butyrate | | |
| Methyl 2-ketoisocaproate | | |
| *n*-Hexyl butyrate | | |
| 3-Methylbutyl caproate | | |
| 3-Methylbutyric acid | | |

garlic enzyme has a broad pH optimum from pH 5 to 8 and may be precipitated at pH 4.0 and redissolved without loss of activity.[667] The onion enzyme is sensitive to acid and is most active at pH 8.8 in pyrophosphate buffer.[402] The basic reaction was outlined by Stoll and Seebeck[668] and is as follows:

$$2RS(O)CH_2 CH - COOH + H_2O \xrightarrow{\text{Alliinase}} 2RS + 2NH_3 + 2CH_3COCOOH$$
$$| $$
$$NH_2$$

Alliin

The primary products of the reaction are believed to be sulfenic acid (RSOH), pyruvic acid, and ammonia. However the sulfenic acid is unstable and immediately gives rise to thiosulfinates which in turn decompose into disulfides, thiosulfonates, trisulfides, etc. If the basic substrate is S-allyl-L-cysteine sulfoxide, the sulfonic acid formed by enzyme action immediately dimerizes to the thiosulfinates (allicin) (Figure 34). Amino acrylic acid is also formed which spontaneously hydrolyzes to ammonia and pyruvic acid. The thiosulfinates are broken down by the catalytic action of cysteine and other thiols as follows:

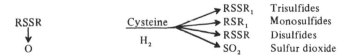

Thus a single enzymic reaction on S-alkyl-cysteine sulfoxide results in many flavor compounds. The flavor compounds produced are not identical for all the bulbs in this particular category. For instance in the case of garlic, the eyes do not water; an effect which is quite characteristic of onions. The major substrate in onion for alliinase is S-1-propenyl-L-cysteine sulfoxide and this leads to the formation of 1-propenylsulfonic acid which isomerizes to thiopropionaldehyde-S-oxide (Figure 35).

The thiopropionaldehyde-S-oxide which is the lachrymatory factor, decomposes to propionaldehyde with elimination of elemental sulfur. The propionaldehyde can dimerize by aldol condensation and lose water to form 2-methyl-pent-2-enal, or it can react with acetaldehyde to form 2-methyl-but-2-enal. These volatile compounds have been isolated from onion.[63]

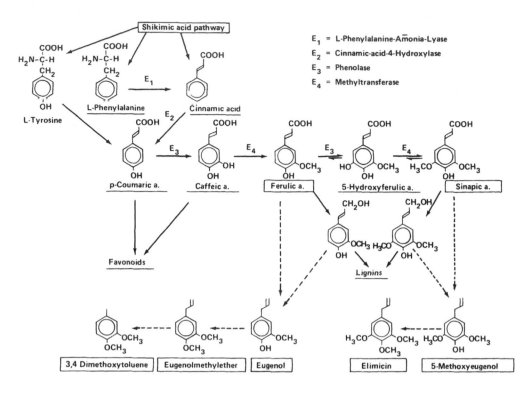

FIGURE 32. Scheme of pathways for formation of phenol ethers in banana. (Reprinted with permission from Tressl, R. and Drawert, F., *J. Agric. Food Chem.*, 21, 562. Copyright 1973 The American Chemical Society.)

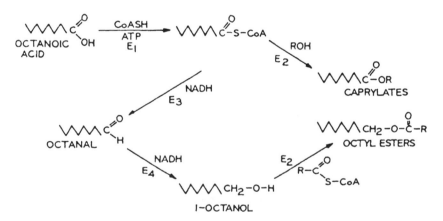

FIGURE 33. React on scheme for conversion of octanoic acid into esters. $E_1$ = Acyl-thiokinase, $E_2$ = Acyl-CoA-alcohol-transacylase, $E_3$ = Acyl-CoA-reductase, $E_4$ = Alcohol-NAD-oxidoreductase. (Reprinted with permission from Tressl, R. and Drawert, F., *J. Agric. Food Chem.*, 21, 564. Copyright 1973 The American Chemical Society.)

Another interesting direct enzymic reaction is that which occurs in mustard and other cruciferous vegetables (cabbages, horseradish, watercress). The pungent taste is caused by isothiocyanate produced when the plant is crushed and an enzyme (myrosinase, merosinigrate glucohydrolase, E.C. 3.2.3.1) acts on the more generally distributed thioglucoside precursors. The thioglucosides yield glucose, potassium hydrogen sulfate, and the pungent isothiocyanate as follows:

$$\overset{\displaystyle SC_6H_{11}O_5}{\underset{\displaystyle NOSO_3K}{RC}} \quad \xrightarrow{\text{Myrosinase}} \quad RNCS + C_6H_{12}O_6 + KHSO_4$$

R may be allyl, 3-butenyl, 3-methylthiopropyl, or 3-methyl sulfinylpropyl. The volatile constituents of cabbage have been documented by Bailey et al.,[29] and further discussion on the myrosinase reaction and its consequence in cooked and dehydrated foods is presented by MacLeod and MacLeod.[432]

*Lipoxygenase Activity in Fruit and Vegetables*

For some years past attention has been focused upon enzymic reactions in certain food products which involve linoleic and linolenic acids as substrates. It is generally accepted that lipoxygenase, a dioxygenase that is distributed widely among plants (Table 15), catalyzes the hydroperoxidation of these *cis-cis*-pentadienes. The unsaturated fatty acids have been shown to be the precursors in the biosynthesis of carbonyls and alcohols in fruit vegetables and plant tissue by Drawert et al.,[167] Kazeniac and Hall,[365] Hatenaka and Ohno,[289] Grosch and Schwencke,[262] Major and Thomas,[439] Tressl and Drawert,[699] Stone et al.,[665] and Singleton et al.[642] The role of lipoxygenase in the production of carbonyl compounds was studied by Grosch and Schwencke,[262] who found a number of volatile and nonvolatile compounds including pentanal, hexanal, hept-2-enal, oct-2-enal, nona-2,4-dienal, and deca-2,4-dienal when soybean lipoxygenase reacted with linoleic acid. Carbonyl compounds produced by cucumber homogenates are also enzymatically formed and a requirement for molecular oxygen was demonstrated by Fleming et al.[198] More recently Pattee et al.[541] found that pentane and hexanal were the major volatile end-products of a peanut lipoxygenase and linoleic acid model system. The question of aldehyde production has received considerable attention. Tressl and Drawert[699] reported a correlation between the production of aldehydes and a decrease in the amounts of linoleic and linolenic acids. Pure lipoxygenase did not produce $C_6$ and $C_9$ aldehydes, but a crude enzyme preparation had high aldehyde activity and labeled linoleic acid was converted by the extract of ripe bananas into hexanal, hexanol, and 12-oxo-*trans*-10-dodecenoic acids. The enzyme responsible for aldehyde production, although only isolated in a crude extract, was named aldehyde-lyase and a reaction scheme (Figure 36) which explains the production of $C_6$ and $C_9$ aldehydes and $C_9$ and $C_{12}$ oxoacids by bananas was outlined. The aldehydes are then either reduced to alcohols or oxidized to carboxylic acid. Reduction of *trans*-2-hexanal to *trans*-2-hexenol by alcohol: NAD oxidoreductase (E.C.1.1.1.1.) in peas has been reported by Eriksson[182] and a similar reaction is reported by Stone et al.[665] for tomatoes. The latter suggest that the alcohol oxidoreductase present in tomatoes may be similar to the alcohol:NAD oxidoreductase present in peas. A reaction scheme by which linolenic and linoleic acids are converted by tomato fruit to aldehydes and alcohols is shown in Figure 37.

There is some question as to whether alcohols are formed from aldehydes by intervention of the alcohol:NAD oxidoreductase, or whether the reverse is the case. The former is more likely under physiological conditions according to Eriksson[182] and more recently, Stone et al.[665] found that the conversion of $^{14}$C-labeled alcohols into the corresponding aldehyde could not be demonstrated. However, Meigh et al.[474] showed that tomato tissues enzymatically produced acetaldehyde, propanal, and acetone from the corresponding alcohol. A similar alcohol-to-aldehyde conversion reaction was noted for peanuts by Singleton et al.[642] Aldehyde formation from amino acids by enzymatic decarboxylation is discussed by Chase,[107] but this mechanism would not account for the formation of acetaldehyde and propanal.

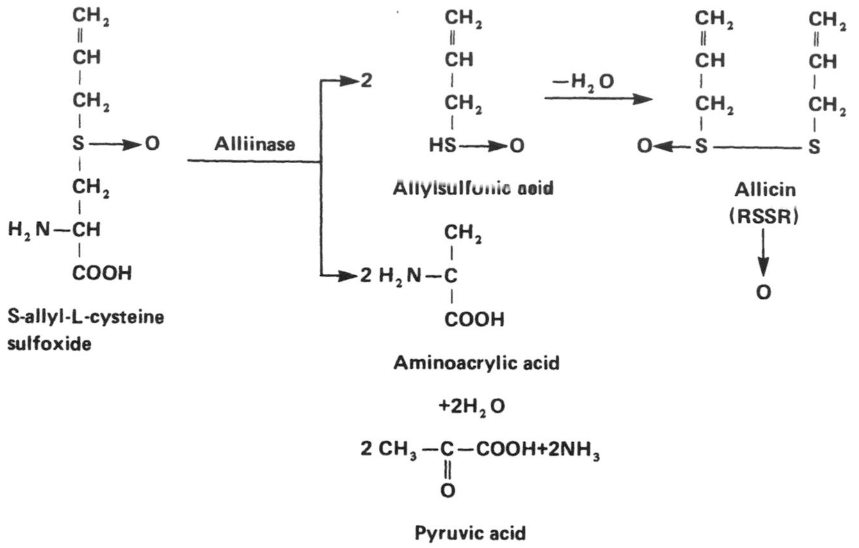

FIGURE 34.    The alliinase reaction.[668]

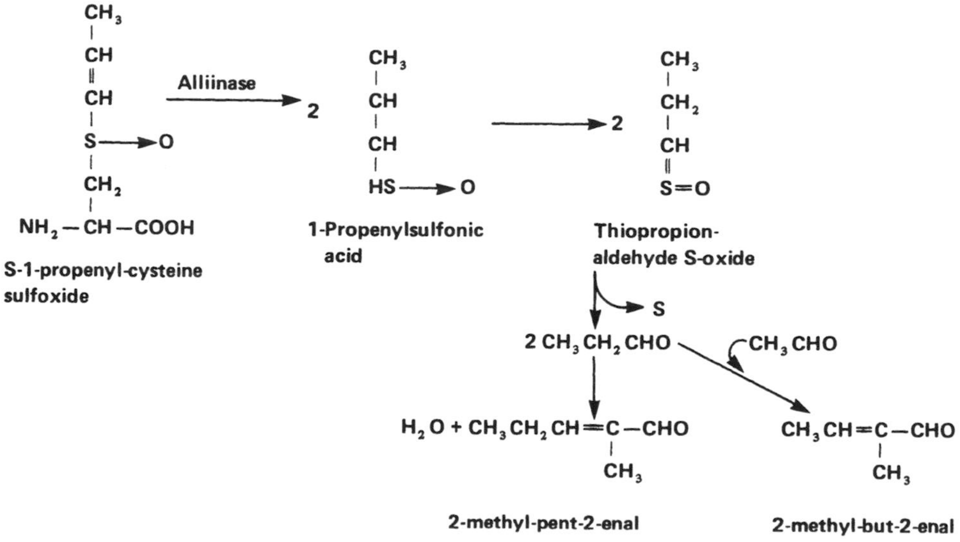

FIGURE 35.    The metabolism of S-1-propenyl L-cysteine sulfoxide.

## Practical Importance of Lipoxygenase Activity

Lipoxygenase is of practical importance to the food scientist since it promotes the peroxidation of polyunsaturated fatty acids and can affect taste, odor and color. The role of lipoxygenase in off-flavor development in soybean meal has been reviewed by Smith and Circle[650] and a correlation between intensity of bitterness and lipoxygenase activity in soybean was noted by Rackis et al.[578] The connection between off-flavor and lipoxygenase in green peas has been extensively studied. Siddigi and Tappel[638] implicated lipoxygenase in the production of off-flavor components in underblanched peas and Eriksson[181] substantiated the role of lipoxygenase in off-flavor production and pointed out that lipoxygenase activity produced aldehydes which served as substrates for alcohol dehydrogenase. *Cis*-3-hexanal, a product of lipoxygenase action, is considered responsible for the "green" flavor of string beans[298] and the enzyme is also

Table 15

PLANTS CONTAINING
LIPOXYGENASE[26]

| | |
|---|---|
| Apple (fruit) | Peas (seed) |
| Barley (seed) | Peanut (seed) |
| Beans (seed) | Potatoes (tubers) |
| Cauliflower (florets) | Pumpkin (seed) |
| Chlorella (whole cell) | Rape (seed) |
| Eggplant (fruit) | Squash (seedling) |
| Flax (seed) | Soybean (seed) |
| Maize (germ) | Sunflower (seed) |
| Olive (seed) | Tomato (fruit) |
| | Wheat (seed) |

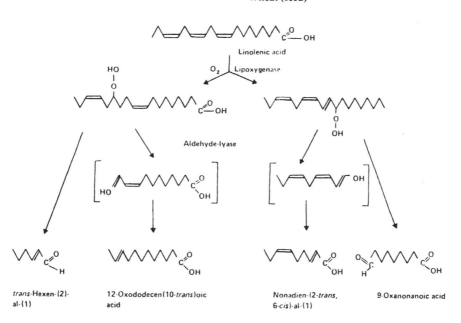

FIGURE 36. Reaction scheme for enzymatic splitting of linolenic acid into aldehydes and ox-oacids. (Reprinted with permission from Tressl, R. and Drawert, F., *J. Agric. Food Chem.*, 21, 564. Copyright 1973 The American Chemical Society.)

associated with off-flavors in unblanched sweet corn,[726] and the cardboard flavor of barley preparations.[247]

*Peroxidase Reactions and Off-flavor*

Peroxidases are distributed widely in plant tissue and, like lipoxygenase, polyphenoloxidase and glucose oxidase are usually intracellular. Peroxidase is a rather interacting enzyme in that it plays an important role in the development and senescence of plant tissue.[494] It has been proposed that peroxidase functions in the degradation of chlorophyll[733] and induces off-flavor development in raw and unblanched vegetables.[351] Peroxides, like most heme pigments, catalyzes the peroxidative degradation of unsaturated fatty acids, yielding carbonyl compounds which contribute to off-flavor[685] and the enzyme is active at sub-zero temperatures as low as −18°C.[587]

The enzyme is one of the most heat-stable enzymes in plants and it is generally accepted that if peroxidase is destroyed, it is quite unlikely that other enzyme systems will have survived. Considerable work has been done on regeneration of peroxidase,[426,615,782] which is considered to be complex as demonstrated by spectral changes, and does not follow either first or second order kinetics.[426]

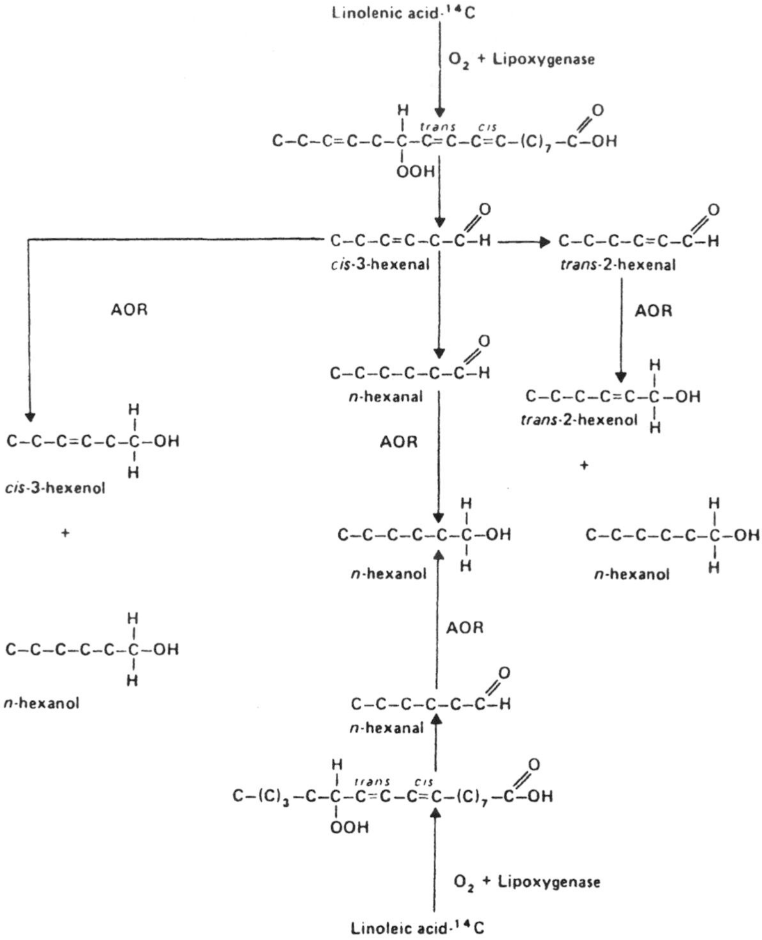

Linolenic acid-$^{14}$C

$O_2$ + Lipoxygenase

FIGURE 37.   Aldehyde and alcohol formation in tomato from linolenic and lino-leic acid. AOR = Alcohol Oxydoreductase. (Reprinted from Stone, E. J., Hall, R. M., and Kazeniac, S. J., *J. Food Sci.*, 40(6), 1141, 1975. Copyright © by Institute of Food Technologists.

Peroxidase activity is used extensively as an indicator for the effectiveness of sub-sterilizing heat treatments,[90] and Bruemmer et al.[86] noted a significant negative corre-lation between peroxidase activities and flavor scores of high- and low-yield orange juices and suggested the potential use of peroxidase activity as an "index of adverse flavor" of orange juice.

## ADDED ENZYMES

### Pectic and Cell Modifying Enzymes

Commercial pectolytic enzyme preparations have been used extensively in the fruit juice industry since the early part of this century. The last 20 years have shown a trend toward the production of specific enzyme preparations for different food processes and products. The application of some of these enzymes are discussed below, but for more detailed information the following references should be consulted: Reed,[587] Char-ley,[106] Fogarty and Ward,[199,200] MacMillan and Sheiman,[433] and Durr and Schobiner.[171]

### Clarification of Fruit Juices

Clarification or dehazing of fruit juices is achieved by enzymic de-esterification of pectin. The resulting low methoxy pectin is precipitated by $Ca^{2+}$ and removed by filtration. Endo[179] studied the clarification mechanism of apple juice with fungal enzymes and found both PE and PG to be responsible. The application of commercial enzyme preparations is not always feasible. For example, accelerated clarification of lemon and lime juice is slow and incomplete because the low pH (1.7 to 2.8) reduces the effectiveness not only of the native pectinesterase, but also of most commercial clarifying enzymes. Krop and Pilnik[397] and Baker[30] used the products of enzyme action, namely polygalacturonic acid to clarify orange juice and lime juice respectively. Pectic enzymes are also used to clarify musk and wine.[128,587] In the case of soft drinks, regulations have been introduced in Germany preventing the use of artificial colors or clouding agents in liquid citrus products.[106] A Danish company produced an enzyme preparation, Pectolase® D.E.10, which degrades the flavedo, albedo, and other cell tissue from citrus fruits, yielding an extract rich in color which is then used to color the juices while at the same time avoiding any off-flavor development. The use of an immobilized multipectic enzyme system was recently outlined by Young[777] for the clarification and reduction of viscosity of apple juice. Unripe fruit and most fruits at the start of the season usually contain some starch. The presence of starch causes turbidity in juices during storage and consequently must be removed. This is done by using an amylase system. However, most amylases do not function economically at temperatures above 30°C and at the pH of most juices. Grampp[246] reports on the production of a fungal $\alpha$-amylase from *Aspergillus niger* which is thermostable and has a temperature optimum of 45 to 50°C — the temperature used in the hot clarification process of apple juice. This author also discusses the use of a fungal pectolytic enzyme preparation (Rohapeet D), produced by *A. niger,* for clarification of apple juice concentrates. The enzyme preparations contain mainly polygalacturonase and pectinmethylesterase activity (70 to 80% of the total activity); only 20 to 30% of its pectolytic activity comes from pectate lyase. The reaction is carried out at 45 to 50°C, at which temperature pectinases are three to four times more active than at 30°C. The high enzymatic activity results in a shorter reaction time and an improved quality product. The application of immobilized enzymes in wine production have also been reported from Russia.[544]

*Improving Yield of Juice*

The juices of some fruits are readily extractable by pressing and filtering. However, improved yields of juice from grapes and blackberries has been achieved by using pectolytic enzymes.[106] This process has a three-fold effect, i.e., improved yield, color, and flavor. Yields of citrus oils from lemon and oranges can be increased considerably by using pectic enzymes.[552] Bolin et al.[66] outlined the use of a pectinolytic enzyme (Pectinol R10) to improve yield, storage stability, color, and flavor of prune juice. Another important consideration not heretofore mentioned is the reduced energy consumption when enzymic methods are used for cell disintegration.

*Production of Purees*

A pectin glycosidase can be used for the maceration of fruit and vegetable tissue to mono-cell suspensions.[106] This process is essential for the production of high Brix staple purees without the browning action of polyphenoloxidase connected with mechanical disintegration. In a recent article Termote et al.,[693] discussed the application of hydrolyzates of pectic acid, prepared by enzymatic action, for the stabilization of cloud in pectinesterase active orange juice. This is perhaps an example of inhibition by the presence of excess reaction product.

*Cleaning Citrus Peel*

Pectolytic enzymes may be used to remove loosely adhering pulp and membrane tissues from citrus peels. The cleaned peels are then suitable for use in soft drinks, candies, and marmalades.

### Miscellaneous Applications

Pectolytic enzymes have been used for cereal bran extraction,[653] treatment of coffee bean,[433] and peeling tomatoes.[670] Low methoxy pectins for sugar free or low sugar jellies[422] may be prepared, not only by partial acid or alkaline hydrolysis of the methyl ester bonds in pectin, but also by the use of fungal pectin esterase.[651]

### Cellulases and Hemicellulases

Cellulase preparations have been used to produce sugars[131,233,440,475] and proteins.[709] This type of enzyme has been used to increase the digestibility and nutritional value of coconut where the major obstacle to its use in human foods is its very high fiber content.[581] The use of cellulolytic enzyme preparations in wine production has also been reported.[700]

Hemicellulases are used to breakdown coffee gums which cause liquid coffee concentrates to gel.

### Flavor Enzymes

The concept of restoring flavor compounds lost during processing of foods through introduction of flavor forming enzymes has attracted considerable interest over the years. According to Hewitt et al.,[299] heating steps in food processing causes loss of natural flavor components. These steps also destroy the enzymes which normally convert nonvolatile flavor precursors to volatile flavor substances. The typical flavor could be regenerated by adding enzymes derived from the same species. In a typical experiment Hewitt et al.[299] prepared a blanched and dehydrated watercress which was quite flavorless on rehydration. However, when a tasteless and odorless enzyme preparation from another member of the Brassica family was added, the typical odor and taste of watercress was restored. The "flavorase" concept of Hewitt et al.[299] was further studied by Schwimmer[616] using a variety of processed vegetables. He found that the quality of enzyme-treated processed food approached that of fresh vegetable but was not identical with it and in general, addition of enzymes tended to overemphasize certain notes of the natural flavor. However, in a previous study, it was found that those samples treated with the enzymes were preferred to control samples without enzyme treatment. In a more recent study, Gremli and Wild[258] found that it was not possible to restore exactly the same flavor as originally present in fresh tomatoes. However, the undesirable hay-note of spray-dried tomato powder was masked with an enzymatically produced fresh note.

Although the principle of restoring a fresh flavor to a processed food product by the addition of enzymes is feasible, it does not seem to have found widespread application. The preparation of the enzyme from natural products obviously presents economic problems. Another problem may be the requirement to sell the processed food and enzyme preparation in two separate containers. Specific inactivation of undesirable enzymes in the preparation is impossible and according to Gremli and Wild,[258] "it is almost a matter of chance whether a fully balanced flavor can be restored with an enzyme preparation".

The "flavorase" concept is, however, feasible where it is sufficient to form a single typical flavor compound by direct enzymic conversion. Thus, Bailey et al.[29] showed that allyl isothiocyanate could be regenerated by enzymatic action in dehydrated cabbage. Similar work was reported recently by Schwimmer and Friedman.[621]

### Debittering Citrus Products

Citrus fruits contain two distinctly different classes of bitter compounds: flavonoids and limonoids.

The flavonoids are ubiquitous constituents of the plant kingdom and are present in high concentration in all citrus fruit; they are distributed throughout the fruit but occur in highest concentration (up to 2%) in the albedo layer. The clear juice of most citrus fruits contains only a low level of flavonoids but commercial preparations of juice are usually contaminated with some rag and pulp and unless these are removed quickly, excessive bitterness will result. Flavonoids consist of one of a range of aglycone moieties attached to one of two disaccharides: neohesperidose and rutinose, both of which contain glucose and rhamnose but differ in the type of glycocidic linkage:

Rhamnose · Glucose
Neohesperidose

Rhamnose · Glucose
Rutinose

The most common aglycone moiety is naringenin which on condensation with neohesperidose yields naringin, the most common flavonoid in citrus fruits.

Rhamnose · Glucose · Naringenin
Prunin
Naringin

Naringin is intensely bitter but neither prunin or naringenin are bitter. In 1955 an enzyme, commercially known as nargininase, was discovered by Japanese workers. Numerous patents for the preparation of naringinase, mostly from *A. niger* or *Concilla diplodiella,* have been taken out.[105]

Commercial naringinase contains a variety of enzymes including:

1.   A pectinase which must be inactivated by differential thermal inactivation or fractionation in alcohol solutions
2.   A rhaminosidase which hydrolyzes naringin to rhamnose and prunin and which is sufficient to reduce the bitterness of naringin
3.   A glucosidase which hydrolyzes prunin to glucose and naringenin

Soluble naringinase has had limited application in debittering citrus juices and canned citrus pieces. The enzyme has also been immobilized, but has had limited success because of relatively poor stability, especially at the natural pH of citrus juices and because the optimum pH (5 to 6) of the immobilized enzyme necessitates neutralization of the juice for best hydrolysis. Chandler and Nicol[105] were not very optimistic about the commercial future of naringinase and appeared to feel that careful selection of fruit and better control of extraction pressures would be more profitable, at least in the immediate future.

An interesting use of naringin is in manufacture of the intensely sweet β-neohesperidin dihydrochalcone for use as a nonnutritive sweetener.

The dominant limonoid in citrus fruit is limonin, which is only slightly soluble in water and occurs predominantly in the albedo, and its hydroxy acid derivative, limonoic acid, which is water soluble and nonbitter. Limonoid bitterness is avoided if only juice sacks are pressed but in practice it is impossible to exclude albedo particles completely.

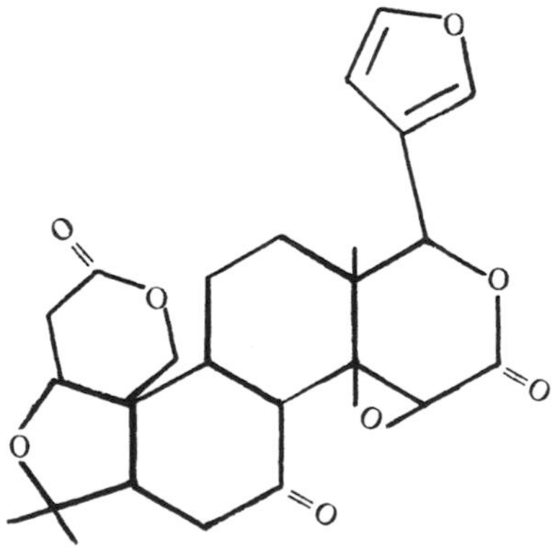

Limonin 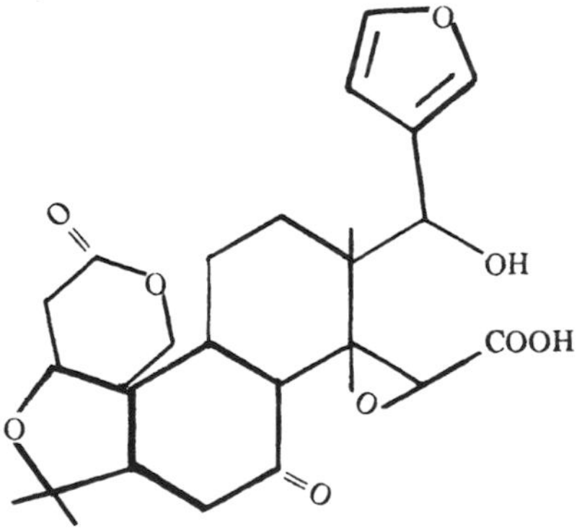                                   Limonoic Acid

Enzymes capable of converting limonin to nonbitter limonoic acid are secreted by the soil bacterium *Arthobacter globiformis* or *Pseudomonas* spp. when grown on a medium containing limonoate ion as sole source of carbon. These enzymes are not at present satisfactory for commercial use because:

1.   They require NAD as cofactor.
2.   Their pH optimum is at 8 to 9, which necessitates neutralization and reacidification of citrus juice for effective enzyme action.
3.   Limonin is required in the bacterial medium, which increases the cost of enzyme production.

Citrus albedo contains a limonin-degrading enzyme, also with a high pH optimum. This enzyme may have potential as a debittering agent in isolated preparations or its activity may be controlled in vivo by ethylene treatment of the fruit, but this latter has the major disadvantage of causing the development of off-flavors if even a slight excess of ethylene is used.

## MISCELLANEOUS APPLICATIONS

The application of enzymes to a wide variety of relatively minor food processes have been suggested and some are of fairly major industrial significance. As most of these applications do not fit readily into the major food commodities discussed above and in many instances are applicable to a number of commodities, we have grouped them together as miscellaneous applications.

### Protein Hydrolyzates

The manufacture of protein hydrolyzates is a well-established process for the utilization of protein-rich food wastes (e.g., meat scrap) and the conversion of nonconventional food proteins (e.g., fish waste, vegetable proteins) into acceptable products. Within the term hydrolyzate are two distinguishable processes: (1) extensive hydrolysis of proteins for such applications as comminuted meats, soups, gravies, flavorings, and dietetic foods; such applications amount to 30 M lb per annum in the U.S. alone according to Connell,[125] who includes useful information on numerous applications and (2) limited hydrolysis with the objective of improving the functionality of the protein.

#### Extensive Hydrolyzates

A major portion of protein hydrolyzates is traditionally prepared from soya, gluten, milk proteins, meat scrap, and fish proteins by acid hydrolysis.[60,563] Neutralization of acid hydrolyzates results in a high salt content (35 to 50%, solids basis). For certain applications (soups, gravies, condiments) a high salt content is not objectionable, but for such applications as dietetic foods and food supplementation it may not be tolerable. Further, acid hydrolysis causes total or partial destruction of some amino acids.

Enzymatic hydrolysis is a viable alternative to acid hydrolysis, but has the serious disadvantage that combinations of certain enzymes and certain substrates give rise to bitter peptides the level of which may be reduced by treating hydrolyzates with activated carbon, although this was considered to be impractical.[491] It now appears that there is a fairly good agreement that the higher the content of hydrophobic amino acids in a protein, the more likely it is that its hydrolyzate will be bitter-tasting. Ney[511] suggested that hydrophobicity was the only factor determining whether or not a peptide would be bitter; of 66 peptides tested, all peptides with an average hydrophobicity <1300 were nonbitter, while those with an average hydrophobicity >1400 were all bitter. However, other factors in addition to hydrophobicity appear to be important in determining bitterness; Kirimura et al.,[379] and Fujimaki et al.[225] isolated peptides with hydrophobicity values <1300 which were bitter. Sullivan and Jago[676] compared the structures of a number of bitter peptides and concluded that the presence of a hydrophobic C-terminal residue as well as high average hydrophobicity was an important feature of bitter peptides.

Apparently then, it is important to select the proper enzyme-substrate combination for the production of protein hydrolyzates by enzymatic means. However, it is possible to eliminate bitterness. Arai et al.[11] describe the use of an acid carboxypeptidase A from Aspergillus species for the debittering of soya protein hydrolyzates. The same group of workers later developed the plastein reaction as a means of eliminating bitterness (to be discussed later). Bitterness is also a problem in certain varieties of cheese due to excessive or imbalanced proteinase and peptidase activity.[425,677]

A number of applications of enzymes in the preparation of protein hydrolyzates are described in detail by Wieland.[760]

*Limited Hydrolyzates*

Many of the novel food proteins prepared from vegetable sources have poor functionality mainly because of poor solubility; further, many proteins which in the native state have good functional properties may lose these following denaturation during processing. A number of approaches have been adopted to improve the functionality of proteins; these include chemical modification of amino acid residues, alkali treatment, and limited proteolysis.

A very wide range of reagents have been investigated for the chemical modification of proteins.[193,473] While the principal application of most of these reagents is for use as probes for study of protein and enzyme structure, some have been used to modify food proteins.[210] Many of these reagents are toxic and are obviously unsuitable for food applications; others are unsuitable for commercial-scale food applications on the basis of cost and availability; even though some reagents have shown promise in laboratory-scale investigations, few if any are yet used on a commercial scale. Hydrogen peroxide treatment of milk for bread manufacture might be regarded as an exception (cf. dairy section). Further, many modifying agents react with essential amino acid residues rendering them resistant to digestive enzymes and thereby reducing the biological value of the protein.

Sodium hydroxide is commonly used in food processing for peeling, neutralizing deodorizing, solubilizing, and texturizing proteins, especially vegetable proteins. However, NaOH at the concentration (0.1 $N$) and temperature ($>60°C$) of normal usage causes a number of major chemical changes in the protein and probably other food constituents, e.g., hydrolysis of peptide bonds; hydrolysis of the guanidino group of arginine; racemization; some destruction of cysteine, cystine, serine, and threonine; elimination of certain side-chain groups (phosphate, sulphydryl, glycosyl) with the concomitant formation of unsaturated side-chains, mostly dehydrolalanine; and reaction of dehydroalanine with various other protein side groups (lysine, ornithine, cysteine, histidine, tryptophan) to form new amino acids, frequently with reduction of the biological value of the protein. These latter reactions (elimination of side-groupings and formation of new amino acids) have been reviewed by Sen et al.[624] and Whitaker and Feeney.[756] It would therefore seem desirable to avoid treatment of foods at high pH and high temperatures, and limited proteolysis by enzymes appears to offer an alternative. Various aspects of the production of enzymic protein hydrolyzates are reviewed by Adler-Nissen.[2,3]

Fish protein concentrate appears to be the most widely studied substrate for enzymatic modification probably because enzymatic hydrolysis does not lead to bitterness and large amounts of high quality raw material are available. Fish protein concentrate is potentially a very valuable and extensive source of animal protein, but its functional properties are limited, due mainly to poor solubility.[118] The proteolytic activity of 20 commercially available enzymes on fish protein was studied by Hale;[273] ficin had the highest initial activity but pronase and pepsin caused the most extensive hydrolysis; various microbial proteinases gave the least hydrolysis. The high activity of pronase and pepsin were confirmed by Cheftel et al.,[108] who established various parameters for a continuous enzyme recycling process for fish protein concentrate as an alternative to the alkaline process investigated by Tannenbaum et al.,[683,684] In this study the protein was fairly extensively hydrolyzed, the average molecular weight of the peptides formed was $<2000$. "Limited proteolysis" of fish protein concentrate is described by Spinelli et al.,[660] as a means of preparing fish protein isolates (sacroplasmic and myofibrillar fractions) with better functionality than isolates prepared by chemical fractionation alone.[659] The fish protein concentrate was first hydrolyzed with Rhozyme® P-11, precipitated with polyphosphate to free the protein of nonprotein nitrogen and extracted with isoproponol to remove fat. The product was reported to have good functional properties and fairly good storage stability. This and further work on the modifying the functional properties of fish protein is reviewed by Spinelli et al.[658]

The effectiveness of bromelain, pronase, and ficin in producing soluble fish protein concentrates is described by Hevia et al.;[297] pronase was most effective, but ficin which had been activated with cysteine was as active at 40°C, as was pronase at 50°C. The nutritive value of enzymatic fish protein hydrolyzates was found to be very high[32,775] and this type of product was considered to be a very suitable supplement for cereal products. The enzyme used to prepare the hydrolyzates was not stated but Tarky et al.,[690] reported that enzymatic hydrolyzates of fish protein prepared with pepsin was deficient in tryptophan, presumably due to destruction of this amino acid at the low pH values used. A five to six fold reduction in the concentration of mercury in soluble fish protein concentrate following treatment with proteolytic enzymes was reported by Archer et al.;[15] the mercury was concentrated in the insoluble fraction.

Proteolysis of vegetable material to increase soluble protein was investigated by Sreekantiah et al.,[669] and the enzymatic refining of unconventional proteins to separate protein from nucleic acid and undesirable flavors was studied by Bednarski et al.;[43] both groups report favorable results.

The recovery of protein from the raw material and products of meat-rendering plants was studied by Criswell et al.[130] and Connelly et al.[126] Treatment of meat scrap with a number of commercial proteinases permitted the recovery of a high quality protein in good yield (bromelain gave best results), but apart from amino acid composition, functionality is not reported.

A product with beef-extract type flavor was produced by fermenting reconstituted skim milk powder with the proteolytic microorganism *P. fluorescens.*[114] The product performed well in nutritional trials and it is suggested that it would be suitable for such products as gravies, soups, and bouillon. No attempt was made to isolate the enzyme(s) responsible but presumably an enzyme preparation from this organism may also yield a satisfactory product.

Casein is notorious for its propensity to yield very bitter hydrolyzates with a variety of enzymes, a characteristic apparent even at the low level of proteolysis which occurs in Cheddar and Gouda cheese.[423] It has been suggested that β-casein, which is more hydrophobic that $\alpha_{si}$-casein, is the principal source of bitter peptides in Cheddar cheese.[209,676] This has been confirmed by Clegg et al.,[115] who identified a peptide containing residues 53 to 79 of the β-casein as the peptide responsible for the bitter flavor of papain digests of casein, although Pelissier and Manchon[546] reported that with most proteinases bovine $\alpha_{si}$-casein is more susceptible to bitterness than bovine β-casein. The same authors reported that whole goat and sheep caseins are less likely to develop bitterness than cows casein. A procedure for removing the bitter taste from ficin/pepsin or papain hydrolyzates of egg white protein or casein using an exopeptidase, leucine amino peptidase, from kidney was developed by Clegg and McMillan[116] and scaled up by Clegg et al.[117] Presumably the exopeptidase completely hydrolyzed the bitter peptides to amino acids; pronase (a broad specificity proteinase from *Streptomyces gresius)* reduced the bitterness of ficin/pepsin or papain hydrolyzates, but did not eliminate it. The objective of the study was to prepare hydrolyzates suitable for patients with digestive disorders, e.g., cystic fibrosis, and preliminary feeding trials with rats showed that the biological value of debittered hydrolyzates was comparable with that of undigested casein.[117] The use of casein hydrolyzates for various special dietary applications was reviewed by Manson.[443]

A method for the production of acid-soluble casein, free of bitterness, by controlled proteolysis was described by Haggett.[272] Partial (8% $\alpha$-amino $N$) hydrolysis of whey protein by trypsin was studied by Jost and Monti;[353] thermal denaturation of the protein before digestion improved hydrolysis. The authors did not refer to the flavor of the product.

By performing the proteolysis of soya protein isolate in an ultrafiltration cell, it is possible to prepare a peptide-rich permeate free of bitter taste;[599] few details of the method are given. A similar technique is also reported by Iacobucci et al.[328] and Myers et al.[493] The principle of an ultrafiltration reactor for continuous protein hydrolysis by enzymes was described by Viniegra-Gonzales.[718] The modification of soya protein by limited proteolysis (with a number of animal, plant, and microbial proteinases) to produce a product with good gelling properties and which might be suitable as an egg-white substitute was described by Pour-El and Swenson.[561] Apparently reduction of protein size by proteolysis and reduction of disulfide groups by treatment with cysteine are necessary to produce a soya protein with gelling properties. The modified protein was not as effective as egg white but the authors considered that further research may produce an acceptable product. The use of proteolysis to modify soya protein for the fortification of breakfast cereal blends is described by Marshall[459] but few details are provided.

### The Plastein Reaction

One of the interesting and perhaps very significant outcomes of research in protein hydrolyzates has been the plastein reaction. It appears to have been recognized for about 100 years that proteinases were capable of synthesizing peptide bonds as well as hydrolyzing them. The synthetic activity of proteinases is troublesome in the production of protein hydrolyzates by enzyme catalysis and much of the early research was concerned with the mechanism by which proteinases catalyzed peptide synthesis;[153-156,719,721,722,761] the term "plastein" was applied to high molecular weight polypeptides synthesized in such reactions.

The significance of the plastein reaction to food science was not appreciated until 1970 when a group at the University of Tokyo used it to debitter enzymatic hydrolyzates of soya protein.[225,772-774] They were successful in this objective but the plastein reaction was seen to have potential far beyond the debittering of protein hydrolyzates, which have been exploited primarily by the Tokyo group, whose work has been reviewed by Fujimaki et al.,[223,224] Arai et al.,[12,13] Eriksen and Fagerson,[183] and Yamashita et al.[769]

All proteinases which have been investigated appear to catalyze the plastein reaction for which three principal conditions, significantly different from those for peptide hydrolysis by the same enzymes, are required:

1.  The best substrate appears to be a mixture of small peptides (tetra, penta, or hexa), preferably produced by enzymatic hydrolysis; esters of amino acids but not free amino acids are also incorporated into plasteins.
2.  A high concentration (20 to 40%) of peptides is required for synthesis; at <7.5% substrate concentration, hydrolysis rather than synthesis occurs.
3.  Regardless of the pH optimum of the proteinase for hydrolysis, the pH optimum for plastein formation is in the range pH 4 to 7.

Resynthesis of peptide bonds can occur either by transpeptidation or by condensation, the contribution of each mechanism depending on the particular circumstances. During proteolysis by most proteinases an acyl-enzyme intermediate is formed following which the acyl group is transferred to a nucleophile, usually water, but in resynthesis the acyl group is transferred to another nucleophile, e.g., the amino group of an amino acid or peptide; whether transfer will be to water or amino group depends on their relative concentrations and pH. In the condensation reaction it appears that an acyl-enzyme complex is formed with the free carboxyl group of a peptide and the acyl group is then transferred to a nucleophile.

Plasteins have low solubility in water and this lack of solubility appears to be the driving force for the synthetic reaction. Hydrophilic hydrolyzates are not effective substrates for plastein formation because the plasteins formed are soluble in water; very hydrophobic hydrolyzates are also poor substrates because the plastein is too insoluble and precipitates out of solution before significant synthesis can occur.[21,22] Arai et al.,[12,13] introduced a term, $\beta/\alpha$ ratio, which is related to the extent of plastein formation and may be useful to predict the degree of synthesis which is likely to occur; $\beta$ is a measure of the insolubility of the plastein and $\alpha$ is a measure of plastein production. For hydrophilic hydrolyzates, e.g., casein, $\alpha = 40\%$ and $\beta/\alpha = 0.28$; for a hydrophobic hydrolyzate, e.g., zein, $\alpha = 57\%$ and $\beta/\alpha = 0.87$, while for ovalbumin $\alpha = 90\%$ and $\beta/\alpha = 0.49$. Arai et al.[12,13] found that maximum plastein formation occurs when $\beta/\alpha \approx 0.5$ and suggests that hydrolyzates from different sources should be mixed to obtain this value.

While the original interest of the Tokyo group in the plastein reaction was in the debittering of protein hydrolyzates, this was quickly overshadowed by more significant applications. The more important of these is the improvement of the nutritional value of plant proteins by incorporation of methionine, lysine, and tryptophan, in which these proteins are deficient, into the plastein.[224] The plasteins so produced are not organoleptically inferior and their nutritional value is very similar to that of the World Health Organization (WHO) reference protein. The formation of peptide bonds by condensation of free amino acids is strongly endothermic ($\Delta F = 4$ Kcal/mole) while the energy required for peptide bond formation between two peptides is $\Delta F = 0.4$ Kcal/mole. In order to obtain satisfactory incorporation of amino acids into a plastein it was necessary to add them as ethyl esters to the hydrolyzate. This development could have immense significance as a means of increasing the world supply of high quality protein.

Soya isolate is insoluble in the pH range 3 to 6 which severely restricts its application in acid foods; an ordinary plastein had improved solubility at acid pH values but was less soluble than soy isolate at pH values >7. By enriching the protein hydrolyzate with Glu-$\alpha$O-Et the resulting plastein was very soluble over the pH range 1 to 11.[12,13] Synthesis of a low-phenylalanine plastein suitable for patients suffering from phenylketonuria is described by Yamashita et al.[770]

The Tokyo group[14,224] have also demonstrated the usefulness of the plastein reaction for deodorizing, removal of off-flavors, decolorizing, and defatting vegetable protein preparations, many of which, especially single cell proteins, are difficult to purify by conventional means.

Recent work by v. Hofsten and Lalasidis[308] suggests that plastein formation is due principally to the formation of noncovalent bonds, mostly through hydrophobic interactions, although electrostatic interactions may also be involved. These authors could not detect condensation reactions which would be expected to lead to a decrease in ninhydrin-reacting groups and such reactions were considered to play a minor role in plastein formation. At high pH values hydrolysis was the dominant reaction catalyzed by alkaline proteinases even at very high substrate concentrations, but there appeared to be a shift toward transpeptidation as the pH was decreased to neutral or slightly acid values, accompanied possibly by a shift in specificity to peptide bonds involving hydrophobic residues. v. Hofstein and Lalasidis[308] consider that plastein formation might best be described as a kind of rearrangement where the equilibrium is influenced by the formation of peptides tending to form insoluble complexes. Chromatography of plasteins dissolved in 50% acetic acid, 8 $M$ urea or 6 $M$ guanidine showed that plasteins were mixtures of low molecular weight peptides which presumably were held together in the plastein by predominantly hydrophobic bonds. In view of this information it will be interesting to see how the debittering effect of plastein formation can be explained; presumably the ethyl esters of amino acids added to hydrolyzates are also attached to the plastein by noncovalent bonds.

### Other Protein Modifications

A variety of enzyme-catalyzed modifications of proteins are discussed by Whitaker.[755] Most of the reactions reviewed occur in vivo and are not yet of industrial significance but they demonstrate possible potential applications for enzymes in food technology.

The modification of proteins resulting from enzymatic reactions, many of them secondary changes and many of them discussed in other sections of this review were discussed by Richardson.[594]

### Use of Invertase in Candy Manufacture

Liquid center candies contain a core of invert sugar syrup (>79% sugar) the osmotic pressure of which is high enough to prevent fermentation but which is still fluid. Since it is not possible to enrobe a liquid syrup in chocolate, a fondant consisting of liquid syrup (67 to 68% sucrose), crystalline sucrose, and invertase is coated with chocolate. Some dissolved surcorse is hydrolyzed to glucose and fructose which have higher solubility than sucrose; additional sucrose dissolves and is in turn hydrolyzed. The process continues, perhaps for several weeks until the syrup becomes saturated with invert sugar (82 to 83% solids). Maturation time may be regulated by adjusting the level of invertase added to the fondant, and the facility to vary maturation time permits the manufacture of liquid center candies to be spread more uniformly over time without the risk of product deterioration.

### Glucose Oxidase

Glucose oxidase catalyze the oxidation of glucose to gluconic acid (via glucono-δ-lactone) in the presence of molecular oxygen. FAD is an essential prosthetic group and $H_2O_2$ is formed as a second product. $H_2O_2$ may accumulate but is usually reduced to $H_2O$ and $O_2$ by catalase present as a contaminant in the glucose oxidase preparation or added separately.

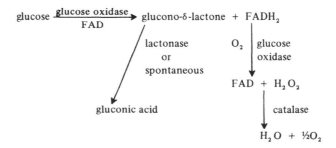

Glucose oxidase is produced commercially from a wide variety of molds, usually *A. niger*, *P. notatum*, or *P. glaucum*. It has a pH optimum at 5.5 and exhibits a very high degree of specificity for d-glucose which makes it a very useful reagent for the assay of glucose in the presence of other sugars.

Glucose oxidase has two principal applications in the food industry: (1) removal of residual oxygen and (2) removal of residual glucose. These applications, which have changed little in the past 10 years, have been reviewed by Underkofler[705] and Reed.[587]

Although eggs contain only a very low level of free sugars, these react with the proteins, especially in dehydrated egg products, through Maillard browning reactions resulting in deterioration of color, solubility, and whippability. Glucose may be removed by fermentation with yeast or bacteria but this approach obviously leads to microbiological problems. Treatment of the liquid egg products with glucose oxidase-catalase prior to drying is a more controllable process and has the added advantage of reducing microbial counts due to the action of the $H_2O_2$ produced in the reaction.[553,602]

Removal of oxygen by treatment with glucose oxidase is probably its most important food application. Low levels of oxygen lead to deterioration in a variety of products: discoloration in white wines due to polyphenoloxidase activity, skunkiness in beer, loss of ascorbic acid in fruit juices,[701] oxidation of lipids in high fat products, e.g., mayonnaise and butter.[380] In wines and fruit juices, oxidation may be prevented by treatment with $SO_2$ or metabisulfide, but treatment with glucose oxidase is more effective[533] and may also be more attractive because of legislation pertaining to the use of $SO_2$. Oxidation of lipids may be retarded or prevented by the use of chemical antioxidants if such are permitted by legislation but treatment with glucose oxidase offers an alternative. Lipid oxidation in whole milk powder is also a serious problem which may be solved by glucose oxidase. With dehydrated foods, glucose oxidase is ineffective if added directly to the product because of the absence of water. To overcome this a packet, impermeable to water but permeable to $O_2$, containing glucose, glucose oxidase, and buffer, is placed in the can prior to sealing and the ensuing enzymatic reaction effectively removes head-space oxygen.

Most of the recent research on glucose oxidase has been concerned with immobilizing and utilizing glucose oxidase-catalase dual systems. Early studies used organic supports but more recent investigations have employed inorganic supports of various forms: silica-alumina, nickel-silica-alumina, nickel-kieselgur, porus glass, and titania.[23,68,69,257,293,450,477,502] The application of glucose oxidase-catalase to foods was not studied in the above investigations. Obviously immobilized glucose oxidase is suitable only for liquid products (wines and fruit juices). Glucose oxidase bound in polyacrylamide gels gave satisfactory results for oxygen removal from apple and cherry juice.[395]

An alternative approach is described by Fresnel and Trosset:[216] glucose in an aqueous medium was brought into contact with an electrode which contained glucose oxidase immobilized on a conducting support; the requisite oxygen was generated electrolytically on the electrode.

## Minor Applications of Lipases

A number of minor applications of lipases in food processing are cited by Seitz:[623] refinement of rice flavor (lipolysis followed by treatment with an oxidizing agent); modification of soybean milk; preparation of smoked carp; and hydrolysis of trace amounts of lipid in egg white (which impairs its whippability).

## Flavor Potentiators

It has been recognized since 1913 that the principal flavor component of bonito (a flavoring additive used in Japan) was the histidine salt of inosine monophosphate (IMP). In 1951 it was shown that only 5′ IMP was flavorful; the 2′ or 3′ nucleotides are not effective. 5′-Guanosine monophosphate (GMP) has a lower flavor threshold than IMP and both, along with monosidum glutamate, are widely used flavor enhancers.

The nucleotides can be prepared commercially by:

1. Extraction from animal tissue especially fish (e.g., press juice from fish canneries or fish meal plants); proteolysis of the tissue protein improves recovery of nucleotides.
2. Biosynthesis by cultures of *B. subtilis* or *A. aerogenes;* large quantities of nucleotides accumulate in the growth medium.

3.     Chemical synthesis.
4.     Enzymatic hydrolysis of ribonucleic acids. Any type of RNA will do but yeast or bacterial biomass are most convenient; these microorganisms contain a high level of nucleic acid, removal of which improves their biological value for animal feed. The selection of enzyme source is very important because it must be free of phosphate mono- and di-esterases which yield 2′ or 3′ nucleotides. An enzyme preparation from *P. citrinum* or some streptomyces species is satisfactory.

The topic has been well reviewed by Kuninaka et al.[401] and Kuninaka.[400] Production of another type of flavor enhancer is described by Jaeggi et al.[333] A milk product, in particular a fermented product such as yogurt, is subjected to hydrolysis by proteinases of vegetable or animal origin (papain, trypsin), neutralized, heat-sterilized, and dried. The desired aroma is formed when the product is heated at temperature normally used in nonenzymic reactions. In the presence of cysteine, heating produces an aroma with intense meat character. The product is suitable for meat-like products made from natural or synthetic proteins as well as soups, sauces, etc. at a rate of 0.2 to 4%.

## Production of L-Amino Acids

Chemical synthesis of amino acids yields a racemic mixture, but only the L-isomer is biologically active; the D-isomers may in fact be antimetabolites. Aminoacylase is an enzyme capable of deacylating acylated L-amino acids but not the D-isomer derivatives. The amino acid mixture is first acylated and then treated with aminoacylase (now available in immobilized form) which yields a mixture of L-amino acid and acyl D-amino acid which can be readily separated by solubility differences.[111]

$$
\underset{\text{Acyl DL-Amino acids}}{R-\overset{\overset{O}{\|}}{C}-\underset{\underset{H}{|}}{\overset{\overset{R}{|}}{N}}-\underset{\underset{H}{|}}{\overset{\overset{O}{\|}}{C}}-C-OH} \xrightarrow[\text{Amino acylase}]{H_2O} \underset{\text{L-Amino acid}}{H_2N-\underset{\underset{H}{|}}{\overset{\overset{R}{|}}{C}}-\overset{\overset{O}{\|}}{C}-OH} + \underset{\text{Acyl-D-Amino acid}}{HO-\overset{\overset{O}{\|}}{C}-\underset{\underset{H}{|}}{\overset{\overset{R}{|}}{C}}-\underset{\underset{H}{|}}{N}-\overset{\overset{O}{\|}}{C}-R}
$$

Trypsin has a somewhat similar application in the production of lysine from DL-lysine raceinates.[482] L-lysine is methylated by reaction with methanol in HCl, the L-lysine ester is hydrolyzed by immobilized trypsin which is unable to hydrolyze the ester of D-lysine. L-lysine is precipitated from methanol and the D-isomer racemized and recycled.

## Utilization Of Cellulose

According to Skinner[644] plants produce $10^{11}$ tons of cellulose per annum. Since cellulose is composed primarily of glucose, there has long been considerable interest in producing glucose commercially from cellulose; the glucose could be used directly, isomerized to fructose/glucose syrups, or used as a feed-stock for the production of ethanol and other chemicals by fermentation or for the production of single-cell biomass. Although cellulose is recycled naturally through the action of microorganisms, it has been surprisingly difficult to isolate microorganisms capable of secreting a cellulase suitable for commercial exploitation. The U.S. Army Natick Development Center has recently isolated an organism, *Trichoderma viride,* which appears to be suitable and is operating a small prepilot plant facility to produce glucose from newspaper using a cellulase from *T. viride.* It is planned to scale up production to 500 tons of waste paper per day by 1980.[644]

## Detoxification of Foods

Plants contain a variety of substances which are themselves toxic to humans or are precursors of toxins.[412] Some of these compounds, e.g., phytate, have been considered previously; other substances, e.g., lactose and stachyose, which may not be considered as actual toxins, exhibit antimetabolic activity in certain circumstances.

Many cruciferous plants contain thioglycosides which are precursors of goiterogenic substances, mostly isothiocyanates, which are formed from the thioglycoside by an enzyme, myrosinase.

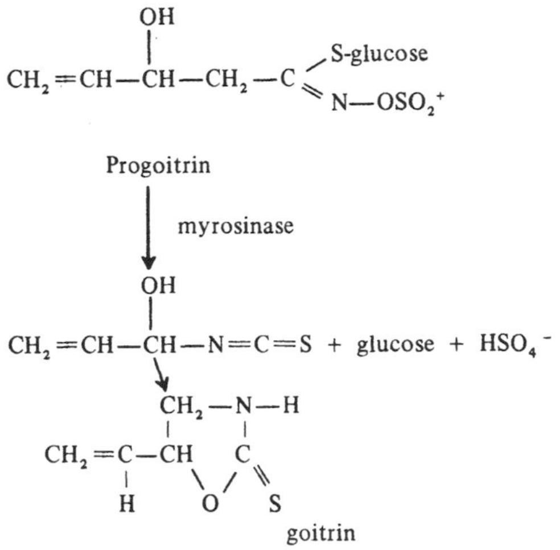

$$CH_2=CH-\overset{\overset{\displaystyle OH}{|}}{CH}-CH_2-C\overset{S\text{-glucose}}{\underset{N-OSO_2^+}{\diagdown}}$$

Progoitrin

$$\downarrow \text{ myrosinase}$$

$$CH_2=CH-\overset{\overset{\displaystyle OH}{|}}{CH}-N=C=S \ + \ glucose \ + \ HSO_4^-$$

$$CH_2=\overset{|}{\underset{H}{C}}-CH \quad \overset{CH_2-N-H}{\underset{O \quad S}{C}}$$

goitrin

Formation of isothiocyantes may be prevented by inactivating myrosinase, and preformed toxins may be removed by extraction with water or alkali. The possibility exists that a heat-inactivated meal may come in contact with an active source of myrosinase resulting in toxin production. It is best to degrade the thioglycoside completely prior to heat treatment, followed by extraction of the goiterogenic products.

Many legumes contain cyanogenetic glycosides, e.g., linamarin, which release HCN following the action of $\beta$-glucosidases, e.g., linamarinase:

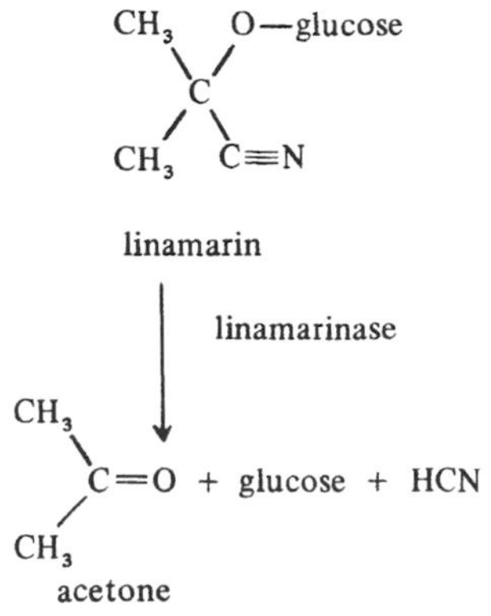

$$\overset{CH_3}{\underset{CH_3}{\diagup}}C\overset{O-glucose}{\underset{C\equiv N}{\diagdown}}$$

linamarin

$$\downarrow \text{ linamarinase}$$

$$\overset{CH_3}{\underset{CH_3}{\diagdown}}C=O \ + \ glucose \ + \ HCN$$

acetone

Toxicity is best overcome by fermenting the crushed product during which the glycosidic is completely degraded and the HCN formed is volatilized during subsequent cooking.

These and other examples of the use of enzymes in detoxification are discussed by Liener.[413]

## Hydrolysis of Oligosaccharides

Small oligosaccharides, e.g., raffinose and stachyose, cause problems for certain food industries:

1. Reduced recovery of sucrose from sugar beet
2. Flatulence in soya bean products

An α-galactosidase from *A. saitoi* has been investigated as a means of hydrolyzing these oligosaccharides and eliminating their effects.[673,678] Immobilized α-galactosidase is now used commercially for the treatment of sugar syrups from beet.

# REFERENCES

1. **Adams, J. B. and Blundstone, H. A. W.**, *The Biochemistry of Fruit and Vegetables*, Hulme, A. C., Ed., Vol. 2, Academic Press, London, 1971.
2. **Adler-Nissen, J.**, *J. Agric. Food Chem.*, 24, 1090, 1976.
3. **Adler-Nissen, J.**, *Process Biochem.*, 12(6), 18, 1977.
4. **Albershein, P., Neukom, H., and Deuel, H.**, *Helv. Chim. Acta*, 43, 1422, 1960.
5. **Allen, J. C. and Humphries, C.**, *J. Dairy Res.*, 44, 495, 1977.
6. **Allen, W. G. and Dawson, H. G.**, *Food Technol. (Chicago)*, 29(5), 70, 1975.
7. **Amoa, B. and Muller, H. G.**, *Cereal Chem.*, 53, 365, 1976.
8. **Anderson, J. A.**, Ed., *Enzymes and Their Role in Wheat Technology*, Interscience, New York, 1946.
9. **Anderson, M. L. and Ravesi, E. M.**, *J. Food Sci.*, 35, 551, 1970.
10. **Anti, A. W.**, *Candy Ind. and Confect. J.*, 135(4), 25, 1970.
11. **Arai, S., Noguchi, M., Kurosawa, S., Kato, H., and Fujimaki, M.**, *J. Food Sci.*, 35, 392, 1970.
12. **Arai, S., Yamashita, M., and Fujimaki, M.**, *Cereal Foods World*, 20, 107, 1975.
13. **Arai, S., Yamashita, M., Aso, K., and Fujimaki, M.**, *J. Food Sci.*, 40, 342, 1975.
15. **Archer, M. C., Stillings, B. R., Tannenbaum, S. R., and Wang, D. I.**, *J. Agric. Food Chem.*, 21, 1116, 1973.
16. **Arima, S., Shimazaki, K., Yamazumi, T., and Kamamaru, Y.**, *Jpn. J. Dairy Sci.*, 23, A83, 1974.
17. **Arnold, R. G., Shahani, K. M., and Dwivedi, B. K.**, *J. Dairy Sci.*, 58, 1127, 1975.
18. **Ashengreen, N. H.**, *Process Biochem.*, 10(4), 17, 1975.
19. **Ashmore, C. R., Parker, W., and Doerr, L.**, *J. Anim. Sci.*, 34, 46, 1972.
20. **Ashoor, S. H., Sair, R. A., Olson, N. F., and Richardson, T.**, *Biochim. Biophys. Acta*, 229, 423, 1971.
21. **Aso, K., Yamashita, M., Arai, S., and Fujimaki, M.**, *Agric. Biol. Chem.*, 37, 2505, 1973.
22. **Aso, K., Yamashita, M., Arai, S., and Fujimaki, M.**, *Agric. Biol. Chem.*, 38, 679, 1974.
23. **Atallah, M. T., and Hultin, H. O.**, *J. Food Sci.*, 42, 7, 1977.
24. **Aurand, L. W., Chu, T. M., Singleton, J. A., and Shen, R.**, *J. Dairy Sci.*, 50, 465, 1967.
25. **Awad, A., Powrie, W. D., and Fennema, O.**, *J. Food Sci.*, 34, 1, 1969.
26. **Axelrod, B.**, *Adv. Chem. Ser.*, 136, 324, 1974.
27. **Babel, F. J. and Hammer, B. W.**, *J. Dairy Sci.*, 28, 201, 1945.
28. **Bailey, M. E. and Kim, M. K.**, 20th Eur. Meeting Meat Res. Workers, Dublin, September 15 to 20, 1974, 36.
30. **Baker, R. A.**, *J. Food Sci.*, 41, 1198, 1976.
31. **Baldwin, E.**, *Dynamic Aspects of Biochemistry*, 3rd ed., Cambridge University Press, London, 1957.
32. **Ballester, D., Yanez, E., Brunser, O., Stekel, P., Chadud, P., Castano, G., and Monckeberg, F.**, *J. Food Sci.*, 42, 407, 1977.
33. **Barker, S. A.**, *Process Biochem.*, 10(10), 39, 1975.
34. **Barman, T. E.**, *Enzyme Handbook*, Springer-Verlag, New York, 1969.
35. **Barman, T. E.**, *Enzyme Handbook*, Suppl. 1, Springer-Verlag, New York, 1974.
36. **Barnes, M. F. and Patchett, B. J.**, *J. Food Sci.*, 41, 1392, 1976.
37. **Barrett, A. J. and Dingle, J. T.**, *Tissue Proteinases*, North-Holland, Amsterdam, 1971.
38. **Barrett, A. J.**, *Lysosomes: A Laboratory Handbook*, Dingle, J. T., Ed., North-Holland, Amsterdam, 1972.

39. **Barrett, A. J.**, Proteases and Biological Control, in *Cold Spring Harbor Conf. Cell Proliferation,* Vol. 2, Reich, E., Rikin, D. B., and Shaw, E., Eds., Cold Spring Harbor Laboratory, New York, 1975.

40. **Bartolome, L. G. and Hoff, J. E.**, *J. Agric. Food Chem.,* 20, 266, 1972.

41. **Bate-Smith, E. C.**, *Adv. Food Res.,* 1, 1, 1948.

42. **Beck, C. I. and Scott, D.**, *Adv. Chem. Ser.,* 136, 1974.

43. **Bednarski, W., Poznanski, S., Jedrychowski, L., Leman, J., and Szezepaniak, M.**, *J. Milk Food Technol.,* 39, 521, 1976.

44. **de Becze, G. I.**, *Crit. Rev. Food Technol.,* 1, 479, 1970.

45. **Bendall, J. R.**, *The Physiology and Biochemistry of Muscle as a Food,* Briskey, E. J., Cassens, R. G., and Trautman, J. C., Eds., University of Wisconsin Press, Madison, 1966.

46. **Bendall, J. R.**, *J. Sci. Food Agric.,* 17, 333, 1966.

47. **Bendall, J. R.**, *Muscles, Molecules and Movement,* Heineman Educational, London, 1969.

48. **Bendall, J. R.**, *The Structure and Function of Muscle,* Vol. 2, 2nd ed., Bourne, C. H., Ed., Academic Press, New York, 1973.

49. **Bendall, J. R. and Wismer-Pedersen, J.**, *J. Food Sci.,* 27, 144, 1962.

50. **Bendall, J. R. and Lawrie, R. A.**, *Anim. Breed. Abstr.,* 32, 1, 1964.

51. **Bender, A. E.**, *Meat,* Cole, D. A. and Lawrie, R. A., Eds., Butterworths, London, 1975.

52. **Bergemeyer, H. U.**, *Methods of Enzymatic Analysis,* Academic Press, New York, 1965.

53. **Berthet, J., Berthet, L., Applemans, F., and de Duve, C.**, *Biochem. J.,* 50, 182, 1951.

54. **Berthet, J. and de Duve, C.**, *Biochem. J.,* 50, 170, 1951.

55. **Beuchat, L. R.**, *J. Agric. Food Chem.,* 21, 453, 1973.

56. **Biale, J. B.**, *Science,* 146, 880, 1964.

57. **Bingham, E. W., Jasewiez, L., and Zittle, C. A.**, *J. Dairy Sci.,* 44, 1247, 1961.

58. **Bingham, E. W. and Zittle, C. A.**, *Arch. Biochem. Biophys.,* 101, 471, 1963.

59. **Birch, G. G. and Green, L. F.**, *Molecular Structure and Function of Food Carbohydrates,* Applied Science, London, 1973.

60. **Bliss, M. J.**, *Encyclopedia of Chemical Technology,* Vol. 2, Interscience, New York, 1953, 212.

61. **Bodwell, C. E. and Pearson, A. M.**, *J. Food Sci.,* 29, 602, 1964.

62. **Bodwell, C. W., Pearson, A. M., and Fanelli, R. A.**, *J. Food Sci.,* 30, 944, 1965.

63. **Boelens, M., de Valoic, P. J., Wobben, H. J., and Van den Gen, A.**, *J. Agric. Food Chem.,* 19, 984, 1971.

64. **Boerhinger-Mannheim**, Food Analysis Manual, Boerhinger-Mannheim, GmGH, Germany, 1971.

65. **Bohler, P., Kirschke, H., Langner, J., Ansorge, S., Wiederanders, B., and Hanson, H.**, *Tissue Proteinases,* Barrett, A. J. and Dingle, J. T., Eds., North-Holland, Amsterdam, 1971.

66. **Bolin, H. R., Stafford, A. E., and Fuller, G.**, *Food Prod. Dev.,* 9(7), 92, 1975.

67. **Borgstrom, G.**, *Principles of Food Science,* Vol. 2, Macmillan, New York, 1968.

68. **Bouin, J. C., Atallah, M. T., and Hultin, H. O.**, *Biotechnol. Bioeng.,* 17, 1783, 1975.

69. **Bouin, J. C., Dudgeon, P. H., and Hultin, H. O.**, *J. Food Sci.,* 41, 886, 1976.

70. **Bourne, G. H.**, Ed., *The Structure and Function of Muscle,* Vols. 1—4, 2nd ed., Academic Press, New York, 1973.

71. **Bouma, J. M. W. and Gruber, M.**, *Biochim. Biophys. Acta,* 89, 545, 1964.

72. **Bouton, P. E., Howard, A., and Lawrie, R. A.**, Special Report No. 66, Food Invest. Board, London, 1957.

73. **Boyer, P. D.**, *The Enzymes,* Academic Press, New York, 1970.

74. **Bradley, H. C.**, *Physiol. Rev.,* 18, 173, 1938.

75. **Branaman, G. A., Pearson, A. M., Magee, W. T., Griswold, R. M., and Brown, G. A.**, *J. Anim. Sci.,* 21, 321, 1962.

76. **Bray, R. W.**, *J. Anim. Sci.,* 25, 838, 1966.

77. **Brignon, G., Ribadeau-Dumas, B., and Mercier, J.**, *FEBS Lett.,* 71(1), 111, 1976.

78. **Briskey, E. J.**, Proc. Campbell Soup Co., Meat Tenderness Symp., Camden, New Jersey, 1963.

79. **Briskey, E. J.**, *Adv. Food Res.,* 13, 89, 1964.

80. **Briskey, E. J. and Fukazawa, T.**, *Adv. Food. Res.,* 19, 279, 1971.

81. **Briskey, E. J. and Lister, D.**, *The Pork Industry: Problems and Progress,* Toppel, D. G., Ed., Iowa State University Press, Ames, 1969.

82. **Briskey, E. J., Cassens, R. G., and Trautman, J. C.**, Eds., *The Physiology and Biochemistry of Muscle as a Food,* University of Wisconsin Press, Madison, 1966.

83. **Briskey, E. J., Cassens, R. G., and Marsh, B. B.**, Eds., *The Physiology and Biochemistry of Muscle as a Food,* Vol. 2, University of Wisconsin Press, Madison, 1970.

84. **Brown, R. J. and Swaisgood, H. W.**, *J. Dairy Sci.,* 58, 796, 1975.

85. **Bruce, H. M. and Callow, R. W.**, *Biochem. J.,* 28, 517, 1934.

86. **Bruemmer, J. H., Roe, B., Bowen, E. R., and Buslig, B.**, *J. Food Sci.,* 41, 186, 1976.

87. Bryce, W. W., *IFST(U.K.), Proc.*, 8(2), 75, 1975.
88. Buchanan, R. A., Bready, B. J. S., and Marston, P. E., *Proc. 19th Int. Dairy Congr.*, IE, 457, 1970.
89. Buckley, D. J., Gann, G. Z., Price, J. P., and Spink, G. C., *J. Food Sci.*, 39, 825, 1974.
90. Burnette, F. S., *J. Food Sci.*, 42, 1, 1977.
91. Burt, J. R., *Process Biochem.* 12(1), 32, 1977.
92. Burt, J. R., Strond, G. D., and Jones, N. R., *Freezing and Irradiation of Fish*, Kreuzer, R., Ed., Fishing News (Books), London, 1969.
93. Busch, W. A., Stromer, M. H., Goll, D. E., and Suzuki, A., *J. Cell Biol.*, 52, 367, 1972.
94. Butler, L. G., Squires, R. G., and Kelly, S. J., *Sugar Azucar*, 72(4), 31, 1977.
95. Carson, J. F., *The Chemistry and Physiology of Flavours*, Schultz, H. W., Day, E. A., and Libbey, L. M., Eds., AVI Publishing, Westport, Conn., 1967.
96. Carse, W. A., *Annu. Res. Rep.*, Meat Industry Research Institute, New Zealand, 1972, 32.
97. Cassens, R. G., *The Physiology and Biochemistry of Muscle as a Food*, Briskey, E. J., Cassens, R. G., and Trautman, J. C., Eds., University of Wisconsin Press, Madison, 1966.
98. Cassens, R. G., Ed., *Muscle Biology*, Vol. 1, Marcel Dekker, New York, 1972.
99. Cassens, R. G., Geisler, F., and Kolb, Q., Eds., *Proc. Pork Quality Symp.*, University of Wisconsin Press, Madison, 1972.
100. Cassens, R. G., Marple, D. N., and Eikelenboom, G., *Adv. Food Res.*, 21, 71, 1975.
101. Chandan, R. C. and Shahani, K. M., *J. Dairy Sci.*, 46, 275, 1963.
102. Chandan, R. C. and Shahani, K. M., *J. Dairy Sci.*, 47, 471, 1964.
103. Chandan, R. C., Parry, R. M., Jr., and Shahani, K. M., *Biochim. Biophys. Acta*, 110, 389, 1965.
104. Chandan, R. C., Parry, R. M., Jr., and Shahani, K. M., *J. Dairy Sci.*, 51, 606, 1968.
105. Chandler, B. V. and Nicol, K. J., *CSIRO Food Res. Q.*, 35, 79, 1975.
106. Charley, V. L. S., *Chem. Ind.*, 20, 635, 1969.
107. Chase, T., *Adv. Chem. Ser.*, 136, 241, 1974.
108. Cheftel, C., Ahern, M., Wang, D. I. C., and Tannenbaum, S. R., *J. Agric. Food Chem.*, 19, 155, 1971.
109. Cheryan, M., Van Wyk, P. J., Olson, N. F., and Richardson, T., *Biotechnol. Bioeng.*, 17, 585, 1975.
110. Cheryan, M., Van Wyk, P. J., Richardson, T., and Olson, N. F., *Biotechnol. Bioeng.*, 18, 273, 1976.
111. Chibata, I., *Conversion and Manufacture of Foodstuffs by Micro-organisms*, Proc. Int. Symp. Conv. Manuf. Microorganisms, Saikon Publishing, Tokyo, 1971.
112. Chichester, C. O., Ed., *The Chemistry of Plant Pigments*, Academic Press, New York, 1972.
113. Chu, H. D., Leader, J. G., and Gilbert, S. C., *J. Food Sci.*, 40, 641, 1975.
114. Claydon, T. J., Mickelsen, R., Pinkston, P. J., and Fish, N. L., *Food Technol.*, 22, 215, 1968.
115. Clegg, K. M., Lim, C. L., and Manson, W., *J. Dairy Res.*, 41, 283, 1974.
116. Clegg, K. M. and McMillan, A. D., *J. Food Technol.*, 9, 21, 1974.
117. Clegg, K. M., Smith, G., and Walker, A. L., *J. Food Technol.*, 9, 425, 1974.
118. Cobb, B. F., III and Hyder, K., *J. Food Sci.*, 37, 743, 1973.
119. Coggins, C. W. and Knapp, J. C. F., *Date Grow Inst. Rep.*, 46, 11, 1969.
120. Cohen, C., *Sci. Am.*, 233, 36, 1975.
121. Cohn, J. A., Hirsch, J. G., and Wiener, E., *Lysosomes*, de Reuch, A. V. S. and Cameron, M. P., Eds., Little, Brown, Boston, 1963.
122. *Cold Spring Harbor Symp. Quant. Biol., Vol. 37,* The Mechanism of Muscle Contraction, Cold Spring Harbor, New York, 1972.
123. Colwick, S. P. and Kaplan, N. O., Eds., *Methods in Enzymology*, Academic Press, New York, 1960.
124. Commission on Enzyme Nomenclature, *Enzyme Nomenclature*, Elsevier, Amsterdam, 1973.
125. Connell, J. E., *Can. Food Ind.*, 20(2), 23, 1966.
126. Connelly, J. J., Vely, V. G., Miuk, W. H., Sachel, G. F., and Litchfield, J. H., *Food Technol.*, 20, 829, 1966.
127. Cooke, R. D. and Caygill, J. C., *Trop. Sci.*, 16, 149, 1974.
128. Cordonnier, R. and Marteau, G., *Bull. OIV.*, 49, 490, 1976.
129. Couteaux, R., *The Structure and Function of Muscle*, Vol. 2 (Part 2), 2nd ed., Bourne, G. H., Academic Press, New York, 1973.
130. Criswell, L. G., Litchfield, J. H., Vely, V. G., and Sachsel, G. F., *Food Technol.*, 18, 1493, 1964.
131. Crocco, S. C., *Food Eng.*, 47(7), 54, 1975.
132. Crocker, E. C., *Food Res.*, 13, 179, 1948.
133. Crystall, B. B. and Hagyard, C. J., Annu. Res. Rep., Meat Industry Research Institute, New Zealand, 1973, 38.
134. Cuq, J. L., Prolansal, M., Guilleno, F., and Cliften, C., *J. Food Sci.*, 38, 11, 1973.
135. Dalfour, A., Jolles, J., Alais, C., and Jolles, P., *Biochim. Biophys. Res. Commun.*, 19, 452, 1965.

136. Dalrymple, R. H. and Kelly, R. F., *J. Anim. Sci.*, 29, 120, 1969.
137. Davey, C. L. and Dickson, R. M., *J. Food Sci.*, 35, 56, 1970.
138. Davey, C. L. and Gilbert, K. V., *J. Food Sci.*, 31, 135, 1966.
139. Davey, C. L. and Gilbert, K. V., *J. Food Sci.*, 34, 69, 1969.
140. Davey, C. L. and Gilbert, K. V., *J. Food Sci.*, 33, 2, 1968.
141. Davies, D. T. and Law, A. J. R., *J. Dairy Res.*, 44, 447, 1977.
142. Day, E. A., Flavour Chemistry, in *Advances in Chemistry Series No. 56,* American Chemical Society, Washington, D.C., 1966.
143. Dayton, W. R., Goll, D. E., Stromer, M. H., Reville, W. J., Zeece, M. G., and Robson, R. M., in *Cold Spring Harbor Conference on Cell Proliferation,* Vol. II, Proteases and Biological Control, Cold Spring Harbor, New York, 1975.
144. Dayton, W. R., Goll, D. E., Zeece, M. G., Robson, R. M., and Reville, W. J., *Biochemistry,* 15, 2150, 1976.
145. Dayton, W. R., Reville, W. J., Goll, D. E. and Stromer, M. H., *Biochemistry,* 15, 2159, 1976.
146. Dean, R. W. and Ball, C. O., *Food Technol.,* 14, 271, 1960.
147. de Duve, C. and Wattiaux, R., *Annu. Rev. Physiol.,* 28, 435, 1966.
148. de Fremey, D., *The Physiology and Biochemistry of Muscle as a Food,* Briskey, E. J., Cassens, R. G., and Trautman, J. C., Eds., University of Wisconsin Press, Madison, 1966.
149. de Koning, P. J., Int. Dairy Fed. Annu. Bull., Part 4, 1972.
150. Denault, L. J. and Underkofler, L. A., *Cereal Chem.,* 40, 618, 1963.
151. Denton, A. E., Beuk, J. F., Hogan, J. M., and McBrady, W. T., U.S. Patent 3,098,014, 1963.
152. Desmazeaud, M., Drapron, R., and Ribadeau-Dumas, B., *Aliment. Vie,* 63(3), 190, 1975.
153. Determann, H., Bonhard, K., Kohler, R., and Wieland, T., *Helv. Chim. Acta,* 46, 2498, 1963.
154. Determann, H. and Kohler, R., *Justus Liebigs Ann. Chem.,* 690, 197, 1965.
155. Determann, H., Eggenschwiller, S. and Michel, W., *Justus Liebigs Ann. Chem.,* 690, 183, 1965.
156. Determann, H., Heuer, J., and Janorek, D., *Justus Liebigs Ann. Chem.,* 690, 189, 1965.
157. Deuel, H. and Stutz, E., *Adv. Enzymol.,* 20, 341, 1958.
158. Dewdney, P. A., *Nutr. Food Sci.,* 33, 20, 1973.
159. Dickinson, D. B. and McCollum, J. P., *Nature (London),* 203, 525, 1964.
160. Dilley, D. R., *Nature (London),* 196, 387, 1962.
161. Dilley, D. R., *The Biochemistry of Fruits and Their Products,* Vol. 1, Hulme, A. C., Ed., Academic Press, New York, 1970.
162. Dilley, D. R., *J. Food Sci.,* 37, 518, 1972.
163. Dingle, J. T. and Fell, H. B., *Lysosomes in Biology and Pathology,* Vols. 1 and 2, North-Holland, Amsterdam, 1969.
164. Dixon, M. and Webb, E. C., *Enzymes,* 3rd ed., Academic Press, New York, 1974.
165. Doesburg, J. J., *Pectin Substances in Fresh and Preserved Fruit and Vegetables,* Inst. Res. Storage Processing Hortic. Produce., Wageningen, The Netherlands, 1965.
166. Downey, W. K., Proc. 19th Int. Dairy Congr., New Delhi, B, 323, 1974.
167. Drawert, F., Heiman, W., and Emberger, R., *Anal. Chem.,* 694, 200, 1966.
168. Dreyfus, J. C., Kruh, J., and Schapira, G., in *Protein Metabolism,* Grass, G. F., Ed., Springer-Verlag, Berlin, 1962.
169. Drissen, F. M. and Stadhouders, J., *Neth. Milk Dairy J.,* 28, 130, 1974.
170. Dulley, J. R., *J. Dairy Res.,* 39, 1, 1972.
171. Dürr, P. and Schobinger, U., *Alimenta,* 15, 143, 1976.
172. Dwivedi, B. K., *Crit. Rev. Food Technol.,* 3(4), 457, 1973.
173. Dwivedi, B. K., *Crit. Rev. Food Technol.,* 5, 487, 1975.
174. Dwivedi, B. K. and Kinsella, J. E., *J. Food Sci.,* 39, 620, 1974.
175. Ebashi, S. and Kodama, A., *J. Biochem. (Tokyo),* 60, 733, 1966.
176. Ebashi, S. and Nonamura, Y., *The Structure and Function of Muscle,* Vol. 3, 2nd ed., Bourne, G. H., Ed., Academic Press, New York, 1973.
177. Eigel, W. N., *Int. J. Biochem.,* 8, 187, 1977.
178. Eigel, W. N., *J. Dairy Sci.,* 60, 1399, 1977.
179. Endo, A., *Agric. Biol. Chem.,* 29, 229, 1965.
180. Eriksson, C. E., *J. Dairy Sci.,* 53, 1649, 1970.
181. Eriksson, C. E., *J. Food Sci.,* 32, 438, 1967.
182. Eriksson, C. E., *J. Food Sci.,* 33, 525, 1968.
183. Eriksen, S. and Fagerson, I. S., *J. Food Sci.,* 41, 490, 1976.
184. Ernstrom, C. A. and Wong, N. P., *Fundamentals of Dairy Chemistry,* Webb, B. H., Johnson, A. H., and Alford, J. A., Eds., AVI Publishing, Westport, Conn., 1974.
185. Eskin, N. A. M., Henderson, H. M., and Townsend, R. J., *Biochemistry of Foods,* Academic Press, New York, 1971.

186. Eskin, N. A. M., Grossman, S., and Pinsky, A., *Crit. Rev. Food Sci. Nutr.*, 9, 1, 1977.
187. Evans, R. B. and Wurtzburg, O. B., in *Starch: Chemistry and Technology*, Vol. 2, Whistler, R. C. and Paschall, E. P., Eds., Academic Press, New York, 1967.
188. Farnham, M. G., U.S. Patent 2,531,329, 1950.
189. Farnham, M. G., U.S. Patent 2,794,743, 1957.
190. Farrell, H. M., Jr. and Thompson, M. P., *Fundamentals of Dairy Chemistry*, 2nd ed., Webb, B. H., Johnson, A. H., and Alford, J. A. Eds., AVI Publishing, Westport, Conn., 1974.
191. Farris, P. L., *Starch: Chemistry and Technology*, Part 1, Whistler R. C. and Paschall, E. P., Eds., Academic Press, New York, 1965.
192. Faulkner, J. A., *The Physiology and Biochemistry of Muscle as a Food*, Part 2, Briskey, E. J., Cassens, R. G., and Marsh, B. B., Eds., University of Wisconsin Press, Madison, 1970.
193. Feeney, R. E. and Whitaker, J. R., Eds., *Food Proteins: Improvement through Chemical and Enzymatic Modification*, Adv. Chem. Ser. No. 160, American Chemical Society, Washington, D.C., 1977.
194. Fennema, O. R., Ed., *Principles of Food Science, Part 1. Food Chemistry*, Marcel Dekker, New York, 1976.
195. Ferrier, L. K., Richardson, T., Olson, N. F., and Hicks, C. L., *J. Dairy Sci.*, 55, 726, 1972.
196. Fink, A. L. and Hay, G. W., *Can. J. Biochem.*, 47, 135, 1969.
197. Finkle, B. J., U.S. Patent 3,126,287, 1964.
198. Fleming, H. P., Cobb, W. Y., Etchells, J. L., and Bell, T. A., *J. Food Sci.*, 33, 572, 1968.
199. Fogarty, W. M. and Ward, O. P., *Process Biochem.*, 7(8), 13, 1972.
200. Fogarty, W. M. and Ward, O. P., *Prog. Ind. Microbiol.*, 13, 59, 1974.
201. Foltmann, B., *Milk Proteins: Chemistry and Molecular Biology*, Vol. 2, McKenzie, H. A., Ed., Academic Press, New York, 1971.
202. Forrest, J. C., Aberle, E. D., Hedrick, H. B., Judge, M. D., and Merkel, R. A., *Principles of Meat Science*, Freeman, San Francisco, 1975.
203. Forrest, J. C., Gundlach, R. F., and Briskey, E. J., Proc. Res. Council Amer. Meat Inst. Found., Univ. of Chicago, 1963, 81.
204. Forrest, J. C., Will, J. A., Schmidt, G. R., Judge, M. D., and Briskey, E. J., *J. Appl. Physiol.*, 24, 33, 1968.
205. Foster, E. M., Nelson, F. E., Speck, M. C., Doctseh, R. N., and Olson, J. C., *Dairy Microbiology*, Prentice-Hall, Englewood Cliffs, N.J., 1958.
206. Fox, P. F. and Kosikowski, F. V., *J. Dairy Sci.*, 50, 1183, 1967.
207. Fox, P. F. and Tarassuk, N. P., *J. Dairy Sci.*, 51, 826, 1968.
208. Fox, P. F., *Industrial Aspects of Biochemistry*, Spenser, B., Ed., North-Holland, Amsterdam, 1974.
209. Fox, P. F. and Walley, B. F., *J. Dairy Res.*, 38, 165, 1971.
210. Fox, P. F., The use of milk and dairy products in non-dairy foods, in *Factors Affecting Milk Composition*, Moore, J. H., Ed., International Dairy Federation, Brussels, Doc. 125, 1980.
211. Fox, P. F., *Dairy Sci. Abstr.*, 40, 727, 1978.
212. Franzini-Armstrong, C., in *The Structure and Function of Muscle*, Vol. 2, Part 2, Bourne, G. H., Ed., 2nd ed., Academic Press, New York, 1973.
213. Fraser, D. I., Pitts, D. P., and Dyer, W. J., *J. Fish, Res. Board Can.*, 25, 239, 1968.
214. Fraser, D. I., Simpson, S. G. and Dyer, W. J., *J. Fish. Res. Board Can.*, 25, 817, 1968.
215. Frazier, W. C., *Food Microbiology*, 2nd ed., McGraw-Hill, New York, 1967.
216. Fresnel, J. M. and Trosset, D., Swiss Patent 564,602, 1975; *Food Sci. Technol. Abstr.*, 8, 12T 676, 1976.
217. Frenkel, C., Klein, I., and Dilley, D. R., *Phytochemistry*, 8, 994, 1969.
218. Fruton, J. S., Irving, G. W., and Bergman, M., *J. Biol. Chem.*, 141, 763, 1941.
219. Fuchs, F., *Annu. Rev. Physiol.*, 36, 461, 1974.
220. Fukawaza, T. and Briskey, E. J., *The Physiology and Biochemistry of Muscle as a Food*, Part 2, Briskey, E. J., Cassens, R. G., and Marsh, B. B., Eds., University of Wisconsin Press, Madison, 1970.
221. Fukazawa, T. and Yasui, T., *Biochim. Biophys. Acta*, 140, 534, 1967.
222. Fullbrook, P. D., *IFST (U.K.) Proc.*, 9(3), 105, 1976.
223. Fujimaki, M., Arai, S. and Yamashita, M., Enzymatic protein hydrolysis and plastein synthesis: their application to producing acceptable proteinacrous food materials, in *Conversion and Manufacture of Foodstuffs by Microorganisms*, Proc. Int. Symp. Conv. Manuf. Microorganisms, Saikon Publishing, Tokyo, 1971.
224. Fujimaki, M., Arai, S., and Yamashita, M., *Food Proteins: Improvement Through Chemical and Enzymatic Modification*, Feeney, R. E. and Whitaker, J. R., Eds., American Chemical Society, Washington, D.C., 1977.
225. Fujimaki, M., Yamashita, M., Okazawa, Y., and Arai, S., *J. Food Sci.*, 35, 215, 1970.
226. Fujimaki, M., Yamashita, M., Arai, S., and Kato, M., *Agric. Biol. Chem.*, 34, 1325, 1970.
227. Gams, Th. C., *Gordian*, 76(7/8), 210, 1975.

228. Gams, Th. C., *Die Sträke*, 28(10), 344, 1976.
229. Gams, Th. C., *Getreide Mehl Brot.*, 30(5), 113, 1976.
230. Gawron, O., Grelecki, C. J., and Duggan, M., *Arch. Biochem. Biophys.*, 44, 455, 1953.
231. Geddes, W. F., *Cereal Chem.*, 27, 14, 1950.
232. Geddes, W. F., *Food Technol.*, 11, 441, 1950.
233. Ghose, T. K., *Biotechnol. Bioeng.*, 11, 239, 1969.
234. Giddings, G. G., *Crit. Rev. Food Technol.*, 5, 143, 1974.
235. Giddings, G. G., *Crit. Rev. Food Sci. Nutr.*, 9, 81, 1977.
236. Goldspink, G. and McLoughlin, J. V., *Irish J. Agric. Res.*, 3, 9, 1964.
237. Goll, D. E., *Proc. 21st Annu. Recip. Meat Conf.*, Natl. Livestock Meat Board, Chicago, 1968, 16-46.
238. Goll, D. E., Arakawa, N., Stromer, M. H., Busch, W. A., and Robson, R. M., in *The Physiology and Biochemistry of Muscle as a Food*, Part 2, Briskey, E. J., Cassens, R. G., and Marsh, B. B., Eds., University of Wisconsin Press, Madison, 1970.
239. Goll, D. E., Stromer, M. H., Robson, R. M., Temple, J., Eason, B. A., and Busch, W. A., *J. Anim. Sci.*, 33, 963, 1971.
240. Goll, D. E., Robson, R. M., Temple, J., and Stromer, M. H., *Biochim. Biophys. Acta*, 226, 433, 1971.
241. Goll, D. E., Stromer, M. A., Olson, D. G., Dayton, W. R., Suzuki, A., and Robson, R. M., *Proc. Meat Ind. Res. Conf.*, American Meat Institute Foundation, Washington, D.C., 1974.
242. Goodwin, T. W., Ed., *Chemistry and Biochemistry of Plant Pigments*, Academic Press, New York, 1965.
243. Gordon, W. G. and Groves, M. L., *J. Dairy Sci.*, 58, 574, 1975.
244. Gordon, W. G. and Kalan, E. B., *Fundamentals of Dairy Chemistry*, 2nd ed., Webb, B. H., Johnson, A. H., and Alford, J. A., Eds., AVI Publishing, Westport, Conn., 1974.
245. Govindarajan, S., *Crit. Rev. Food Technol.*, 4, 117, 1973.
246. Grampp, E., *Food Technol.*, 31(11), 38, 1977.
247. Graveland, A., Pesman, L., and Van Erde, P., *Tech. Quart.*, 9, 97, 1972.
248. Greaser, M. L., *Proc. 27th Annu. Recip. Meat Conf.*, American Meat Science Association, 1974, 337.
249. Greaser, M. L., Cassens, R. G., Briskey, E. J., and Hoekstra, W. G., *J. Food Sci.*, 34, 120, 1969.
250. Greaser, M. L., Cassens, R. G., Hoekstra, W. G., and Briskey, E. J., *J. Food Sci.*, 34, 633, 1969.
251. Green, M. L., *Neth. Milk Dairy J.*, 27, 278, 1973.
252. Green, M. L., *J. Dairy Res.*, 44, 159, 1977.
253. Green, M. L. and Crutchfield, G., *Biochem. J.*, 115, 183, 1969.
254. Green, R. G., Carlson, W. E., and Evans, C. A., *J. Nutr.*, 23, 165, 1942.
255. Greenbank, G. R. and Pallansch, M. J., *J. Dairy Sci.*, 45, 958, 1962.
256. Greenfield, P. F. and Laurence, R. L., *Food Technol. Aust.*, 26, 509, 1974.
257. Greenfield, P. F. and Laurence, R. L., *J. Food Sci.*, 40, 906, 1975.
258. Gremli, H. and Wild, J., *Proc. 4th Inst. Congr. Food Sci. Tech.*, 1, 158, 1974.
259. Groninger, H. S., *Arch. Biochem. Biophys.*, 108, 175, 1964.
260. Groninger, H. S. and Spinelli, J., *J. Agric. Food Chem.*, 16, 97, 1968.
261. Gross, H., Bell, R. L., Fischer, F., and Redfern, S., *Cereal Sci. Today*, 12, 394, 1967.
262. Grosch, W. and Schwencke, D., *Lebensm. Wiss. Technol.*, 2, 109, 1969.
263. Grosch, W. and Schwartz, J. M., *Lipids*, 6, 351, 1971.
264. Groves, M. L., *Milk Proteins: Chemistry and Molecular Biology*, McKenzie, H. A., Ed., Academic Press, New York, 1971.
265. Gudnason, G. V. and Shipe, F., *J. Dairy Sci.*, 45, 1440, 1962.
266. Guildbault, G. G., *Enzymatic Methods of Analysis*, Pergamon Press, Elmsford, N.Y., 1970.
267. Gutmann, H. and Fruton, J. S., *J. Biol. Chem.*, 174, 851, 1948.
268. Guy, E. J., Vettel, H. E. and Pallansch, M. J., *J. Dairy Sci.*, 52, 432, 1969.
269. Haard, N. F., *Crit. Rev. Food Technol.*, 2, 305, 1971.
270. Haard, N. F., in *Principles of Food Science, Part I, Food Chemistry*, Fennema, O. R., Ed., Marcel Dekker, New York, 1976.
271. Haga, T., Yamamoto, M., Maruyana, K., and Noda, H., *Biochim. Biophys. Acta*, 127, 128, 1966.
272. Haggett, T. O. R., *Proc. 18th Int. Dairy Congr.*, B(5), 339, 1970.
273. Hale, M. B., *Food Technol.*, 33, 107, 1969.
274. Hall, J. T., *Proc. Pork Quality Symp.*, Cassens, R. G., Geisler, F., and Kolb, Q., Eds., University of Wisconsin Press, Madison, 1972.
275. Hall, C. B. and Mullins, J. T., *Nature (London)*, 206, 638, 1965.
276. Hamdy, M. K., May, K. N., and Powers, J. J., *Proc. Soc. Exp. Biol. Med.*, 108, 185, 1961.
277. Hansen, P. M. T. and Black, D. H., *J. Food Sci.*, 37, 452, 1970.

278. Harris, R. S. and von Loesecke, E., Eds., *Nutritional Evaluation of Food Processing*, AVI Publishing, Westport, Conn., 1973.

279. Harper, W. J., *J. Dairy Sci.*, 40, 556, 1957.

280. Harper, W. J. and Gould, I. A., *J. Dairy Sci.*, 38, 87, 1955.

281. Harper, W. J. and Long, J. E., *J. Dairy Sci.*, 39, 129, 1956.

282. Harte, B. R. and Stein, C. M., *J. Dairy Sci.*, 60, 1266, 1977.

283. Hasegawa, S., Maier, V. P., Kaszychi, H. P., and Grawford, J. K,, *J. Food Sci.*, 34, 525, 1969.

284. Hasegawa, S. and Nagel, C. W., *Arch. Biochem. Biophys.*, 124, 513, 1968.

285. Hasegawa, S. and Smolensky, D. C., *J. Food Sci.*, 36, 966, 1971.

286. Hashimoto, Y., FAO Symp. Significance Fundamental Res. Utiliz. Fish, Husum, Germany, 1964, WP/11/6.

287. Hasselbach, W. and Makinose, M., *Biochem. Biophys. Res. Commun.*, 7, 132, 1962.

288. Hatanaka, C. and Ozawa, J., *Agric. Biol. Chem.*, 28, 627, 1964.

289. Hatenaka, A. and Ohno, M., *Agric. Biol. Chem.*, 35, 1044, 1971.

290. Havel, R. J., *The Physiology and Biochemistry of Muscle as a Food*, Part 2, Briskey, E. J., Cassens, R. G., and Marsh, B. B., Eds., University of Wisconsin Press, Madison, 1970.

291. Henderson, D. W., Goll, D. E., and Stromer, M. H., *Am. J. Anat.*, 128, 117, 1970.

292. Herbert, R. A. and Shewan, J. M., *J. Sci. Food Agric.*, 27, 89, 1976.

293. Herring, W. M., Laurence, R. L., and Kittrell, J. R., *Biotechnol. Bioeng.*, 14, 1975, 1972.

294. Herrington, B. L., *J. Dairy Sci.*, 37, 775, 1954.

295. Hers, H. G., de Wulf, H., and Stalmans, W., *FEBS Lett.*, 12, 73, 1970.

296. Hessel-de-Heer, J. C. M., Schmidt, G. R., Sybesma, W., and van der Wal, P. G., Eds., *Proc. 2nd Int. Symp. Condition Meat Qual. Pigs*, Wageningen, The Netherlands, 1971.

297. Hevia, P., Whitaker, J. R., and Olcolt, H. S., *J. Agric. Food Chem.*, 24, 383, 1976.

298. Hewitt, E. J., *J. Agric. Food Chem.*, 11, 14, 1963.

299. Hewitt, E. J., Mackey, D. A. M., Konigsbacher, S., and Hassenstrom, T., *Food Technol.*, 10, 487, 1956.

300. Herz, K. O. and Chang, S. S., *Adv. Food Res.*, 18, 1, 1970.

301. Hicks, C. L., Ferrier, L. K., Olson, N. F., and Richardson, T., *J. Dairy Sci.*, 58, 19, 1975.

302. Hidalgo, J. and Gamper, E., *J. Dairy Sci.*, 60, 1515, 1977.

303. Hildebrand, F. C., *Enzymes and Their Role in Wheat Technology*, Anderson, J. A., Ed., Interscience, New York, 1946.

304. Hiltz, D. F., Dyer, W. J., Nowlan, S., and Dingle, J. R., *Fish Inspection and Quality Control*, Kreuzer, R., Ed., Fishing News (Books), London, 1971.

305. Hinton, D. M. and Pressey, R., *J. Food Sci.*, 39, 783, 1974.

306. Hobson, G. E., *Biochem. J.*, 92, 324, 1964.

307. Hobson, G. E., *J. Food Sci.*, 33, 588, 1968.

308. v. Hofsten, B. and Lalasidis, G., *J. Agric. Food Chem.*, 24, 461, 1976.

309. Holmes, D. G., Duersch, J. W., and Ernstrom, C. A., *J. Dairy Sci.*, 60, 862, 1977.

310. Hoover, W. J., *Food Process.*, 25(10), 67, 1964.

311. Howe, M. and Glick, D., *Cereal Chem.*, 23, 360, 1946.

312. Hsu, C. P., Deshpande, S. N., and Desrosier, N. W., *J. Food Sci.*, 30, 583, 1965.

313. Huang, H. T., *Nature (London)*, 177, 39, 1956.

314. Huang, H. T., *J. Agric. Food Chem.*, 3, 141, 1955.

315. Huang, H. T. and Dooley, J. G., *Biotechnol. Bioeng.*, 18, 909, 1976.

316. Huang, F. L. and Tappel, A. L., *Biochim. Biophys. Acta*, 236, 739, 1971.

317. Huffman, D. L., Palmer, A. Z., Carpenter, J. W., Hargrove, D. D., and Kroger, M., *J. Anim. Sci.*, 26, 290, 1967.

318. Hulme, A. C., *The Biochemistry of Fruit and their Products*, Vol. 1, Academic Press, New York, 1970.

319. Hulme, A. C., *The Biochemistry of Fruit and their Products*, Vol. 2, Academic Press, New York, 1971.

320. Hulme, A. C., Jones, J. D., and Wooltorton, L. S. C., *Proc. R. Soc. London Ser. B.*, 158, 514, 1963.

321. Hulme, A. C. and Wooltorton, L. S. C., *Nature (London)*, 196, 388, 1962.

322. Hultin, H. O., *J. Food Sci.*, 37, 524, 1972.

323. Hultin, H. O., *Principles of Food Science, Part II, Food Chemistry*, Fennema, O. R., Ed., Marcel Dekker, New York, 1976.

324. Hunter, A. C., Wilson, J. M., and Greig, G. W., *J. Soc. Dairy Technol.*, 21, 139, 1968.

325. Huston, R. B. and Krebs, E. G., *Biochemistry*, 7, 2116, 1968.

326. Hwang, Q. S., Ramachandran, K. S., and Whitney, R. McL., *J. Dairy Sci.*, 50, 1723, 1967.

327. Hyde, R. B. and Morrison, J. W., *Am. Potato J.*, 41, 163, 1964.

328. Iacobucci, G. A., Myers, M. J., Emi, S., and Myres, D. V., 4th Int. Food Sci. Technol. Congr., Madrid, 1974; Adler-Nissen, J., *J. Agric. Food Chem.*, 24, 1090, 1976.
329. I.D.F. Proc. Lipolysis Symp., Cork, Ireland, 1975, Downey, W. K. and Cogan, T. M., Eds., Doc. No. 86, International Dairy Federation, Brussels.
330. Inesi, G., Millman, M., and Eletr, S., *J. Mol. Biol.*, 81, 483, 1973.
331. Ioannou, J., Chism, G., and Haard, N. F., *J. Food Sci.*, 38, 1022, 1973.
332. Isherwood, F. A., *Recent Advances in Food Science, Vol. 3, Biochemistry and Biophysics*, Leitch, J. M. and Rhodes, D. N., Eds., Butterworths, London, 1963.
333. Jaeggi, K., Krasnohajew, V., Weber, P., Wild, J., Givaudan, L., and Cie, S. A., Br. Patent 1,449,279, 1976; *Food Sci. Technol. Abstr.*, 9, 8 T456, 1977.
334. Jahns, F. D., Howe, J. L., Coduri, R. J., and Rand, A. G., *Food Technol.*, 30(7), 27, 1976.
335. James, W. O., *Plant Respiration*, Oxford University Press, Oxford.
336. Janolino, V. G. and Swaisgood, H. E., *J. Biol. Chem.*, 250, 2532, 1975.
337. Jay, J. M., *Modern Food Microbiology*, D-Van Nostrand, New York, 1970.
338. Jaynes, T. A., and Nelson, O. E., *Plant Physiol.*, 47, 629, 1971.
339. Jensen, R. G., *J. Dairy Sci.*, 47, 210, 1964.
340. Johnson, H. A., *Fundamentals of Dairy Chemistry*, Webb, B. H., Johnson, A. H., and Alford, J. A., Eds., AVI Publishing, Westport, Conn., 1974.
341. Johnson, A. E., Nursten, H. E., and Williams, A. A., *Chem. Ind. Week*, 21, 556, 1971.
342. Johnson, A. E., Nursten, H. E., and Williams, A. A., *Chem. Ind. Week*, 43, 1212, 1971.
343. Johnson, A. R. and Vickery, J. R., *J. Sci. Food Agric.*, 15, 695, 1964.
344. Jolles, P. and Jolles, J., *Nature (London)*, 192, 1187, 1961.
345. Jolly, R. C. and Kosikowski, F. V., *J. Dairy Sci.*, 58, 846, 1975.
346. Jolly, R. C. and Kosikowski, F. V., *J. Dairy Sci.*, 58, 1272, 1975.
347. Jones, J. G., *IFST (U.K.) Proc.*, 9(3), 99, 1976.
348. Jones, N. R., *Proc. 11th Int. Congr. Refrig.*, Munich, 1963, 917.
349. Jones, N. R. and Murray, J., *J. Sci. Food Agric.*, 15, 684, 1964.
350. Joseph, R. L. and Saunders, W. G., *Biochem. J.*, 100, 827, 1966.
351. Joslyn, M. A., *Adv. Enzymol. Relat. Subj. Biochem.*, 9, 613, 1949.
352. Joslyn, M. A., *Adv. Food Res.*, 11, 1, 1962.
353. Jost, R. and Monti, J. C., *J. Dairy Sci.*, 60, 1387, 1977.
354. Judge, M. D., Briskey, E. J., Cassens, R. G., Forrest, J. C., and Meyer, R. K., *Am. J. Physiol.*, 214, 146, 1968.
355. Kaminogawa, S., Mizobuchi, H., and Yamauchi, K., *Agric. Biol. Chem.*, 36, 2163, 1972.
356. Kaminogawa, S., Sato, F., and Yamuchi, K., *Agric. Biol. Chem.*, 35, 1465, 1971.
357. Kaminogawa, S. and Yamauchi, K., *Agric. Biol. Chem.*, 38, 2343, 1974.
358. Kaminogawa, S. and Yamauchi, K., *Agric. Biol. Chem.*, 36, 255, 1972.
359. Kaminogawa, S., Yamauchi, K., and Tsugo, T., *Jpn. J. Zootech. Sci.*, 40, 559, 1969.
360. Kang, C. K. and Rice, E. E., *J. Food Sci.*, 35, 563, 1970.
361. Kano, T., Kakuma, F., Homma, M., and Fukuda, S., *Biochim. Biophys. Acta*, 88, 155, 1964.
362. Kassemsarm, B., Sanz-Perez, B., Murray, J., and Jones, N. R., *J. Sci. Food Agric.*, 15, 763, 1963.
363. Kastenschmidt, L. L., *The Physiology and Biochemistry of Muscle as a Food*, Part 2, Briskey, E. J., Cassens, R. G., and Marsh, B. B., Eds., University of Wisconsin Press, Madison, 1970.
364. Kastenschmidt, L. L., Hoekstra, W. G., and Briskey, E. J., *Nature (London)*, 212, 288, 1966.
365. Kazeniac, S. and Hall, R. M., *J. Food Sci.*, 35, 519, 1970.
366. Kennedy, J. F., *Adv. Carbohydr. Chem. Biochem.*, 29, 306, 1973.
367. Kennedy, M. G. H. and Isherwood, F. A., *Phytochemistry*, 14, 667, 1975.
368. Kent, N. L., *Technology of Cereals*, Pergamon Press, Oxford, 1970.
369. Kent-Jones, D. W. and Amos, A. J., *Modern Cereal Chemistry*, Northern Publishing, London, 1957.
370. Kertesz, Z. I., *The Pectic Substances*, Interscience, London, 1951.
371. Khan, A. W., and van den Berg, L., *J. Food Sci.*, 29, 49, 1964.
372. Khan, A. W. and Nakamura, R., *J. Food Sci.*, 35, 266, 1970.
373. Kidd, F. and West, C., *Rep. Food. Invest. Board for 1923*, 1924, 27.
374. Kidd, F. and West, C., *Proc. R. Soc. Ser. B*, 106, 93, 1930.
375. Kiermeier, F. and Petz, E., *Z. Lebensm. Unters. Forsch.*, 132, 342, 1967.
376. Kiermeier, F. and Petz, E., *Z. Lebensm. Unters. Forsch.*, 134, 97, 1967.
377. Kiermeier, F. and Petz, E., *Z. Lebensm. Unters. Forsch.*, 134, 149, 1967.
378. Kinsella, J. E. and Hwang, D. H., *Crit. Rev. Food Sci. Nutr.*, 8(2), 191, 1977.
379. Kirimura, J., Shimiza, A., Kimizuka, A., Ninomiya, T., and Katsuya, N., *J. Agric. Food Chem.*, 17, 689, 1969.
380. Kiss, E., *Tejipar*, 24(3), 53; *Food Sci. Technol. Abstr.*, 9, 5P770, 1977.
381. Kitchen, B. J., Taylor, G. C., and White, I. C., *J. Dairy Res.*, 37, 279, 1970.

382. Kleinschmidt, A. W., Higashiuchi, K., Anderson, R., and Ferrari, C. G., *Bakers Dig.*, 37(5), 44, 1963.
383. Kleter, G., *Neth. Milk Dairy J.*, 30, 254, 1976.
384. Kolattukudy, P. E., *Lipids*, 5, 259, 1970.
385. Kohn, R. R., *Lab. Invest.*, 20, 202, 1969.
386. Koller, A., Ph.D. dissertation No. 3774, E.H.T., Zurich, 1966.
387. Kooi, E. R. and Smith, R. J , *Food Technol.*, 36(9), 57, 1972.
388. Korus, R. A. and Olson, A. C., *J. Food Sci.*, 42, 258, 1977.
389. Kosikowski, F. V., *J. Food Sci.*, 58, 994, 1975.
390. Kosikowski, F. V., U.S. Patent 3,975,544, 1976; *Food Sci. Technol. Abstr.*, 9, 4P630, 1977.
391. Kosikowski, F. V. and Iwasaki, T., *J. Food Sci.*, 58, 963, 1975.
392. Koszalka, T. R. and Miller, L. L., *J. Biol. Chem.*, 235, 665, 1960.
393. Koszalka, T. R. and Miller, L. L., *J. Biol. Chem.*, 235, 669, 1960.
394. Kneen, E. and Sandstedt, R. M., *Enzymes and Their Role in Wheat Technology*, Anderson, J. A., Ed., Interscience, New York, 1946.
395. Kreen, M. I., Kestner, A. I., and Kask, K. A., Food Sci. Technol. Abstr., 7, 3L309, 1975.
396. Kretovich, V. L., Yarovenko, V. L., Mikeladze, V. M., Tokareva, R. R., Livshits, D. B., Salmanova, L., Datunashvili, E. N., and Vedernikova, E. I., *Enzyme Preparations in the Food Industry*, Pischechevaya Promyshlenmost (in Russian), 1976.
397. Krop, J. J. P. and Pilnik, W., *Lebensm. Wiss. Technol.*, 7, 62, 1974.
398. Kuehler, C. A. and Stine, C. M., *J. Food Sci.*, 39, 379, 1974.
399. Kundig, H. and Somogyi, J. C., *Vit. Res.*, 37, 476, 1967.
400. Kuninaka, A., *Conversion and Manufacture of Foodstuffs by Microorganisms*, Proc. Int. Symp. Conv. Manuf. Microorganisms, Saikon Publishing, Tokyo, 1971.
401. Kuninaka, A., Kibi, M., and Sakaguchi, K., *Food Technol.*, 18, 287, 1964.
402. Kupiecki, F. P. and Virtanen, A. I., *Acta Chem. Scand.*, 14, 1913, 1960.
403. Kushmerick, M. J. and Davies, R. D., *Biochim. Biophys. Acta*, 153, 279, 1968.
403a. Anon., *Proc. Int. Symp. Conversion Manuf. Foodstuffs Microorganisms*, Saikon Publishing, Tokyo, 1971.
404. Landmann, W. A., Proc. Meat Tenderness Symp., Campbell Soup Co., Camden, N.J., 1963.
405. Lardy, H. A., *The Physiology and Biochemistry of Muscle as a Food*, Briskey, E. J., Cassens, R. G., Trautmann, J. C., Eds., University of Wisconsin Press, Madison, 1966.
406. Lawrence, R. C. and Hawke, J. C., *J. Gen. Microbiol.*, 46, 65, 1967.
407. Lawrence, R. C. and Hawke, J. C., *J. Gen. Microbiol.*, 51, 289, 1968.
408. Lawrie, R. A., *Meat Science*, 3rd ed., Pergamon Press, Oxford, 1979.
409. Layrisse, M., Martinez-Torres, C., and Walker, R., *Am. J. Clin. Nutr.*, 25, 401, 1972.
410. Lea, C. H., *J. Soc. Chem. Ind.*, 56, 376T, 1937.
411. Lerner, A. B. and Fitzpatrick, T. B., *Physiol. Rev.*, 30, 91, 1950.
412. Liener, I. E., Ed., *Toxic Constituents in Plant Foodstuffs*, Academic Press, New York, 1969.
413. Liener, I. E., *Food Proteins: Improvement Through Chemical and Enzymatic Modification*, Feeney, R. E. and Whitaker, J. R., Eds., American Chemical Society, Washington, D.C., 1977.
414. Linko, Y. Y., Pohjola, L., and Linko, P., *Process Biochem.*, 12(6), 14, 1977.
415. Lister, D., *The Physiology and Biochemistry of Muscle as a Food, Part 2*, Briskey, E. J., Cassens, R. G., and Marsh, B. B., Eds., University of Wisconsin Press, Madison, 1970.
416. Lister, D., E.E.A.P. Pig Commission, 1972.
417. Lister, D. and Ratcliff, P. W., Proc. 2nd Int. Symp. Cond. Meat Qual. Pigs, Hessel-de-Heer, J. C. M., Schmidt, G.R., Sybesma, W., and vander Wal, P. G., Eds., Wageningen, The Netherlands, 1971.
418. Locker, R. H., *Food Res.*, 25, 304, 1966.
419. Locker, R. H. and Hagward, C. J., *J. Sci. Food Agric.*, 14, 787, 1963.
420. Locker, R. H., Davey, C. L., Nottingham, P. M., Haughey, D. P., and Law, N. H., *Adv. Food Res.*, 21, 157, 1975.
421. Looney, N. E. and Patterson, M. E., *Nature (London)*, 214, 1245, 1967.
422. Lopez, A. and Li-Hsiang, Li, *Food Technol.*, 22, 1023, 1968.
423. Lovern, J. A. and Olley, J., *J. Food Sci.*, 27, 551, 1962.
424. Lowey, S., Slayter, H. S., Weeds, A. G., and Baker, H., *J. Mol. Biol.*, 42, 1, 1969.
425. Lowrie, R. J. and Lawrence, R. C., *N.Z. J. Dairy Sci. Technol.*, 7, 51, 1972.
426. Lu, A. T. and Whitaker, J. R., *J. Food Sci.*, 39, 1173, 1974.
427. Luck, H., *Dairy Sci. Abstr.*, 18, 32, 1956.
428. Lutola-Bosa, A. J. and MacRae, H. F., *J. Food Sci.*, 34, 401, 1969.
429. Lyster, R. L. J., *J. Dairy Res.*, 39, 279, 1972.
430. Mackinlay, A. G. and Wake, R. G., *Biochim. Biophys. Acta*, 104, 167, 1965.
431. Mackinlay, A. G. and Wake, R. G., *Milk Proteins: Chemistry and Molecular Biology*, McKenzie, H. A., Ed., Academic Press, New York, 1971.

432. MacLeod, A. J. and MacLeod, G., *J. Food Sci.*, 35, 739, 1970.

433. MacMillan, J. D. and Sheiman, M. I., *Adv. Chem. Ser.*, 136, 101, 1974.

434. Macy, R. L., Naumann, H. D., and Bailey, M. E., *J. Food Sci.*, 35, 78, 1970.

435. Maga, J. A., *Crit. Rev. Food Technol.*, 5(4), 443, 1975.

436. Maga, J. A., *Crit. Rev. Food Sci. Nutr.*, 6, 153, 1975.

437. Maga, J. A., *Crit. Rev. Food Sci. Nutr.*, 6, 241, 1975.

438. Maga, J. A., *Crit. Rev. Food Sci. Nutr.*, 7, 147, 1976.

439. Major, R. T. and Thomas, M., *Phytochemistry*, 11, 611, 1972.

440. Mandels, M., Hontz, L. and Nystrom, J., *Biotechnol. Bioeng.*, 16 1471, 1974.

441. Mangino, M. E. and Brunner, J. R., *J. Dairy Sci.*, 60, 841, 1977.

442. Manners, D. T., *Adv. Carbohydr. Chem.*, 17, 371, 1962.

443. Manson, W., Submission to IDF Group D3, Sept. 10, 1976.

444. Manson, W., Carolan, T., and Annan, W. D., *Eur. J. Biochem.*, 78, 411, 1977.

445. Manyua, J. K., *Milchwissenschaft*, 29, 737, 1974.

446. Manyua, J. K., *Milchwissenschaft*, 30, 730, 1975.

447. Mapson, L. W., *Nutrition (London)*, 19, 123, 1965.

448. Mapson, L. W., Swain, T., and Tomalin, A. W., *J. Sci. Food Agric.*, 14, 673, 1963.

449. Markakis, P., *Crit. Rev. Food Technol.*, 4, 437, 1974.

450. Markey, P. E., Greenfield, P. F., and Kittreal, J. R., *Biotechnol. Bioeng.*, 17, 285, 1975.

451. Markower, R. and Schwimmer, S., U.S. Patent 2,738,280, 1956.

452. Marsh, B. B. and Thompson, J. F., *J. Sci. Food Agric.*, 9, 417, 1958.

453. Marsh, B. B. and Leet, N. G., *J. Food Sci.*, 31, 450, 1966.

454. Marsh, B. B., *Meat*, Cole, D. J. A. and Lawrie, R. A., Eds., Butterworths, London, 1975.

455. Marshall, J. J., *Wallerstein Lab. Commun.*, 35, 49, 1972.

456. Marshall, J. J., *Die Starke*, 27(11), 377, 1975.

457. Marshall, R. O. and Kooi, E. R., *Science*, 125, 648, 1957.

458. Martens, R. and Naudts, M., *Annu. Bull. Int. Dairy Fed.*, Doc. 91, 1976.

459. Marshall, W. E., *Biotechnol. Bioeng.*, 18, 921, 1976.

460. Matsui, T., Shimizu, C., and Matsuura, F., *Bull. Jpn. Soc. Sci. Fish.*, 41, 761, 1975.

461. Matz, S. A., *The Chemistry and Technology of Cereals as Food and Feed*, AVI Publishing, Westport, Conn., 1959.

462. Matz, S. A., *Cereal Technology*, AVI Publishing, Westport, Conn., 1970.

463. McChance, R. A. and Widdowson, E. M., *J. Physiol.*, 101, 44, 1943.

464. McChance, R. A. and Widdowson, E. M., *J. Physiol.*, 101, 304, 1943.

465. McFeeters, R. F. and Chichester, C. O., Abstr. Pacific Slope Biochem. Conf., 1968, 58.

466. McGillivray, W. A., *N.Z. J. Dairy Sci. Technol.*, 7, 61, 1972.

467. McGlasson, W. B., *The Biochemistry of Fruit and their Products*, Vol. 1, Hulme, A. C., Ed., Academic Press, New York, 1970.

468. McKenzie, H. A., *Milk Proteins: Chemistry and Molecular Biology*, Vols. 1 and 2, Academic Press, New York, 1971.

469. McLoughlin, J. V., Proc. 9th Conf. Eur. Meat Res. Workers, Budapest, September 4 to 11, 1963.

470. McLoughlin, J. V., Proc. 17th Annu. Recip. Meat Conference, Wisconsin, June 10 to 12, 1964.

471. McLoughlin, J. V., *J. Food Sci.*, 35, 717, 1970.

472. McLoughlin, J. V. and Tarrant, P. J. V., *Recent Points of View on the Condition and Meat Quality of Pigs for Slaughter*, Sybesma, W., van der Wal, P. G., and Walstra, P., Eds., I.V.O. Zeist, The Netherlands, 1969.

473. Means, G. E. and Feeney, R. E., *Chemical Modification of Proteins*, Holden-Day, San Francisco, 1971.

474. Meigh, P. F., Pratt, H. K., and Cole, C., *Nature (London)*, 211, 419, 1966.

475. Menezes, H. C. de, Menezes, T. J. B. de, and Boas, H. V., *Biotechnol. Bioeng.*, 15, 1723, 1973.

476. Messer, M., Anderson, C. M., and Hubbard, L., *Gut*, 5, 295, 1964.

477. Messing, R. A., *Biotechnol. Bioeng.*, 16, 897, 1974.

478. Mitchell, J. H. and Henick, A. S., *Autoxidation and Antioxidants*, Vol. 2, Lundberg, W. O., Ed., Interscience, New York, 1962.

479. Miyada, D. S. and Tappel, A. L., *Food Res.*, 21, 217, 1956.

480. Miyauchi, D., Eklund, M., Spinelli, J., and Stoll, N., Summary Report for Division of Isotope Development, U.S. AEC Contract No. AT (49-11)-2058, U.S. Atomic Energy Commission, 1964.

481. Monsan, P. and Durand, G., *Ind. Aliment Agric.*, 93(5), 543, 1976.

482. Monsan, P. and Mazarguil, H., Colloq. Soc. Fr. Microbiol, Paris; Monsan, P. and Durand, G., *Ind. Aliment Agric.*, 93(5), 543, 1976.

483. Montreuil, J., *Ann. Nutr. Aliment.*, 25, A1, 1971.

484. Moran, F., Nasuno, S., and Starr, M. P., *Arch. Biochem. Biophys.*, 125, 734, 1968.

485. Moskowitz, G. J., Shen, T., West, I. R., Cassaigne, R., and Feldman, L. I., *J. Dairy Sci.*, 60, 1260, 1977.
486. Mulder, E. G., *Plant Soil*, 2, 59, 1949.
487. Muneta, P. and Walradt, J., *J. Food Sci.*, 33, 606, 1968.
488. Murphy, J. F. and Murphy, R. E., U.S. Patent 3,159,487, 1964.
489. Murray, D. G., *Food Eng.*, 41(5), 78, 1969.
490. Murray, D. G., *Food Eng.*, 41(6), 87, 1969.
491. Murray, T. K. and Baker, B. E., *J. Sci. Food Agric.*, 3, 170, 1952.
492. Murray, J. M. and Weber, A., *Sci. Am.*, 230, 58, 1974.
493. Myers, D. V., Ricks, E., Myers, M. J., Wilkinson, M., and Iacobucci, G. A., 5th Int. Food Sci. Technol. Congr., Madrid, 1974; Adler-Nissen, J., *J. Agric. Food Chem.*, 24, 1090, 1976.
494. Nagle, N. E. and Haard, N. F., *J. Food Sci.*, 40, 576, 1975.
495. Nagai, Y. and Funahashi, S., *Agric. Biol. Chem.*, 26, 794, 1962.
496. Naguib, K. and Hussein, L., *Milchwissenschaft*, 27, 758, 1972.
497. Naudts, M., *Annu. Bull. Int. Dairy Fed.*, 7, 1, 1969.
498. Nauss, K. M. and Davies, R. E., *J. Biol. Chem.*, 241, 2918, 1966.
499. Neal, G. E., *J. Sci. Food Agric.*, 16, 604, 1965.
500. Needham, D. M., *Machina Carnis*, Cambridge University Press, 1971.
501. Neelakanten, S., Shahani, K. M., and Arnold, R. G., *Food Prod. Dev.*, 5(7), 52, 1971.
502. Nelboeck, M. and Jaworek, D., *Chimica*, 29(3), 109, 1975.
503. Nelson, J. H., *Food Prod. Dev.*, 4(1), 53, 1970.
504. Nelson, J. H., *J. Agric. Food Chem.*, 18, 567, 1970.
505. Nelson, J. H., *J. Am. Oil Chem. Soc.*, 49, 559, 1972.
506. Nelson, J. H., *J. Dairy Sci.*, 58, 1739, 1975.
507. Neukom, H., *Schweiz, Landwirtsch. Forsch.*, 2, 112, 1963.
508. Neukom, H., *Kirk-Othmer Encycl. Chem. Tech.*, 14, 436, 1967.
509. Newbold, R. P., *The Physiology and Biochemistry of Muscle as a Food*, Briskey, E. J., Cassens, R. G., and Trautman, J. C., Eds., University of Wisconsin Press, Madison, 1966.
510. Newbold, R. P. and Lee, C. A., *Biochem. J.*, 97, 1, 1965.
511. Ney, K. H., *Z. Lebensm. Unters. Forsch.*, 147, 64, 1971.
512. Nickerson, T. A., *Fundamentals of Dairy Chemistry*, Webb, B. H., Johnson, A. H., and Alford, J. A., Eds., AVI Publishing, Westport, Conn., 1974.
513. Nicolaysen, R. and Njaa, L. R., *Acta Physiol. Scand.*, 22, 246, 1950.
514. Nielands, J. B. and Stumpf, P. K., *Outlines of Enzyme Chemistry*, John Wiley & Sons, New York, 1958.
515. Noomen, A., *Neth. Milk Dairy J.*, 29, 153, 1975.
516. Novikoff, A. B., *Lysosomes*, Ciba Foundation Symp., de Reuck, A. V. S. and Cameron, M. P., Eds., Little, Brown, Boston, 1963.
517. Novikoff, A. B., Essner, E., and Quintana, N., *Fed. Proc.*, 23, 1010, 1964.
518. Nursten, H. E., *The Biochemistry of Fruit and their Products*, Vol. 1, Hulme, A. C., Ed., Academic Press, New York, 1970.
519. Offer, G., *Companion to Biochemistry*, Bull, A. T., Lagnado, J. R., Thomas, J. D., and Tipton, K. F., Eds., Longman Group, London, 1974.
520. Ohad, I., Friedberg, I., Ne'eman, Z., and Schramm, M., *Plant Physiol.*, 47, 465, 1971.
521. Ohren, J. A. and Tuckey, S. L., *J. Dairy Sci.*, 47, 679, 1964.
522. Oi, S., Yamazaki, O., Sawada, A., and Satomura, Y., *Agric. Biol. Chem.*, 33, 729, 1969.
523. O'Keeffe, R. B., Fox, P. F., and Daly, C., *J. Dairy Res.*, 43, 97, 1976.
524. O'Keeffe, A. M., Fox, P. F., and Daly, C., *J. Dairy Res.*, 45, 465, 1978.
525. O'Leary, P. A. and Fox, P. F., *Irish J. Agric. Res.*, 12, 267, 1973.
526. O'Leary, V. S. and Woychik, J. H., *J. Food Sci.*, 41, 791, 1976.
527. Olley, J. and Duncan, W. R. H., *J. Sci. Food Agric.*, 16, 99, 1965.
528. Olson, A. C. and Cooney, C. L., *Immobilized Enzymes in Food and Microbial Processes*, Plenum Press, New York, 1974.
529. Olson, D. G., Parrish, F. C., Jr., Dayton, W. R., and Goll, D. E., *J. Food Sci.*, 42, 117, 1977.
530. Olson, D. G., Parrish, F. C., Jr., and Stromer, M. H., *J. Food Sci.*, 41, 1036, 1976.
531. Olson, N. F. and Richardson, T., *J. Dairy Sci.*, 58, 1117, 1975.
532. Osman, E. M., *Starch: Chemistry and Technology*, Whistler, R. L., and Paschall, E. F., Ed., Academic Press, New York, 1965.
533. Ough, C. S., *Am. J. Enol. Vitic.*, 26(1), 30, 1975.
534. Paez, L. E. and Hultin, H. O., *J. Food Sci.*, 35, 46, 1970.
535. Pang, C. Y. and Markakis, P., *Nature (London)*, 199, 597, 1963.
536. Pantastico, E. B., Ed., *Postharvest Physiology, Handling and Utilization of Tropical and Subtropical Fruits and Vegetables*, AVI Publishing, Westport, Conn., 1975.

537. Parry, R. M., Jr., Chandan, R. C., and Shahani, K. M., *Arch. Biochem. Biophys.*, 103, 59, 1969.
538. Patel, C. V., Fox, P. F., and Tarassuk, N. P., *J. Dairy Sci.*, 51, 1879, 1968.
539. Patel, R. B., Michelson, R., and Johnson, R. A., *Cereal Sci. Today*, 12, 377, 1967.
540. Patil, S. K., Finney, K. F., Shogren, M. D., and Tsen, C. C., *Cereal Chem.*, 53(3), 347, 1976.
541. Pattee, H. E., Singleton, J. A., and Johns, E. B., *Lipids*, 9, 302, 1974.
542. Patterson, R. L. S., *J. Sci. Food Agric.*, 19, 31, 1968.
543. Patterson, R. L. S., *Meat*, Cole, D. J. A. and Lawrie, R. A., Eds., Butterworths, London, 1975.
544. Pavlenko, N. M., *Food Sci. Technol. Abstr.*, 8, 7H 1262, 1976.
545. Pearse, K. N., *J. Dairy Res.*, 43, 27, 1976.
546. Pelissier, J. P. and Manchon, P., *J. Food Sci.*, 41, 231, 1976.
547. Penny, I. F., Voyle, C. A., and Lawrie, R. A., *J. Sci. Food Agric.*, 15, 559, 1964.
548. Peppler, H. J., Dooley, J. G., and Huang, H. T., *J. Dairy Sci.*, 59, 859, 1976.
549. Perry, S. V., *Progr. Biophys. Mol. Biol.*, 17, 325, 1967.
549a. Phelan, J. A., personal communication.
550. Phelan, J. J., Stevens, F. M., McNicholl, B., Fottrell, P. F., and McCarthy, C. F., *Clin. Sci. Mol. Biol.*, 53, 35, 1977.
551. Pilnik, W. and Voragen, A. G. J., *The Biochemistry of Fruit and Vegetables*, Vol. 1, Hulme, A. C., Ed., Academic Press, New York, 1970.
552. Platt, W. C. and Poston, A. L., U.S. Patent 3,058,887, 1962.
553. Plotka, A. and Wos, Z., *Postepy Drobiarstiva*, 12(2), 71, 1970; *Food Sci. Technol. Abstr.*, 4, 4Q49, 1972.
554. Polock, C. J. and Rees, T., *Phytochemistry*, 14, 613, 1975.
555. Pomeranz, Y., *Wheat: Chemistry and Technology*, American Association of Cereal Chemists, St. Paul, Minn., 1971.
556. Pomeranz, Y., *Food Technol.*, 18, 682, 1964.
557. Pomeranz, Y., *Brot Gebaeck*, 20(3), 40, 1966.
558. Pomeranz, Y., Rubenthaler, G. L., and Finney, K. F., *Food Technol.*, 20(3), 327, 1966.
559. Ponting, J. D., *Food Enzymes*, Schultz, H. W., Ed., AVI Publishing, Westport, Conn., 1966.
560. Porter, K. R. and Franzini-Armstrong, C., *Sci. Am.*, 212, 72, 1965.
561. Pour-El, A. and Swenson, T. S., *Cereal Chem.*, 53, 438, 1976.
562. Pratt, D. B., Jr., *Wheat: Chemistry and Technology*, Pomeranz, Y., Ed., American Association of Cereal Chemists, St. Paul, Minn., 1970.
563. Prendergast, K., *Food Trade Rev.*, 44(1), 14, 1974.
564. Pressey, R., *Arch. Biochem. Biophys.*, 113, 667, 1966.
565. Pressey, R., *Plant Physiol.*, 42, 1780, 1967.
566. Pressey, R., *Plant Physiol.*, 43, 1430, 1968.
567. Pressey, R., *J. Food Sci.*, 37, 521, 1972.
568. Pressey, R., *Amer. Chem. Soc.*, 172, AGFD 22, 1976.
569. Pressey, R. and Avants, J. K., *Plant Physiol.*, 52, 252, 1973.
570. Pressey, R. and Avants, J. K., *J. Food Sci.*, 40, 937, 1975.
571. Pressey, R. and Shaw, R., *Plant Physiol.*, 41, 1657, 1966.
572. Pressey, R., Hinton, D. M., and Avants, J. K., *J. Food Sci.*, 36, 1070, 1971.
573. Price, J. F. and Schweigert, B. S., Eds., *The Science of Meat and Meat Products*, W. H. Freeman, San Francisco, 1971.
574. Pritchard, E. I., *Inst. Food Sci. Technol. Proc.*, 4, 118, 1971.
575. Protein Advisory Group, Low Lactase Activity and Milk Intake, Bull. No. 2, 7, 1972.
576. Pyler, E. J., *Bakers Dig.*, 43(2), 36, 1969.
577. Pyler, E. J., *Bakers Dig.*, 43(4), 46, 1969.
578. Rackis, J. J., Honig, D. H., Sessa, D. J., and Moser, H. A., *Cereal Chem.*, 49, 586, 1972.
579. Rand, A. G., Jr., *J. Food Sci.*, 37, 698, 1972.
580. Rand, A. G., Jr., and Hourigan, J. A., *J. Dairy Sci.*, 58, 1144, 1975.
581. Ramamurti, K. and Johan, D. S., *Nature (London)*, 198, 481, 1963.
582. Ranhotra, G. S. and Loewe, R. J., *J. Food Sci.*, 40, 940, 1975.
583. Randall, C. J. and MacRae, H. F., *J. Food Sci.*, 32, 182, 1967.
584. Reddy, V., *Neth. Milk Dairy J.*, 27, 355, 1973.
585. Reddi, P. K., Constantinides, S. M., and Dymsza, H. A., *J. Food Sci.*, 37, 643, 1972.
586. Reed, G., *Am. Soc. Bakery Engineers Bull.*, 171, 691, 1963.
587. Reed, G., *Enzymes in Food Processing*, 1st and 2nd eds., Academic Press, New York, 1966, 1975.
588. Reed, G., *Cereal Foods World*, 21(11), 578, 1976.
589. Reed, G. and Thorn, J. A., *Wheat: Chemistry and Technology*, Pomeranz, Y., Eds., American Association of Cereal Chemists, St. Paul, Minn., 1971.
590. Reiser, R., *J. Am. Oil Chem. Soc.*, 26, 116, 1949.

591. Reiter, B., Sorokin, Y., Pickering, A., and Hall, A. J., *J. Dairy Res.*, 36, 65, 1969.
592. Rhodes, M. J. C., *The Biochemistry of Fruits and their Products*, Vol. 1, Hulme, A. C., Ed., Academic Press, New York, 1970.
593. Richardson, T., *Principles of Food Science, Part I, Food Chemistry*, Fennema, O. R., Ed., Marcel Dekker, New York, 1976.
594. Richardson, T., *Food Proteins: Improvement Through Chemical And Enzymatic Modification*, Feeney, R. E. and Whitaker, J. R., Eds., American Chemical Society, Washington, D.C., 1977.
595. Richardson, G. H., Nelson, J. H., and Farnham, M. G., *J. Dairy Sci.*, 54, 643, 1971.
596. Richardson, T. and Olson, N. F., *Immobilized Enzymes in Food and Microbial Processes*, Olson, A. C. and Cooney, C. L., Eds., Plenum Press, New York, 1974.
597. Roadhouse, C. L. and Henderson, J. L., *Bull. Calif. Agric. Exp. Stn.*, 595, 5, 1935.
598. Rombouts, F. M. and Pilnik, W., *Crit. Rev. Food Technol.*, 3, 1, 1972.
599. Roozen, J. P. and Pilnik, W., *Process Biochem.*, 8(7), 24, 1973.
600. Rorem, E. S. and Schwimmer, S., *Experimentia*, 19, 150, 1963.
601. Rosensweig, N. S., *J. Dairy Sci.*, 52, 585, 1969.
602. Rudavskaya, A. B. and Orlova, N. Y., *Tovarovedeni*, 6, 67, 1973; *Food Sci. Technol. Abstr.*, 5, 10Q 139, 1973.
603. Russo, J. R., *Food Eng. Int.*, 1(5), 37, 1976.
604. Sayre, R. N., Kiernat, B., and Briskey, E. J., *J. Food Sci.*, 29, 175, 1964.
605. Sacher, J. A., Hatch, M. D., and Glasziou, K. T., *Plant Physiol.*, 38, 348, 1963.
606. Sair, R. A., Lister, D., Moody, W. G., Cassens, R. G., Hoekstra, W. G., and Briskey, E. J., *Am. J. Physiol.*, 218, 108, 1970.
607. Sakamura, S., Shibusa, S., and Obata, Y., *J. Food Sci.*, 31, 317, 1961.
608. Salunkhe, D. K. and Do, J. Y., *Crit. Rev. Food Sci. Nutr.*, 8, 161, 1976.
609. Salunke, D. K. and Wu, M. J., *Crit. Rev. Food Technol.*, 5, 15, 1974.
610. Sanderson, G. W. and Graham, H. N., *J. Agric. Food Chem.*, 21, 576, 1973.
611. Schmidt, G. R., Cassens, R. G., and Briskey, E. J., *J. Food Sci.*, 35, 571, 1970.
612. Schopes, R. K. and Lawrie, R. A., *Nature (London)*, 197, 1202, 1963.
613. Schultz, H. W., *Food Enzymes*, AVI Publishing, Westport, Conn., 1960.
614. Schutte, L., *Crit. Rev. Food Technol.*, 4, 457, 1974.
615. Schwimmer, S., *J. Biol. Chem.*, 154, 487, 1944.
616. Schwimmer, S., *J. Food Sci.*, 28, 460, 1963.
617. Schwimmer, S., *Starch Round Table*, Corn Industries Res. Foundation, Pocono Manor, Pa., 1965.
618. Schwimmer, S., *Lebensm. Wiss. Technol.*, 2, 97, 1969.
619. Schwimmer, S., *J. Food Sci.*, 37, 530, 1972.
620. Schwimmer, S. and Burr, H. K., in *Potato Processing*, Talburt, W. E. and Smith, O., Eds., 2nd ed., AVI Publishing, Westport, Conn., 1967.
621. Schwimmer, S. and Friedman, M., *Flavour Ind.*, 3, 137, 1972.
622. Scott, R., *Process Biochem.*, 7(11), 33, 1972.
623. Seitz, E. W., *J. Am. Oil Chem. Soc.*, 51(2), 12, 1974.
624. Sen, L. C., Gonzalez-Flores, E., Feeney, R. E., and Whitaker, J. R., *J. Agric. Food Chem.*, 25, 623, 1977.
625. Shahani, K. M., *J. Dairy Sci.*, 49, 907, 1965.
626. Shahani, K. M., Arnold, R. G., Kilara, A., and Dwivedi, B. K., *Biotechnol. Bioeng.*, 18, 891, 1976.
627. Shahani, K. M., Harper, W. J., Jensen, R. G., Parry, R. M., Jr., and Zittle, C. A., *J. Dairy Sci.*, 56, 531, 1973.
628. Shankaranarayana, M. L., Raghavan, R., Abraham, K. O., and Natarajan, C. P., *Crit. Rev. Food Technol.*, 4, 395, 1974.
629. Sharp, J. G., Proc. 5th Meeting Eur. Meat Res. Workers, Paris, September 7 to 12, 1959.
630. Sharp, J. G., *J. Sci. Food Agric.*, 14, 468, 1963.
631. Sharp, J. G. and Marsh, B. B., Spec. Rep. Food Invest. Bd., Paper No. 58, London, 1953.
632. Shellenberger, J. A., *Cereal Sci. Today*, 16(4), 114, 1971.
633. Shipe, W. F., Lee, E. C., and Senyk, G. F., *J. Dairy Sci.*, 58, 1123.
634. Shestakov, S. D., Proc. 8th Meeting Eur. Meat Res. Workers, Paper No. 21, Moscow, 1962.
635. Schormuller, J., *Adv. Food Res.*, 16, 231, 1968.
636. Shukla, T. P., *Crit. Rev. Food Technol.*, 5(3), 325, 1975.
637. Shrikhande, A. J., *Crit. Rev. Food Sci. Nutr.*, 7, 193, 1976.
638. Siddigi, H. H. and Tappel, A. L., *Arch. Biochem. Biophys.*, 60, 91, 1956.
639. Siebert, G., *Experientia*, 14, 65, 1958.
640. Siebert, G., *Fish in Nutrition*, Heew and Kruezer, R., Eds., Fishing News (Books), London, 1962.
641. Silberstein, O., *Bakers Dig.*, 35(6), 44, 1961.
642. Singleton, J. A., Pattee, H. E., and Sanders, T. H., *J. Food Sci.*, 41, 148, 1976.

643. Sinnhuber, R. O. and Landers, N. K., *J. Food Sci.*, 29, 190, 1964.
644. Skinner, K. J., *Chem. Eng. News*, 53(33), 22—29, 32—41, 1975.
645. Skupin, J., Rosinska, K., Skupin, A., and Warchalewski, J., *Bull. Pol. Acad. Sci. Ser. Sci. Biol.*, 14, 397, 1966.
646. Slattery, C. W., *J. Dairy Sci.*, 59, 1547, 1976.
647. Slump, P. and Schreuder, H. A. W., *J. Sci. Food Agric.*, 24, 657, 1973.
648. Smith, O., *Potato Processing*, Talburt, W. E. and Smith, O., Eds., 2nd ed. AVI Publishing, Westport, Conn., 1967.
649. Smith, D. S., *Muscle*, Academic Press, New York, 1972.
650. Smith, A. K. and Circle, S. J., *Rep. 52nd Conv. Am. Soybean Assoc.*, Chemical Technical Institute, Columbus, Ohio, 1972.
652. Snoke, J. E. and Neurath, H., *J. Biol. Chem.*, 187, 127, 1950.
653. Societe Biscuits Brun, Cereal Bran Extractions, Br. Patent 1,140,123, 1969.
654. Solov'ev, N. I., *The Ripening of Meat: Theory and Practice of the Process*, Vols. 1 and 2, Haugh, B. and Ingram, M., Trans. Nat. Lending Library Sci. Technol., Yorkshire, England, 1966.
655. Sommer, N. F., Buchanan, R. J., and Fortlage, R. J., *Calif. Agric.*, 28, 8, 1974.
656. Spencer, B., *Industrial Aspects of Biochemistry*, North Holland, Amsterdam, 1973.
657. Spinelli, J., *J. Food Sci.*, 32, 38, 1967.
658. Spinelli, J., Groninger, H., Koury, B., and Miller, R., *Process Biochem.*, 10(10), 31, 1975.
659. Spinelli, J., Koury, B., and Miller, R., *J. Food Sci.*, 37, 599, 1972.
660. Spinelli, J., Koury, B., and Miller, R., *J. Food Sci.*, 37, 604, 1972.
661. Stadhounders, J. and Mulder, H., *Neth. Milk Dairy J.*, 14, 141, 1966.
662. Stadhounders, J. and Veringa, H. A., *Neth. Milk Dairy J.*, 27, 77, 1973.
663. Stauffer, C. E. and Glass, R. L., *Cereal Chem.*, 16, 319, 1966.
664. Strauss, W., *Enzyme Cytology*, Roodgn, D. B., Ed., Academic Press, New York, 1967.
665. Stone, E. J., Hall, R. M., and Kazeniac, S. J., *J. Food Sci.*, 40, 1138, 1975.
666. Stoll, A. and Seebeck, E., *Helv. Chim. Acta*, 31, 189, 1948.
667. Stoll, A. and Seebeck, E., *Helv. Chim. Acta*, 32, 197, 1949.
668. Stoll, A. and Seebeck, E., *Adv. Enzymol. Relat. Subj. Biochem.*, 11, 377, 1951.
669. Sreekantiah, K. R., Ebine, H., Obta, T., and Nakano, M., *Food Technol. (Chicago)*, 23, 1055, 1969.
670. Straniero, D., *Food Eng.*, 28, 58, 1956.
671. Stromer, M. H., Goll, D. E., and Roth, L. E., *J. Cell Biol.*, 34, 431, 1967.
672. Sybesma, W., van der Wal, P. G., and Walstra, P., Eds., *Recent Points of View on the Condition and Meat Quality of Pigs for Slaughter*, I. V. O. Zeist, The Netherlands, 1969.
673. Sugimoto, H. and van Buren, J. P., *J. Food Sci.*, 35, 655, 1970.
674. Sullivan, B., *Enzymes and Their Role in Wheat Technology*, Anderson, J. A., Eds., Interscience, New York, 1946.
675. Sullivan, B., *Cereal Chem.*, 25(6), 16, 1948.
676. Sullivan, J. J. and Jago, G. R., *Aust. J. Dairy Technol.*, 27, 98, 1972.
677. Sullivan, J. J., Mou, L., Rood, J. I., and Jago, G. R., *Aust. J. Dairy Technol.*, 28, 20, 1973.
678. Suzuki, H., Ozawa, Y., Ohta, H., and Yoshida, H., *J. Agric. Biol. Chem.*, 33, 501, 1969.
679. Swaisgood, H. E., *Crit. Rev. Food Technol.*, 3(4), 375, 1974.
680. Tager, J. M. and Biale, J. B., *Plant Physiol.*, 10, 79, 1957.
681. Takahashi, K., Fukazawa, T. and Yasui, T., *J. Food Sci.*, 32, 409, 1967.
682. Tang, N. Y. and Hilker, D. M., *J. Food Sci.*, 35, 676, 1970.
683. Tannenbaum, S. R., Ahern, M., and Bates, R. P., *Food Technol.*, 24, 604, 1970.
684. Tannenbaum, S. R., Bates, R. P., and Broadfeld, L., *Food Technol.*, 24, 607, 1970.
685. Tappel, A. L., *Lipids and their Oxidation*, Schultz, H. W., Day, E. A., and Sinnhuber, R. O., Eds., AVI Publishing, Westport, Conn., 1962.
686. Tappel, A. L., Zalkin, H., Caldwell, K. A., Desei, I. D., and Shibko, S., *Arch. Biochem. Biophys.*, 93, 340, 1962.
687. Tarr, H. L. A., *Can. Inst. Food Technol. J.*, 2, 42, 1969.
688. Tarassuk, N. P., *Creamery Co-operator*, Nov., 5, 1941.
689. Tarassuk, N. P. and Frankel, E. N., *J. Dairy Sci.*, 40, 418, 1957.
690. Tarky, W., Agarwala, O. P., and Pigott, G. M., *J. Food Sci.*, 38, 917, 1973.
691. Tayama, N., *Advances in Enzymic Hydrolysis of Related Materials*, Reese, E. J., Ed., Macmillan, New York, 1963.
692. Taylor, M. J., Richardson, T., and Olson, N. F., *J. Milk Food Technol.*, 39(12), 864, 1976.
693. Termote, F., Rombouts, F. M., and Pilnik, W., *J. Food Biochem.*, 1, 15, 1977.
694. Thomas, M., *Plant Physiology*, 4th ed., J & A Churchill, London, 1956.
695. Ting, Chao-Yun, Montgomery, M. W., and Anglemier, A. F., *J. Food Sci.*, 33, 617, 1968.
696. Topel, D. G., Ed., *The Pork Industry: Problems and Progress*, Iowa State University Press, Ames, 1968.

697. Towle, G. A. and Christensen, D., *Industrial Gums*, Whistler, R. I., Ed., 2nd ed., Academic Press, New York, 1973.
698. Tracey, M. V., *J. Sci. Food Agric.*, 15, 607, 1964.
699. Tressl, R. and Drawert, F., *J. Agric. Food Chem.*, 21, 560, 1973.
700. Tsakov, D., Valichkov, A., Spirn, N., and Penkov, I., *Food Sci. Technol. Abstr.*, 8, 7H 1260, 1976.
701. Tschagowadse, S. K. and Bakuradse, N. S., *Lebensm Ind.*, 19(7), 287, 1972.
702. Tsen, C. C., *Cereal Chem.*, 42, 86, 1965.
703. Tuma, H. J., *Dissert. Abstr.*, 24, 1563, 1963.
704. Tuma, H. J., Henrickson, R. L., Stephens, D. F., and Moore, R., *J. Anim. Sci.*, 21, 848, 1962.
705. Underkofler, L. A., *Soc. Chem. Ind. London Chem. Eng. Group Proc.*, 11, 72, 1961.
706. Underkofler, L. A., Enzymes, in *CRC Handbook of Food Additives*, Furia, T. E., Ed., CRC Press, Boca Raton, Fla., 1968.
707. Underkofler, L. A., Barton, R. B., and Rennert, S. S., *Appl. Microbiol.*, 6(3), 212, 1958.
708. Underkofler, L. A., Denault, L. J., and Hou, E. F., *Die Starke*, 6, 179, 1965.
709. Updergraff, D. M., *Biotechnol. Bioeng.*, 13, 77, 1971.
710. U.S. Patent 2,903,362, 1959.
711. Vaheri, M. and Kauppinen, V., *Process Biochem.*, 12(6), 5, 1977.
712. van der Bergh, S. G., *Proc. 2nd Int. Symp. Cond. Meat Qual. Pigs*, Hessel-de-Heer, J. M. C., Schmidt, G. R., Sybesma, W., and vander Wal, P. G., Eds., Wageningen, The Netherlands, 1971.
713. von Loesecke, H., *Nutritional Evaluation of Food Processing*, Harris, R. S. and von Loesecke, H., Eds., 2nd ed., AVI Publishing, Westport, Conn., 1973.
714. van Logtestijn, J. G., Sybesma, W., and van Gils, J. H. J., *Arch. Lebensmittelhyg.*, 3, 55, 1970.
715. Venugopal, B., Ph.D. thesis, University of Missouri, Columbia, Mo., 1970.
716. Vernon, L. P. and Seeley, G. R., Eds., *The Chlorophylls*, Academic Press, London, 1966.
717. Villadsen, K. J. S., *DECHEMA Monogr.*, 70, 135, 1972.
718. Viniegra-Gonzales, G., Proc. 9th Int. Congr. Nutr., Mexico City, 3, 91, September 3 to 9, 1972.
719. Virtanen, A. I., *Makromol. Chem.*, 6, 94, 1951.
720. Virtanen, A. I. and Matikkala, E., *Acta Chem. Scand.*, 13, 1898, 1959.
721. Virtanen, A. I., Lacksonen, T., and Kantola, M., *Acta Chem. Scand.*, 5, 316, 1951.
722. Virtanen, A. I., Kerkkonen, H. K., Loaksonen, T., and Hakala, M., *Acta Chem. Scand.*, 3, 520, 1949.
723. Visser, F. M. W., *Neth. Milk Dairy J.*, 31, 210, 1977.
723a. Visser, F. M. W., *Neth. Milk Dairy J.*, 31, 265, 1977.
724. Voragen, A. G. J. and Pilnik, W., *Dtsch. Lebensm. Rundsch.*, 66, 325, 1970.
725. Voragen, A. G. J. and Pilnik, W., *Z. Lebensm. Unters. Forsch.*, 142, 346, 1970.
726. Wagenknecht, A. C., *Food Res.*, 24, 539, 1959.
727. Wagenknecht, A. C., Scheiner, S. M., and van Buren, J. P., *Food Technol.*, 14, 47, 1960.
728. Wager, H. G., *J. Sci. Food Agric.*, 15, 245, 1964.
729. Waldt, L. M., *Cereal Sci. Today*, 10, 447, 1965.
730. Waldt, L. M., *Bakers Dig.*, 42(5), 64, 1968.
731. Waldt, L. M., *Wallerstein Lab. Commun.*, 32(107), 39, 1969.
732. Walker, A. R. P., *Lancet*, 11, 244, 1957.
733. Walker, G. C., *J. Food Sci.*, 29, 383, 1964.
734. Walker, P. G. and Levy, G. A., *Biochem. J.*, 49, 28, 1951.
735. Weber, A. and Murray, J. M., *Physiol. Rev.*, 53, 612, 1973.
736. Walker, S. M. and Schrodt, G. R., *Nature (London)*, 211, 935, 1966.
737. Walters, C. L. and Taylor, A., *Food Technol. (Chicago)*, 17, 354, 1963.
738. Wallenfels, K. and Malhota, O. P., *Adv. Carbohydr. Chem.*, 16, 239, 1961.
739. Walters, C. L., Burger, T. H., Jewell, G. G., Lewis, D. F., and Parke, D. V., *Z. Lebensm. Unters. Forsch.*, 158, 193, 1975.
740. Wang, H., Weir, C. E., Birkner, M., and Ginger, B., Proc. 9th Res. Conf., Am. Meat Institute, 1957.
741. Warner, R. C. and Polis, E., *J. Am. Chem. Soc.*, 67, 529, 1945.
742. Weber, R., *Lysosomes*, Ciba Foundation Symposium de Reuch, A. V. S. and Cameron, M. R. J., Eds., Churchill, London, 1963.
743. Weetal, H. M., *Food Prod. Dev.*, 7(3), 46, 1973.
743a. Weetal, H. M., *Food Prod. Dev.*, 7(4), 49, 1973.
744. Weetall, H. H., *Process Biochem.*, 10(6), 3, 1975.
745. Weetall, H. H., *Cereal Foods World*, 21(11), 581, 1976.
746. Weetal, H. H., Havewala, N. B., Pitcher, W. P., Jr., and Yaverbaum, S., *Biotechnol. Bioeng.*, 16, 295, 1974.
747. Weinberg, B. and Rose, D., *Food Technol.*, 14, 376, 1960.
748. West, R. L., Moeller, P. W., Link, B. A., and Landmann, W. A., *J. Food Sci.*, 39, 29, 1974.

749. Whelan, W. J., *Nature (London)*, 190, 954, 1961.
750. Whistler, R. L. and Paschall, E. F., *Starch: Chemistry & Technology*, Vols. 1 and 2, Academic Press, New York, 1965, 1967.
751. Whitaker, J. R., *Adv. Food Res.*, 9, 1, 1959.
752. Whitaker, J. R., *Principles of Enzymology for the Food Sciences*, Marcel Dekker, New York, 1972.
753. Whitaker, J. R., *Food Related Enzymes*, American Chemical Society, Washington, D.C., 1974.
754. Whitaker, J. R., *Adv. Food Res.*, 22, 73, 1976.
755. Whitaker, J. R., *Food Proteins: Improvement Through Chemical and Enzymatic Modification*, Feeney, R. E. and Whitaker, J. R., Eds., American Chemical Society, Washington, D.C., 1977.
756. Whitaker, J. R. and Feeney, R. E., *Protein Crosslinking: Nutritional and Medical Consequences*, Friedman, M., Ed., Plenum Press, New York, 1977.
757. Whiting, G. C., *The Biochemistry of Fruit and their Products*, Vol. 1, Hulme, A. C., Ed., Academic Press, New York, 1970.
758. Whitney, R. McL., Brunner, J. R., Ebner, K. E., Farrell, H. M., Jr., Josephson, R. V., Morr, C. V., and Swaisgood, H. E., *J. Dairy Sci.*, 59, 785, 1976.
759. Wichser, F. W., *Bakers Dig.*, 26(1), 8, 1952.
760. Wieland, H., *Enzymes in Food Processing and Products*, Noyes Data, Park Ridge, N.J., 1972.
761. Wieland, T., Determan, H., and Albrealt, E., *Justus Liebigs Ann. Chem.*, 633, 185, 1960.
762. Wierzbicki, L. E. and Kosikowski, F. V., *J. Dairy Sci.*, 56, 1182, 1972.
763. Wilkie, D. R., *Muscle*, Edward Arnold.
764. Wiseman, A., *Handbook of Enzyme Biotechnology*, Halsted Press, New York, 1975.
765. Worth, H. G. J., *Chem. Rev.*, 67, 465, 1967.
766. Wrench, P. M., *J. Sci. Food Agric.*, 16, 51, 1965.
767. Wright, D. G. and Rand, A. G., Jr., *J. Food Sci.*, 38, 1132, 1973.
768. Yamauchi, K. and Kaminogawa, S., *J. Agric. Biol. Chem.*, 36, 249, 1972.
769. Yamashita, M., Arai, S., and Fujimaki, M., *J. Agric. Food Chem.*, 24, 1100, 1976.
770. Yamashita, M., Arai, S., and Fujimaki, M., *J. Food Sci.*, 41, 1029, 1976.
771. Yamauchi, K., Kaminogawa, S., and Tsugo, T., *Jpn. J. Zootech. Sci.*, 40, 551, 1969.
772. Yamashita, M., Arai, S., Gonda, M., Kato, H., and Fujimaki, M., *J. Agric. Biol. Chem.*, 34, 1333, 1970.
773. Yamashita, M., Arai, S., Matsuyama, J., Gonda, M., Kato, H., and Fujimaki, M., *J. Agric. Biol. Chem.*, 34, 1484, 1970.
774. Yamashita, M., Arai, S., Matsuyama, J., Kato, H., and Fujimaki, M., *J. Agric. Biol. Chem.*, 34, 1492, 1970.
775. Yanez, E., Ballister, D., Moncheberg, F., Hiemlich, W., and Rutman, M., *J. Food Sci.*, 41, 1289, 1976.
776. Yang, H. Y. and Steele, W. F., *Food Technol.*, 12, 517, 1958.
777. Young, L. S., *Dissert, Abstr. Int.*, B37, 1166, 1976.
778. Young, M., *Annu. Rev. Biochem.*, 38, 913, 1969.
779. Yudkin, J., *Physiol. Rev.*, 29, 389, 1949.
780. Zender, R., Lataste-Dorolle, C., Collet, R. A., Rowinski, P., and Mouton, R. F., *Food Res.*, 23, 305, 1958.
781. Zikakis, J. P., Rzucidlo, S. J., and Biassotto, N. O., *J. Dairy Sci.*, 60, 533, 1977.
782. Zoueil, M. E. and Esselen, W. B., *Food Res.*, 24, 119, 1959.

# EFFECT OF PROCESSING ON NUTRITIVE VALUE OF FOOD: IRRADIATION

## H. F. Kraybill

## INTRODUCTION

In order to preserve food and prevent bacterial spoilage, man, through his innovativeness and quest for his survival, has developed methods that increase the shelf life of various foods and provide a constant resource when environmental and climatic conditions preclude accessibility. These methods include sun-drying or dehydration, salting, pickling, and natural freezing. One of the earliest preservation methods was that of drying with solar energy, practiced by native tribes in North and South America. Early settlers on this continent consumed large quantities of salted meats; however, the principle of pickling tissues was known to the early Egyptians, as evidenced by their preservation of human remains. During the Napoleonic era, Nicholas Appert introduced thermal processing, or canning, which is still widely practiced today.[1-4]

Although freezing is an old method of preservation, the fullest potential of this technique had to await the development of freezer equipment, which took place in the U.S. over the last 40 years. In less developed countries of the world, freezer preservation is still uncommon. Combinations of methods have also been applied, and during World War II, spray and roller-drying (thermal methods) and lyophilization or freeze-drying were resorted to for preservation of serum, biologicals, and food.[3]

As a result of a wide-scale program on peaceful uses of atomic energy, a comprehensive research and development project was instituted in the U.S. and Europe to determine how ionizing radiation or nuclear energy can be used to preserve foods, agricultural commodities, and pharmaceuticals and to sterilize medical supplies.[4] Radiation sterilization dates back to the discovery of ionizing radiations by Roentgen[5] and Becquerel[6] in 1895 and to some of the initial research on bactericidal properties of such radiations, which was reported shortly thereafter.[7,8]

Development of radiation sources between 1930 and 1940 and the availability after 1950 of increasing quantities of spent fuel rods and radioactive isotopes from nuclear reactors disclosed new potentials for the beneficial use of such energy sources.[9] Although one might contend that the nutritive value of foods processed by radiation does not differ markedly from that of foods processed by other methods of preservation, it is difficult to find a comprehensive evaluation on all food processing methods and their comparable effects on nutrient value (starting with identical resource material or foods to be processed). For example, Raica et al.,[10] in discussing the relative values for nutrient content of thermally and radiation-processed foods, indicate that the data on nutritional quality are not always in agreement because there is a lack of standardization in food selection, preparation, packaging, radiation techniques, and the subsequent handling prior to analysis. Perhaps some of this variation is inevitable, since the nutrient content of food is a highly variable commodity, depending upon seasonal and geographical factors and perishability. When following a systematic approach, one should use a standard source of a food of known origin and identical methods of handling and preparation, allowing only the method of processing to vary. Adhering to this method could allow analytical values on nutrient content to be derived, and data so obtained might provide a more accurate comparison between nutritive values of various foods processed by the methods described above. Therefore, it should be kept in mind that the data reported herein are only as accurate as those reported in the literature.

## TYPES OF RADIATION AND TERMS OF REFERENCE

Emerging largely from a program on peaceful uses of atomic energy, a process was developed to preserve foods by ionizing radiation. Foods so processed are referred to as "irradiated foods."

It was recognized simultaneously that the sterilization or pasteurization effect, to inhibit the development of spoilage bacteria, could be accomplished by three main forms of ionizing radiation: gamma rays similar to X-rays of $^{60}$Cobalt or $^{137}$Cesium sources, and electrons or X-rays produced by electrons in an X-ray target. Thus generally available sources of radiant energy were gamma radiation, sources from radioisotopes, and electron beam radiation from high energy machines such as a linear accelerator or other modifications of electron beam generators. The gamma sources of relatively low energy rays (1.17 to 1.33 MeV) act directly on a target such as food or, by conversion of beta particles, are transformed by Bremsstrahlung into X-rays. Machine sources such as the cascade generator (Cockroft Walton® machine), resonant transformer, or capacitors produce energies less than 5 MeV, but the Van de Graaf generator and Linac (linear accelerator) can develop higher energies in the region beyond 10 MeV. The problem arises at least beyond 10 MeV, at which level some induced radioactivity can occur as a result of a gamma-n reaction in food elements. Thus, high energy sources that create the neutron activation problem have only been used experimentally and are not advocated for commercial application.[11]

Primary or secondary electrons arising from the gamma or X-rays that hit water molecules and/or targets within the food itself produce activated molecules; consequently, bacteria, viruses, and even enzymes become inactivated. In essence, for purposes of spoilage prevention and shelf-life extension, this process accomplishes what thermal processing (canning) has achieved for years. Because it does so without significant rise in temperature and little chemical change, it has been termed cold sterilization. Many potential applications of food irradiation have become apparent, and the following terminology is frequently used.[12]

**Radappertization or sterilization** — The process of foods which are stable at room temperature (not requiring refrigeration), wherein all vegetative forms of bacteria or fungi are destroyed or there is complete inactivation of all resting spores of public health significance, e.g., *Clostridium botulinum* spores). Any storage effects in food would be comparable chemically to those, for example, on macro- and micronutrients in thermal or heat processed foods.

**Radurization** — Foods may have a prolonged storage life in the fresh state by some inactivation of spoilage bacteria through exposure of food to ionizing radiation. Because such foods do not attain commercial sterility, they must be protected by refrigeration if spoilage reduction and quality are required. Doses are generally below 1 Mrad, and the process is comparable to pasteurization.

**Radicidation** — A term proposed by international experts in the radiation treatment relevant to destruction of nonspore-forming pathogenic organisms. Doses are generally below 1 Mrad, and the process is analogous to pasteurization.

Beyond these preservation processes, ionizing radiation, has been used for disinfection or the sexual sterilization of various insects or parasites within bulk or packaged forms of food. This process is quite useful for stored cereal products or grains. Another practical application is the use of ionizing radiation for sprout inhibition in bulk-stored potatoes and onions, a process currently being used in several countries.

There is no adequate standard for comparison of radiation processing with other types of food processing. As regards the *extent* of processing and its effect upon food constituents, radiation sterilization is comparable to canning or the thermal processing of foods. With respect to appearance and textures, however, radiation-sterilized foods are more comparable to unprocessed foods. Because the public has accepted thermally processed foods for more than 100 years now, it is logical to compare any relative destructive effect on nutritive value to heat-processed or canned foods.

In general, for radappertization (sterilization) or radiation processing of foods, a dose of two to five million rad (Mrad) is used.* The higher dose — 5 Mrad — is used to ensure protection from botulism. When foods are pasteurized or radurized in order to extend their shelf life, doses of less than 1 Mrad are common (usually between 0.4 and 0.6). Comparative evaluations on the effects of processing on the nutrient content of foods are usually referenced to whole foods or nutrients within a given food rather than to isolated nutrients present as solids or in aqueous solutions. Data on the latter cannot always be extrapolated to situations for intact food, but some comparative data are useful to indicate a protective effect on nutrients from other nutrients or organic molecules in food, a situation which does not prevail in pure solutions.

## EFFECT OF RADIATION PROCESSING ON MACRONUTRIENTS

### Proteins and Amino Acids

In spite of the fact that few of the chemical bonds in irradiated materials become broken, in the case of proteins, denaturation, degradation, and polymerization occur. Proteins show the influence of aggregation reflected by an increase in viscosity of irradiated protein solutions. For example, Kraybill and co-workers[13] studied the effects of irradiation of milk protein at high dosage levels (6 to 10 Mrad) and noted a marked alteration in serological activity or reduction in antigenicity in guinea pigs sensitized to this type of protein. (Table 1).

Irradiation of free amino acids or peptides results in deamination and decarboxylation. Amino acids in protein, as they occur in peptide linkages, are more resistant than the amino acids in five solutions.[14] Some proteins, e.g., beef protein, may yield ammonia and at least six amines, predominantly methylamine and ethylamine.[15] The sulfur-containing amino acids yield methylmercaptan, hydrogen sulfide, methyl disulfide, and isobutyl mercaptan.[16] These degradation products formed at ambient temperatures are identified and those molecular species associated with objectionable odors and tastes are characterized. While this was true for earlier techniques in radiation processing, later procedures using inert atmospheres and temperatures as low as −196°C circumvent the detection of these objectionable off-flavor, off-odor compounds. One of the carbonyl compounds mentioned earlier, 3-methyl-thio-propionaldehyde, is only one of a whole series of compounds identified as volatiles in concurrent radiation and distillation of beef protein at a dose of 5 Mrad.[17,18]

Some amino acid mixtures lose glutamic acid and serine after radiation processing. The influence of salt, pH, temperature, and oxygen or, more specifically, the lack of a protective mechanism of inert gases at low temperature, influences the extent of radiation damage. Current technologies use more innovative procedures in the radiation processing of food proteins. Thus, one cannot extrapolate findings from tests of model systems to explain effects observed in whole food, in which protective mechanisms are present. Metta and Johnson[19] studied the effect of radiation processing on the nitrogen metabolism of raw and radiation-sterilized beef (Table 2). Additionally, they determined the biological value and coefficients of apparent and true digestibility of heat-treated and radiation-processed milk (Table 3). In further studies, these researchers demonstrated the comparative effects of thermal and heat processing on the nutritive value of lima bean and pea protein[20] (Table 4).

* 1 Mrad = 100 erg of energy absorbed per gram of matter.

Table 1
MEAN LETHAL SHOCKING DOSE FOR MILK-
SENSITIZED GUINEA PIGS CHALLENGED
WITH GAMMA IRRADIATED AND RAW
SKIM MILK

| Series | Radiation dose ($10^6$ rad) | No. of animals tested | $LSD_{50}$ Protein N per 0.5 ml dose | Ratio of control to irradiated sample |
|--------|------|------|------|------|
| 1 | 0 | 66 | 36 ± 7 | 1:0.8 |
|   | 0.475 | 66 | 29 ± 4 | |
| 2 | 0 | 77 | 32 ± 4 | 1:2 |
|   | 2.79 | 87 | 64 ± 11 | |
| 3 | 0 | 64 | 69 ± 16 | 1:9 |
|   | 5.58 | 50 | 602 ± 270 | |
| 4 | 0 | 60 | 37 ± 4 | 1:31 |
|   | 9.30 | 55 | 1157 ± 422 | |

From Kraybill, H. F., Reed, M. S., Linder, R. O., Harding, R. S., and Issac, G. J., *J. Allergy*, 30(4), 342, 1959. With permission.

Table 2
DIGESTION AND NITROGEN METABOLISM
DATA OF RAW AND RADIATION-
STERILIZED BEEF

|  | Raw beef | Radiation sterilized |
|--------|------|------|
| Apparent digestibility (%) | 91.8 | 92 |
| True digestibility (%) | 100 | 100 |
| Nitrogen balance (mg/g N intake) | 578 | 591 |
| Biological value (%) | 78 | 78 |

From Metta, V. C. and Johnson, B. C., *J. Nutr.*, 59, 479, 1956. With permission.

A radiation dose of up to 10 Mrad has little effect on the digestibility or biological value of food proteins. The loss of biological value of milk protein at very high doses, i.e., beyond 6 Mrad, is due to sulfur amino acid destruction.[21] Similarly, the loss of biological value for pea and lima bean protein is also probably due to the destruction of sulfur amino acids. Radiation treatment does not cause as great an improvement in the biological value of lima bean protein as does heat processing. This may be accounted for by the fact that heat has a greater destructive effect on trypsin inhibitor, which was shown to be present in lima beans by Borchers and Ackerson.[22] Ley et al.[23] radiation sterilized (radappertized) a rat diet (which included soya bean, meat, bone, and fish meals as protein sources) with radiation doses ranging from 0.5 to 7.0 Mrad. As indicated in Table 5, the radiation treatment did not adversely effect the digestibility or biological value of protein. Read and co-workers[24] fed an irradiated diet of nine foods to rats, and when compared to a control or nonradiation-processed composite diet, no variation in the percentage of protein availability occured.

Ley et al.[23] also found that there was no significant alteration in the levels of amino acids in the protein of a rat diet when the diet was irradiated or radiation sterilized. Of course, the protective action of amino acids within the mixture or other constituents

Table 3
AVERAGE BIOLOGICAL VALUES AND
COEFFICIENTS OF APPARENT AND TRUE
DIGESTIBILITY OF PROTEIN FOR VARIOUS
RAW, HEAT-STERILIZED, AND RADIATION-
STERILIZED MILK

|  | Condensed raw milk | Heat sterilized | Radiation sterilized |
|---|---|---|---|
| Apparent digestibility (%) | 86.4 | 85.2 | 85.3 |
| True digestibility (%) | 97.8 | 96.7 | 96.9 |
| Biological value (%) | 89.5 | 84.3 | 81.8 |

From Metta, V. C. and Johnson, B. C., *J. Nutr.*, 59, 479, 1956.
With permission.

Table 4
EFFECT OF HEAT AND RADIATION
PROCESSING ON THE NUTRITIVE VALUE OF
LIMA BEAN AND PEA PROTEIN

|  | Raw | Heat processed | Radiation processed |
|---|---|---|---|
| Pea protein |  |  |  |
|     Apparent digestibility (%) | 84 | 84 | 83 |
|     True digestibility (%) | 92 | 91 | 91 |
|     Biological value (%) | 58 | 58 | 51 |
| Lima bean protein |  |  |  |
|     Apparent digestibility (%) | 61 | 68 | 61 |
|     True digestibility (%) | 68 | 77 | 70 |
|     Biological value (%) | 48 | 64 | 47 |

*Note:* Biological value $= \dfrac{\text{Nitrogen utilized}}{\text{Nitrogen absorbed}} \times 100.$

From Metta, V. C., Norton, H. W., and Johnson, B. C., *J. Nutr.*,
63, 143, 1957. With permission.

may have been partially responsible for these results. The amino acid composition of irradiated and nonirradiated diets is given in Table 6.

There are other reports on the effects of ionizing radiation on protein quality in various products such as fruits. For example, when radiation was used for disinfestation of mangoes and papayas, no significant effect on nutritive value of protein moiety was noted.[25] Apple and grape juices have been treated at radiation doses of 0.8 Mrad with no alteration in amino acid levels.[26] Similarly, orange juice processed at 1.0 Mrad showed no alteration in amino acid composition.[27]

Some changes in the viscosity of protein solutions exposed to 0.25 Mrad do occur: Meats appear to have a reduced water-holding capacity, which may be due to the alteration in the affinity of denatured proteins for water.[28]

## Carbohydrates

Fundamental changes that can occur in carbohydrates are similar to those that do take place in proteins, e.g., changes resulting from the influence of air and water and the associated reactions from radiolysis, which are decomposition (degradation and splitting) and synthesis (cross-linking polymerization). Hexoses are degraded by dehy-

Table 5

RADIATION PROCESSING EFFECT ON
DIGESTIBILITY AND BIOLOGICAL
VALUE OF PROTEIN COMPONENTS
IN A STANDARDIZED RAT DIET

| Radiation dose | True digestibility (%) | Biological value (%) | Net protein utilization (%) |
|---|---|---|---|
| 0 | 85.6 | 80.5 | 68.9 |
| 0.5 | 83.6 | 75.8 | 63.5 |
| 1.0 | 86.5 | 81.7 | 70.6 |
| 2.5 | 87.0 | 78.1 | 68.0 |
| 3.5 | 84.8 | 77.3 | 65.4 |
| 7.0 | 85.3 | 76.4 | 65.2 |

From Ley, F. J., Bleby, J., Coates, M. E., and Patterson, J. S., *Lab. Anim.*, 3, 221, 1969. With permission.

Table 6

COMPARISON OF AMINO ACID
COMPOSITION OF PROTEIN IN
UNIRRADIATED AND RADIATION-
PROCESSED RAT DIET

| Amino acid | Unirradiated diet (g/16 g N) | Irradiated diet dose (7 Mrd g/16 g N) |
|---|---|---|
| Asparagine | 8.85 | 8.38 |
| Alanine | 5.61 | 5.54 |
| Arginine | 6.04 | 6.05 |
| Cystine | 1.34 | 1.44 |
| Glutamic acid | 15.70 | 15.61 |
| Glycine | 5.82 | 5.79 |
| Histidine | 2.29 | 2.37 |
| Isoleucine | 3.99 | 3.99 |
| Leucine | 7.44 | 7.47 |
| Lysine | 5.72 | 5.82 |
| Methionine | 2.33 | 2.11 |
| Phenylalanine | 4.12 | 4.28 |
| Serine | 4.17 | 4.16 |
| Threonine | 3.80 | 3.73 |
| Tryptophane | 1.16 | 1.32 |
| Tyrosine | 3.28 | 3.38 |
| Valine | 4.78 | 4.68 |

From Ley, F. J., Bleby, J., Coates, M. E., and Patterson, J. S., *Lab. Anim.*, 3, 221, 1969. With permission.

drogenation, and complex polysaccharides exhibit a break in the glycosidic linkage. Effects produced by irradiation are continued during storage. This is, of course, dependent upon the presence of water and temperature, as indicated above. Some properties are altered slightly; for instance, loss in gelation and some browning occurs, the latter being accentuated in the presence of protein, in which case interaction produces polymers. Of course, the browning reaction also occurs in heat-processed foods.[12,29]

Although the findings from radiation treatment of pure solutions or systems cannot be extrapolated to effects on whole foods, it is interesting to note that the reducing

## Table 7
## RESULTS OF EXPERIMENTS ON METABOLIZABLE ENERGY OF
## UNPROCESSED AND IRRADIATED RAT DIETS

|  | Diet 1 | | Diet 2 | | Diet 3 | |
|---|---|---|---|---|---|---|
|  | Nonprocessed | Irradiated | Nonprocessed | Irradiated | Nonprocessed | Irradiated |
| Gross energy (cal/100 g diet) | 353.61 | 356.43 | 212.97 | 213.28 | 274.80 | 276.31 |
| Metabolizable energy (cal/100 cal gross energy intake) | 89.6 | 90.1 | 89.2 | 89.0 | 92.3 | 91.4 |

### Metabolizable Energy of Nutrients (cal/g)

|  | Nonprocessed | Irradiated |
|---|---|---|
| Casein (protein) | $4.56 \pm 0.298$ | $4.51 \pm 0.220$ |
| Lard (fat) | $8.82 \pm 0.314$ | $8.87 \pm 0.391$ |
| Carbohydrate | $3.87 \pm 0.196$ | $3.78 \pm 0.299$ |

From Johnson, B. C., *Atomic Energy and Agriculture,* Comar, C. W., Reitemier, R. F., Tukey, H. B., Patrick, M., and Trum, B. F., Eds., American Association for the Advancement of Science Publ. No. 49, Westview Press, Washington, D.C., 1957, 391. With permission.

## Table 8
## COMPOSITION OF RAT DIETS
## USED IN METABOLIZABLE
## ENERGY EXPERIMENTS

|  | Diet 1 (g) | Diet 2 (g) | Diet 3 (g) |
|---|---|---|---|
| Casein | 30 | 14 | 20 |
| Lard | 40 | 10 | 30 |
| Carbohydrate | 23 | 69 | 43 |
| Mineral mix 446 | 4 | 4 | 4 |
| Barium sulfate | 2 | 2 | 2 |
| Sodium chloride | 1 | 1 | 1 |
| Water | 80 | 100 | 100 |
| Total | 180 | 200 | 200 |

From Johnson, B. C., *Atomic Energy and Agriculture,* Comar, C. W., Reitemier, R. F., Tukey, H. B., Patrick, M., and Trum, B. F., Eds., American Association for the Advancement of Science Publ. No. 49, Westview Press, Washington, D.C., 1957, 391. With permission.

ability of glucose decreased by 2 to 14% when treated at 10 to 100 Mrad.[30] Sucrose at 50% concentration in solution can be decomposed into reducing sugars at 100 Mrad.[31]

Polysaccharides such as cellulose and starch are depolymerized by irradiation, as was sucrose. For example, Lawton et al.[32] found that wood cellulose irradiated at 6.5 to 7.5 Mrad had a greatly increased level of water-soluble solids, forming pertoses and reducing sugars. Simple depolymerization can occur with dextrans and starch,[33] and it is possible to degrade cellulose to digestible sugars by radiation doses up to 100 Mrad.[34] While it may seem to have commercial applications, such large scale radiation processing would be economically prohibitive due to the exposure time and amount of radiation energy required.[12]

The metabolizable energy of carbohydrates is not appreciably affected by radiation processing. Metta[35] studied the effects of a radiation dose of 3 Mrad on the energy value of synthetic rations containing 50 to 70% water. No changes in metabolizable energy of carbohydrate, i.e., starch plus glucose, occurred, irrespective of whether the carbohydrates were irradiated separately in the presence of water or as part of the total ration (Table 7).

Table 8 shows three diets containing various levels of protein (casein), fat (lard), and carbohydrate (starch, sucrose, and amidex). These diets, both nonprocessed and irradiated, were fed to rats and the metabolizable energy was measured; results are given in Table 7. The metabolizable energy of the carbohydrate component of the diet was not altered by irradiation when compared to a nonprocessed ration. Additionally, as previously mentioned, Read et al.[24] found that radiation processing has no effect on protein availability of a composite diet whether nonprocessed or irradiated at 5.58 Mrad.

Other feeding experiments with rats fail to show any effect of radiation processing on energy utilization. Examples of such studies are those on irradiated potatoes (10 to 100 krad) fed at levels of 72% in diet[37] and studies on the energy availability of starch in corn of nonprocessed and irradiated diets.[38]

Therefore, whether radiation processing is used for radappertization or sterilization of laboratory rations; for composite diet of human foods; or for insect disinfestation of grains and fruits, for mold inhibition (fruits), retardation of ripening (fruits), or sprout inhibition (tubers); there is no detrimental effect on the metabolizable energy furnished by the carbohydrates in the ration, diet, or food.

## Lipids

The effect of radiation on fats is similar to that of autoxidation with hydroperoxides among the initial products formed during irradiation. The reaction chains in the formation of peroxides during irradiation are shorter than in autoxidation, since free radical concentrations are higher. The radiation dose determines the concentration of peroxides formed, while interestingly enough, more peroxides are formed at the lower dose rates. Therefore, peroxides, formed as they sometimes are in lipid spoilage in foods on standing, are of fleeting existence and are transformed into other carbonyls such as aldehyde or ketones or, ultimately, free fatty acid. Irradiated unsaturated fatty acids show changes in double bond configuration. Following protein irradiation, when physical properties are altered as previously discussed, lipids do not show changes such as alteration in melting point or dielectric constants even at high doses of irradiation.[12,39]

It has been observed that animal fats are more susceptible to radiation-induced chemical changes than are vegetable fats. These alterations can, of course, be reduced by low temperature processing and exclusion of oxygen, i.e., the use of inert gases. Some investigators have debated the prevalence of hydroperoxides when lipids are irradiated.[40] They only seem to be formed if the peroxide numbers of fats reach a value of 100 or above, which is not attained at radappertization doses of 2.8 to 5.6 Mrad.[41] Thus, the irradiation or peroxidative effect on lipids could involve transformation of some essential fatty acids, thereby inducing nutrient deficiency.[42] (This subject will be discussed in more detail later.)

The rate of digestion and absorption of highly oxidized, degraded, or polymerized lipids can be a problem, and the literature is replete with references to the toxic effects of highly oxidized fats and oils. One of the first specific studies on irradiated lard involved a product with a high peroxide number, thus suggesting that there may have

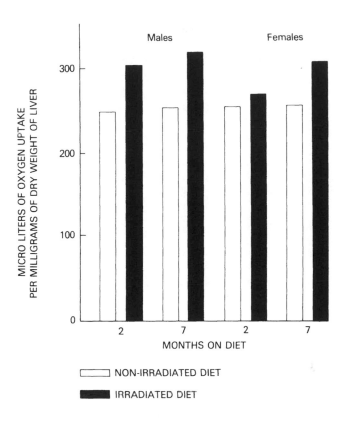

FIGURE 1. Liver cytochrome: oxidase activities in rats maintained on irradiated and nonirradiated diets.

been reduced acceptability. Monty et al.[44] noted that fats irradiated at 5 Mrad had a slightly reduced rate of digestion and absorption. In general, however, this had no nutritional significance.

As indicated previously, fats having peroxide values of $\leqslant 100$ are not harmful,[45,46] but the highly polymerized fats may be toxic.[47,48] Thus, to the extent that such compounds could be formed in very high levels and reduce the total amount of fat per se, which is available solely as an energy source, it is inconceivable that such a mechanism or event would markedly reduce the total available energy.

Investigating protein and carbohydrate availability after radiation processing of rations and foods, Read and co-workers[24] also found that the availability of fat derived from food components irradiated at a dose of 5.58 Mrad was 95.8%, compared to 94.8% for nonirradiated control fat. Corn oil irradiated at doses of 2.79 and 5.58 Mrad was also fed to rats by Moore,[49] who reported that radiation processing does not adversely alter the digestibility of corn oil.

A study that may serve as a reference point for data on humans was performed at Fitzsimons Army Hospital, Army Medical Nutrition Laboratory. Plough et al.[50] fed human volunteers in a metabolic ward pork irradiated at a dose of 2.79 Mrad and stored for 1 year at room temperature. They found that the digestibility values for irradiated fat (in pork) were not different than those obtained for the nonirradiated fat.

Several tissue enzymes have been measured, e.g., xanthine oxidase, cytochrome oxidase, succinic dehydrogenase, and alkaline phosphatase, to indicate the course of lipid and protein metabolism in animals fed irradiated and nonirradiated diets. During 2 and 7 month feeding experiments in which rats were fed irradiated and nonirradiated

Table 9
LIPASE ACTIVITY ON FAT FROM ROOM
TEMPERATURE-STORED BEEF STERILIZED
BY THERMAL OR IONIZING ENERGY
COMPARED TO FAT FROM FROZEN-STORED
ENZYME-INACTIVATED CONTROL BEEF

|  | Peroxide value (meq/ kg extracted fat) | Relative activity | |
| --- | --- | --- | --- |
|  |  | 10 min | 24 hr |
| Control | 1.34 | 100 | 100 |
| Thermal treated | 1.32 | 95 | 78 |
| Electron irradiated | 1.60 | 93 | 75 |
| $^{60}$Cobalt irradiated | 2.20 | 90 | 77 |

*Note:* Radiation dose 4.6 to 7.1 Mrd at $-30°C$; extracted control
fat irradiated to 5 Mrad. at $0°C$; beef homogenized and extracted with $CHCL_3$ and $CH_3OH$.

From Raica, N., Scott, J., and Nielsen, W., *Radiat. Res. Rev.*, 3,
447, 1972. With permission.

Table 10
EFFECT OF GAMMA IRRADIATION ON VITAMIN
A AND CAROTENOIDS IN MILK AND MILK
PRODUCTS

|  | Irradiation time (hr) | | | | |
| --- | --- | --- | --- | --- | --- |
|  | 0 | 1 | 3 | 6 | 12 |
| Vitamin A (% destruction) |  |  |  |  |  |
| Milk | — | 31.0 | 46.0 | 70.0 | 35.0 |
| Evaporated milk | — | 9.0 | 16.0 | 35.0 | 66.0 |
| Butter | — | 3.3 | 2.2 | 1.4 | 0.9 |
| Cheese (cheddar) | — | 7.0 | 32.0 | 47.0 | — |
| Cream | — | 10.0 | 17.0 | 31.0 | — |
| Carotenoids (% destruction) |  |  |  |  |  |
| Milk | — | 5.3 | 26.0 | 40.0 | 45.0 |
| Evaporated milk | — | 8.0 | 17.0 | 27.0 | 49.0 |

Reprinted with permission from Kung, H. C., Gaden, E. L., and King,
C. G., *J. Agric. Food Chem.*, 1(2), 142, 1953. Copyright by the American
Chemical Society.

diets, respectively, a slight increase in activities for cytochrome oxidase in the livers of
rats fed the irradiated diet was noted.[51] These findings suggest that radiation processed
diets have some effect on lipid metabolism, since Kunkel and Williams[52] have noted a
marked increase in cytochrome activity in rats fed a fat-deficient diet. In other words,
radiation processing could have an effect on the essential unsaturated fatty acids altered by oxidative effects of radiation, which is in turn reflected in the increase in
cytochrome oxidase activity (Figure 1).

Raica and co-workers[10] have reported extensively on the instability of irradiated fats
and oils and on the work of the U.S. Army Medical Nutrition Laboratory in exploring
the effects of radiation upon corn oil, cooking oils, and beef fat. They found that
retinyl acetate, when added to irradiated corn oil immediately after irradiation, is stable for 24 hr. However, they also noted that when it is irradiated in oil sealed under

air or nitrogen, retinyl acetate is largely destroyed. Raica et al. further observed that cooking oils (corn, peanut, cottonseed, and soybean) irradiated at 5 Mrad do not significantly reduce the in vitro lipase initial hydrolysis rate of the treated oils. Peanut oil seemed to be the most stable to irradiation. However, when it was heated to attain a peroxide value of 24 meq/k the lipase activity was reduced to about 20% of a control value. Irradiated triolein and trilinolein were hydrolyzed by lipase at about 90% the rate of that of control or nonirradiated triglycerides.

Extracting fat from irradiated and nonirradiated (sterilization dose) beef samples, Raica et al. found that the irradiated beef fat had only a slightly inhibitory effect on lipase as compared to nonirradiated beef fat. Also, when there is prolonged exposure to solvents, fats from thermally treated and irradiated beef did significantly inhibit lipase activity. Thus, there are probably lipase-inhibiting substances in lipids that are formed during either thermal or radiation processing. Results of the studies by Raica and co-workers[10] on the lipase activity of fat from room temperature-stored beef (sterilized by thermal or ionizing energy) compared to fat from frozen-stored, enzyme-inactivated control beef are given in Table 9.

Despite these slight variations in effects resulting from the processing of fats by irradiation or through heating, it may be concluded that irradiation applied at doses below 7 Mrad (sterilization maximum range) should not result in any overall loss in energy value or a reduction in digestibility great enough to imply a loss in nutritive value.

## EFFECT OF RADIATION TREATMENT ON MICRONUTRIENTS

### Fat-Soluble Vitamins

*Vitamin A and Carotene*

Kung and co-workers[53] demonstrated that vitamin A and carotenoids are sensitive to destruction within the time period required for sterilization in milk or milk fat. Their experiments involved treatment of whole and evaporated milk, butter, and cheese at 80,000 R/hr for periods of up to 12 hr. The percentages of destruction of vitamin A and carotenoids in these products within a given period of time are shown in Table 10. The total radiation dose for the 12-hr range, required for sterilization of mixed bacterial cultures, was between 1.0 and 1.5 Mrad using [60]Cobalt as the radiation source.

The destruction reaction follows a first-order reaction, and it is apparent that fresh milk, which has more water molecules than other dairy products, reflects a higher percentage destruction of vitamin A with time than either evaporated milk, butter, cheese, or cream. The percentage destruction of carotenoids does not appear as great as that for vitamin A. In tests on margarine conducted by the same investigators, the destructive effect on vitamin A did not seem as great as it was in milk fat. This is apparently due to protective compounds in margarine.

Thomas and Calloway[54] have shown in their studies on vegetables (green beans, carrots, and corn) that beta-carotene levels are not appreciably effected after radappertization (sterilization) followed by cooking or heating. The radiation dose used was 4.8 Mrad. Beta-carotene values for the vegetables processed are shown in Table 11.

The destructive effect of radiation may be indirect; free radicals in the solvent or the oxidized components, e.g., peroxides or carbonyls in the medium, react with the vitamins and other biologically active materials. Therefore, it is important during observations on experimental animal response to ascertain whether the observed aberrant physiological effect is really a manifestation of a toxic reaction to the radiation endproduct or merely a reflection of a nutrient deficiency induced by radiation processing.

As indicated previously, other components in a food may provide a protective mech-

Table 11
EFFECT OF FREEZING,
RADAPPERTIZATION, AND
THERMAL PROCESSING ON BETA-
CAROTENE LEVELS IN SOME
VEGETABLES[54]

| Vegetable | Beta-carotene levels (mg/100 g dry wt) | |
| --- | --- | --- |
| | As processed | As served |
| Green beans | | |
| Initial frozen | 1.6 | — |
| Radappertized | 2.7 | 3.4 |
| Canned (thermal) | 3.8 | 4.9 |
| Carrots | | |
| Initial frozen | 129 | — |
| Radappertized | 112 | 131 |
| Canned (thermal) | 143 | 167 |
| Corn | | |
| Initial frozen | 1.6 | — |
| Radappertized | 0.9 | 0.4 |
| Canned (thermal) | 1.3 | 0.9 |

Table 12
PROTECTIVE EFFECT OF ALPHA-
TOCOPHEROL ON CAROTENE AND VITAMIN A
ACETATE IRRADIATED IN ISOOCTANE
SOLUTIONS[a]

| Indicator | Atmosphere | Dose at $10^5$ rad protective effect[b] | | | |
| --- | --- | --- | --- | --- | --- |
| | | 0.93 | 1.86 | 3.72 | 7.44 |
| Carotene | Air | 0.6 | 0.9 | 0.6 | 1.1 |
| | $N_2$ | 0.7 | 1.0 | 0.6 | 0.9 |
| Vitamin A acetate | Air | 0.2 | 0.5 | 0.7 | 0.5 |
| | $N_2$ | 0.6 | 0.3 | 0.8 | 0.4 |

[a] Concentrations: alpha-tocopherol $1 \times 10^{-4}$ *M*; carotene $1 \times 10^{-4}$ *M*; vitamin A acetate $8.5 \times 10^{-5}$ *M*.
[b] See definition in text.

Reprinted with permission from Knapp, F. W. and Tappel, A. L., *J. Agric. Food Chem.*, 9(6), 430, 1961. Copyright by the American Chemical Society.

anism. For example, carotene destruction can be minimized by the addition of ascorbic acid and alpha-tocopherol (vitamin E). Knapp and Tappel[55] have demonstrated the protective effect of alpha-tocopherol on carotene and vitamin A acetate when these vitamins are irradiated in an isooctane solution in the presence of air or an atmosphere of nitrogen. The protective effect is defined as the ratio of the does absorbed by the protector per concentration of protector divided by the dose absorbed by the indicator per concentration of indicator. These values are given in Table 12. Certainly, carotene is more stabilized than vitamin A, and alpha-tocopherol protects vitamin A acetate and carotene. Vitamin A acetate is twice as stable to ionizing radiation as carotene.

The presence of vitamin E or alpha-tocopherol seems to negate any comparative effect of air or oxygen and nitrogen, since vitamin E in the system acts as a protector to vitamin A acetate and carotene.

Knapp and Tappel also reported on the effects of radiation on vitamin D in salmon oil.[55] They noted that this vitamin is apparently unaffected by ionizing radiation. Here again, the protective effect of some of the sterols in the oil may be operable, since these sterols could be converted to vitamin D-like substances. Vitamin E in the salmon oil could have provided some protection. One might infer, however, that insofar as foods are concerned, the vitamin D reduction (such as occurs in fishery products) would not be significant.

### Vitamin K

The synthesis of vitamin K by microorganisms in the intestinal tract is usually adequate in animals. Because of this mechanism, vitamin K deficiency in animals and man is not encountered. However, during an experimental program designed to establish the wholesomeness of irradiated beef, an extensive program supported by the Department of Defense in the mid 1950s, there was a high incidence of hypoprothombinemia in rats fed irradiated beef diets. These findings led to a series of research projects that added much to our understanding of vitamin K metabolism.[56]

Estrogens apparently decrease the need for vitamin K, since male rats fed an irradiated beef diet and not practicing coprophagy (recycling of feces) are quite susceptible to vitamin K deficiency and thus hemorrhagic diathesis. The age of the animal as well as its gender are also important factors.[57] Beef treated at a sterilizing dose of 6 Mrad and fed to rats resulted in almost a cessation of coprophagy, whereas a 3 Mrad-treated beef diet did not produce such a pronounced effect.[12] Vitamin A plays a role in the hemorrhagenicity of certain diets, and the type of protein in the diet relates to acceleration of hypoprothrombinemia. DL-Methionine has a sparing effect on vitamin K.[12]

Richardson et al.[58] discovered that no vitamin K destruction occurred when a diet containing dehydrated alfalfa leaf meal or fresh spinach was irradiated. Metta et al.[56] found that the irradiated beef diet at 35% dry weight, caused internal hemorrhages in rats and, ultimately, death in less than 8 weeks. Thus a diet low in vitamin K, or producing a vitamin K deficiency such as that produced by the specific beef diet but not by irradiated alfalfa leaf meal diet, leads to a hemorrhagic syndrome in male rats. Addition of vitamin K to the diet of course, eliminated the syndrome.

Judging from these observations, it becomes apparent that intestinal synthesis or absorption of vitamin K may not be adequate to prevent a deficiency when the diet consumed has been irradiated and therefore has an insufficient amount of this vitamin. Accordingly, Richardson and co-workers[58] compared the relative vitamin K activity of frozen, irradiated, and heat-processed foods and found no significant differences in vitamin K activity (using the chick assay procedure) for spinach, broccoli, cabbage, asparagus, and green beans either initially or after 9 and 15 months of storage following either of the three processing procedures (Table 13). Although there appears to be some variation in their results, they attributed most of it to variation in the assay procedure.

Investigators researching the hemorrhagic syndrome have speculated that this condition may have developed because: (1) vitamin K antagonists might be formed in the beef due to radiation processing, (2) coprophagy; which provides an important source of vitamin K to the rat, might be reduced due to presence of irradiated beef, or (3) vitamin K is destroyed by the radiation process. Whatever the mechanism, beef irradiated at the 6 Mrad dose reduced the vitamin K activity enough to render nutritionally inadequate those diets that depend solely upon the radiation-processed beef as a source of vitamin K. The same result could be achieved even with a synthetic diet of amino

Table 13
INFLUENCE OF FREEZING, HEAT
PROCESSING AND RADIATION
STERILIZATION ON VITAMIN K
ACTIVITY OF CERTAIN FOODS[a]

| | | | Processing methods | |
| | | | Radiation (Mrad) | |
| Food | Frozen | Thermal | 2.79 | 5.58 |
|---|---|---|---|---|
| Asparagus | 33 | 41 | 37 | 46 |
| Broccoli | 63 | 68 | 74 | 44 |
| Cabbage | 56 | 54 | 78 | 56 |
| Green beans | 28 | 28 | 20 | 58 |
| Spinach | 93 | 125 | 227 | 198 |

[a]    Average K activity in micrograms per 100 g of food.

Adapted from Richardson, L. R., Wilkes, S., and Ritchey, S. J., *J. Nutr.*, 73(4), 369, 1961. With permission.

acids if the rat is prevented from practicing coprophagy.[59] In a practical sense, man would not experience such vitamin K deficiencies because a wide spectrum of foods in the diet would furnish enough vitamin K over and above any decreased level resulting from irradiation of beef or other natural foodstuffs.

When untreated beef was fed to rats, none of the animals developed a prolonged prothrombin time regardless of whether coprophagy was prevented or allowed. This suggests that there is a sufficient level of vitamin K in the G.I. tract and that coprophagy is not required to enhance its intake. Thus, the primary cause of the hemorrhagic diathesis in the male rat is destruction of vitamin K in beef by irradiation, with an increased effect at the higher radiation dose of 5 to 6 Mrad.

Knapp and Tappel[55] have concluded that the vitamin reacts to alkyl radicals more than it does to peroxides, while others have speculated that destruction of the vitamin may thus proceed through a reductive attack by alkyl radicals or hydrogen atoms. Thus, a saturation of double bonds in the case of menadione (vitamin K) results in a reduction or etherification of the benzoquinone moiety.

*Vitamin E (Alpha-tocopherol)*
Vitamin E is the most sensitive of the fat-soluble vitamins to irradiation, exceeding the sensitivity of the others as follows:

Vitamin E > Carotene > Vitamin A > Vitamin D > Vitamin K

Lipids form peroxides when irradiated; thus, any peroxidized compounds or hydroxy-hydroperoxides have an antagonistic or destructive effect upon an antioxidant and essential reproductive vitamin such as vitamin E.

Perhaps the first observation of this destructive effect on vitamin E was made in 1948 by DaCosta and Levenson,[60] who found that reproductive failure occurred when a diet exposed to capacitron irradiation was fed to female rats. This important work, recognized by toxicologists conducting studies on irradiated foods, was overlooked by some investigators. As a result, poor reproduction was observed in test animals because

Table 14

VITAMIN E STABILITY IN FOODS AND
DIET AS INFLUENCED BY RADIATION
DOSE AND CONDITIONS OF PACKING

| Food or diet | Radiation dose (Mrad) | Destruction of vitamin (%) |
|---|---|---|
| Rolled oats | 0[a] | 26 |
|  | 0.1[a] | 85 |
| Milk, raw | 0 |  |
|  | 0.08 | 29 |
|  | 0.24 | 40 |
|  | 0.48 | 61 |
| Chick diet | 2.0 | 68 |
|  | 3.0 | 69 |
|  | 5.0 (in air)[b] | 51 |
|  | 5.0 (in a vacuum)[b] | 10 |

[a]  Product stored for 8 months.
[b]  Sealed in container with air space or evacuated prior
to radiation treatment.

of the failure to provide a vitamin E supplement. Later, to obviate any variant effect of vitamin E deficiency, supplementation was practiced by those conducting toxicity studies on irradiated foods.

Raica et al.,[10] reporting work performed by Diehl,[61] indicated that vitamin E was quite labile in rolled oats after a radiation treatment of only 0.1 Mrad followed by an 8-month storage period. For example, immediately after radiation treatment at 0.1 Mrad, the vitamin E retention was 80%, which decreased to 15% after 8 months of storage. The control rolled oats sample, on the other hand, retained 44% of its vitamin E following 8 months of storage. Thus, during storage, the presence of peroxides in the product has a great destructive effect on this antioxidant vitamin.

Kung et al.[53] observed a similar destructive effect on alpha-tocopherol in raw whole milk when it was irradiated at 80,000 R/hr for 1, 3, 6, and 12 hr, the values decreasing from 119 gammas per 100 m$\ell$ of milk prior to irradiation to 47 gammas per 100 m$\ell$ of milk after 6 hr of radiation treatment. This represents a progressive percentage of destruction from 0 to 29 to 40 to 61% at 0, 1, 3, and 6 hr, respectively.

Josephson et al.,[62] analyzing the work of other researchers, showed that radiation with $^{60}$Cobalt gamma source has an effect on vitamin E retention of various diets for the chick, guinea pig, cat, and mouse. In a chick diet treated at 2 and 5 Mrad, it is interesting to note that whereas gamma irradiation at 2 or 3 Mrad resulted in only a 32 and 31% retention of vitamin E, respectively, a similar diet packed under air and under vacuum had a 49 and 90% retention rate, respectively. Values for vitamin E retention and destruction in foods and diets under variant conditions are reported in Table 14.

## Water-Soluble Vitamins

As indicated earlier, the radiosensitivity of the micronutrients (including water-soluble vitamins) differs, depending on whether they are in pure solution, in a food, or protected by other chemicals in food, including the mutual protective action of vitamins. Free radicals, peroxides, and carbonyls react with the vitamins.

### Thiamin

Thiamin appears to be the most labile of the B vitamins. It acts as a scavenger for the radicals produced in water and, in the process, is destroyed. Thiamin is destroyed in meat at room temperature when it is irradiated to the same extent as it is during heat sterilization. In the frozen state or under an inert atmosphere at low temperature, the vitamin destruction is quite small. Thiamin destruction in thermally processed foods is approximately 65%, whereas in radiation-processed food it is 63%.[2] Ziporin et al.[63] and Wilson[65] conducted some of the earliest extensive studies on thiamin. While the above value of 65% was cited for thiamin destruction, some investigators reported that there was as much as 95% destruction of this vitamin by radappertization.

In studies by Ziporin and co-workers[63] a range of thiamin destruction from 70 to 95% was noted in haddock, beef, turkey, ham, bacon, peaches, powdered milk, and beets (Table 15). These researchers also found that the radiosensitivity of this vitamin in foods was less than in pure solution and that it is degraded into pyrimidine and thiazole moieties. The thiazole underwent further degradative changes at high doses of irradiation. The relative percentages of destruction of thiamin in eight foods as determined by Ziporin et al.,[63] and Day et al.[64] on beef are reported in Table 15. The effect of radiation dose and temperature on destruction of thiamin in irradiated beef is shown in Figures 2 and 3.[65]

Destruction of thiamin appears to be greatest in foods that have a relatively high level of that vitamin. Low-temperature (−80°C) radiation of meat appears to protect against the destruction of thiamin resulting in a retention rate of as high as 85%, compared to 2% retention at ambient temperature.[54]

Measurements on nutrient content have also been made on standard wheat mixtures used for baking that were irradiated with a $^{60}$Cobalt gamma irradiation source at 75,000 rad and then stored. Wheat is irradiated at this level for the purpose of disinfestation, a process that was accepted by the U.S.S.R. in 1959, the U.S. in 1963, and Canada in 1969. According to a report of the Institute for Radiation Technology, Karlsruhe, West Germany, the thiamin content of wheat was not reduced even after 24 months of storage.[66] Values on irradiated and nonirradiated wheat used in the making of bread are shown in Table 16.

*Riboflavin*

Vitamin $B_2$, or riboflavin, is not as radiation labile as thiamin. Some of the earliest studies of this vitamin, as well as of niacin and ascorbic acid, were conducted by Proctor and Goldblith,[69] who used soft X-rays to study the effects of irradiation at doses ranging from 100,000 to 400,000 R on these vitamins in pure solutions, either alone or in combination. For example, at a dose of 250,000 R, the riboflavin concentration in solution was decreased from 50 gammas per milliliter to 44.8 gammas per milliliter, with a retention value, therefore, of 89.6%. The niacin showed a retention of 100% at a radiation dose of 400,000 R, while ascorbic acid in solution irradiated at 100,000 R retained only 17.1% of the vitamin.

The greater the dilution, the more sensitive were the vitamins to ionizing radiation. If niacin and ascorbic acid were mixed in solution, then niacin had a sparing effect on ascorbic acid. Ribloflavin was protected by oxalic acid from the effect of ionizing radiation.

As stated previously, vitamins in dry state or in a substrate such as food are protected. For example, Day et al.[67] have observed that riboflavin in beef is fairly resistant to irradiation, since only about 8% was destroyed by the irradiation process. Heat processing of beef apparently has a greater destructive effect than radiation processing at either 2.8 or 5.6 Mrad.[42] Thomas and Josephson[68] have reported that low temperature radiation sterilization (radappertization) of pork results in a very high retention of riboflavin. (The low temperature was −80°C and the radiation dose was 4.5 Mrad.) For example, when pork is irradiated at an ambient temperature at 4.8 Mrad, the

Table 15
THIAMIN CONTENT (μg/g) IN
VARIOUS IRRADIATED AND
NONIRRADIATED FOODS[62,63]

| | Radiation dose (Mrad) | | |
|---|---|---|---|
| | 0 | 2.79 | 5.58 |
| Haddock | 0.11 | 0.035 | 0.026 |
| Turkey | 0.14 | 0.034 | 0.033 |
| Ham | 8.15 | 1.03 | 0.31 |
| Bacon | 3.03 | — | 0.21 |
| Peaches | 0.79 | 0.045 | 0.017 |
| Milk (powdered) | 1.53 | 1.96 | 1.90 |
| Beets | 0.48 | 0.23 | 0.12 |
| Beef | 0.24 | 0.057 | 0.037 |
| Beef[62] | 1.05 | 0.45 | — |

Table 16
THIAMIN CONTENT IN BREAD MADE
FROM IRRADIATED AND
UNIRRADIATED WHEAT AFTER
VARYING PERIODS OF STORAGE

| | Average thiamin content of bread (μg/100 g bread) | |
|---|---|---|
| Storage time | Unirradiated | Irradiated |
| Initial value | 249 | 281 |
| 6 Months of storage | 226 | 209 |
| 12 | 241 | 246 |
| 18 | 194 | 225 |
| 24 | 222 | 236 |

From Schönborn, W. and Ehrhardt, G. (1974) Technical Report IFIP-R 16, International Project in the Field of Food Irradiation, Federal Research Centre for Nutrition, Karlsruhe, F. R. Germany. With permission.

riboflavin retention is 50%, whereas at low temperature radiation processing, the retention rate is 78%, compared to 81% for thermal processing. As is true for some of the other B vitamins, Thomas and Calloway[54] have noted further losses in riboflavin after radiation-processed meats are cooked.

Ziporin et al.,[63] in studies on the eight foods previously mentioned, found that riboflavin was substantially reduced in turkey at radiation doses of 2.79 and 5.58 Mrad, the greater destruction occurring at the higher radiation dose (Table 17). For the other foods mentioned (haddock, beef, ham, bacon, peaches, beets and powdered milk), the reduction of riboflavin content was not significant. The reasons for the variation in turkey were not given.

*Niacin*

Like the other B vitamins, niacin in pure solution is more sensitive to radiation than it is when present in food. However, it is far less radiosensitive than thiamin or riboflavin. Goldblith et al.[69] have shown that niacin at a concentration of 100 gammas per milliliter when irradiated in aqueous solution at a dose of $0.17 \times 10^6$ rep, showed de-

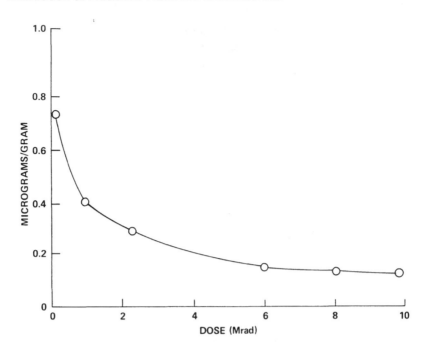

FIGURE 2.    Effect of irradiation dose on the destruction of thiamin in beef processed at room temperature. (Data from Reference 65.)

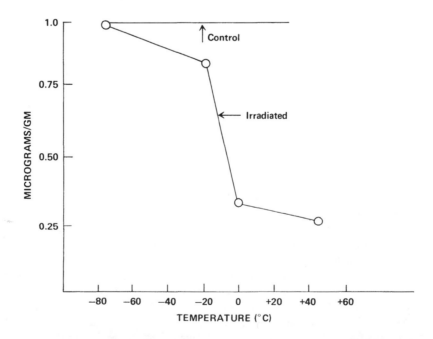

FIGURE 3.    Effect of temperature on the destruction of thiamin in beef irradiated at 1 Mrad. (Data from Reference 65.)

carboxylation to the extent of 28%. Splitting of the pyridine ring did not occur until the radiation dose was increased to $0.66 \times 10^6$ rep using a cathode ray source. Thus, the splitting of the pyridine ring required much more radiation energy than is required for decarboxylation.

Table 17
RIBOFLAVIN LEVELS AND PERCENT
REDUCTION IN FOODS EXPOSED TO
VARIANT DOSES OF GAMMA RADIATION

| Food (μg/g) | Radiation dose (Mrad) | | | Maximum percent decrease |
|---|---|---|---|---|
| | 0 | 2.79 | 5.58 | |
| Haddock | 0.71 | 0.76 | 0.68 | 4.2 |
| Beef | 1.86 | 1.76 | 1.79 | 3.7 |
| Turkey | 2.05 | *1.50* | *1.03* | 50.0 |
| Ham (fresh) | 1.65 | 1.86 | 1.62 | 1.8 |
| Bacon | 1.11 | — | 1.03 | 7.2 |
| Peaches | 0.26 | 0.32 | 0.27 | — |
| Milk (powdered) | 12.6 | 13.9 | 14.3 | — |
| Beets | 0.50 | 0.43 | 0.45 | 10.0 |

*Note:* Italicized values indicate greatest percent destruction of vitamin $B_2$ for the particular protein food.

From Ziporin, Z. Z., Kraybill, H. F., and Thack, H. J., *J. Nutr.*, 63(2), 201, 1957. With permission.

Ziporin et al.[63] reported that there was no significant loss in niacin for seven of eight foods (mentioned earlier) irradiated at 2.79 and 5.58 Mrad. The exception was peaches, which showed a 50% loss. Since ascorbic acid is usually added to this fruit prior to freezing or canning, it is possible that the commercial-grade product might account for the destruction of niacin because, while radioprotective for ascorbic acid, niacin is in turn more readily degraded in the presence of vitamin C.

Niacin in beef is very resistant to the effects of gamma radiation at doses of up to 4 Mrad.[67] Gamma irradiation of bleached, enriched, hard wheat flour at a dose of 30 to 50 krad caused no significant loss of niacin. Earlier work was confirmed by the International Project in Field of Food Irradiation even at doses of up to 75 krad.[66] Brooke et al.[70] reported no significant loss in niacin content of clams processed at a radiation dose of 450 krad. Similarly, oysters irradiated at 0.2 Mrad showed no significant loss of niacin.[71]

*Pyridoxine (Vitamin $B_6$)*

Day and co-workers[67] reported that pyridoxine in beef is more radiosensitive than riboflavin. At a radiation dose of 3.2 Mrad, they found that 24% of this vitamin was destroyed. By irradiating pork at a temperature of −80°C, a high retention of pyridoxine was achieved even at a radiation dose of 4.5 to 4.8 Mrad.[54,68] However, some of the results on pyridoxine are variable. For example, Brin et al.[72] reported pyridoxine retentions in pork ranging from 50 to 100%. These investigators indicated that pyridoxine is stable in irradiated pork that is subsequently cooked.

Day and co-workers[67] reported that supplementation of a rat diet with penicillin could exert a sparing effect on the pyridoxine requirement of the rat, as shown by increased growth rate and increased level of pyridoxine in the liver. This finding is important in the microbiological assay for pyridoxine in diets in which irradiated beef is incorporated.

As was the case with thiamin, Richardson et al.[73] found that irradiated beef liver, boned chicken, cabbage, and green beans showed a significant drop in pyridoxine content (40 to 60%) when stored for 15 months. Heat processing of foods also caused a similar decrease. In contrast, irradiated sweet potatoes and lima beans did not change

Table 18
EFFECT OF RADIATION PROCESSING,
HEAT PROCESSING, AND STORAGE ON
PYRIDOXINE ACTIVITY COMPARED TO
FROZEN CONTROL FOODS[58]

| Food | Storage period (months) | Activity retained (%) | | |
|---|---|---|---|---|
| | | Heat processed | Irradiated | |
| | | | 2.8 | 5.6 |
| Beef liver | 0 | 29 | 100 | 82 |
| After storage | 15 | 13 | 53 | 57 |
| Bonded chicken | 0 | 57 | 68 | 63 |
| After storage | 15 | 61 | 85 | 54 |
| Cabbage | 0 | 94 | 63 | 53 |
| After storage | 15 | 70 | 62 | 52 |
| Green beans | 0 | — | 67 | 44 |
| After storage | 15 | — | 66 | 62 |
| Sweet potatoes | 0 | — | 52 | 24 |
| After storage | 15 | — | 53 | 32 |

in their pyridoxine activity after 15 months of storage. The effects of irradiation treatment and storage on the pyridoxine activity of six foods are shown in Table 18. The vitamin $B_6$ activities of these foods after irradiation and storage were compared to control samples of frozen foods at each corresponding storage period.

The destructive effect of thermal processing (canning) on pork and the constituent B vitamins (thiamin, riboflavin, niacin, and pyridoxine) is shown in Figure 4. For comparative purposes, the percent of destruction of these vitamins by radiation sterilization at doses of 4.5 and 4.8 Mrad under ambient temperatures and in a frozen state ($-80°C$) are also given. It is obvious from this figure that it is advantageous to use low temperatures during radiation processing in order to increase the retention of these vitamins.[42,63,68] Other vitamins in this class, e.g., biotin, choline, folic acid, inositol, and pantothenic acid, have not been studied sufficiently under variant radiation conditions and heat processing to furnish comparative data.

*Vitamin $B_{12}$ (Cobalamin)*

This antipernicious anemia vitamin, isolated and studied extensively in 1949, was also examined in 1951 by Markakis[74] to ascertain the effects of high energy electrons on this vitamin in pure solution. These investigators found that radiation doses of 2500, 4500, 8100 and 14,600 rep caused retention levels of 68, 52, 35, and 21%, respectively, when the concentration in solution was 10 $\mu g/m\ell$. However, when the concentration was increased to 15 $\mu g/m\ell$, the retention values were 77, 67, 52, and 32%, respectively. As might be expected, when radiation treatment was applied to this vitamin in a food such as milk, the retention values were higher, even if the radiation doses were higher than those given above. For example, when raw whole milk containing $4.9 \times 10^{-3}$ $\mu g/m\ell$ of this vitamin was used and radiation doses of 50,000, 100,000, 250,000 and 500,000 rep were applied, the retention rates were 100, 75, 67, and 69%, respectively. The effect of heat processing on this vitamin in pure solution or in milk was not determined.

Liuzzo et al.[71] noted that vitamin $B_{12}$ losses were not extensive in oysters irradiated at a dose of 0.2 Mrad to extend their shelf life.

*Pantothenic Acid*

Thomas and Josephson[68] and Thomas and Calloway[54] determined the percentage

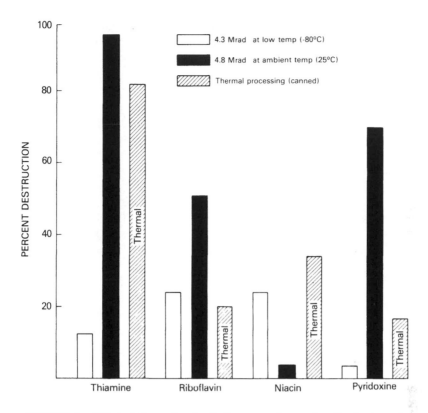

FIGURE 4. Effect of thermal and radiation processing on the vitamins in pork (radiation processing at ambient temperature and frozen temperatures). (Data from References 42 and 68.)

retention of pantothenic acid in pork that was irradiated at ambient temperature at a dose of 4.8 Mrad. They found that 32% of this vitamin was retained. When pork was canned or thermally processed, the retention percentage was slightly higher (43%). Josephson et al.[62] found that there was a high retention of this vitamin in various animal diets when they were irradiated at various doses. For example, in a chick diet, 95 and 92% of the vitamin was retained at radiation doses of 2 and 3 Mrad, respectively. When the diet was air-packed and vacuum-packed and then irradiated at 5 Mrad, the retention value was about 100%. In a guinea pig diet irradiated at a 2.5-Mrad dose, the retention was 79%, while a cat diet treated at the same dose had a retention value of 88%.

*Folacin (Pterolyglutamic Acid)*

This chick vitamin and bacterial growth factor was elucidated as a single substance or factor in 1941. Shefner and Spector[75] found no destruction of this vitamin when pork was irradiated at 5.58 Mrad, and Richardson[76] showed that irradiated diets fed to chicks caused no significant decrease in folacin activity.

*Biotin*

Biotin, a component of the enzyme carbonyl phosphate synthetase, is an essential nutrient for man and is widely distributed in animal and vegetable products. Luizzo et al.[71] found no extensive loss of this vitamin in oysters irradiated at 0.2 Mrad. Josephson et al.,[62] reporting data of Ley[77] and Coates et al.,[78] found that biotin was not destroyed appreciably in various diets. For example, in chick diets irradiated at 2 and 3 Mrad, the retention was 79%. However, when the radiation dose was increased to 5

Mrad in an air-packed or vacuum-packed container, the retention increased to 100%. Guinea pig and cat diets irradiated at 2.5 Mrad had retention values for this vitamin of over 100%.

### Choline

Choline analogues have been examined by Lemmon and co-workers[79] for sensitivity to electrons and gamma rays. Choline chloride was more sensitive than other similar compounds. (The other analogues of choline chloride were 60 to 90% more resistant.)

### Ascorbic Acid (Vitamin C)

Studies in 1949 by Proctor and Goldblith[80] showed that ascorbic acid in pure solution, when treated with X-rays, is the most sensitive vitamin. The amount of destruction increased with increased dose and time. The greater the dilution, the greater the radiosensitivity. Although niacin alone is much more radioresistant than ascorbic acid, these investigators found that in a mixture of the two there is a greater destruction of the niacin and sparing of the ascorbic acid. It was stated that niacin competed more successfully for the molecules of activated water, while ascorbic acid had a protective effect on riboflavin in pure solution. The relative destructive effects of irradiation on ascorbic acid in pure solution as compared to niacin and riboflavin are shown in Table 19.

Some comparative data on the destructive effects of radappertization (radiation sterilization) and thermal processing of green beans, carrots, and corn were reported by Thomas and Calloway.[54] Reduced ascorbic acid was almost completely oxidized, however, as shown in Table 20, the canning or thermal treatment of these foods was equally destructive.

As stated earlier, the vitamin C loss at a low radiation dose, especially in foods, is minimal. This has been shown in the case of potatoes treated at 10 krad to prevent sprouting, with a loss of about 15% according to some investigators.[62] However, McKinney[81] reported no loss of vitamin C in potatoes subjected to radiation treatment.

Radiation treatment has been applied to fruits to increase shelf life, for deinfestation, and to inhibit surface molds. This type of processing, achieved at dose ranges of 100 to 400 krad, is perhaps one of the most promising radiation processing technologies. Dennison and Ahmed[82] and Wenkam and Moy[83] have studied the effects of radiopasteurization on the ascorbic acid level in oranges, tangerines, tomatoes, and papayas. In essence, they noted that these items treated at radiation doses ranging from 40 to 300 krad had retentions varying from 72 to 100%, dependent upon the fruit and the radiation dose.

It was mentioned previously that Kung and co-workers[53] in their work on radiation treatment of milk, found that ascorbic acid, vitamin E, and vitamin A were destroyed to a greater extent than riboflavin in this liquid food. Additionally, Ziporin et al.[63] observed that the excessive loss in niacin in peaches (about 48% at 2.79 Mrad and 56% at 5.58 Mrad) was due to the additive effect of ascorbic acid, a vitamin included in all commercially packed fruits to prevent browning. This interactive effect was noted earlier in work of Proctor and Goldblith.[80]

### Inositol

None of the reports on the bioassay of foods that have been frozen, irradiated, or heat treated mention the effect of radiation on this vitamin. Inositol is known to be very stable chemically. However, Day et al.[67] did report some values for inositol in beef that was irradiated at a dose of 3.0 Mrad. The analysis of several samples at various times showed no difference between the level of inositol in frozen beef and the level in the radiation-sterilized beef. These workers indicate that such results would

## Table 19
### RELATIVE RADIOSENSITIVITIES OF ASCORBIC ACID, NIACIN, AND RIBOFLAVIN WHEN EXPOSED TO VARIANT RADIATION DOSES IN SOLUTION

| Vitamin | Dosage (rad) | Concentration ($\mu$g/m$l$) | Retention of vitamin (%) |
|---------|--------------|------------------------------|---------------------------|
| Ascorbic acid | 10,000 | 100 | 98.0 |
| | 25,000 | 100 | 85.6 |
| | 50,000 | 100 | 68.7 |
| | 150,000 | 100 | 19.8 |
| | 200,000 | 100 | 3.5 |
| Niacin | 400,000 | 50 | 100.0 |
| Riboflavin | 250,000 | 50 | 89.6 |
| Niacin (alone) | 400,000 | 10 | 72.0 |
| Niacin plus oxalic acid | 400,000 | 10 | 34.5 |
| Niacin plus ascorbic acid | 400,000 | 10 | 14.0 (niacin) |
| | | | 71.8 (ascorbic acid) |

From Proctor, B. E. and Goldblith, S. A., *Nucleonics*, 5, 56, 1949. With permission.

## Table 20
### RELATIVE EFFECTS OF RADIATION AND THERMAL PROCESSING ON VITAMIN C IN SOME VEGETABLES[54]

| Item | Ascorbic acid (mg/100 g) | |
|------|---------|-------|
| | Reduced | Total |
| Green beans | | |
|   Frozen | 40.0 | 53.3 |
|   Irradiated (4.8 Mrad) | 0 | 39.2 |
|   Thermal | 0 | 14.7 |
| Carrots | | |
|   Frozen | 46.9 | 46.9 |
|   Irradiated (4.8 Mrad) | 0 | 36.5 |
|   Thermal | 10.9 | 21.7 |
| Corn | | |
|   Frozen | 28.4 | 28.4 |
|   Irradiated (4.8 Mrad) | 10.1 | 20.1 |
|   Thermal | 12.6 | 16.8 |

be in accordance with the concept in that secondary reactions are chiefly responsible for nutrient destruction. Since there are no secondary reactions, this vitamin is relatively nonradiosensitive.

## NUTRIENTS, PROCESSING, AND EFFECT ON PHYSIOLOGICAL PERFORMANCE

The availability or nonavailability of nutrients in a mammalian system may be associated, on a long- or short-term basis, with any physiological performance. Beyond the nutrient depletion is the aspect of overt toxicity. It is not within the scope of this chapter to discuss the broad category of probable toxicological effects of radiolytic products (radiation processing) or thermal degradation products (thermal processing) that may be formed in processing. Differentiation of nutrient depletion effects from a toxic effect may not always be easily elucidated.

Table 21

EFFECT OF RADIATION TREATMENT OF SEMISYNTHETIC
DIET ON GROWTH AND FERTILITY OF THE ALBINO RAT

|  | Control unirradiated diet | Irradiated diet |
|---|---|---|
| Days on each diet | 540 | 540 |
| Average final weight (g) | | |
| First generation (males) | 430 | 440 |
| First generation (females) | 285 | 295 |
| Reproduction | | |
| Number of litters (four generations) | 105 | 66 |
| Number of sterile males (four generations) | 1 | 6 |
| Longevity | | |
| Total number of living males (all generations) | 293 | 140 |
| Total number of living females (all generations) | 304 | 180 |

From DaCosta, E. and Levenson, S. M., U.S. Army Med. Nutr. Lab. Rep. No. 89,
U.S. Army Surgeon General, Chicago, 1951. With permission.

In the development of experimental studies on irradiated foods and diets, it became evident that the destruction of vitamin E in some instances and the nonavailability of vitamin K due to lack of G.I. synthesis described earlier could lead to reproductive problems and hemorrhagic diathesis. Some of these events may be unique for irradiation treatment; however, pyrolysis products formed through heating can contribute similar molecular species in the degradative process.

One of the first classical studies, frequently overlooked, is that of DaCosta and Levenson,[60] who demonstrated that feeding an irradiated semisynthetic diet to rats produces a loss in fertility and a significant decrease in life span. Recognition of this finding in 1951 prompted investigators to add appropriate amounts of vitamin E to experimental diets. The loss in fertility and decrease in life span was attributed to the loss of radiolabile vitamin E, probably induced by the formed hydroxyhydroperoxides (Table 21).

The fact that such occurrences were not restricted to treatment of semisynthetic diets was later shown by Poling et al.[84] in a 2-year feeding experiment on irradiated beef administered to male and female rats (radiation dose = 2 Mrad). These investigators noted that the males being fed a nonirradiated-beef diet (about 50% solids) survived an average of $614 \pm 18.8$ days as compared with a survival time of $581 \pm 24.9$ days for animals receiving the irradiated-beef diet. For female rats, the comparable figures were $685 \pm 14.7$ days and $612 \pm 21.8$ days, respectively.

As indicated previously, no other observations relevant to growth and reproduction in animals fed irradiated foods have been reported. However, such findings may have been obviated in many experimental studies because nonirradiated vitamin supplements were added to all diets.

Brownell[85] compared the mortality rate and life span of rats raised on a diet containing either 50% irradiated, heat-processed, or nonirradiated heat-processed beef. The life span of rats on thermally processed beef was comparable to that of rats receiving radiation-processed beef (Table 22). These findings were reported by Kraybill and Hays[86] in 1956.

Such longevity studies need to be confirmed for a wider variety of irradiated foods and diets with and without vitamin supplementation. For many years, it has been assumed that, whereas studies on the physiological effects of vitamins E and K may have experimental interest, in actual human dietary situations these events would not be relevant. Some researchers have argued that because man consumes a wide variety of

Table 22
MORTALITY AND LIFESPAN OF RATS MAINTAINED ON DIET OF 50%
IRRADIATED HEAT-PROCESSED BEEF COMPARED WITH RATS
MAINTAINED ON 50% NONIRRADIATED HEAT-PROCESSED BEEF[86]

| | Males | | Females | |
|---|---|---|---|---|
| | Nonirradiated beef | Irradiated beef | Nonirradiated beef | Irradiated beef |
| Number of rats started | 31 | 31 | 31 | 31 |
| Survival (weeks) | | | | |
| 0—32 | 31 | 30 | 31 | 31 |
| 33—64 | 28 | 27 | 29 | 28 |
| 65—81 | 22 | 23 | 24 | 26 |
| 82—104 | 9 | 8 | 12 | 17 |
| Average number of weeks survival | $90.7 \pm 13.8$ | $93.0 \pm 13.4$ | $92.2 \pm 12.9$ | $94.7 \pm 13.6$ |

foods rich in vitamins K and E, vitamin depletion severe enough to alter physiological performance would not be encountered, since unprocessed foods are significant components of the diet. Nevertheless, more experimental studies in this area would provide a greater element of public health assurance.

## SUMMARY

Of all food components, including macro- and micronutrients, vitamins are most affected by ionizing radiation, since they are, in general, the most radiosensitive. Of these, some of the fat-soluble (e.g., vitamins E and K) and water-soluble vitamins (e.g., ascorbic acid and thiamin) appear to be the most radiosensitive. Nevertheless, vitamin losses as a result of radiation processing are comparable to the losses caused by canning or thermal processing of foods. The micronutrients (vitamins) receive some protective effect from other chemical constituents and the interactant vitamins themselves. It is therefore quite unlikely that nutrient loss would be significant in the human diet, and hence there would be no influence on physiological performance and human nutritional status.

In countries in which radiation-processed foods could eventually comprise a major portion of the diet, special consideration would have to be given and epidemiological observations made in relation to particular foods if the nutrient value of the diet as a whole could be effected. Of course, this specification would probably be applicable even if the sole dietary source were thermally processed foods. National nutritional surveys would certainly provide some unequivocal evidence in this regard so that special groups in the population such as infants, the elderly, and those on restricted diets would be adequately protected. After all the studies supported through contractual projects by the Department of Defense and the Energy Research and Development Administration (formerly the Atomic Energy Commission) over the last 25 years, radiation-processed foods are still considered to be safe and nutritionally adequate.

Recent developments in radiation-processing technology as contrasted with results of the earliest studies, have shown some marked advantages in low-temperature irradiation. Even with an inert atmosphere (exclusion of oxygen), low-temperature irradiation aids materially in reducing radiolytic products or degradative changes, which of course enhances organoleptic properties and consumer acceptance. Additionally, destruction of nutrients is minimized.

While continuing progress may be made in improvement of this unique technology of food preservation from various research efforts, it is most likely that the product quality or the nutritional value will be improved. Some areas require further exploration. For example, the stability of nutrients during long storage periods should be examined, and more data on the added nutrient losses resulting from superimposed cooking processes are needed. The fact that some vitamins can be at least partially destroyed through contact with a medium containing radiolysis products would suggest that there is a need for study on added vitamin losses. More extensive data also need to be acquired on the comparative effects of thermal processing and radiation processing of various foods in terms of their influence on reproductive performance and survival or life span.

Information acquired over the years on wholesomeness would appear to indicate that radiation-processed foods could assume a place in our society at some point in the future. Beyond this, the use of low-dose radiation for shelf-life extension, deinfestation, and sprout inhibition would appear to be one of the most significant advances in the peaceful use of atomic energy.

Within the last 10 years, newer processing techniques are used based on low-temperature frozen foods that are radappertized, resulting in minimum destruction of nutrients. Thus, nutrient values for earlier studies reflect a much greater degree of vitamin destruction.

# REFERENCES

1. Kraybill, H. F., *J. Home Econ.,* 50(9), 695—700, 1958.
2. Kraybill, H. F., *J. Assoc. Food Drug Off.,* 20, 171—180, 1956.
3. Kraybill, H. F., *Nutr. Rev.,* 13(7), 193-195, 1955.
4. Kraybill, H. F., Radiation and appraisal, in *Funeral Directors Review,* Higgins, Chicago, 1960.
5. Roentgen, W. C., *Ann. Phys. Leipzig),* 64, 1, 1898.
6. Becquerel, H., *C. R. Acad. Sci., Ser. D.,* 122, 501, 1895.
7. Pacinotti, G. and Porcalli, V., cited in Buchanan, R. E. and Fulmer, E. T., *Physiology and Biochemistry of Bacteria,* Vol. 2, Williams & Wilkins, Baltimore, 1898, 188.
8. Prescott, S. C., *Science,* 20, 246-248, 1904.
9. Report on Radiation Preservation of Foods, Publ. No. 1273, National Academy of Sciences/National Research Council, Washington, D.C., 1965.
10. Raica, N., Scott, J., and Nielsen, W., *Radiat. Res. Rev.,* 3, 447-457, 1972.
11. Kraybill, H. F. and Brunton, D. C., *J. Agric. Food Chem.,* 8, 349-356, 1960.
12. Kraybill, H. F. and Whitehair, L. A., *Ann. Rev. Pharmacol.,* 7, 357—380, 1967.
13. Kraybill, H. F., Read, M. S., Linder, R. O., Harding, R. S., and Issac, G. J., *J. Allergy,* 30(4), 342-351, 1959.
14. Johnson, B. C., FAO Report on Evaluation of the Wholesomeness of Irradiated Foods, Brussels, October 23-30, 1961, 61-74.
15. Burks, R. E., Baker, E. B., Clarks, P., Esslinger, J., and Lacey, J. C., *J. Agric. Food Chem.,* 7, 778-782, 1959.
16. Merritt, C., Bresnick, S. R., Bazinet, M. L., Welsh, J. T., and Angeline, P., *J. Agric. Food Chem.,* 7, 784-787, 1959.
17. Wick, E. L., Yamanishi, T., Wertheim, L. C., Hoff, J. E., Proctor, B. E., and Goldblith, S. A., *J. Agric. Food Chem.,* 9, 289-293, 1961.
18. Merritt, C., *Radiat. Res. Rev.,* 3, 353-368, 1972.
19. Metta, V. C. and Johnson, B. C., *J. Nutr.,* 59, 479, 1956.
20. Metta, V. C., Norton, H. W., and Johnson, B. C., *J. Nutr.,* 63, 143, 1957.
21. Tsien, W. S. and Johnson, B. C., *J. Nutr.,* 68, 419-428, 1959.
22. Borchers, R. and Ackerson, C. W., *J. Nutr.,* 41, 339, 1950.
23. Ley, F. J., Bleby, J., Coates, M. E., and Patterson, J. S., *Lab Anim.,* 3, 221-254, 1969.
24. Read, M. S., Kraybill, H. F., Worth, W. S., Thompson, S. W., and Isaac, G. J., *Toxicol. Appl. Pharmacol.,* 3, 153, 1961.
25. Loaharanu, P., *Use of Irradiation to Solve Problems in the International Fruit Trade,* International Atomic Energy Agency, Vienna.
26. Funes, F., *Ann. Inst. Nac. Invest. Agron.,* 19, 63—82, 1970.

27. Obara, T., Shimotsuura, A., Shimazu, F., and Watanabe, W., *Radioisotopes,* 7, 127-132, 1958.
28. Bellamy, W. D., Pultz, W., Mendenhall, R. M., and Clark, L. B., *Radiat. Res.,* 5(4), Abstr. 10 and 67, 1956.
29. LaFontaine, A., Deschreides, A., and Bugyaki, L., FAO Report on Evaluation of the Wholesomeness of Irradiated Foods, Brussels, Oct. 23-30, 1961, 97-112.
30. Saeman, F. S., Millett, A., and Lawton, E. J., *Ind. Eng. Chem.,* 44, 2848, 1952.
31. Proctor, B. E. and Goldblith, S. A., *Adv. Food Res.,* 3, 119, 1951.
32. Lawton, E. J., Bellamy, W. D., Hungate, R. E., Bryant, M. P., and Hall, E., *Science,* 113, 380, 1951.
33. Price, F. P., Bellamy, W. D., and Lawton, E. J., *J. Phys. Chem.,* 58, 821, 1954.
34. Wolfrom, M. L., Brinkley, W. W., and McCabe, L. J., unpublished data, 1954.
35. Metta, V. C., unpublished data, 1955.
36. Johnson, B. C., *Atomic Energy and Agriculture,* Comas, C. L., Reitemier, R. F., Tukey, H. B., Patrick, M., and Trum, B. F., Eds., American Association for the Advancement of Science Publication No. 49, Washington, D. C., 1957, 391—414.
37. Lang, K. and Bassler, K. H., in *Proc. Symp. Food Irradiation,* International Atomic Energy Agency, Vienna, 1966.
38. Saint Lebe, L., Berger, G., Mucchielli, A., and Coquet, B., in *Proc. Conf. Radiation Preservation of Food,* International Atomic Energy Agency, Vienna, 1973. (In French.)
39. Partmann, W., FAO Report on Evaluation of the Wholesomeness of Irradiated Foods, Brussels, 1962, 75-96.
40. Newman, A. A., *Food Manufac.,* 33, 374-378 and 422-425, 1958.
41. Andrews, J. S., Mead, J. F., and Griffith, W. H., *Fed. Proc. Fed. Am. Soc. Exp. Biol.,* 15, 918-920, 1956.
42. Kraybill, H. F., *Int. J. Appl. Radiat. Isot.,* 6, 233-254, 1959.
43. Schreiber, M. and Nasset, E. S., *J. Appl. Physiol.,* 14, 639, 1959.
44. Monty, K. J., Tappel, A. L., and Groninger, H. S., *J. Agric. Food Chem.,* 9, 55-58, 1961.
45. Mead, J. F. and Griffith, W. H., unpublished data, 1955.
46. Quachenbush, F. W., *Oil Soap (Chicago),* 22, 336, 1945.
47. Kraybill, H. F. and Nielsen, H. W., *Commer. Fish. Rev.,* 9 (10), 7—15, 1947.
48. Crampton, E. W., Common, R. H., Farmer, F. A., Berryhill, F. M., and Wiseblatt, I., *J. Nutr.,* 44, 177, 1951.
49. Moore, R. O., Contract Final Report to Dept. of Army (DA-49-007-MD-787), Department of Agriculture and Biochemistry, Ohio State University Research Foundation, Columbus; Defense Documentation Center, Alexandria, Va.
50. Plough, I. C., Wholesomeness of Irradiated Foods, Tech. Rep. No. 204, U.S. Army Medical Nutrition Laboratory, Fitzsimons Army Hospital, Denver, 1957.
51. Kraybill, H. F. and Read, M. S., *Proc. Conf. Radioactive Isotopes in Agriculture,* U.S. Atomic Energy Commission Rep. No. TID 7512, U.S. Government Printing Office, Washington, D. C., 1956, 227-282.
52. Kunkel, H. O. and Williams, J. N., *J. Biol. Chem.,* 189, 755, 1951.
53. Kung, H. C., Gaden, E. L., and King, C. G., *J. Agric. Food Chem.,* 1(2), 142-144, 1953.
54. Thomas, M. H. and Calloway, D. H., *J. Am. Diet. Assoc.,* 39, 105—110, 1961.
55. Knapp, F. W. and Tappel, A. L., *J. Agric. Food Chem.,* 9(6), 430-433, 1961.
56. Metta, V. C., Mameesh, M. S., and Johnson, B. C., *J. Nutr.,* 69, 18-22, 1959.
57. Mellette, S. J. and Leone, L., *Fed. Proc. Fed. Am. Soc. Exp. Biol.,* 19, 1045-49, 1960.
58. Richardson, L. R., Wilkes, S., and Ritchey, S. J., *J. Nutr.,* 73(4), 369-373, 1961.
59. Mameesh, M. S., Metta, V. C., Rama Rao, P. B., and Johnson, B. C., *J. Nutr.,* 44, 165-170, 1962.
60. DaCosta, E. and Levenson, S. M., Effect of Diet Exposed to Capacitron Irradiation on the Growth and Fertility of the Albino Rat, U.S. Army Medical Nutrition Laboratory Rep. No. 89, U.S. Army Surgeon General, Chicago, 1951.
61. Diehl, J. F., *Fed. Proc. Abstr.,* 28, 305, 1969.
62. Josephson, E. S., Thomas, M. H., and Calhoun, W. F., Effects of treatment of foods with ionizing radiation, in *Nutritional Evaluation of Food Processing,* 2nd ed., Harris, R. S. and Karmas, E., Eds., AVI, Westport, Conn., 1975, 393-411.
63. Ziporin, Z. Z., Kraybill, H. F., and Thack, H. J., *J. Nutr.,* 63(2), 201-210, 1957.
64. Day, E. J., Alexander, H. D., Sauberlich, H. E., and Salmon, W. D., J. Nutr., *62(1), 107—118,*
65. Wilson, G. M., *J. Sci. Food Agric.,* 10, 295-299, 1959.
66. Schönborn, W. and Ehrhardt, G., Technical Report IFIP-R 16, International Project in Field of Food Irradiation, Federal Research Center for Nutrition, Karlsruhe, West Germany, 1974.
67. Day, E. J., Alexander, H. D., Sauberlich, H. E., and Salmon, W. D., *J. Nutr.,* 62(2), 27-38, 1957.
68. Thomas, M. H. and Josephson, E. S., *Sci. Teach.,* 37(3), 59-63, 1970.

69. Goldblith, S. A., Proctor, B. E., Hogness, J. R., and Langham, W. H., *J. Biol. Chem.*, 179(3), 1163-1167, 1949.

70. Brooke, R. O., Raves, E. M., Gadbois, D. F., and Steinberg, M. A., *Food Technol. (Chicago)*, 18, 1060-1064, 1964.

71. Liuzzo, J. A., Barone, W. B., and Novak, A. F., *Fed. Proc. Abstr.*, 25, 722, 1966.

72. Brin, M., Ostashever, A. S., Tai, M., and Kalensky, H., *J. Nutr.*, 75(2), 35-42, 1961.

73. Richardson, L. R., Wilkes, S., and Ritchey, S. J., *J. Nutr.*, 73(4), 363-368, 1961.

74. Markakis, P. C., Goldblith, S. A., and Proctor, B. E., *Nucleonics*, 9, 71—82, 1951.

75. Sheffner, A. L. and Spector, H., Action of ionizing radiations on vitamins, sterols, hormones and other physiologically active compounds, in Radiation Preservation of Food, U.S. Army Quartermaster Corps, U. S. Government Printing Office, Washington, D.C., 1957.

76. Richardson, L., Progress Report U.S. Army Surgeon General, Contract No. DA 49-007-MD-582, Defense Documentation Center, Alexandria, Va., 1955.

77. Ley, F. J., *Food Irradiat. Inform.*, 1, 8-22, 1972.

78. Coates, M. E., Fuller, R., Harrison, G. F., Lev, M., and Suffolk, S. F., A comparison of the growth of chicks in the Gustafsson germ and in a conventional environment, with free apparatus and without dietary supplements of penicillin, *Br. I. Nutr.*, 17, 141-150, 1963.

79. Lemmon, R. M., Mazzetti, F., and Parsons, M. A., University of California Radiation Laboratory Report No. UCRL 3068, U.S. Atomic Energy Commission Contract No. W—7405 eng-48, Berkeley July 1955.

80. Proctor, B. C. and Goldblith, S. E., *Nucleonics*, 5, 56-62, 1949.

81. McKinney, F. E., *Isot. Radiat. Technol.*, 9, 188-193, 1971.

82. Dennison, R. A. and Ahmed. E. M., *Isot. Radiat. Technol.*, 9, 194-200, 1971-72.

83. Wenkam, N. S. and Moy, A. P., Atomic Energy Commission Contract Rep. No. UH-235-P-5-4, University of Hawaii, Honolulu, 1968, 126-135.

84. Poling, C. E., Warner, W. D., Humberg, R. F., Reber, E. F., Urbain, W. M., and Rice, E. E., *Food Res.*, 20, 193, 1955.

85. Brownell, L. E., personal communication, 1956.

86. Kraybill, H. F. and Hays, S. B., Effect on longevity of feeding foods sterilized and preserved by ionizing radiation, in Proc. 1st Pan Am. Gerontol. Congress, Mexico City, September 15-22, 1956.

# EFFECT OF PROCESSING ON NUTRITIVE VALUE OF FOOD: MICROWAVE COOKING

## Barbara P. Klein

## INTRODUCTION

The use of microwave appliances for home and institutional preparation of foods has grown considerably over the past 30 years. Projections indicate that over four million units will be in homes in the U.S. by 1980.[26] Because of this rapid increase in the numbers of these ovens being used, it is essential to estimate the impact they will have on nutrient intakes.

In microwave heating, nonionizing electromagnetic waves vibrating at microwave frequencies create temperature rises when absorbed by certain materials. The heating depends on the presence of polar molecules within the absorbing medium. Dipolar molecules, such as water, in dielectric substances respond to the field caused by the microwaves. The heat that builds up in a food dielectric is due to friction caused by rapidly turning and twisting dipole molecules.[33] Comprehensive reviews of microwave heating theory have been presented by Van Zante[38] and Copson[16] and will not be discussed here.

Current regulations of the Federal Communications Commission provide certain frequencies for industrial, scientific, and medical (ISM) uses of microwaves. The frequencies that may be used for microwave heating are 915 ± 25, 2,450 ± 50, 5,800 ± 75, and 22,125 ± 125 megacycles per sec or megahertz (MHz). The first two frequencies are most commonly used for microwave ovens in the U.S.

Microwave ovens are either of the consumer/domestic or commercial type. They may use either 110/120 or 220/240 V AC, 60 Hz. Oven nameplates generally state the wattage requirements or power input. Available cooking power or wattage output is sometimes given. Cooking power or output indicates the speed of heating within the microwave oven; this is information that would be useful to the consumer or researcher. Nominal wattage outputs of consumer microwave ovens are between 400 and 1000 W; commercial ovens range from 600 to 3000 W. In the data given in the tables, the brand of microwave oven used, microwave frequency, and available cooking power are given whenever possible.

Assessment of the reported work on nutrient retention in microwave-heated food is complicated by a variety of factors. Studies prior to 1960 were generally performed using commercial microwave or electronic ovens. Wave frequency, power input and output, voltage requirements, or oven size were not consistently reported. In addition, cooking parameters, such as final internal temperatures of food, mass, load size, and amount of water added were not well-controlled. Direct comparisons of nutrient retention when foods are cooked by different methods are therefore not always possible.

## MEAT PRODUCTS

Most of the research on microwave heating effects on nutrients in meats has centered about vitamin losses, particularly of the B-complex vitamins. Fenton[20] summarized the findings of early workers on the nutrient content of meats cooked by microwave and conventional methods. Lachance[25] reported later studies as well. No consistent trends were observed in retention of B vitamins during meat preparation by various cooking methods. In addition, results have been reported in a variety of ways: percent retention, concentration of nutrients on an "as determined" basis or on a moisture-free, or moisture- and fat-free basis. The latter two are not useful from the practical stand-

Table 1

EFFECT OF MICROWAVE AND CONVENTIONAL HEATING ON THIAMIN, RIBOFLAVIN, AND NIACIN CONTENT AND RETENTION OF MEATS

| Food | Method of cooking | Thiamin | | Riboflavin | | Niacin | | Ref. |
|---|---|---|---|---|---|---|---|---|
| | | μg/g | Percent retention | μg/g | Percent retention | μg/g | Percent retention | |
| Beef patties | Microwave[a] | 0.72 | 88 | 0.95 | 88 | — | — | 31 |
| | Panbroiled | 0.79 | 96 | 0.94 | 88 | — | — | 31 |
| Beef patties | Microwave[b] | — | 77 | — | 99 | — | 89 | 37 |
| | Grilled | — | 55 | — | 105 | — | 91 | 37 |
| Beef patties, frozen cooked from thawed state | Microwave[b] | 1.0[c] | 77 | 2.1[c] | 80 | — | — | 9 |
| | Panbroiled | 0.9 | 81 | 2.3 | 81 | — | — | 9 |
| | Ovenbroiled | 1.0 | 81 | 2.2 | 80 | — | — | 9 |
| Beef patties, frozen cooked from frozen state | Microwave[b] | — | 84 | — | 69 | — | — | 9 |
| | Panbroiled | — | 84 | — | 87 | — | — | 9 |
| | Ovenbroil | — | 89 | — | 84 | — | — | 9 |
| Pork patties | Microwave[b] | — | 91 | — | 87 | — | 81 | 37 |
| | Grilled | — | 79 | — | 102 | — | 84 | 37 |
| Pork patties, frozen cooked from thawed state | Microwave[b] | 6.2[c] | 94 | 2.1[c] | 92 | 36.7[c] | 99 | 10 |
| | Panbroiled | 6.3 | 86 | 2.3 | 84 | 33.9 | 104 | 10 |
| | Ovenbroiled | 6.9 | 89 | 2.0 | 81 | 34.6 | 99 | 10 |
| Pork patties, frozen cooked from frozen state | Microwave[b] | — | 85 | — | 87 | — | 94 | 10 |
| | Panbroiled | — | 85 | — | 95 | — | 96 | 10 |
| | Ovenbroiled | — | 83 | — | 84 | — | 88 | 10 |
| Pork patties | Microwave[d] | 15.88[e] | 54 | — | — | — | — | 2 |
| | Conventional electric | 15.42 | 54 | — | — | — | — | 2 |

| | | | | | | | | |
|---|---|---|---|---|---|---|---|---|
| Lamb patties, frozen cooked from thawed state | Microwave[b] | 1.0[c] | 84 | 1.6[c] | 57 | — | — | 11 |
| | Panbroiled | 1.1 | 84 | 1.5 | 51 | — | — | 11 |
| | Ovenbroiled | 0.9 | 80 | 1.5 | 44 | — | — | 11 |
| Lamb patties, frozen cooked from frozen state | Microwave[b] | — | 82 | — | 45 | — | — | 11 |
| | Panbroiled | — | 88 | — | 60 | — | — | 11 |
| | Ovenbroiled | — | 94 | — | 61 | — | — | 11 |
| Beef roasts | Microwave[b] | — | 63 | — | 84 | — | 73 | 37 |
| | Conventional electric | — | 75 | — | 90 | — | 81 | 37 |
| Beef roasts | Microwave[f] | 0.52 | 58 | — | — | — | — | 24 |
| | Conventional gas | 0.60 | 80 | — | — | — | — | 24 |
| Beef roasts | Microwave[f] | 0.68 | 67 | — | — | — | — | 24 |
| | Conventional electric | 0.71 | 86 | — | — | — | — | 24 |
| Beef roasts | Microwave[g] | 0.89 | 61 | 2.00 | 98 | 46.54 | 94 | 4 |
| | Microwave[h] | 0.74 | 49 | 1.73 | 83 | 43.44 | 86 | 4 |
| | Conventional gas | 0.92 | 69 | 1.79 | 99 | 43.94 | 104 | 4 |
| Pork chops | Microwave[d] | 16.62[e] | — | — | — | — | — | 2 |
| | Microwave, institutional[d] | 20.80 | — | — | — | — | — | 2 |
| | Conventional | 16.62 | — | — | — | — | — | 2 |
| Pork roasts | Microwave[i] | 12.89 | 60 | — | — | — | — | 24 |
| | Conventional gas | 11.50 | 61 | — | — | — | — | 24 |
| Pork roasts | Microwave[e] | 14.78 | 73 | 2.32 | 81 | 41.31 | 87 | 4 |
| | Microwave[k] | 14.48 | 67 | 2.52 | 82 | 59.06 | 79 | 4 |
| | Conventional gas | 17.51 | 72 | 2.97 | 96 | 46.01 | 101 | 4 |
| Lamb roasts | Microwave[j] | 1.13 | 57 | 1.78 | 75 | — | — | 30 |
| | Conventional | 0.98 | 54 | 1.85 | 84 | — | — | 30 |

## Table 1 (continued)
## EFFECT OF MICROWAVE AND CONVENTIONAL HEATING ON THIAMIN, RIBOFLAVIN, AND NIACIN CONTENT AND RETENTION OF MEATS

| Food | Method of cooking | Thiamin | | Riboflavin | | Niacin | | Ref. |
| | | µg/g | Percent retention | µg/g | Percent retention | µg/g | Percent retention | |
|---|---|---|---|---|---|---|---|---|
| Lamb roasts | Microwave[g] | 1.96 | 52 | 3.78 | 88 | 44.56 | 71 | 4 |
| | Microwave[h] | 2.10 | 49 | 3.24 | 73 | 36.67 | 64 | 4 |
| | Conventional | 1.93 | 52 | 4.03 | 98 | 43.14 | 86 | 4 |
| Beef loaves | Microwave[i] | 0.70 | 80 | — | — | — | — | 24 |
| | Conventional gas | 0.64 | 76 | — | — | — | — | 24 |
| Beef loaves | Microwave[j] | 0.8 | 69* | — | — | — | — | 43 |
| | Conventional electric | 0.9 | 82 | — | — | — | — | 43 |
| Beef (85%)-soy flour (15%) loaves | Microwave[j] | 1.0 | 65* | — | — | — | — | 43 |
| | Conventional electric | 1.0 | 76 | — | — | — | — | 43 |
| Beef (85%)-soy concentrate (15%) loaves | Microwave[j] | 0.9 | 67* | — | — | — | — | 43 |
| | Conventional electric | 0.9 | 75 | — | — | — | — | 43 |
| Pork loaves, frozen cooked from thawed state | Microwave[b] | 5.9[c] | 71 | 2.6* | 85 | 40.9* | 88 | 10 |
| | Conventional | 5.6 | 60 | 2.9 | 89 | 46.5 | 97 | 10 |
| Pork loaves, frozen cooked from frozen state | Microwave[b] | — | 61 | — | 77 | — | 94 | 10 |
| | Conventional | — | 59 | — | 88 | — | 100 | 10 |
| Ham loaves | Microwave[i] | 6.78 | 87 | 0.64 | 86 | — | — | 24 |
| | Conventional gas | 6.19 | 91 | 0.63 | 92 | — | — | 24 |
| Turkey breast | Microwave[i] | 0.37 | 79 | — | — | — | — | 5 |
| | Conventional gas | 0.45 | 79 | — | — | — | — | 5 |

a Radarange® 3000 MHz, 2.0 kw.

b Radarange® specifications not known.

c Average content for meat cooked from thawed and frozen state.

d Radarange® 450 W cooking power.

e Expressed on moisture and fat-free basis.

f Hotpoint® 10 RE 1, 2450 MHz, 735 W cooking power.

g Litton® 70/50 2450 MHz, 1054 W cooking power.

h Amana Radarange® RR-2, 2450 MHz, 492 W cooking power.

i Whirlpool® W5750880-H, 2450 MHz.

j 2450 MHz, 1190 W cooking power.

k Retention expressed on dry-weight basis.

l Amana Radarange® RR-2, 2450 MHz, 675 W cooking power (nominal).

Table 2
EFFECT OF MICROWAVE AND CONVENTIONAL HEATING ON VITAMIN B-6 CONTENT AND
RETENTION OF MEATS

| Food | Method of cooking | Internal temperature | Vitamin B-6 | | | | |
|------|-------------------|----------------------|-------------|---|---|---|---|
| | | | "As determined" (µg/g) | Moisture-free basis (µg/g) | Moisture and fat-free basis (µg/g) | Percent retention | Ref. |
| Chicken breasts | Microwave[a] | — | — | 18.5 | — | 91 | 42 |
| | Conventional | — | — | 16.7 | — | 83 | 42 |
| Turkey breast | Microwave[b] | 75°C | 5.9 | 16.7 | — | — | 6 |
| | | 85°C | 5.7 | 15.9 | — | — | 6 |
| | Conventional electric | 75°C | 5.3 | 16.5 | — | — | 6 |
| | | 85°C | 5.0 | 15.5 | — | — | 6 |
| Turkey breast, cooked and reheated | Microwave[b] | — | 3.79 | — | 11.78 | — | 19 |
| | Conventional electric | — | 3.69 | — | 12.12 | — | 19 |
| Pork roasts | Microwave[b] | 75°C | 5.1 | 12.3 | — | — | 7 |
| | | 85°C | 5.2 | 12.6 | — | — | 7 |
| | Conventional electric | 75°C | 4.8 | 13.2 | — | — | 7 |
| | | 85°C | 5.3 | 14.4 | — | — | 7 |

[a]   Litton® 550, 2450 MHz, 1250 W cooking power.
[b]   Amana Radarange® RR-2, 2450 MHz, 675 W cooking power (nominal).

point of determining nutrient intakes. They may be used, however, to determine the extent of vitamin destruction during heating.

In the data given below, only studies that reported percent retention of nutrients are used. Microwave cooking methods which included a prebrowning step or simultaneous use of thermal and microwave energy are not included in the tables because the data are so sparse. Thiamin, riboflavin, and niacin content and retention in meats are shown in Table 1. Vitamin B-6 values are given in Table 2.

## Thiamin

Results of early studies of microwave effects on thiamin content and retention of meats are contradictory. Proctor and Goldblith[31] found that thiamin retention was slightly less in microwave-cooked (MC) beef patties than in pan-broiled patties. The findings of Thomas et al.[37] indicated that thiamin retention was higher in MC beef or pork patties than in grilled patties.

Causey et al.[9-11] investigated the effects of different thawing and cooking methods, including microwave, on frozen meats. Beef, pork, and lamb patties were prepared by several different procedures. No consistent relationships between thiamin retention in microwave and conventionally prepared meat patties were noted. Thiamin content of patties thawed before and during cooking did not vary much, so the values given in Table 1 are averages for the two thawing methods. Thiamin retentions ranged from 77 to 89% for beef patties, 83 to 94% for pork, and 80 to 94% for lamb patties. Unlike the findings of Thomas et al.,[37] differences in thiamin retention among cooking methods were not significant. Causey et al.[9-11] also used a prebrowning plus microwave treatment. They noted that the use of a browning step improved the palatability of MC meat patties, but the vitamin retention was similar to the other cooking methods. In the same study, pork loaves prepared by microwave and conventional methods were similar in thiamin content, but the method of thawing affected the thiamin retention.

In 1959, Apgar et al.[2] compared the effects of microwave and conventional cooking on pork patties, roasts, and chops. No significant differences in thiamin content on a dry, fat-free basis due to cooking method were observed, except in pork chops prepared in an institutional microwave oven. The differences in content were small, 0.2 to 0.4 mg, and probably of no practical importance.

The published studies of thiamin retention in ground meat patties were done prior to 1959. In the last two decades, emphasis has been on larger cuts of meat or meat loaves, since savings in time and energy used for cooking may be more significant with greater load size. In that same period, changes in oven specifications such as power output into the heating cavity have occurred. Later reports include more information on oven type and power levels, making it easier to compare findings.

When larger pieces of meat are heated in the microwave oven, certain problems are encountered. Both the geometry of the meat and its mass affect the rate of heat transfer. In the study done by Thomas et al.[37] the temperature rise after removal from the oven which occurs in MC meat was not considered. Higher thiamin retention occurred in conventionally cooked (CC) beef roasts, and the MC roasts were noted to be overcooked and dehydrated on the outside. This might have affected thiamin content and retention, particularly of the outer layers of the meat. When the final postcooking temperature rise was taken into account by Kylen et al.,[24] the differences in thiamin retention between microwave and conventionally cooked beef roasts were about the same; approximately 20% less thiamin was retained in the MC roasts in the two series of beef roasts. In pork roasts the same relationship was not found. About the same retention, approximately 60%, occurred with both cooking methods. Noble and Gomez[30] found that thiamin retention was similar in MC and CC lamb roasts.

Only one comparison of beef, pork, and lamb roasts cooked by microwave and conventional methods was found in the literature.[4] Minor differences in thiamin retention were noted between beef and lamb but not pork roasts cooked conventionally and electronically with 1054 W of cooking power. However, significantly less thiamin was retained in all roasts cooked at lower microwave power (492 W) than in those conventionally roasted. Based on this study,[4] thiamin retention in roasts appears to be affected as much by the microwave cooking power as by the source of the heating energy.

When Kylen et al.[24] prepared beef loaves conventionally and with microwave heating, thiamin retention was slightly higher (80%) in the MC loaves than in the CC loaves (76%). In ham loaves, however, 87% of the thiamin was retained in the MC products and 91% in the CC. Ziprin and Carlin[43] found that thiamin retention was lower in beef and beef-soy loaves cooked in microwave ovens when retention was expressed on a dry weight basis. This study suggested that there may be more thiamin destruction in microwave-heated foods, but this point needs further clarification. The effects of microwave and conventional heating on turkey breasts were investigated in one study.[5] No differences in thiamin content on retention were obtained.

The results of all of these studies indicate that there are thiamin losses in meats during microwave cooking. The values in Table 1 are for meat only. In those studies which reported total thiamin losses, most of the thiamin could be found in the meat and drippings. Decreases in thiamin content seem to be comparable in microwave and conventionally prepared meats, but the results are not consistent. Clearly, thiamin retention depends on cooking time, meat mass, internal temperature, and kind of meat as well as on the oven type and amount of microwave power used for cooking. The differences in the amounts of thiamin per serving are minor and are probably not important in terms of dietary intake of this nutrient.

In the investigations cited previously, the microwave frequency used was 2450 MHz, as far as can be determined. Only one report in which microwave frequency was 915 MHz was found.[27] In this study, microwave and thermal energy were used simultaneously. These investigators determined thiamin and riboflavin retention in three kinds of meat cooked — wrapped in film bags and unwrapped — in conventional gas, electric, and microwave-thermal ovens. The results are difficult to interpret, however. The percent thiamin retention on a dry weight basis ranged from 117 to 139% for turkey breast rolls, 21 to 44% for beef arm roasts, and 70 to 270% for pork loin roasts cooked in film bags. Thiamin retention in unwrapped roasts ranged from 91 to 154% for turkey, 38 to 90% for beef, and 143 to 169% for pork. The authors suggested that a variation in thiamin content in meat muscles, sampling procedures, and basis for reporting results may have affected the findings. The need for uniform methodology is emphasized by reports such as this.

## Riboflavin

In many of the studies of thiamin retention in meats, riboflavin content and retention were also reported. Similarly inconsistent trends with different cooking methods were noted.

No differences in riboflavin content and retention of MC and CC beef patties were found by Proctor and Goldblith,[31] but the riboflavin content was considerably less than values reported by later workers. Thomas et al.[37] indicate that riboflavin retention was approximately 100% in both MC and CC beef patties, but about 15% less riboflavin was retained in MC than in CC pork patties. Causey et al.[9-11] reported lower riboflavin retention in MC beef and lamb patties thawed before cooking and higher retention in thawed MC pork patties. The riboflavin content of the meats cooked by the various methods was not significantly different, but these investigators suggested that the riboflavin assay was not always reliable.

In the study done by Thomas et al.,[37] 6% lower riboflavin retention was found in

MC than in CC beef roasts. Noble and Gomez[30] reported approximately the same variation in riboflavin retention in lamb roasts; 75% retention in MC and 84% in CC meat. Riboflavin content was not different in MC and CC turkey breasts, although retention was slightly lower in MC roasts.[5]

Baldwin et al.[4] showed that, as with thiamin, riboflavin retention was not consistently correlated with energy source. Although riboflavin retention was not different in beef roasts cooked in the 1054 W microwave and conventional ovens, it was lower in the 492 W microwave oven. With pork and lamb, riboflavin retention was lower in both microwave ovens. No significant differences in the riboflavin content of the meats cooked by different methods were obtained.

In the work of McMullen and Cassilly,[27] riboflavin content and retention in turkey, pork, and beef roasts, cooked in oven film bags and uncovered in three different types of oven, did not vary significantly. Armbruster and Haefele[3] also found that the use of plastic film covers on microwave-cooked chicken breasts did not affect riboflavin content.

Meats, in general, are not considered important sources of riboflavin in the U.S. dietary. One serving of meat contributes approximately 10% of the Recommended Dietary Allowance for the reference man.[28] Since the concentration of riboflavin per 100 g of meat is about the same whether microwave or conventional heating is used, the increased application of microwave cookery should cause no problems with the intake of this nutrient.

## Niacin

The effect of different meat preparation methods on niacin content and retention is less marked than for thiamin and riboflavin. Thomas et al.[37] and Causey et al.[10] found little difference in niacin retention in the meats they examined which could be attributed to the kind of oven used.

Baldwin et al.[4] noted that the niacin retention was significantly lower in beef and pork roasts cooked in the 492 W microwave oven than in a conventional oven. This was not true of lamb roasts, although niacin retention was slightly less at the low microwave power level. In spite of the differences in niacin retention, niacin content did not differ significantly. These investigators did point out, however, that the niacin content of all the meats tested was lower than that given by Watt and Merrill,[39] indicating the need for updating food composition information.

## Vitamin B$_6$

The heat stability of vitamin B$_6$ has been questioned, but it is now considered to be relatively stable. Muscle meats are considered good sources of vitamin B$_6$ or pyridoxine, but the effects of cooking procedures have been examined in only a few products (Table 2).

In 1972, Wing and Alexander[42] determined vitamin B$_6$ content and retention in MC and CC chicken breasts. On a dry weight basis, pyridoxine was significantly lower in conventionally prepared chicken. Total percent retention in meat and drippings and retention in the chicken meat only was less than in microwave-processed chicken, but the percent retained in the drippings was higher. This study suggested that vitamin B$_6$ was not as stable during microwave as during conventional heating.

However, a series of studies from one laboratory showed no marked destruction of vitamin B$_6$ during microwave cooking and reheating of turkey breasts[6,19] or pork roasts.[7] Because there was more moisture lost during microwave cooking, pyridoxine concentration tended to be higher in MC meat when expressed on the "as determined" basis. When turkey and pork roasts were cooked to two different internal temperatures, 75 and 85°C, vitamin B$_6$ content was lower at the higher temperature. This may indicate that there is some destruction of $B_6$ with more heating. However, Engler and Bowers,[19] as well as Wing and Alexander,[42] pointed out that differences between birds were greater than those attributable to cooking treatment.

### Other Nutrients

In meat cooking studies, only a few other nutrients have been examined. Causey et al.[10,11] determined lysine content in beef and lamb patties. In the beef patties, 89% of the lysine was retained in the meat, and in lamb, 92%. Differences due to cooking methods were not significant.

Free amino acid content tended to be lower in microwave than in conventionally prepared meats in the study by Baldwin et al.[4] Greater amounts of free valine and leucine were found in lamb, beef, and pork cooked conventionally, but other amino acids varied with the species of meat.

Mineral content of meat and drippings was also determined by Baldwin et al.[4] Although there was a trend toward lower mineral retention in MC meats, the differences were not always significant. Phosphorus and iron retention in CC beef and iron retention in CC lamb were significantly higher than in the microwave heated meats.

### Other Considerations

Watt and Murphy[40] pointed out that the data available for minerals and vitamins in different meat species was limited and out of date. Baldwin et al.[4] indicated that there were differences between their values and those presented by Watt and Merrill.[39] Changes in meat composition have undoubtedly occurred over the years and nutrient content should be reassessed as well as the effects of cooking procedures.

Little or no data are available for other vitamins or minerals in microwave-cooked meats. Certain nutrients which may be limited in modern diets have received little attention. Some workers[15,32] suggested that folacin was the least stable of the B vitamins during cooking. Interest in this nutrient is increasing, and further studies should be forthcoming.

Although the reported work indicates that microwave heating is comparable to conventional cooking procedures with respect to retention of certain nutrients, essentially no work on other meats, eggs, fish, or milk products has been done. Systematic investigations to confirm earlier findings using modern microwave appliances and including other vitamins and trace minerals are needed.

## PREPARED FOODS

The use of microwave energy for heating or reconstitution of frozen and refrigerated prepared foods has important implications for the food service industry. Rapid heating methods that conserve food quality and nutrient content would be useful in fast-food operations and institutional settings. There is some evidence that foods that are refrigerated or frozen and then reheated retain vitamins well, but the evidence is not conclusive.[29,41] Relatively few studies of nutrient retention during microwave reheating of prepared foods have been reported. Data from these investigations are shown in Table 3.

In a study using partially or fully cooked vegetables, Causey and Fenton[12] showed that ascorbic acid retention was not significantly affected by the reheating method and averaged 65% for all methods. The reheating procedures included a Maxon® oven, conventional household oven, microwave appliance, double boiler, and immersion in boiling water. Causey and Fenton[13] also prepared four frozen, cooked products and then reheated them. Thiamin retention in the reheated foods which included four different meat entrees — chicken on rice, paprika chicken, spaghetti and meatballs, and

Table 3
EFFECT OF HEATING METHODS ON VITAMIN CONTENT AND RETENTION OF FRESH OR FROZEN PREPARED FOODS

| Food | Method of heating | Thiamin (mg/100 g) | Percent retention | Riboflavin (mg/100 g) | Percent retention | Ascorbic acid (mg/100 g) | Percent retention | Ref. |
|---|---|---|---|---|---|---|---|---|
| Green beans, frozen partially cooked | Microwave[a] | — | — | — | — | — | 67 | 12 |
| | Maxon® oven, 300°F | — | — | — | — | — | 71 | 12 |
| | Conventional oven, 400°F | — | — | — | — | — | 75 | 12 |
| | Double boiler | — | — | — | — | — | 59 | 12 |
| | Immersion in boiling water | — | — | — | — | — | 76 | 12 |
| Swiss chard, frozen cooked | Microwave[a] | — | — | — | — | — | 85 | 12 |
| | Maxon® oven, 300°F | — | — | — | — | — | 66 | 12 |
| | Conventional oven, 400°F | — | — | — | — | — | 64 | 12 |
| | Double boiler | — | — | — | — | — | 79 | 12 |
| Broccoli, frozen | Microwave[a] | — | — | — | — | — | 85 | 12 |
| | Maxon® oven, 300°F | — | — | — | — | — | 91 | 12 |
| | Conventional oven, 400°F | — | — | — | — | — | 74 | 12 |
| | Double boiler | — | — | — | — | — | 79 | 12 |
| | Immersion in boiling water | — | — | — | — | — | 82 | 12 |
| Creamed chicken on rice, frozen | Microwave[a] | — | 99 | — | — | — | — | 13 |
| | Maxon® oven, 300°F | — | 89 | — | — | — | — | 13 |
| | Conventional oven, 400°F | — | 93 | — | — | — | — | 13 |
| Paprika chicken and gravy, frozen | Microwave[a] | — | 101 | — | — | — | — | 13 |
| | Maxon® oven. 300°F | — | 114 | — | — | — | — | 13 |
| | Conventional oven, 400°F | — | 105 | — | — | — | — | 13 |
| | Double boiler | — | 135 | — | — | — | — | 13 |
| | Immersion in boiling water | — | 130 | — | — | — | — | 13 |

## Table 3 (continued)
## EFFECT OF HEATING METHODS ON VITAMIN CONTENT AND RETENTION OF FRESH OR FROZEN PREPARED FOODS

| Food | Method of heating | Thiamin (mg/100 g) | Percent retention | Riboflavin (mg/100 g) | Percent retention | Ascorbic acid (mg/100 g) | Percent retention | Ref. |
|---|---|---|---|---|---|---|---|---|
| Spaghetti and meatballs, frozen | Microwave[a] | — | 105 | — | — | — | — | 13 |
| | Maxon® oven, 300°F | — | 118 | — | — | — | — | 13 |
| | Conventional oven, 400°F | — | 93 | — | — | — | — | 13 |
| | Double boiler | — | 97 | — | — | — | — | 13 |
| | Immersion in boiling water | — | 113 | — | — | — | — | 13 |
| Ham patties, frozen | Microwave[a] | — | 95 | — | — | — | — | 13 |
| | Maxon® oven, 300°F | — | 88 | — | — | — | — | 13 |
| | Conventional oven, 400°F | — | 100 | — | — | — | — | 13 |
| | Double boiler | — | 111 | — | — | — | — | 13 |
| | Immersion in boiling water | — | 125 | — | — | — | — | 13 |
| Beef stew, frozen | Microwave[c] | 0.093 | 95 | — | — | — | — | 22 |
| | Infrared oven | 0.089 | 91 | — | — | — | — | 22 |
| | Immersion in boiling water | 0.083 | 85 | — | — | — | — | 22 |
| | Fresh-held at 180°F 3 hr | 0.062 | 63 | — | — | — | — | 22 |
| Chicken à la king, frozen | Microwave[c] | 0.078 | 94 | — | — | — | — | 22 |
| | Infrared oven | 0.075 | 90 | — | — | — | — | 22 |
| | Immersion in boiling water | 0.072 | 87 | — | — | — | — | 22 |
| | Fresh-held at 180°F 3 hr | 0.052 | 63 | — | — | — | — | 22 |
| Shrimp Newburg, frozen | Microwave[c] | 0.086 | 92 | — | — | — | — | 22 |
| | Infrared oven | 0.082 | 88 | — | — | — | — | 22 |
| | Immersion in boiling water | 0.080 | 86 | — | — | — | — | 22 |
| | Fresh-held at 180°F 3 hr | 0.061 | 66 | — | — | — | — | 22 |

| | | | | | | | |
|---|---|---|---|---|---|---|---|
| Peas in cream sauce,[b] frozen | Microwave[c] | 0.105 | 93 | — | — | — | — | 22 |
| | Infrared oven | 0.104 | 92 | — | — | — | — | 22 |
| | Immersion in boiling water | 0.098 | 87 | — | — | — | — | 22 |
| | Fresh-held at 180°F 3 hr | 0.086 | 76 | — | — | — | — | 22 |
| Beef stew[d] | Microwave[c] | 0.087 | 94 | — | — | — | — | 22 |
| | Infrared oven | 0.083 | 89 | — | — | — | — | 22 |
| Chicken à la king[d] | Microwave[c] | 0.076 | 94 | — | — | — | — | 22 |
| | Infrared oven | 0.072 | 89 | — | — | — | — | 22 |
| Shrimp Newburg[d] | Microwave[c] | 0.080 | 91 | — | — | — | — | 22 |
| | Infrared oven | 0.076 | 86 | — | — | — | — | 22 |
| Peas in cream sauce[d] | Microwave[c] | 0.110 | — | — | — | — | 22 | 22 |
| | Infrared oven | 0.107 | 89 | — | — | — | — | 22 |
| Peas in cream sauce[d] | Microwave[c] | 0.110 | 92 | — | — | — | — | 22 |
| | Infrared oven | 0.107 | 89 | — | — | — | — | 22 |
| Mashed potatoes | Freshly prepared | 0.163[c] | 100 | 0.255[c] | 100 | 7.47[c] | 100 | 1 |
| | Held at 180°F 3 hr | 0.133 | 82 | 0.248 | 97 | 2.96 | 40 | 1 |
| | Convection oven | 0.144[c] | 88 | 0.246[c] | 96 | 2.67[c] | 36 | 1 |
| | Infrared oven | 0.145 | 89 | 0.239 | 94 | 1.75 | 24 | 1 |
| Frozen, reheated, Held ½ hr at 180°F | Steamer | 0.141 | 86 | 0.236 | 93 | 3.09 | 41 | 1 |
| | Microwave[g] | 0.150 | 92 | 0.246 | 96 | 1.80 | 24 | 1 |
| Peas and Onions | Freshly prepared | 1.32[c] | 97 | 0.566[c] | 94 | — | — | 1 |
| Held ½ hr at 180°F | Infrared oven | 1.27 | 93 | 0.569 | 95 | — | — | 1 |
| | Steamer | 1.09 | 80 | 0.545 | 91 | — | — | 1 |
| | Microwave[g] | 1.23 | 90 | 0.560 | 93 | — | — | 1 |

## Table 3 (continued)
## EFFECT OF HEATING METHODS ON VITAMIN CONTENT AND RETENTION OF FRESH OR FROZEN PREPARED FOODS

| Food | Method of heating | Thiamin | | Riboflavin | | Ascorbic acid | | Ref. |
|---|---|---|---|---|---|---|---|---|
| | | (mg/100 g) | Percent retention | (mg/100 g) | Percent retention | (mg/100 g) | Percent retention | |
| Carrots | Freshly prepared | 0.395ᶜ | 97 | — | — | — | — | — |
| | Held at 180°F 3 hr | 0.339 | 83 | — | — | — | — | — |
| | Convection oven | 0.373ᶜ | 92 | — | — | — | — | 1 |
| | Infrared oven | 0.389 | 96 | — | — | — | — | 1 |
| | Steamer | 0.363 | 89 | — | — | — | — | 1 |
| | Microwaveᵍ | 0.396 | 97 | — | — | — | — | 1 |
| Pot roast and gravy | Freshly prepared | 0.144ᶠ | 99 | 0.810ᶠ | 89 | — | — | 1 |
| | Held at 180°F 3 hr | 0.121 | 83 | 0.745 | 82 | — | — | 1 |
| | Convection oven | 0.126ᶠ | 87 | 0.826ᶠ | 91 | — | — | 1 |
| | Infrared Oven | 0.126 | 87 | 0.838 | 93 | — | — | 1 |
| | Steamer | 0.121 | 83 | 0.774 | 86 | — | — | 1 |
| | Microwaveᵍ | 0.127 | 88 | 0.801 | 89 | — | — | 1 |
| Beans and frankfurters | Freshly prepared | 0.393ᶜ | 96 | 0.221ᶜ | 97 | — | — | 1 |
| | Held at 180°F 3 hr | 0.333 | 82 | 0.216 | 95 | — | — | 1 |
| | Convection oven | 0.377ᶜ | 93 | 0.221ᶜ | 97 | — | — | 1 |
| | Infrared oven | 0.383 | 94 | 0.227 | 97 | — | — | 1 |
| | Steamer | 0.357 | 88 | 0.211 | 93 | — | — | 1 |
| | Microwaveᵍ | 0.367 | 90 | 0.226 | 99 | — | — | 1 |
| Fried fish | Freshly prepared | 0.250ᶠ | 104 | — | — | — | — | 1 |
| | Held at 180°F 3 hr | 0.186 | 77 | — | — | — | — | 1 |
| | Convection oven | 0.241 | 100 | — | — | — | — | 1 |
| | Infrared oven | 0.231 | 96 | — | — | — | — | 1 |
| | Steamer | 0.215 | 89 | — | — | — | — | 1 |
| | Microwaveᵍ | 0.231 | 96 | — | — | — | — | 1 |

[a] Radarange®, specifications unknown.
[b] Prepared in laboratory (Reference 22).
[c] Radarange Mark VI®-Ten, 2450 MHz, 650 W cooking power.
[d] Commercially frozen product.
[e] Expressed on moisture-free basis.
[f] Expressed on moisture and fat-free basis.
[g] Philips® Model 1104, 2450 MHz, 2.1 kW.

ham patties — was generally high, ranging from 88 to 135%. No significant differences due to reheating method were observed, however.

Kahn and Livingston[22] compared thiamin retention in four frozen, prepared products reheated by three high-speed heating techniques: microwave and infrared ovens, and immersion heating. The products (beef stew, chicken à la king, shrimp Newburg, and peas in cream sauce) were prepared in the laboratory. Commercial samples of similar products were also tested. Thiamin retention in the products which were freshly prepared and held for 1, 2, and 3 hr at steam table temperature, 180°F, was also determined. Only the retention values for the 3-hr holding period are shown in Table 3. In all four products, the rapid heating resulted in considerably higher thiamin retention than after the 3-hr holding period. Foods held for a shorter period also retained less thiamin than those heated rapidly. The commercial samples were heated by microwave and infrared processes, and thiamin retention was comparable, although slightly higher in microwave-heated samples.

A more extensive study of reheated frozen food was done by Ang et al.[1] In this investigation, six different foods were examined and the effects on several vitamins of "conventional institutional handling" and "convenience food systems" were compared. The "conventional institutional handling" involved the preparation of the foods followed by holding periods at 180°F of ½, 1½, and 3 hr. The "convenience food systems" included reheating the frozen products by convection, infrared, or microwave ovens, or in a steamer, all followed by a ½ hr holding period. Ascorbic acid, thiamin, and riboflavin were determined. In general, thiamin retention varied from product to product but was retained best in the freshly prepared product that was held for only ½ hr. The fast reconstitution methods were all comparable, with the exception of the steamer-heated foods. Riboflavin retention was over 90% in most reheated foods, indicating that it is a relatively stable vitamin. Ascorbic acid, which was determined only in mashed potatoes, was extremely unstable during all of the rapid heating processes as well as during holding.

These findings suggest that the use of rapid reconstitution methods, including microwave heating, are probably justified in institutional settings because of the convenience. Foods may be prepared in advance of serving, frozen, and reheated with less loss of nutrients than that which occurs during usual steam-table holding times. More research is indicated, however, particularly when foods are considered good sources of unstable vitamins, such as ascorbic acid.

## FOODS OF PLANT ORIGIN

### Ascorbic Acid

The existing literature regarding ascorbic acid losses during vegetable cookery must be examined carefully before any conclusions can be drawn. Several effects are apparent in the data which are presented in Table 4. The water-to-vegetable ratio used in the cooking procedure is important because losses of ascorbic acid are primarily due to leaching of the vitamin. When the same ratio of water to vegetable is used in microwave and conventional cooking, ascorbic acid losses are approximately the same if cooking times are comparable. Little difference in ascorbic acid retention was seen in broccoli[23,37] green beans, spinach, cabbage, and cauliflower[23] under these conditions. In almost all vegetables cooked in a minimum amount of water, ascorbic acid retention was over 70%. Eheart and Gott[17] noted that when no water or very small amounts were used, ascorbic acid retention was about the same.

If large quantities of water were used for boiling vegetables,[21] however, even though the microwave and conventional cooking times were similar, ascorbic acid retention was lower in the conventionally cooked vegetables.

Table 4

ASCORBIC ACID CONTENT AND RETENTION IN VEGETABLES COOKED BY DIFFERENT METHODS

| Vegetable | Method of cooking | Water: vegetable ratio | Cooking time (min) | Ascorbic acid in vegetable | | | | Ascorbic acid in liquid | | | | Ref. |
|---|---|---|---|---|---|---|---|---|---|---|---|---|
| | | | | Reduced (mg/100 g) | Percent retention | Total (mg/100 g) | Percent retention | Reduced (mg/ml) | Percent retention | Total (mg/ml) | Percent retention | |
| Broccoli | Microwave[a] | 1.5:1 | 5.5 | — | 66 | — | 64 | — | — | — | 23 | 37 |
| | Conventional | 1.5:1 | 7 | — | 61 | — | 60 | — | — | — | 25 | 37 |
| Broccoli | Microwave[b] | 2:1 | 3 | 69.0 | 72.2 | 72.8 | 72 | — | — | — | — | 8 |
| | Conventional | 2:1 | 10 | 56.5 | 59.1 | 61.4 | 60.7 | — | — | — | — | 8 |
| Broccoli, frozen | Microwave[b] | 0.7:1 | 4 | 61.9 | 74.7 | 68.2 | 78.6 | — | — | — | — | 8 |
| | | 0.4:1 | 3 | 57.1 | 104.2 | 61.5 | 102.2 | — | — | — | — | 8 |
| | Conventional | 0.9:1 | 15 | 59.5 | 71.8 | 63.7 | 73.5 | — | — | — | — | 8 |
| | | 0.4:1 | 13 | 47.1 | 86.2 | 48.1 | 80.0 | — | — | — | — | 8 |
| Broccoli, frozen, chopped | Microwave[b] | 0.3:1 | 3 | 51.1 | 98.8 | 56.3 | 97.1 | — | — | — | — | 8 |
| | Conventional | 0.4:1 | 11 | 35.9 | 69.5 | — | — | — | — | — | — | 8 |
| Broccoli | Microwave[c] | 0.4:1 | 5 | — | 87 | — | — | — | 7 | — | — | 21 |
| | Conventional | 5.5:1 | 6.5 | — | 45 | — | — | — | 55 | — | — | 21 |
| Broccoli | Microwave (236 V) | 0.5:1 | 6 | 93.1 | 88 | — | — | — | 8 | — | — | 14 |
| Broccoli | Conventional | 0.7:1 | 10 | 74.8 | 71.8 | — | — | — | 10.5 | — | — | 35 |
| Broccoli, frozen | Microwave (236 V) | No water | 12 | 42.2 | 83 | — | — | — | 5 | — | — | 14 |
| Broccoli, frozen | Conventional | 0.4:1 | 10 | 66.9 | 78 | — | — | — | 18 | — | — | 36 |

Table 4 (continued)
ASCORBIC ACID CONTENT AND RETENTION IN VEGETABLES COOKED BY DIFFERENT METHODS

| Vegetable | Method of cooking | Water: vegetable ratio | Cooking time (min) | Ascorbic acid in vegetable | | | | Ascorbic acid in liquid | | | | Ref. |
|---|---|---|---|---|---|---|---|---|---|---|---|---|
| | | | | Reduced (mg/100 g) | Percent retention | Total (mg/100 g) | Percent retention | Reduced (mg/m$l$) | Percent retention | Total (mg/m$l$) | Percent retention | |
| Broccoli | Microwave[d] | 0.5:1 | 8 | 133 | 79* | — | — | 0.55 | 11* | — | — | 23 |
| | Conventional | 0.5:1 | 10 | 123 | 83 | — | — | 0.54 | 10 | — | — | 23 |
| Broccoli, frozen 4 months | Microwave[d] | 0.25:1 | 6 | 74 | 52* | — | — | 0.41 | 9* | — | — | 23 |
| | Conventional | 0.5:1 | 6 | 66 | 48 | — | — | 0.30 | 12 | — | — | 23 |
| Broccoli, frozen 8 months | Microwave[d] | 0.25:1 | 6 | 63 | 48* | — | — | 0.39 | 7* | — | — | 23 |
| | Conventional | 0.5:1 | 6 | 62 | 47 | — | — | 0.38 | 11 | — | — | 23 |
| Broccoli, frozen | Microwave | No water | 6 | 55.2[i] | 82.2 | — | — | — | — | — | — | 17 |
| | Microwave | 0.2:1 | 6 | | 76.4 | — | — | — | — | — | — | 17 |
| | Conventional | 0.2:1 | 12—13 | | 74.8 | — | — | — | — | — | — | 17 |
| Broccoli | Microwave | 0.7:1 | 11 | 66.0[h] | 56.8 | — | — | — | — | — | — | 18 |
| | Stir-fry | 0.7:1 | 10 | | 76.6 | — | — | — | — | — | — | 18 |
| | Uncovered pot | 4:1 | 15 | 38.2 | 44.8 | — | — | — | — | — | — | 18 |
| | Covered | 0.5:1 | 20 | | 74.2 | — | — | — | — | — | — | 18 |
| Cabbage | Microwave[a] | 2:1 | 6 | — | 57 | — | 59 | — | — | — | 37 | 37 |
| | Conventional | 2:1 | 15 | — | 39 | — | 42 | — | — | — | 31 | 37 |

| Vegetable | Method | Water ratio | Time (min) | | | | | | | | Ref. |
|---|---|---|---|---|---|---|---|---|---|---|---|
| Cabbage | Microwave[b] | No water | 5 | 39.93 | 92.8 | — | — | — | — | — | 8 |
| | Microwave[b] | 3.5:1 | 4 | 36.80 | 85.0 | — | — | — | — | — | 8 |
| | Microwave[t] (in moist cloth) | No water | 5 | 39.77 | 92.4 | — | — | — | — | — | 8 |
| | Microwave (in parchment) | 3:1 | 4 | 34.65 | 79.7 | — | — | — | — | — | 8 |
| | Open pot | 4:1 | 30 | 8.58 | 19.6 | — | — | — | — | — | 8 |
| | Covered pot | 4:1 | 25 | 8.42 | 19.5 | — | — | — | — | — | 8 |
| | Double boiler | No water | 35 | 9.90 | 23.2 | — | — | — | — | — | 8 |
| | Pressure cooker | 1.25:1 | 3 | 21.62 | 50.3 | — | — | — | — | — | 8 |
| Cabbage | Microwave[c] | 0.25:1 | 4 | — | 80 | — | — | — | 4 | — | 21 |
| | Conventional | 5:1 | 6.5 | — | 38 | — | — | — | 37 | — | 21 |
| Cabbage | Microwave[d] | 0.5:1 | 12 | 41 | 72 | — | 0.17 | — | 11 | — | 23 |
| | Conventional | 0.5:1 | 14 | 37 | 69 | — | 0.20 | — | 14 | — | 23 |
| Carrots | Microwave[e] | 0.5:1 | 2.25 | — | 81 | 83 | — | — | — | 15 | 37 |
| | Conventional | 0.6:1 | 9 | — | 73 | 80 | — | — | — | 10 | 37 |
| Cauliflower | Microwave[c] | 0.4:1 | 4.25 | — | 90 | — | — | — | 4 | — | 21 |
| | Conventional | 3.7:1 | 8.5 | — | 73 | — | — | — | 16 | — | 21 |
| Cauliflower | Microwave[d] | 0.5:1 | 8.5 | 76 | 87 | — | 0.14 | — | 6 | — | 23 |
| | Conventional | 0.5:1 | 7.0 | 78 | 92 | — | 0.28 | — | 7 | — | 23 |
| Green Beans | Microwave[d] | 0.5:1 | 12 | 16 | 78* | — | 0.07 | — | 7* | — | 23 |
| | Conventional | 0.5:1 | 14 | 15 | 74 | — | 0.06 | — | 9 | — | 23 |
| Green beans, frozen 4 months | Microwave[d] | 0.4:1 | 8 | 8 | 38* | — | 0.03 | — | 8* | — | 23 |
| | Conventional | 0.4:1 | 8 | 8 | 38 | — | 0.05 | — | 8 | — | 23 |

Table 4 (continued)
ASCORBIC ACID CONTENT AND RETENTION IN VEGETABLES COOKED BY DIFFERENT METHODS

| Vegetable | Method of cooking | Water: vegetable ratio | Cooking time (min) | Ascorbic acid in vegetable | | | | Ascorbic acid in liquid | | | | Ref. |
|---|---|---|---|---|---|---|---|---|---|---|---|---|
| | | | | Reduced (mg/100 g) | Percent retention | Total (mg/100 g) | Percent retention | Reduced (mg/ml) | Percent retention | Total (mg/ml) | Percent retention | |
| Green beans, frozen 8 months | Microwave[d] | 0.4:1 | 8 | 6 | 28[c] | — | — | 0.03 | 6[c] | — | — | 23 |
| | Conventional | 0.4:1 | 8 | 6 | 30 | — | — | 0.04 | 5 | — | — | 23 |
| Green beans | Microwave | 0.8:1 | 10 | 4.7[f] | 58.9 | — | — | — | — | — | — | 18 |
| | Stir-fry | 0.5:1 | 15 | | 57.5 | — | — | — | — | — | — | 18 |
| | Ucovered pot | 4:1 | 20 | | 59.6 | — | — | — | — | — | — | 18 |
| | Covered pot | 0.5:1 | 20 | 6.2 | 76.0 | — | — | — | — | — | — | 18 |
| Peas, frozen | Microwave[a] | No water | 3.75 | 20.2 | 83 | — | — | — | — | — | — | 34 |
| | Conventional | 0.1:1 | 9 | 19.7 | 86 | — | — | — | — | — | — | 34 |
| Peas, frozen | Microwave[b] | 0.3:1 | 3 | 13.22 | 84.8 | 13.52 | 81.3 | — | — | — | — | 8 |
| | Conventional | 0.3:1 | 8 | 12.85 | 82.5 | 14.26 | 85.7 | — | — | — | — | 8 |
| Peas, frozen | Microwave[b] | 6:7 | 1 | 8.15 | 96.6 | 9.32 | 84.4 | — | — | — | — | 8 |
| | Microwave[b] | No water | 1 | 11.7 | 105.3 | 13.5 | 95.0 | — | — | — | — | 8 |
| | Conventional | 6:7 | 6 | 6.14 | 77.8 | 6.29 | 62.8 | — | — | — | — | 8 |
| Peas | Microwave[d] (boiling water) | 0.5:1 | 7 | 30 | 74 | — | — | 0.38 | 17 | — | — | 23 |
| | Microwave[d] (cold water) | 0.5:1 | 10 | 30 | 74 | — | — | 0.41 | 15 | — | — | 23 |
| | Conventional | 0.5:1 | 12 | 29 | 73 | — | — | 0.38 | 23 | — | — | 23 |
| Peas, frozen | Microwave | No water | 6 | 11.1[f] | 65.0 | — | — | — | — | — | — | 17 |
| | Microwave | 0.2:1 | 6 | — | 62.3 | — | — | — | — | — | — | 17 |
| | Conventional | 0.2:1 | 12 | — | 68.4 | — | — | — | — | — | — | 17 |

| | | | | | | | | | | | | | | |
|---|---|---|---|---|---|---|---|---|---|---|---|---|---|---|
| Potatoes | Microwave[a] | 1.2:1 | 6 | — | 93 | — | 81 | — | — | — | — | — | 13 | 37 |
| | Conventional | 1.2:1 | 18 | — | 88 | — | 76 | — | — | — | — | — | 18 | 37 |
| Potatoes, six | Microwave[a] | — | 8 | — | — | — | 53 | — | — | — | — | — | — | 37 |
| | Baked | — | 39 | — | — | — | 47 | — | — | — | — | — | — | 37 |
| Potatoes | Microwave | No water | 7 | 9.7[f] | 74.4 | — | — | — | — | — | — | — | — | 17 |
| | Microwave | 0.2:1 | 7 | — | 76.5 | — | — | — | — | — | — | — | — | 17 |
| | Conventional | 0.2:1 | 25—30 | — | 79.9 | — | — | — | — | — | — | — | — | 17 |
| Soybeans, green | Microwave[d] | 10:1 | 17.5 | 20 | 76 | — | — | 0.30 | 10 | — | — | — | — | 23 |
| | Conventional | 0.5:1 | 20 | 20 | 79 | — | — | 0.25 | 11 | — | — | — | — | 23 |
| Spinach | Microwave[d] | No water | 7 | 42 | 56[e] | — | — | 0.31 | 9[e] | — | — | — | — | 23 |
| | Conventional | No water | 7 | 52 | 61 | — | — | 0.44 | 5 | — | — | — | — | 23 |
| Spinach, frozen 4 months | Microwave[d] | 0.15:1 | 10 | 25 | 26[e] | — | — | 0.20 | 5[e] | — | — | — | — | 23 |
| | Conventional | 0.5:1 | 7 | 21 | 22 | — | — | 0.14 | 10 | — | — | — | — | 23 |
| Spinach, frozen 8 months | Microwave[d] | 0.15:1 | 10 | 20 | 23[e] | — | — | 0.13 | 5[e] | — | — | — | — | 23 |
| | Conventional | 0.5:1 | 7 | 16 | 20 | — | — | 0.09 | 8 | — | — | — | — | 23 |
| Spinach, frozen | Microwave | No water | 6 | 26.9[g] | 67.2 | — | — | — | — | — | — | — | — | 17 |
| | Microwave | 0.2:1 | 6 | 22.0 | 64.7 | — | — | — | — | — | — | — | — | 17 |
| | Conventional | 0.2:1 | 12 | 22.0 | 49.3 | — | — | — | — | — | — | — | — | 17 |

a Radarange®, specifications unknown.
b Radarange® 1161, 2450 MHz, 1500 W cooking power.
c Whirlpool® W575880-4, 2450 MHz.
d Hotpoint® 10 RE 1, 2450 MHz, 735 W cooking power.
e Retention determined on the fresh, raw weight basis.
f Average ascorbic acid content for vegetables cooked by all three methods.
g Average ascorbic acid content for vegetables cooked with and without water in microwave oven.
h Average ascorbic acid content for vegetables cooked by all methods except in uncovered pot.
i Average ascorbic acid content for vegetables cooked by all methods except in covered pot.

In a study of several vegetables, Campbell et al.[8] found that ascorbic acid retention was greater with microwave than with other heating methods. Approximately the same amount of water was used with all procedures, but the cooking time was less in the microwave method. Chapman et al.[14] observed the same trend in ascorbic acid retention in broccoli.

Eheart and Gott[19] found that when broccoli was cooked by a stir-frying method, ascorbic acid retention was higher than when it was cooked by microwaves or in large amounts of water. Using small amounts of water in conventional cooking resulted in less loss of ascorbic acid than microwave cooking. In green beans the minimum amount of water resulted in the highest ascorbic acid retention.

Thomas et al.[37] and Kylen et al.[23] pointed out that the amount of water and, to a lesser extent, the cooking time affect ascorbic acid losses in vegetables more than the source of energy for the heating. If short cooking times and small amounts of water are used more ascorbic acid will be retained in any cooking method.

Studies in which the ascorbic acid retention and content of the cooking liquid were determined[21,23,37] showed that total ascorbic acid retention was generally about 90% after cooking. Therefore, ascorbic acid appeared to be relatively heat stable, although it was easily leached into the cooking water. When larger proportions of water were used,[21] a higher percentage of ascorbic acid was found in the cooking liquid, which emphasizes the importance of using minimum amounts of water in vegetable cookery.

Most of the studies reported retention in frozen vegetables on the basis of ascorbic acid content of the frozen raw vegetable. Kylen et al.[23] found that ascorbic acid retention as percent of that in the fresh raw vegetable decreased markedly when vegetables were kept frozen for 4 or 8 months. Spinach, in particular, retained only a small fraction, 20%, of its original ascorbic acid after 8 months. However, the method by which the vegetables were cooked, microwave or conventional, did not significantly affect ascorbic acid content.

**Other Nutrients**

In only one investigation was the thiamin and riboflavin retention in vegetables determined. Thomas et al.[37] found no difference between microwave and conventional cooking with respect to the retention of these vitamins. If the cooking water was included, thiamin retention was approximately 100% and that of riboflavin, 90%. Since vegetables are not good sources of these two vitamins, providing less than one tenth of the daily allowances, few researchers have included their determination in vegetable studies.

Many vegetables are considered good sources of carotene, a precursor of vitamin A. Thomas et al.[37] noted a 20 to 30% increase in carotene in cooked vegetables which they attributed to a loss of carotene in the raw sample due to enzymatic activity, or difficulty in extracting carotene from raw samples. Chapman et al.[14] found great variability in carotene content of raw broccoli. The amount of carotene in microwave-cooked fresh broccoli was 90 to 105% of the raw value, while in cooked frozen broccoli, it was 67 to 86% of the thawed raw value.

Eheart and Gott[17] reported that carotene was completely retained in frozen peas cooked by microwaves, with and without water, or by conventional heating. Retentions ranged from 74.8 to 156%, comparable to those reported by Thomas et al.[37] In reheated frozen carrots, carotene retention was over 90%, confirming early findings regarding carotene stability.[1]

**Other Considerations**

Clearly, one of the most important vitamins that vegetables contribute to the diet is ascorbic acid. Because of this, the major emphasis in research has been on losses of this nutrient during cooking procedure. Although there is much data available, caution should be used in interpreting the results. In any future studies of the effects of microwave cookery on water-soluble nutrients, the ratio of water to vegetable should be controlled and a minimum amount of liquid used. If possible, load size should be standardized, and the texture described so that cooking times can be more easily compared. Other nutrients, which may be more limiting in the diet, should also be determined.

No comparisons of different home microwave appliances used in vegetable cookery were found in the literature. Many of the early studies were done using commercial microwave ovens, and in many cases the power output of the ovens was not known. Although ascorbic acid losses do not appear to be directly correlated with the energy source, it may be of interest to see what the effects of different power levels are on this and other unstable nutrients.

## SUMMARY

As the use of microwave appliances for home and institutional food preparation increases, more concern must be directed toward evaluation of the nutritional effects of this trend. Although comparisons of conventional and microwave cooking of food have appeared in the literature since 1948, assessment of the nutrient retention studies is complicated by many factors. Descriptions of microwave ovens, including wave frequency cooking power, oven size, or heating pattern have not been reported consistently. Cooking parameters such as final internal temperature of food, mass, and load size have not always been well controlled.

Cooking procedures have changed over the past 20 years and practices used in some of the early studies may not be consistent with present recommendations. Furthermore, preparation methods appropriate for conventionally cooked foods may not produce the best microwave-heated products. Careful consideration of the sampling and cooking techniques, the rationale for certain cooking procedures, and the way in which results are expressed is essential. Sensory evaluation is also important in these comparative studies, since there is some indication that microwave-heated foods are less acceptable than those conventionally prepared. Institutional as well as home uses of microwave energy must be carefully examined since it appears that microwave heating has great potential in mass feeding systems. Reconstitution of refrigerated and frozen, prepared foods should be compared to traditional heating and holding practices.

In about half of the studies reviewed, nutrient retention was higher in microwave than in conventionally cooked foods, but the data were restricted to relatively few nutrients. Further investigations are necessary to ascertain that other heat-sensitive components are not adversely affected.

## ADDENDUM

Since the initial preparation of this review, reports of studies of nutrient content and retention in foods heated by microwave energy have appeared. Although they are not numerous, it is appropriate that the data be included in this publication. A summary of the data is given in Table 5.

It should be pointed out that, in addition to the previously cited discussion of the effects of microwave heating by Lachance,[25] a comprehensive review has been published by Lorenz.[51] Limited reviews by Decareau[46] and Livingston[50] are also available, but no new data have been added.

Two investigations of the nutrient content of microwave and conventionally cooked beef roasts have been reported.[48,53] Korschgen and Baldwin[48] cooked beef round roasts

## Table 5
## VITAMIN CONTENT AND RETENTION IN FOODS COOKED BY DIFFERENT METHODS

| Food | Method of cooking | Water: vegetable ratio | Cooking time (min) | Ascorbic acid | | Thiamin | | Riboflavin | | Niacin | | Folacin | | Ref. |
|---|---|---|---|---|---|---|---|---|---|---|---|---|---|---|
| | | | | mg/g | %Ret. | µg/g | %Ret. | µg/g | %Ret. | µg/g | %Ret. | µg/g | %Ret. | |
| Beef round roasts | Microwave,ᵃ moist heat | — | — | — | — | 0.48 | 25 | 2.14 | 90 | 35.6 | 52 | — | — | 48 |
| | Conventional, moist heat | — | — | — | — | 0.34 | 19 | 1.89 | 81 | 33.7 | 50 | — | — | 48 |
| Beef round roasts | Microwave,ᵇ dry heat | — | — | — | — | 0.95 | — | — | — | — | — | — | — | 53 |
| | Conventional, dry heat | — | — | — | — | 0.96 | — | — | — | — | — | — | — | 53 |
| Fried chicken | Frozen, unheated | — | — | — | — | 6.1ᵃ | 100 | 6.3ᵃ | 100 | — | — | — | — | 44 |
| | Convection heated, held 3 hr | — | — | — | — | 4.5 | 74 | 5.7 | 90 | — | — | — | — | 44 |
| | Infrared | — | — | — | — | 5.1 | 84 | 5.8 | 92 | — | — | — | — | 44 |
| | Steam | — | — | — | — | 5.5 | 90 | 5.5 | 87 | — | — | — | — | 44 |
| | Microwaveᶜ | — | — | — | — | 5.6 | 92 | 5.8 | 93 | — | — | — | — | 44 |
| Beef-soy patties | Raw, frozen | — | — | — | — | 2.8ᵃ | 100 | 10.5ᵃ | 100 | — | — | — | — | 44 |
| | Char-broiled, frozen | — | — | — | — | 2.4 | 86 | 10.3 | 98 | — | — | — | — | 44 |
| | Convection heated, held 3 hr | — | — | — | — | — | — | — | — | — | — | — | — | 44 |
| | Infrared | — | — | — | — | 2.3 | 81 | 8.4 | 80 | — | — | — | — | 44 |
| | Steam | — | — | — | — | 2.6 | 91 | 9.4 | 90 | — | — | — | — | 44 |
| | Microwaveᶜ | — | — | — | — | 2.4 | 90 | 10.4 | 99 | — | — | — | — | 44 |
| Broccoli, frozen | Microwaveᵈ | No water | 8 | — | — | — | — | — | — | — | — | 1.28 | 55 | 47 |
| | Conventional | 0.4:1 | 5 | — | — | — | — | — | — | — | — | 0.98 | 51 | 47 |
| Green beans, frozen | Microwaveᵈ | No water | 8.5 | — | — | — | — | — | — | — | — | 0.60 | 10 | 47 |
| | Conventional | 0.4:1 | 9 | — | — | — | — | — | — | — | — | 0.52 | 10 | 47 |
| Peas, frozen | Microwaveᵈ | No water | 7 | — | — | — | — | — | — | — | — | 0.99 | 73 | 47 |
| | Conventional | 0.4:1 | 6 | — | — | — | — | — | — | — | — | 1.02 | 84 | 47 |

| | | | | | | | | | | | | | |
|---|---|---|---|---|---|---|---|---|---|---|---|---|---|
| Spinach, frozen | Microwave[a] | No water | 8 | — | — | — | — | — | — | — | 1.78 | 105 | 47 |
| | Conventional | 0.4:1 | 10 | — | — | — | — | — | — | — | 1.72 | 89 | 47 |
| Peas, frozen | Conventional | 1:4 | 8 | .15 | 71 | — | — | — | — | — | — | — | 52 |
| | Microwave[e] | 1:4 | 8 | .16 | 72 | — | — | — | — | — | — | — | 52 |
| | Microwave[c] | No water | 6.5 | .21 | 96 | — | — | — | — | — | — | — | 52 |
| | Microwave[f] | 1:4 | 6 | .17 | 78 | — | — | — | — | — | — | — | 52 |
| | Microwave[f] | No water | 5 | .22 | 101 | — | — | — | — | — | — | — | 52 |
| Sweet potatoes | Baked | — | 75-90 | .23 | — | — | 5.4 | — | 7.8 | — | — | — | 49 |
| | Boiled | — | 40-60 | .22 | — | — | 2.6 | — | 5.4 | — | — | — | 49 |
| | Steamed | — | 40-70 | .23 | — | — | 3.0 | — | 6.5 | — | — | — | 49 |
| | Microwave[g] | — | 18-35 | .21 | — | — | 3.8 | — | 7.4 | — | — | — | 49 |

a    Litton® Model 416, 2450 MHz, 550 W "high," 250 W "simmer."
b    Litton® Model 419, 2450 MHz, 283-317 W "roast," 182-204 W "simmer."
c    Phillips® Model 1104, 2450 MHz, 2.1 kW.
d    Litton® Model 419, 2450 MHz, 585 W.
e    Litton® Model 416, 2450 MHz, 550 W.
f    Litton® Menumaster, 2450 MHz, 1150 W.
g    Litton® 2450 MHz.
h    On fat-free, dry basis.

to an internal temperature of 98°C by a moist-heat microwave method and by braising in a conventional oven at 135°C. No significant differences due to cooking method, in moisture, fat or protein of the meat, thiamin, riboflavin or niacin content of meat plus drippings, were found. Niacin retention was approximately 50% in the cooked roasts. Retentions of thiamin and riboflavin were significantly higher in microwave than conventionally cooked meat, but much lower than previously reported values. Selected minerals were also determined, but only small differences between cooking methods were noted.

Voris and Van Duyne[53] compared top round beef roasts that were dry roasted to an internal temperature of 68.3°C in a microwave oven or conventional oven at 149°C. The microwave roasting was accomplished at low power settings to determine if a palatable product could be achieved with low wattage cooking. Thiamin content was similar in the roasts cooked by the two methods. Retention was not determined.

The effects of microwave heating on different forms of folate in aqueous solutions were studied by Cooper et al.[45] This investigation emphasized the differences in stability of the folate vitamins during heating, either by microwave energy or conventional heat. It is important, therefore, to know which form is present in food. Klein et al.[47] reported that frozen vegetables cooked by microwave and conventional methods were comparable in folacin content. Folate retention in peas, green beans, and spinach ranged from 78 to 105%. Retention of folacin in broccoli was 50 to 59%, which may be a consequence of the form of folate present. The differences between the microwave and conventional methods were small, indicating that folate was equally well-conserved by either procedure.

Mabesa and Baldwin[52] found that frozen peas cooked with and without water in a domestic or institutional microwave oven, or conventionally, varied in ascorbic acid content. The addition of water and the time of cooking influenced the ascorbic acid content and retention in the vegetable, as was noted earlier in this review.

Lanier and Sistrunk[49] compared the effects of baking, boiling, steaming, and microwave heating, as well as canning, on the nutritional quality of sweet potatoes. Ascorbic acid content was significantly lower in canned and microwave cooked sweet potatoes. Total carotenoids were not affected by the cooking procedure. Riboflavin was significantly higher in baked sweet potatoes than in the others. Baked and boiled and microwave cooked sweet potatoes retained the most pantothenic acid, and niacin was highest in baked and microwave heated roots.

Ang et al.[44] showed that riboflavin retention in frozen fried chicken was not significantly affected when heated by methods used in food service operations, including microwave heating. Thiamin retention, however, was highest in microwave heated chicken and lowest in convection heated chicken held for 3 hr. Riboflavin retention was high in beef-soy patties heated and held by a variety of methods, except infrared or steam heated. Over 90% of the thiamin was retained in patties heated by convection, steam, or microwaves, although thiamin retention was significantly lower in microwave and steam heated patties than in the raw meat. The authors suggested that the thiamin loss during microwave cooking of thin patties may be increased due to locally intense hot spots generated during electronic cooking.

## REFERENCES

1. **Ang, C. Y. W., Chang, C. M., Frey, A. E., and Livingston, G. E.,** Effects of heating methods on vitamin retention in six fresh or frozen prepared food products, *J. Food Sci.*, 40, 997, 1975.

2. **Apgar, J., Cox, N., Downey, I., and Fenton, F.,** Cooking pork electronically, *J. Am. Diet. Assoc.,* 35, 1260, 1959.
3. **Armbruster, G. and Haefele, C.,** Quality of foods after cooking in 915 mHz and 2450 mHz microwave appliances using plastic film covers, *J. Food Sci.,* 40, 721, 1975.
4. **Baldwin, R. E., Korschgen, B. M., Russell, M. S., and Mabesa, L.,** Proximate analysis, free amino acid, vitamin and mineral content of microwave cooked meat, *J. Food Sci.,* 41, 762, 1976.
5. **Bowers, J. A. and Fryer, B. A.,** Thiamin and riboflavin in cooked and frozen reheated turkey, *J. Am. Diet. Assoc.,* 60, 399, 1972.
6. **Bowers, J. A., Fryer, B. A., and Engler, P. P.,** Vitamin B₆ in turkey breast muscle cooked in microwave and conventional ovens, *Poult. Sci.,* 53, 844, 1974.
7. **Bowers, J. A., Fryer, B. A. and Engler, P. P.,** Vitamin B₆ in pork muscle cooked in microwave and conventional oven, *J. Food Sci.,* 39, 426, 1974.
8. **Campbell, C. L., Lin, T. Y., and Proctor, B. E.,** Microwave vs. conventional cooking, *J. Am. Diet. Assoc.,* 34, 365, 1958.
9. **Causey, K., Andreas, E. G., Hausrath, E., Along, C., Ramstad, P. E., and Fenton, F.,** Effect of thawing and cooking methods on palatability and nutritive value of frozen ground meat. I. Pork, *Food Res.,* 15, 237, 1950.
10. **Causey, K., Hausrath, M. E., Ramstad, P. E., and Fenton, F.,** Effect of thawing and cooking methods on palatability and nutritive value of frozen ground meat. II. Beef, *Food Res.,* 15, 249, 1950.
11. **Causey, K., Hausrath, M. E., Ramstad, P. E., and Fenton, F.,** Effect of thawing and cooking methods on palatability and nutritive value of frozen ground meat. III. Lamb, *Food Res.,* 15, 256, 1950.
12. **Causey, K. and Fenton, F.,** Effect of reheating on palatability, nutritive value and bacterial count of frozen cooked food. I. Vegetables, *J. Am. Diet. Assoc.,* 27, 390, 1951.
13. **Causey, K. and Fenton, F.,** Effect of reheating on palatability, nutritive value and bacterial count of frozen cooked foods. II. Meat dishes, *J. Am. Diet. Assoc.,* 27, 491, 1951.
14. **Chapman, V. J., Putz, J. O., Gilpin, G. L., and Sweeney, J. P.,** Electronic cooking of fresh and frozen broccoli, *J. Home Econ.,* 52, 161, 1960.
15. **Cheldelin, V. H., Woods, A. A., and Williams, R. J.,** Losses of B vitamins due to cooking of foods, *J. Nutr.,* 26, 477, 1943.
16. **Copson, D. A.,** *Microwave Heating,* AVI Publishing, Westport, Conn., 1975, 1—34.
17. **Eheart, M. S. and Gott, C.,** Conventional and microwave cooking of vegetables. Ascorbic acid and carotene retention and palatability, *J. Am. Diet. Assoc.,* 44, 116, 1964.
18. **Eheart, M. S. and Gott, C.,** Chlorophyll, ascorbic acid and pH changes in green vegetables cooked by stir-fry, microwave and conventional methods and a comparison of chlorophyll methods, *Food Technol.,* 19, 867, 1965.
19. **Engler, P. P. and Bowers, J. A.,** Vitamin B₆ content of reheated, held and freshly cooked turkey breast, *J. Am. Diet. Assoc.,* 67, 42, 1975.
20. **Fenton, F.,** Losses in nutrients during large scale preparation for direct feeding, in *Nutritional Evaluation of Food Processing,* Harris, R. S. and Von Loesecke, H., Eds., John Wiley & Sons, New York, 1960, 391-418.
21. **Gordon, J. and Noble, I.,** Comparison of electronic vs. conventional cooking of vegetables, *J. Am. Diet. Assoc.,* 35, 241, 1959.
22. **Kahn, L. N. and Livingston G. E.,** Effect of heating methods on thiamine retention in fresh or frozen prepared foods, *J. Food Sci.,* 35, 349, 1970.
23. **Kylen, A. M., Charles, V. R., McGrath, B. H., Schleter, J. M., West, L. C., and Van Duyne, F. O.,** Microwave cooking of vegetables, *J. Am. Diet. Assoc.,* 39, 321, 1961.
24. **Kylen, A. M., McGrath, B. H., Hallmark, E. L., and Van Duyne, F. O.,** Microwave and conventional cooking of meat, *J. Am. Diet. Assoc.,* 45, 139, 1964.
25. **Lachance, P.,** Effects of food preparation procedures on nutrient retention with emphasis on food service practices, in *Nutritional Evaluation of Food Processing,* Harris, R. S. and Karmas, E., Eds., AVI Publishing, Westport, Conn., 1975, 463—528.
26. **Litton Microwave Cooking Products,** Microwave oven sales continue to increase, *Food Technol.,* 31(3), 111, 1977.
27. **McMullen E. A. and Cassilly, J. P.,** Thiamin and riboflavin retention in meats cooked uncovered and in oven film, *Home Econ. Res. J.,* 5(1), 33, 1976.
28. **National Academy of Sciences — National Research Council,** Recommended Dietary Allowances, 1974.
29. **Nielsen, L. M. and Carlin, A. F.,** Frozen, precooked beef and beef-soy loaves, *J. Am. Diet. Assoc.,* 65, 35, 1974.
30. **Noble, I. and Gomez, L.,** Vitamin retention in meat cooked electronically. *J. Am. Diet. Assoc.,* 41, 217, 1962.
31. **Proctor, B. E. and Goldblith, S. A.,** Radar energy for rapid food cooking and blanching and its effects on vitamin content, *Food Technol.,* 2, 95, 1948.

32. Schweigert, B. S., Pollard, A. E., and Elvehjem, C. A., The folic acid content of meats and the retention of this vitamin during cooking, *Arch. Biochem.*, 10, 107, 1946.
33. Sherman, V. W., Electronic heat in the food industries, *Food Ind.*, 18, 90, 1946.
34. Stevens, H. P. and Fenton, F., Dielectric vs. stewpan cookery, *J. Am. Diet. Assoc.*, 27, 32, 1951.
35. Sweeney, J. P., Gilpin, G. L., Staley, M. G., and Martin, M. E., Effect of cooking methods on broccoli. I. Ascorbic acid and carotene, *J. Am. Diet. Assoc.*, 35, 354, 1959.
36. Sweeney, J. P., Gilpin, G. L., Martin, M. E., and Dawson, E. H., Effect of cooking time, method and storage on the palatability and nutritive value of frozen broccoli, *J. Am. Diet. Assoc.*, 36, 122, 1960.
37. Thomas, M. H., Brenner, S., Eaton, A., and Craig, V., Effect of electronic cooking on nutritive value of foods, *J. Am. Diet. Assoc.*, 25, 39, 1949.
38. Van Zante, H., *The Microwave Oven*, Houghton Mifflin, Boston, 1973, 79—94.
39. Watt, B. K. and Merrill, A. L., *Composition of Foods*, Agric. Handb. No. 8, U.S. Department of Agriculture, Washington, D.C., 1963.
40. Watt, B. K. and Murphy, E. W., Tables of food composition: scope and needed research, *Food Technol.*, 24, 50, 1970.
41. West, L. C., Titus, M. C., and Van Duyne, F. O., Effect of freezer storage and variations in preparation on bacterial count, palatability and thiamin content of ham loaf, Italian rice and chicken, *Food Technol.*, 13, 323, 1959.
42. Wing, R. W. and Alexander, J. C., Effect of microwave heating on vitamin $B_6$ retention in chicken, *J. Am. Diet. Assoc.*, 61, 661, 1972.
43. Ziprin, Y. A. and Carlin, A. F., Microwave and conventional cooking in relation to quality and nutritive value of beef and beef-soy loaves, *J. Food Sci.*, 41, 4, 1976.
44. Ang, C. Y. W., Basillo, L. A., Cato, B. A., and Livingston, G. E., Riboflavin and thiamine retention in frozen beef-soy patties and frozen fried chicken heated by methods used in food service operations, *J. Food Sci.*, 43, 1024, 1978.
45. Cooper, R. G., Chen, T. S., and King, M. A., Thermal destruction of folacin in microwave and conventional heating, *J. Amer. Diet. Assoc.*, 73, 406, 1978.
46. Decareau, R. V., Do microwaves make food more nutritious?, *Microwave Energy Applications Newsletter*, 10(2), 13, 1977.
47. Klein, B. P., Lee, H. C., Reynolds, P. A., and Wangles, N. C., Folacin content of microwave and conventionally cooked frozen vegetables, *J. Food Sci.*, 44, 286, 1979.
48. Korschgen, B. M. and Baldwin, R. E., Moist-heat microwave and conventional cooking of round roasts of beef, *J. Microwave Power*, 13, 257, 1978.
49. Lanier, J. and Sistrunk, W. A., Influence of cooking method on quality attributes and vitamin content of sweet potatoes, *J. Food Sci.*, 44, 374, 1979.
50. Livingston, G. E., Nutrition aspects of microwave cooking, *Microwave Energy Application Newsletter*, 12(5), 4, 1979.
51. Lorenz, K., Microwave heating of foods, Changes in nutrient and chemical composition, *CRC Crit. Rev. Food Sci. Nutr.*, 7, 339, 1976.
52. Mabesa, L. B. and Baldwin, R. E., Ascorbic acid in peas cooked by microwaves, *J. Food Sci.*, 44, 932, 1979.
53. Voris, H. H. and Van Duyne, F. O., Low wattage microwave cooking of top round roasts: energy consumption, thiamin content and palatability, *J. Food Sci.*, 44, 1447, 1979.

# EFFECT OF HOME PREPARATION PRACTICES ON NUTRITIVE VALUE OF FOOD*

John W. Erdman, Jr. and Edith A. Erdman

## INTRODUCTION

Home preparation practices must be considered in evaluating nutrient losses from foods. The major loss of vitamins and minerals from foods often occurs during final preparation in the home or institution prior to eating.[5] Utilization of proper preparation techniques will lead to maximum nutrient retention in foods as consumed.

The purpose of this chapter is to evaluate various food preparation techniques in relation to nutrient retention in the final product. No attempt will be made to provide extensive tabular data for individual foods. Selected research reports, especially those found in recent literature, are presented to provide a basis for evaluation of each preparation technique. It is hoped that the reader will find these references helpful in selection of preparation methods. Extensive tabular material is found in previous publications.[65,67,91,92,114]

Nutrient profiles of foods are essential (1) for dietitians and physicians to plan menus for both regular and therapeutic diets, (2) to evaluate national and regional household food consumption, and (3) to study an individual's food intake for a relatively brief period or more extended time as an index of the nutritive value of his diet.[119] Good estimates of nutrient content of foods are found in various food composition tables. The most frequently used tables in this country are in the U.S. Department of Agriculture Agricultural Handbook No. 8[170] and U.S. Department of Agriculture Handbook No. 456.[1] The latter revises and updates Handbook No. 8 and expresses nutritive contents of approximately 1500 foods in common household units.

These handbooks contain nutrient levels in both raw and "as consumed" foods. The data are not merely the averages of nutrient profiles from USDA files. Each nutrient level is based on a careful review of information from previous handbooks and new literature and is derived from values that most nearly represent that food year-round and nationwide.[119] Nutrient losses during processing and factors such as storage losses are also taken into account. Only the analyses that follow standard approved methods are incorporated into the USDA handbooks.[45]

The Nutrient Data Research Center of the USDA is currently sponsoring research to establish what changes in nutrient content occur with the processing of foods. Format[7] and guidelines[118] for reporting food composition and nutrient retention data are available.

Compilation of a Nutrient Data Bank began at the USDA in 1972 to integrate data in files of government, public, and private laboratories, with increased emphasis placed on data for processed foods, accelerated rate of data input, and retrieval of data.[71] Computer-stored nutrient data and the anticipated release of updated Handbook No. 8 in looseleaf form will make nutrient retrieval much more rapid.

At this time USDA handbooks provide only nutrient content of foods after selected (common) processes or cooking methods. No attempt is made to differentiate preparation procedures or to assign relative percent retentions to different methods. To evaluate an individual preparation practice, one must search the literature. Unfortunately, much of the nutrient retention literature suffers because of lack of available data, poor design of some of the experiments, and methodology changes over the years. Even

* Reprinted in part from *Food Technol.*, February 1979, 38-48, Copyright © by Institute of Food Technologists. With permission.

with the best intentions, large experimental variability complicates comparison of data from lab to lab. For example, Chan et al.[28] point out that 3 to 23% differences in nutrient analysis can occur due to sampling. In their work, sampling error was significantly greater than experimental error. Murphy et al.[118] further warn that nutrient retentions must be reported as true rather than apparent retentions because apparent retention overestimates retention by assuming that solids are not lost to water or drip during cooking.

With these and other handicaps, this reviewer will devote the remainder of this chapter to an evaluation of home preparation techniques of foods from both animal and vegetable origin and will conclude with a plea for more systematic research upon the subject.

# FOODS OF ANIMAL ORIGIN

## Losses Preparatory to Cooking

Possible losses of nutritional value prior to cooking in foods of animal origin are those from storage conditions, fat trim, and discarded thaw juices.

### Storage Conditions

Foods of animal origin can be stored either refrigerated or frozen for various lengths of time and at various temperatures. Proper storage conditions have minimal adverse effects upon nutrient retention.

Refrigerated storage of ground pork for 2 weeks at 40°F produced less than a 10% loss of thiamin, riboflavin, and pantothenic acid.[142,143] Cold storage of shell eggs from 3 to 12 months resulted in small but significant losses of B vitamins.[52-58] The average loss of the eight B-complex vitamins measured was 6, 11, and 19% after storage periods of 3, 6 to 7, and 12 months, respectively. One-year losses of vitamin $B_6$ (47%), folic acid (27%), and vitamin $B_{12}$ (23%) were high, whereas no measurable losses of choline or biotin were found.

The rate of freezing was not found to have much of an effect upon B-vitamin content of different cuts of beef[95] or pork chops,[94] nor did it have a significant effect upon the flavor or tenderness of beef.[95] A lower freezing rate may increase the drip after defrosting.[78]

Recent work by Kramer et al.[87] demonstrates that fluctuations in freezer storage temperatures, which are probably quite common with the home refrigerator-freezer averaging ±9°F fluctuation each 20 min have detrimental effects on the texture and flavor of frozen prepared foods such as ground beef, with and without textured soy protein (TVP) or with TVP plus yeast single-cell proteins particularly when stored at temperatures above 0°F. They found that, with the possible exception of ascorbic acid and thiamin, the nutritional quality was maintained in constant-temperature frozen storage up to 6 months. Higher storage and fluctuating temperatures both led to destruction of vitamin $B_1$ and C over time. Unsatisfactory packaging materials also have marked adverse effects upon meats stored in fluctuating temperatures.[78]

Engler and Bauers[51] concluded from their review that no consistent trend has been observed with frozen storage time in relation to retention of various B-complex vitamins in meat. Morgan et al.[116] investigated the retention of thiamin, riboflavin, and niacin from chicken tissues after frozen storage of −9°F for up to 1 year. Niacin was retained well for up to 8 months of storage, but some tissues lost 25 to 50% after 1 year. Riboflavin was also well-retained up to 8 months in most cases, while thiamin was stable in two of three lots of small broilers. Millares and Fellers[111] stored both light and dark chicken meat at −0.4°F for 8 months and reported greater losses of thiamin and riboflavin in the dark meat, 42 and 11%, respectively, than the white meat, 12 and 3%. Nicotinic acid was fully retained in both types of meat.

Table 1
RELATIVE SUITABILITY OF FISHERY PRODUCTS FOR
FREEZING AND FROZEN STORAGE

Degree of suitability

| High<br>Storage life of 7 to 12<br>months at 0°F | Moderate<br>Storage life of 5 to 9<br>months at 0°F | Low<br>Storage life of 4 to 6<br>months at 0°F |
| --- | --- | --- |
| Haddock | Ocean perch | Mackerel |
| Cod | Whiting | Tuna |
| Flounders | King, red, or coho salmon | Catfish |
| Hake | Lake herring | Sea herring |
| Shrimp | Red snapper | Spanish mackerel |
| Halibut | Smelt | Pacific sardines |
| King crab | Crawfish | Clams |
| Dungeness crab | Rockfish | Chub |
| Pollock | Carp | Chum or keta salmon |
| Sea scallops | Buffalofish | Whale meat |
| Blue pike | Swordfish | |
| Yellow perch | Pacific oysters | |
| | Alewives | |
| | White bass | |

From Slavin, J. W., *Industrial Fishery Technology*, edited by M. E. Stansby
© 1963 by Litton Educational Publishing, Inc. Reprinted by permission of Van
Nostrand Reinhold Company.

Freezer storage of pork chops for 6 months at 0 or −15°F resulted in loss of 40%
of thiamin, 31% of riboflavin, and no loss of nicotinic acid.[97] Nicotinic acid content
of lamb chops increased in frozen storage, while thiamin and riboflavin decreased,
especially after 3 months storage at 0 or −15°F.[98] Differences in freezing temperatures
had no marked effect on retention of the three vitamins.[97,98] Westerman et al.[172] found
considerable animal variation (as did most other studies reported in this subsection)
in freezing studies with pork, but they found no outstanding losses of thiamin, riboflavin, pantothenic acid, or niacin in frozen storage of up to 72 weeks. Studies with rat
growth assays indicated that $B_6$ retention, after 15 months frozen storage at −4°F, of
beef liver and boned chicken was 82 and 77%, respectively.[144] Kemp et al.[84] compared
thiamin contents of fresh and frozen (120 days at +4°F) normal and PSE (pale, soft
exudative) pork and found lower $B_1$ contents in PSE loins and decreased contents in
both during storage. Breading of meats seems to protect the product during frozen
storage.[78] Breaded meats show very satisfactory storage lifetimes even at temperatures
considerably above −4°F, which is conventionally considered maximum freezer storage
temperature.

Fish are good sources of animal protein, vitamins, and minerals. However, storage
stability of fish is poor for many varieties, especially those with higher polyunsaturated
oil contents. Very little work has been reported concerning nutrient retention during
storage. Slavin[155] has divided fishery products into categories of suitability for freezing
and frozen storage. These categories are presented in Table 1 since this reference is
not readily available. Frozen storage stability depends directly upon the amount of
time stored in ice prior to freezing. For example, Slavin[155] points out that the shelf life
of frozen whiting is 12 months if iced for only 2 days. If iced for 7 days, however, the
shelf life reduced to 2 months at 0°F. Extensive autolysis, bacterial break down, dehydration, and oxidation that reduce fish quality and, presumably, nutritive value occur during ice storage. The shelf life of other products of animal origin are found in
Table 2.

Table 2
SHELF-LIFE FOR RETAIL PRODUCTS
OF ANIMAL ORIGIN

| Product | Days | Months |
|---|---|---|
| Cottage cheese | 10—15 | — |
| Creamed cheese | — | 3 |
| Evaporated milk | — | 12 |
| Fluid milk | 5—7 | — |
| Frozen dinners | — | 6 |
| Frozen foods (general) | — | 12 |
| Frozen lobster | — | 6 |
| Gravy/sauce mixes, dehydrated | — | 12—15 |
| Ice cream | — | 3 |
| Lard | — | 3 |

From *Anon.*, *Food Stability Survey*, Vol. 2, Department of Food Science, Rutgers University, U.S. Government Printing Office, Washington, D.C., 1971.

*Trimming*

The National Association of Meat Purveyors (NAMP)[121] has provided purchasing recommendations for the meat buyers for the food service industry. Their buyer's guide suggests that, unless specified by the purchaser, steaks should not exceed ¾ in. in fat trim at any one point and should average no more than ½ in. in thickness; chops, cutlets, and filets should not exceed 3/8 in. fat at any one point and should average no more than ¼ in. while roasts (disregarding seam fat) can average ¾ in. (1 in. max) or ½ in. (¾ in. maximum). With the decline of local butcher shops and increased purchase of meats from supermarkets, the shopper is more likely to obtain meats that require trimming. In these cases home trimming to NAMP guidelines may result in significant loss of fat and total weight.

Toepfer et al.[158] studied the fat trim from oven roasts in boneless beef cut to U.S. Army specifications (external fat limited to a maximum of ¾-in. thickness) or further trimmed to leave about ¼ in. of fat. The trim amounted to 6% of the average weight of the cuts and consisted mostly of fat (82.6 to 87.5%) and only 2.1 to 4.5% protein.

Leverton and Odell[99] reported results of analysis of common retail meat cuts cooked by usual household methods. They analyzed three different portions of each cut; the extremely lean portion, the lean and marbeled-with-fat portion, and the obviously fat portion. Evaluation of 48 different cuts from each of three carcasses revealed that the composition of separable fat portions of cooked beef, lamb, and pork were similar, but veal was higher in protein. Not many Americans can afford the calories of fat trim, but if consumed, the trim can contain appreciable protein (up to 5%) and ⅓ the phosphorus and magnesium of the lean and marble portions.[99]

*Thawing*

Although vitamins are lost to thaw juices (see below), B vitamins are generally heat stable during thawing of meats. Extensive studies were performed by Causey et al. on the effects of thawing on nutritive value of pork,[24] beef,[25] and lamb.[26] These ground meats were stored frozen (−13°F) for 6 to 18 weeks and thawed during cooking, at room temperature (65 to 75°F) to internal temperature of 37°F, or for the pork, under running cold water (57°F) to an internal temperature of 37°F. No appreciable losses of thiamin, riboflavin, or niacin occurred during thawing of ground pork. Thawing of beef patties prior to cooking had no significant effect upon thiamin, riboflavin, or lysine content in the final cooked product compared to direct cooking of the freezer product. Thawing of lamb prior to cooking resulted in slightly lower thiamin, riboflavin, and lysine levels in the cooked product. The thawing method had no effect upon eventual weight loss of pork, but thawing of beef and lamb resulted in greater weight loss than when meat was cooked from the frozen state.

Westerman et al.[173] also reported little loss of thiamin, riboflavin, or niacin from beef round steaks due to thawing method. They did find that pantothenic acid was better retained in refrigerated and room temperature thawing than under running water at 163°F.

### Thaw Juices

Thaw losses from frozen meats to thaw juices are of significant concern.[75] In one report the percentage weight loss from pork chops varied from 6 to 12%,[134] whereas Toepfer et al.[158] reported an average loss of 4.2% from different beef cuts. Thaw-drip loss from liver slices and pieces that have a large cut-surface area per volume, was reported to be 8 to 15% of initial weight.[86] Total loss of thaw juice from frozen fish ranged from 4.5 to 15.2%.[163] Protein loss from beef to thaw juices was small and followed a similar pattern to weight loss (1.4 to 3.1%), while no fat was found in the thaw juice.[158]

Considerable amounts of B vitamins can be found in the drip from thawed meats.[51] Beef steaks[133] and pork chops[134] were frozen at approximately 0°F and defrosted at room temperature. Beef dripping losses amounted to 12% of thiamin, 10% of riboflavin, 15% of niacin, 9% of pyridoxine, 33% of pantothenic acid, and 8% of the folic acid. Pork drip included losses of 9% of thiamin, 4% of riboflavin, 11% of niacin, 9% of vitamin $B_6$, 7% of pantothenic acid, 6% of vitamin $B_{12}$ and in excess of 7% of five measured amino acids. B-vitamin retention during thawing of chicken broilers was good under most thawing conditions.[153,154]

No reports were found dealing with the effects of retaining thaw juices and adding them to the cooking pan for eventual use in the gravy. Since the thaw juices contain significant quantities of protein and B vitamins, their reuse has nutritional potential. Microbial growth in thaw juices may be high, however, and safety consideration could override nutritional potential of thaw juice reuse.[92]

### Losses in Cooking
#### Broiling

Tucker et al.[160] measured thiamin and riboflavin retention in broiled beef loin-end cut steaks cooked rare to medium to internal temperature of 136°F or medium to well done to 158°F. They found 70% medium-well and 77% for rare-medium retention of thiamin in the cooked meats and 7% in the drippings of both types. Riboflavin retention was higher: 92% for each heat treatment, and 4 to 5% in the drippings. Causey et al.[25] pan and oven broiled ground beef to an internal temperature of 165°F and found retentions of between 80 to 90% of thiamin and riboflavin in the cooked product, while 1 to 3% of the thiamin and 5 to 7% of the riboflavin was found in the drip. Nobel[124] found no difference in thiamin or riboflavin retention in pan- or oven-broiled beef (internal temperature of 160°F). Thiamin retentions were higher in broiled beef loin steaks and one-serving beef patties (78%) than in rib steaks and three-serving patties (62%). Riboflavin retention was good in all beef products, ranging from 84% for one-serving ground beef to 100% for three-serving ground beef. Toepfer et al.[158] reported that broiled steaks on griddle without added fat retained 96.6% protein and 95.8% fat.

Noble[124] also investigated broiling of lamb and pork. Thiamin retention in lamb chops and one-portion ground lamb averaged 66%, while three-portion ground lamb patties averaged 55%. Retention of vitamin $B_1$ in broiled ham slices was 65%, while

Canadian-style bacon was 79%. Riboflavin retention in lamb chops was significantly higher (96%) than the two types of lamb patties (average was 75%). The bacon and ham retained an average of 81% of vitamin $B_2$. Causey et al.[24] found good retention of B vitamins in ground pork patties — 79 to 94% for thiamin, 61 to 95% for riboflavin, and 88 to 104% for niacin. Less than 10% of the initial vitamins was found in the cooking drip. Broiling of lamb patties yielded 80 to 94% retention of thiamin, 40 to 60% retention of riboflavin, and 85 to 98% retention of lysine, with 3 to 8% of the vitamins in the drip.[26]

The effect of electric oven broiling on retention of thiamin, riboflavin, and niacin of pork *gluteus medius* muscle of pale, soft, watery (PSW) or dark, firm, dry (DFD) pork muscles was reported.[110] PSW pork had about twice the niacin content of DFD on both a dry and cooked weight basis. Fresh DFD muscle had slightly higher thiamin and riboflavin content. After broiling 5 min per side, 3 in. from the broiling unit, PSW muscle showed greater exudate formation, more expressible juice, and higher nutrient loss on a fresh weight basis. Evaluation of the total content of the three B vitamins in the cooked products favors neither use of PSW nor DFD meat despite large loss in the drip, but DFD muscles are considered more tender and juicy.[82]

### Braising

Braising, addition of water during cooking of meats, reduces retention of nutrients in cooked meat. In contrast to waterless cooking with 95% retention of protein, Swiss steaks and pot roasts retained only 83.7 and 89.9% of protein, respectively, when they were braised.[158] Less than 70% of the fat was retained in these two braised cuts of beef.

Noble[125] reported data on thiamin, riboflavin, fat, and moisture contents of various cuts of beef, veal, and pork before and after braising. Total weight losses of various cuts ranged from approximately 35 to 40% of uncooked weight, while the cooking liquids leached out 15 to 30% of the thiamin and riboflavin of the beef and veal and 1 to 13% of the thiamin of the pork. Thiamin and riboflavin retentions of various cooked meats were lower than found in the previous subsection on broiled meats. Beef and veal cuts retained less than 50% of the original thiamin and 75% of the riboflavin from the raw meat. Retention of vitamin $B_1$ in pork ranged from 44% of the pork chops to 57% of pork tenderloin. Vitamin $B_2$ retention averaged 73% for different pork cuts. Meyer et al.[108] found only about 55% retention of nicotinic acid and 51% retention of pantothenic acid in braised beef.

The thiamin and riboflavin contents of braised or simmered calf sweetbreads, beef kidney, and lamb and pork heart were presented by Noble.[126] The braised meats as a group, with water amounting to 8% of raw weight, retained a larger proportion of vitamins than did the simmered meats with half their raw weight of water or sweetbreads and kidneys that were with equal amounts. Sweetbreads retained the highest percent thiamin (66% braised and 55% simmered), while beef, veal, and pork heart retained only about 29%. Vitamin $B_2$ retention ranged from 75% for the veal, beef, lamb, and pork hearts to 55% for beef kidney. Total weight loss of the various meats during braising averaged 46% for braising and 40% for simmering.

Meyer et al.[109] reported that braising of beef round roasts by searing each side for 7 min and braising to internal temperature of 210°F resulted in an average retention of 56% of pantothenic acid, 44% of which was recovered in the drip and 49% vitamin $B_6$, 34% of which was transferred to the drip. Much higher retention of these two vitamins was obtained when beef loins were roasted (see below).

### Roasting

Toepfer et al.[158] reported little loss of protein in oven or pot roasting of boneless beef (95.6% retention in the drained roast and 1.8% in drip) except when water was added (89.9% retention and 7.6% loss in drippings). Nobel and Gomez[128] roasted five cuts of beef at 350 or 300°F to internal temperature of 160°F, or in the case of a beef loaf, 167°F. Thiamin and riboflavin analysis of the raw and cooked meats revealed that longer cooking time did not affect thiamin retention. Roasted beef loaf retained an average of 70% of the thiamin, whereas significantly less was retained by the cooked, top round and rib roasts (average was equal to 54%). Rump and tenderloin roasts were intermediate. Roasted beef loaf and top round retained the lowest proportion of riboflavin (about 80%), while rib and rump roasts retained the highest (about 87%).

Thiamin and riboflavin contents in lamb (boned, rolled shoulders, legs, rack roasts, and loin roasts) roasted to either 180 or 174°F internal temperature in a 300°F oven were recorded by Nobel and Gomez.[127] Results showed that longer heating periods did not affect the thiamin retention, nor were there significant differences of vitamin $B_1$ or $B_2$ retention in different cuts. The average vitamin $B_1$ retention was 64%, while riboflavin retention was 89%.

Cover et al.[39] reported that high oven temperatures (400°F vs. 300°F) reduced B vitamins in large-scale cooking of beef and pork roasts. They found that total retentions for meat plus drip were higher for thiamin, pantothenic acid, niacin, and riboflavin for both beef and pork when roasting was done with low rather than high temperatures. Cover et al.[32] obtained similar results with small-scale roast beef. Their retentions in rib roasts, rare and well done, respectively, were for thiamin, 75 and 69%; riboflavin, 83 and 77%; nicotinic acid, 75 and 79%; and pantothenic acid, 91 and 75%. Leeking et al.[96] used large-scale cooking practices (40-lb lots) to roast ham at 300°F to an internal temperature of 170°F. They concluded that the long roasting period of approximately 4 hr was at least partially responsible for low thiamin content found in the cooked ham (0.476 mg/100 g of meat on a wet basis or 1.71 mg/100 g on a moisture-, fat-, chloride-free basis). Roasting beef loins at 300°F to an internal temperature of 158°F resulted in retention of 89% of pantothenic acid (19% in drip) and 72% of vitamin $B_6$ (16% in drip).[109]

Engler and Bowers[49] investigated the vitamin $B_6$ content of muscle and drip from raw and roasted (at 350°F to internal temperature of 176°F) turkey breast and thigh muscle. On a moisture and fat-free basis, uncooked turkey breast muscle and muscle cooked from the partially frozen state had significantly more vitamin $B_6$ than muscle cooked from the thawed state; muscle cooked from the frozen state was intermediate in vitamin $B_6$ content. Roasting reduced vitamin $B_6$ content of thigh muscle, independent of thaw state.

*Frying*

Cooking liver slices in a pan with margarine over a slow gas flame resulted in loss of 15% of the vitamin $B_1$, 6% vitamin $B_2$, and 13% of niacin.[86] Cooking frozen liver slices increased the loss of thiamin and decreased the loss of riboflavin, while niacin results were variable.

*Microwave (Electronic)*

Utilization of microwave cooking in the home has increased dramatically in the last few years. Microwave heating, accomplished by high-energy, electromagnetic radiations, is an extremely efficient process that permits virtually no heat loss.[174] It has been estimated that, although conventional heating produces a coupling efficiency of only a few percent, microwave coupling efficiency is about 80%.[169]

Thomas et al.[159] first reported that thiamin retention was higher in beef and pork patties (77 to 91%) cooked with "high-frequency energy" than in patties that were grilled (55 to 79%), while retentions of niacin (about 90%) and riboflavin (about 100%) were equally stable in both methods of cooking. Kylen et al.[90] cooked beef or pork roasts and beef and ham loaves in a gas oven at 325°F to internal temperatures of 136 to 137°F or in an electronic range to the same internal temperatures. Mean cooking losses were higher for electronic cooking, as drippings were significantly higher for beef and pork roasts prepared in the electronic range. Mean percentage retention of thiamin in the lean portion of beef roasts cooked by microwave were lower (58% to 67%) than oven cooked (80 to 86%), but pork roasts and beef and ham loaves showed similar retentions of vitamin $B_1$ by both cooking methods. No differences in vitamin $B_1$ or $B_2$ retentions were found when cooking lamb roasts or bacon by conventional or microwave procedures.[129]

Bowers and Fryer[14] also compared retention of vitamins $B_1$ and $B_2$ from microwave and gas ovens. In this case, frozen turkey pectoralis muscles were (1) cooked, (2) cooked and reheated after 1 day of refrigerated storage, (3) cooked frozen, or (4) cooked, frozen and reheated. Results showed that the type of oven had no significant effect on vitamin $B_1$ content, but gas-heated turkey meat was higher in vitamin $B_2$ if retentions were placed on a moisture-free, fat-free basis. Wing and Alexander[174] found that chicken breasts heated by microwave radiations (2450 MHz for 1.5 min) retained significantly more vitamin $B_6$ (91%) than breasts roasted in a conventional oven (83%) at 325°F for 45 min. Conventional cooking resulted in significantly larger drip volume and more vitamin $B_6$ in the drip than microwave cooking. Microwave-cooked turkey breast muscle retained significantly more vitamin $B_6$ on a cooked weight basis than did conventionally cooked muscle.[15] However, little difference in vitamin $B_6$ content was found between conventional and microwave cooking of pork muscle.[16]

Baldwin et al.[9] cooked beef, pork, and lamb roasts with two 2450 MHz microwave ranges, one operated at 220 V (1050 W cooking power), and the other at 115 V (492 W power) or with a conventional gas oven (325 ± 5°F). Retention of thiamin, riboflavin, and niacin was less in meat cooked with 115 V than by the other two methods. Baldwin and co-workers also reported that microwave cooking resulted in less formation of free amino acids, without affecting total protein significantly. There was a trend toward less retention of sodium, chloride, phosphorus, and iron in meat cooked by microwaves. Mineral content of microwave-cooked meat was investigated in only one other report,[140] but no relationship of cooking method to mineral retention was made.

Janicki and Appledorf[74] obtained ground beef patties from a fast food chain and either broiled, grill-fried (natural gas at over 700°F), or microwave-cooked (2450 MHz) raw patties or broiled, frozen, and reheated patties with microwave. Lipid analysis showed that the ratio of unsaturated to saturated fatty acids increased during all cooking treatments. Microwave-treated patties had the largest ratio of unsaturated to saturated fatty acids. The authors postulated that the C18:1 and C18:2 fatty acids increased because they are probably more intimately involved as structural components and phospholipids and are less likely to be lost to drip. They concluded that since microwave heating produced patties with less crude fat than the two conventional cooking procedures, this cooking procedure might be recommended for persons on low-fat diets.

Goldblith et al.[61] concluded that microwave energy per se had no effect on destruction of thiamin. Although Van Zante and Johnson[168] found slightly higher retentions of thiamin and riboflavin in conventionally heated aqueous solutions (buffered to simulate the pH of pork) than those heated by microwave, the researchers concluded that the differences in retention were small and of little practical significance. It appears that the increased or decreased losses of nutrients in microwave vs. conventionally cooked meats are largely related to amount of drip and the duration of heating. Published research indicates that microwave cooking of meats is nutritionally equivalent to conventional methods, but more nutrients besides vitamins $B_1$, $B_2$, and $B_6$ must be measured.

### Stewing

Cover et al.[33-38] extensively studied the effects of several stewing methods upon the retention of thiamin, pantothenic acid, niacin, and riboflavin in beef and lamb. They stewed the meat via pressure cooking, boiling, or simmering. In addition, all cooking procedures were tested with or without prior browning of the meat with a small or a large amount of cooking water. The average total retention after stewing was about 50% for thiamin, 75% for pantothenic acid, and 100% or above for niacin and riboflavin. Browning significantly reduced total vitamin content of all four vitamins except niacin in beef. Temperature of cooking and amount of water had minor adverse effects in this study.

### Other Cooking Methods

Cover et al.,[40] using a home process, canned beef and veal in No. 2 and No. 3 tin cans and in pint and quart glass jars (15 psi, 250°F for at least 60 min) and analyzed the contents for thiamin, pantothenic acid, niacin, and riboflavin. Retentions were calculated on dry basis immediately after canning and after storage for 3 months at 95 to 98°F. After canning, losses of vitamin $B_2$ and pantothenic acid were negligible, but vitamin $B_1$ losses were up to 65% and pantothenic acid at about 30%. Only thiamin was further lost during storage. Saftey recommendations for home canning have recently been published.[6]

Little or no published reports were found on the effects of small-scale practices (at home) of pressure cooking, infrared cooking, or broasting (pressure frying) of meat products, nor were reports found on the use of crock pots. Use of crock pots is on the rise, and knowledge of time-temperature nutrient destructions would predict low B vitamin retentions with this cooking method. However, more research is obviously needed on these and other new home practices.

### Summary: Nutrient Stability During Cooking

The major losses of nutrients in cooked animal products are the vitamins lost due to heat destruction and those water-soluble nutrients that leach out into the drip. Reuse of drip, where possible, can conserve small amounts of protein, some minerals, and, in some cases, considerable amounts of B vitamins. Proper choice of cooking method and conditions can reduce heat-induced destruction of vitamins. Little if any of the essential amino acids, tryptophan, methionine, and lysine are destroyed or lost by heat treatment using standard cooking procedures.[151]

Thiamin is unstable in all heating processes. Broiling, frying, and roasting yield 50 to 90% retention of vitamin $B_1$, while braising and home canning can reduce thiamin to less than ½ of the raw product. Rice and Beuk[141] determined the chemical kinetics of thermal destruction of thiamin in pork and found that, at temperatures above 170°, the rate of loss is constant at any given temperature and was proportional to the temperature. The half life of the vitamin heated at 250°F is about ½ hour but at 210°F is over 2 hr. Use of water during cooking increases thiamin leaching into the drip.

Riboflavin is also labile to heat, although not to the extent of thiamin, and can be leached into the drip. Vitamin $B_2$ retention is almost always better than thiamin and ranges from 60 to 100%. Retention of 90 to 100% vitamin $B_2$ in waterless cooking is not uncommon.

Niacin is one of the most heat-stable vitamins, but it is readily lost in leaching. Braising and stewing can result in ⅓ to ½ loss of this vitamin from muscle meat, but nearly all can be recovered in the broth. Combination of drip and meat will usually yield 90 to 100% recovery of niacin, irrespective of cooking treatment.

Pantothenic acid is also readily lost in the drip from cooked meats, especially those heated with water. Braising can result in over 40% loss of pantothenic acid in the drip. This loss is about twice that of roasted meats. Total recovery from meat and drip is usually very good, from 75 to 100%.

Folic acid retention in cooked meats has been reported to be very poor: 5 to 54%[30] and 8 to 67%.[149] These and other published reports preceded newer developments on methodology.[136] Hurdle et al.[73] utilized ascorbic acid as an antioxidant and conjugase to free-bound folate in folate assays of foods. They found that boiling and frying of lamb liver and chicken meat resulted in no loss of the vitamin. Boiled, pasteurized milk lost no folate, but boiled and fried egg yolk lost 70 and 29% of folate, respectively. Systematic studies using standardized procedures are needed to determine folic acid contents and retentions in foods.

The early literature on vitamin $B_6$ retention also reported extremely low retentions in cooked meats. McIntire et al.[105] used a yeast growth assay and showed roasting and broiling produced only 30% retention and braising and stewing only about 18% retention of the vitamin. Rat growth assays published in 1941[70] yielded similar results. Lushbough et al.[101] utilized the *Saccharomyces carlsbergensis* microbiological assay and reported somewhat higher retentions of vitamin $B_6$ in several different types of cooked meat (average 54%). Recent assays have shown much higher retentions in cooked meats. Meyer et al.[109] used *S. carlsbergensis* to measure pyridoxine retention in roasted and braised beef and found 72 and 49% retentions, respectively. Combinations of the vitamin $B_6$ of the meat and the drip for both cooking methods indicated approximately 85% total retention. Bowers and co-workers have published a series of papers[15,16,49,50] on vitamin $B_6$ retention in cooked turkey and pork utilizing the yeast *S. uvarum*. They generally found 70% or more retention of total vitamin $B_6$ after various cooking procedures.

McIntire et al.[105] found that nearly all of the choline was retained in meat, while Schweigert et al.[148] found about 77% retention of biotin in cooked meats. No other publications were found that reported retention of choline or biotin in cooked meats, and none investigated vitamin $B_{12}$.

### Effect of Holding and Reheating Animal Products

Singh et al.[152] showed that riboflavin loss from stored, refrigerated, whole milk was greatest in glass or translucent plastic containers at high light intensities and at higher storage temperatures. Riboflavin losses in containers stored in the dark were insignificant. Retention of vitamin A in margarine and butter exceeded 75% after refrigerated storage (41°F) for 1 year.[44]

Reheating of meat and meat products that have been stored refrigerated or frozen results in excellent retentions of thiamin and riboflavin.[51] Causey and Fenton[27] cooked, froze, and reheated individual servings of four meat recipes (creamed chicken and rice, paprika chicken and gravy, spaghetti and meat balls, and ham patties) by five different cooking methods. No difference in thiamin retention in either of the chicken dishes was noted due to cooking method. Although cooking method affected the thiamin content of the other dishes, little total loss of vitamin $B_1$ was recorded. Vitamin $B_6$ retention in turkey breast muscle reheated by either electric or microwave ovens was evaluated by Engler and Bowers.[50] They found no differences in vitamin $B_6$ when calculated on a basis of cooked weight, but on a moisture-free and fat-free basis, freshly roasted samples contained significantly more vitamin $B_6$ than those that were recooked. These losses were small, and the variation among birds was greater than among treatments.

Turkey muscle, cooked and refrigerated for 1 day and then reheated by microwave or gas oven, was unexpectedly higher in thiamin than muscle that was (1) cooked, (2) cooked and frozen, or (3) cooked, frozen, and reheated.[14] There was no significant effect of cooking and/or storage upon riboflavin except that gas heating resulted in more vitamin $B_2$ retention than microwave cooking. The variations among birds were again greater than among treatments or between ovens.

West et al.[171] reported that thiamin retentions in three frozen precooked foods (Italian rice, chicken, and ham loaf) were very similar to those of freshly prepared products after 2 months of freezer storage (about −4.5°F). Kahn and Livingston[79] found better retention of vitamin $B_1$ in four common, frozen food dishes (beef stew, chicken à la king, shrimp Newburg, and peas in cream sauce) that were prepared, frozen, stored at −10°F, and reheated in a microwave or an infrared oven to 194°F than in the same dishes freshly prepared and held hot at 180°F for 1, 2, or 3 hr.

Nielsen and Carlin[123] investigated thiamin retention in frozen, raw, or precooked all-beef loaves and precooked beef-soy loaves. Precooking to 165°F, freezing, and reheating to 130°F of all beef loaves resulted in 90% retention of vitamin $B_1$ but only 58% retention for thiamin-fortified beef-soy (30% soy) loaves. The authors hypothesized that the synthetic thiamin added to the beef-soy was less heat stable than that naturally occurring in the all-beef loaf. Ziprin and Carlin[178] recently investigated microwave and conventional preparation of cooked beef and beef-soy loaves (15% soy as flour or as a concentrate). In this study the soy substitution (soy was not fortified with thiamin) had no effect on fat or thiamin content or retention. Thiamin retention in beef loin roasts that were held over dry heat (90 min) before and after slicing or refrigerated for 24 hr, sliced, and reheated, was compared to that of roasts cooked to 129°F in a 300°F oven, sliced, and served immediately.[17] Thiamin retention in roasts held unsliced (79.2%) or sliced (76.5%) compared well with roasts served immediately (78.8%). The refrigerated, sliced, and reheated roast beef retained 67.8% vitamin $B_1$. Vail and Westerman[164] found less than 10% further loss of thiamin from roasted pork that was refrigerated overnight and/or reheated.

Canned storage of pork for 1 year at various temperatures[59] showed no significant losses of riboflavin, niacin, or pantothenic acid, but thiamin disappearance increased with time and temperature of storage (80 to 88% loss of 98°F for 1 year, but 0 to 11% at 45°F for 1 year).

## FOODS OF PLANT ORIGIN

### Losses Preparatory to Cooking
Major losses in the nutrient content of plant foods, especially vegetables, can occur due to storage and preparation procedures prior to cooking. Damaging practices include improper storage, washing and soaking, trimming, and chopping.

### *Storage Conditions*
Proper storage conditions of unprocessed cereal grains, vegetables, fruits, and other plant stuffs is a world-wide nutrition problem. The problem is far greater than the loss of a small percentage of the vitamin content; it concerns protection of these foods from invasion by microbes, insects, and rodents.

We must take precautions in the home to prevent deterioration of fresh vegetable products. Storage temperature, humidity, time of storage, and light in some cases directly affect shelf life and, therefore, the nutritional value of fresh foods. Vegetables such as spinach, broccoli, and salad greens must be refrigerated in a vegetable crisper or in moisture-proof bags near freezing to maintain their nutritional values.[161] For example, Van Duyne et al.[166] reported that ascorbic acid content of cabbage did not decrease when freshly harvested heads were stored in closed containers at 31 to 39°F (−0.5 to 4.0°C) for 2 months, or when the heads were kept refrigerated for a week. Carrots, potatoes, and other tubers retain their food value best at cool and moist temperatures. Grains, dry legumes, flours, etc., must be kept cool and dry to prevent microbial attack. When properly stored, grains and legumes are stable for extended periods with no nutrient modifications.

Fresh fruits are particularly vulnerable to spoilage. Many fruits enter a rapid respiratory period known as the climacteric rise following harvesting. Climacteric fruits include apples, apricots, pears, and bananas. These fruits are harvested green and timed to reach the market place at the beginning of their ripening period. When purchased they must be kept cool but not frozen to retard their rate of deterioration. Nonclimacteric fruits such as the citrus fruits and many berries are less perishable than the climacteric fruits and have a longer shelf life.

Very little information has been published on the effects of time of harvest, in relation to maturity of the fruit, on nutritional value of the product. Home gardeners should be encouraged, since at least for the tomato, ripening on the vine results in one quarter to one third more ascorbic acid than picking green and ripening off the vine as are most store-bought, whole tomatoes.[132]

The modern shopper, for better or for worse, is purchasing more and more of the family vegetables and fruits either frozen or canned instead of fresh. Processing plant foods surely extends shelf life and in doing so increases total nutritional value of the products by decreasing spoilage. Processed vegetable products all undergo some heat treatment, however, and thus they cannot be as nutritious as fresh products. Even the avid naturalist cannot obtain a good variety of fresh product year-round for reasonable costs. Therefore, frozen or canned products must be utilized.

Table 3 provides a listing of typical shelf life for various retail foods of plant origin. The reader should keep in mind that shelf life takes into account product safety and appeal and not nutritional value.

One of the best approaches to preserving the quality of processed vegetables is freezing. If the food is properly blanched, quick frozen, and stored, nutrient retention is generally as high or higher than in food preserved by any other technique.[4] The purchaser must assume proper processing, packaging, and handling of frozen foods at point of purchase. At purchase, however, the consumer assumes responsibility. Frozen items should be transferred to suitable cold storage immediately upon arrival home. Derse and Teply[43] investigated the effects of storage conditions on 21 nutrients in frozen green beens, peas, orange juice, and strawberries. With the exception of ascorbic acid in green beans, they found good retention of vitamins after 12 months storage at 0°F (−18°C), the normal temperature of a home freezer. However, they concluded that there appears to be a critical break point in stability of frozen food products not far above 0°F. Bissett and Berry[12] reported 90% or more retention of ascorbic acid in frozen concentrate orange juice after a year at −5°F, but after 8 months at 19°F, only an average of 61% vitamin C remained. Fennema,[60] in reviewing the effects of freeze-preservation on nutrients, points out that exposure of vegetables to 22°F, a temperature equivalent to many freezing compartments of home refrigerators, almost invariably results in greater losses of vitamin C, B carotene, folic acid, and pantothenic acid, but has no significant effect on losses of niacin, riboflavin, thiamin, vitamin $B_6$, or minerals when compared to freezer units of 0°F (−18°C).

The International Institute of Refrigeration in Paris[4] maintains that commercially frozen foods can be adequately stored in home freezers 0°F (−18°C) for up to 3 months. This organization also instructs those who home freeze to utilize foods in perfect condition rather than overripe or bruised products. The food should then be sealed in a container or wrapped in moisture and vapor-proof materials to exclude air.

## Table 3
## SHELF-LIFE FOR RETAIL PRODUCTS OF PLANT ORIGIN

| Product | Days | Weeks | Months |
|---|---|---|---|
| Bread, white (summer) | 2—5 | — | — |
| Bread, white (winter) | 3—7 | — | |
| Bread, white (frozen) | 30+ | — | — |
| Cake, angel or cup | — | 2 | — |
| Canned apricots | — | — | 36 |
| Canned asparagus | — | — | 24 |
| Canned kidney beans | — | — | 36 |
| Canned fruit cocktail | — | — | 36 |
| Canned fruit and vegetable juices | — | — | 24 |
| Canned puddings | — | — | 24 |
| Canned tomatoes | — | — | 30—36 |
| Catsup | — | — | 24 |
| Cereal, ready to eat | — | — | 6—8 |
| Donuts | 1—4 | — | — |
| Dough, refrigerated flours, all purpose | — | 9—10 | — |
| Flours, all purpose | — | — | 15 |
| French/Italian dressings | — | — | 10—12 |
| Frozen foods (general) | — | — | 12 |
| Macaroni (dry) | — | — | 6—8 |
| Margarine | — | — | 2—6 |
| Pizza sauce | — | — | 36 |
| Spaghetti | — | — | 9—12 |
| Sweet or dill pickles | — | — | 12—15 |
| Vegetable oil (liquid) | — | — | 4 |

From *Anon., Food Stability Survey*, Vol. 2, Department of Food Science, Rutgers University, U.S. Government Printing Office, Washington, D.C., 1971.

Canning vegetables and fruits results in significant losses of nutrients. These losses will continue in home storage if canned foods are not stored in cool temperatures (50 to 65°F), and if they are not consumed in a reasonable time period. Significant losses of B-complex vitamins, ascorbic acid, and B carotene occur when canned vegetables and fruits are stored for a year or more at 80°F.[23] Nagy and Smoot[120] studied the retention of ascorbic acid during storage of 14 commercially canned single-strength orange juices stored from 40 to 120°F over 12 weeks. They found that storage temperatures greater than about 80°F markedly decreased the rate of vitamin C retention. Similar results were reported by Lamb et al.[93] for canned tomato juice and tomato paste. Two-year storage studies indicated that ascorbic acid was more stable in tomato juice than paste and storage at 70°F or above resulted in more rapid ascorbic acid loss.

*Washing and Soaking*

Some dry cereal grains and legumes are traditionally soaked for extended periods of time to tenderize them. During soaking the grains or cereals take up water so that there is little leaching of nutrients into the soak water. Rockland et al.[145] found only slight leaching of thiamin, pyridoxine, and niacin but did encounter a 29 to 46% loss of total folacin from dry pinto beans during extensive soaking. Washing losses of processed grains or beans may be considerable. Swaminathan[156,157] found that as much as 60% of the niacin and thiamin was lost when raw-milled rice was washed.

Although soaking and washing of vegetables and tubers before cooking allows for leaching of water-soluble constituents, these losses are minimal. For example, peeled potatoes held at room temperature in cold water, either still or running, for up to 24 hr lost only 13% of their ascorbic acid contents.[18]

*Trimming*

When foods of plant origin are trimmed, the nutrient losses generally exceed the weight losses because the nutrient concentration is usually higher in the outer leaves of vegetables and outer layers of seeds, tubers, and fruits.[91] Outer green leaves of lettuce, although coarser than the tender, inner leaves, have higher calcium, iron, and vitamin A value.[161] Cabbage vitamin C content, on the other hand, is fairly consistent from outer to inner leaves, while cabbage thiamin and riboflavin is in highest concentration in the inner leaves.[175] Sheets[150] reported that the green leaves of cabbage had 21 times the carotene, up to 3 times the iron, and 1.5 times the ascorbic acid as the bleached inner leaves. Trimming losses, therefore, depend upon the variety of the food, season of the year, the condition of the food (bruising decreases nutrient levels and increases the amount of trimming), the trimming habits of the consumer, and the nutrient in question.

Total trimming wastes are quite high when expressed as a percentage of purchase weight. They have been estimated[104] as 21 to 61% in leafy vegetables, 14 to 26% for root vegetables if scraped, and 63 to 71% for fresh peas and broad beans. Andross[3] and Watt and Merrill[170] have published tables including refuse losses of fruits and vegetables.

*Chopping, Slicing, Mashing, Etc.*

Many plant foods require some type of home process to reduce them to cooking and eating size. The harshness of the procedures can vary from chopping into large slices to a fine puree. To different degrees, all of these procedures damage and rupture cells, exposing the contents for nutrient destruction.

Van Duyne et al.[166] found only a 6% reduction in ascorbic acid content of cabbage due to shredding and allowing it to stand for 1 hr in air or 1 to 3 hr in water. Munsell et al.[117] investigated the effects of large-scale preparation practices upon vitamin retention in cabbage and coleslaw. Their practices are not dissimilar to home practices. They found that the cutting method and holding for 22 hr at room temperature had little effect upon total ascorbic acid, thiamin, riboflavin, niacin, or carotene content of cabbage or coleslaw. However, there was great destruction of reduced ascorbic acid (up to 52%). Millross et al.[112] found that washing spring cabbage after shredding resulted in a 35 to 37% loss of vitamin C.

In a review by Harris[67], cucumbers reportedly retained 78% of their ascorbic acid during slicing, 67 to 65% after standing for 1 hr, and 59 to 51% after standing for 3 hr. Grated radish lost 27% of thiamin in 24 hr at 50°F, while grated sweet potatoes lost 21% thiamin.[91] Ascorbic acid retention in tomato pulp was good for 4 hr but was only 60% after 24 hr storage.[69] Bananas that were sliced and exposed at room temperature, lost almost 50% of their ascorbic acid in 5 hr,[68] while quartered apples lost 20% in 1 to 2 hr and 33% in 3 hr.[22]

**Losses During Cooking**

Major losses in nutritive value of plant foods can occur during cooking processes. Excessive heat and overuse of cooking water can result in destruction of 50% of some heat-labile and water-soluble nutrients. The USDA[161] recommends, for example, that the best method of cooking vegetables to preserve their nutritive value is to cook them only until tender in just enough water to prevent scorching. Use of pans with tight-fitting lids is also suggested to lessen cooking time and water use.

When home-scale portions of plant foods are cooked, nutrient losses vary according to: the type of food, amount of cooking water, the time of cooking, type of equipment, and the nutrient in question.[92] In addition, leaching and heat destruction will increase with increased food surface area. Fine chopping or slicing of vegetables prior to cooking increases vitamin losses. A variety of cooking procedures are utilized in the home. Choice of home process can directly effect the nutrient intake of a family.

*Boiling*

Perhaps the most utilized cooking procedure for foods of plant origin is boiling. This is where overuse of water and cooking time takes its toll in labile nutrients. Harris and Levenberg[67] and Lachance and Erdman[92] presented extensive tabular data on nutrient retention in boiled cereals, vegetables, fruits, and legumes. The reader should consult these references for information on specific foods and nutrients.

Krehl and Winters[88] published possibly the most exhaustive paper concerned with retention of five vitamins and three minerals in 12 commonly used vegetables cooked by four different cooking methods. Family-size portions of the individual vegetables were cooked by: (1) pressure cooking with ½ cup added water, (2) cooking (boiling) with water to cover, (3) cooking (boiling) with ½ cup water, and (4) cooking (waterless) with no added water (except for the water clinging to vegetable from rinsing). Their results showed that the average retention of the minerals calcium, iron, and phosphorus was only about 75% when the vegetables were cooked covered with water, while 85% of the minerals were retained after pressure cooking or cooking with minimal water (½ cup), and over 90% were recovered from waterless cooking. The same type of results was reported for the retention of the vitamins: thiamin, riboflavin, niacin, ascorbic acid, and carotene. There was about a 10% reduction in vitamin retention when comparing waterless to pressure cooking or cooking with ½ cup water, and an additional 10% loss when the vegetables were cooked covered with water. It was concluded that the greatest loss of nutritive value was due to water leaching. Hewston et al.[72] also reported results of a comprehensive study on the effect of home preparation practices on the vitamin and mineral content of some 20 common foods. They concluded that the retentions were lowest when the volume of the cooking water was large, the time of cooking was long, and the size of particles was small.

More recently, Gordon and Noble[64] looked at ascorbic acid retention, flavor, and color of four serving portions of six vegetables cooked by pressure saucepan, waterless method, or boiling water to cover. They reported that vegetables cooked in sufficient boiling water to cover were milder in flavor and greener than those cooked by the other methods. However, this method of cooking produced the lowest retention of ascorbic acid in four of the six vegetables. A pressure saucepan proved to retain the most ascorbic acid in five of the six vegetables.

Sodium bicarbonate can be added to vegetables during boiling to tenderize and bring out the green color. Beans are also soaked and cooked in bicarbonate solution to decrease cooking time[137] and increase tenderness.[122] However, sodium bicarbonate is particularly destructive to thiamin. Aughey and Daniel[8] found that the use of small concentrations of sodium bicarbonate markedly increased the destruction of thiamin in simmered green peas (12%) and boiled snap beans (41%) but had no significant effect upon vitamin $B_1$ content of boiled navy beans. In a study of sodium bicarbonate use in a preparation of soy milk, Bankhead et al.[10] found very large losses of thiamin (50%) and small losses of pantothenic acid (12%) attributable to the base.

Choice of cooking equipment can effect nutrient retention. Boiled parsnips retained more vitamin C in enamel (84%) and pyrex (81%) pans than in stainless steel (66%) and aluminum (71%).[21] According to Harris and Levenberg,[67] van der Lann and Van der Mijll Dekker[165] reported that glass, stainless steel, aluminum, enamel, and similar equipment had no measurable effect on nutrient content of cooked foods, whereas copper, brass, and monel could be quite destructive.

The cooking water from boiled vegetables often contains large percentages of the raw vegetable nutrients, especially when the vegetables have a large surface area or are cut into small pieces. For example, Munsell et al.[17] prepared boiled cabbage until done in a large-scale process and found more thiamin, riboflavin, and ascorbic acid in the cooking water than in the cabbage. Meiners et al.[106] investigated the content of nine minerals in raw and cooked lots of ten different mature dry legumes. Cooking times ranged from 30 to 140 min, and the total deionized water added was about four times the weight of the dry beans. They found that mineral retention in cooked beans was only one third to one half of the value of the raw beans.

The practice of saving vegetable cooking waters for soups is deserting the younger generations. This is unfortunate since we are probably pouring more nutrients down the drain each day than some less fortunate people consume. In one report Meredith et al.[107] found that more than half of the lysine and isoleucine from canned turnip greens would be lost if the canning liquid were discarded.

The modern supermarket provides the shopper with convenient boil-in-the-bag vegetables as well as frozen vegetables that direct us to add a tablespoon or so of water prior to boiling. These products are great nutrient savers and are competitively priced. On the other hand, if one grows or purchases fresh vegetables, these should be cooked in minimal water or preferably steamed.

The use of "hard" or "soft" water for cooking vegetables affects mineral retention in the final product. Marston et al.[102] investigated the phosphorus, calcium, and magnesium content of boiled cabbage, carrots, and broccoli as affected by: (1) distilled water, (2) hardness (150 ppm magnesium and 160 ppm calcium), and (3) 60 ppm sodium tripolyphosphate. They found that the vegetable cooked with high amounts of calcium and magnesium retained more of these two minerals, while phosphorus content of the cooking water did not significantly effect retention of minerals.

*Steam and Pressure Cooking*

Invariably, improved retentions of nutrients are obtained when vegetables are steam cooked rather than boiled. Steaming reduces leaching and also reduces the time required to cook plant foods. Munsell et al.[117] compared the vitamin contents of boiled cabbage with cabbage steamed in a vegetable steamer or steamed in a pot held above boiling water. Although Munsell's group utilized large-scale preparation methods, they clearly showed that retentions of carotene, thiamin, riboflavin, and ascorbic acid doubled with use of either steaming method rather than boiling water.

As mentioned above, Gordon and Noble[64] found that pressure saucepan cooking of six vegetables led to more retention of ascorbic acid in five of six vegetables tested when compared to boiling and waterless cooking. Gordon and Noble[62] earlier compared ascorbic acid retention in 11 vegetables cooked by a steamer, pressure saucepan, tightly covered saucepan, and boiling. All steaming methods produced significantly higher vitamin C retentions (69% average) than boiling (45%). Within the steaming methods there were no differences of loss rate. Kamalanathan et al.[81] measured the retention of ascorbic acid, thiamin, calcium, iron, and phosphorus in three native Indian vegetables as affected by boiling, steaming, pressure cooking, or panning. They concluded that pressure cooking was the best for vitamin and mineral retention. Additions of ammonia bicarbonate to broccoli prior to steam blanching increased its greenness compared to the control blanched product and produced no differences in retention of seven minerals and total ascorbic acid.[130]

*Frying*

With the exception of the potato, few vegetables are commonly fried in the home.

Pan or stir frying of mixed vegetables or oriental meat-vegetable dishes is becoming more popular but still lags far behind other cooking methods. Frying vegetables alleviates the problem of water leaching of vitamins and minerals but increases the chance of heat destruction of heat-labile vitamins such as ascorbic acid. One must be reminded, however, that frying increases the caloric value and therefore decreases the nutrient density (nutrient per calorie) of the product, since fried foods retain cooking oil.

There are many reports in the literature that point to loss of ascorbic acid during frying of potatoes. One of the most recent works[46] demonstrates that during frying, reduced ascorbic acid is readily oxidized to dehydro-ascorbic acid, but the further hydrolysis of dehydro-ascorbic acid to the nonactive diketo form is slow, probably due to dehydration of the potatoes during frying. Therefore, even frying for 30 min at 284°F retains 80% or more of the total ascorbic acid, but all of it is in the dehydro form. Domah's group, in the same publication,[46] points out that boiling the potatoes for 25 min results in rapid destruction of the dehydro form and results in only about 50% retention of total ascorbic acid.

Eheart and Gott[48] compared the retention of ascorbic acid in broccoli and green beans cooked by four cooking methods:

1.    Chinese stir-fry (1 in. pieces of vegetables cooked at 350°F while stirring with 10 m*l* of cooking oil, the heat reduced to 250°F, and enough water added to prevent browning)
2.    Microwave
3.    Boiling in uncovered pot with four parts water
4.    Boiling covered with one-half part water

Stir-frying proved to be as good as the covered, low-water method and better than microwave and uncovered, high-water method with broccoli but ranked lower than the covered, low-water method and equivalent to the other methods with green beans. Perhaps the poor retention of vitamin C in green beans (57.5%) as compared to broccoli (76.6%) was caused by the 5-min frying in the case of the beans and 1-min fry in the case of the broccoli. Cheldelin et al.[30] fried onions in an open pan for 20 min and found 74% retention of riboflavin. Published data are not available (especially using current analytical methodologies) on the effects of frying on retention of other micronutrients.

Some research has been published dealing with degradation, oxidation, and polymerization of constituents of cooking oils. Prolonged use and reuse of cooking oils is most common in restaurants and cafeterias and probably not much of a problem in the home. Overuse of frying oils should be discouraged, however, since fresh vegetable oils are adsorbed to fried food; for example, one tablespoon of oil is consumed with 20 small french fries,[162] and prolonged frying can alter the oil's chemical makeup and nutritional value.

Kilgore and Bailey[85] reported a decrease in linoleic acid, an essential fatty acid, in fats used in frying potatoes. The precentages of linoleic acid, expressed as percentages of total fatty acids, in the fresh fats were safflower oil, 72.0; corn oil, 57.2; cottonseed oil, 55.5; and shortening, 30.2. After the fats had been used for intermittent frying periods totaling 7½ hr, during which 10 lb of potatoes were fried, the percent losses of linoleic acid were safflower, 6.2; corn, 6.3; cottonseed, 11.0; and shortening, 2.7. The result of linoleic acid loss is not only a decrease of this essential fatty acid but a decrease in the polyunsaturated/saturated fatty acid ratio of the oil.

Yuki and Ishikawa[176] reported the changes in total tocopherol (vitamin E) contents of nine vegetable frying oils after simulated deep fat frying conditions. After 10 hr of frying, they found from 91.2% (safflower oil) to 53.5% (corn oil) retention for unsaturated oils but only 32.6% (palm oil) to nondetectable levels (coconut oil) in saturated oils as determined by thin-layer and gas chromatography.

*Baking: Vegetables and Fruits*

Most published research dealing with baking of either vegetables or fruits deals with potatoes. If those results can be extended to other baked vegetables and fruits, then this cooking procedure seems to be more destructive compared to other cooking methods.

Kahn and Halliday[80] investigated ascorbic acid retention in fried, steamed, and baked potatoes. They found no loss of vitamin C in steamed, whole potatoes but 20% loss in potatoes boiled in their skins or pared and cut, then baked. Fried potatoes lost 23% of their ascorbic acid content, while pared, halved, steamed and mashed potatoes lost 29%. Vitamin $B_6$ and niacin retention in boiled half and baked whole potatoes were determined in three varieties grown in four states.[131] Baking losses (9% for vitamin $B_6$ and 4% for niacin) were less than boiling losses (20 and 18%, respectively). However, the total recovery of vitamin $B_6$ and niacin was greater for boiled half than baked whole potatoes when one adds the amounts of the nutrients that had been leached into the cooking water. Pearson and Luecke[135] found less retention of thiamin (92.3 vs. 75.5), riboflavin (103.2 vs. 88.6), nicotinic acid (100.6 vs. 85.1), and pantothenic acid (99.9 vs. 76.8) in sweet potatoes that were baked instead of boiled in their skins. Approximately 80% of the ascorbic acid content of apples was lost when corded apples were baked with sugar for up to 90 min at 400°F or when apples were incorporated into a pie and baked.[41]

*Baking: Bread*

Choice of flour for baked goods can affect nutrient content of the product. Utilizing results reported by Moran,[113] one can calculate that from 80 to 95% of seven B-complex vitamins and vitamin E are retained in whole wheat flour (95% extract), while only 15 to 60% are retained in white flour (70% extract) when compared to wheat. Enrichment returns some but not all of the nutrients.

Nutrient destruction in bread or baked goods is primarily related to the temperature and duration of the oven exposure during the baking process and the pH of the dough or batter. Mixing, fermentation, and make-up phases do not appear to significantly alter nutrient retention. In fact, fermentation can increase B complex vitamin content due to synthesis by yeast.[103] Fermentation may also make minerals such as calcium and iron more available because of hydrolysis of phytic acid complexes.[138] These mineral inositol-phosphate complexes can prevent mineral absorption. They can also be attacked by natural wheat phytases or by yeast phytases.[139]

Thiamin is quite labile during baking, due both to heat duration and alkalinity. When rolls and breads were baked to pale, medium-brown, or dark-brown crust colors (400°F), thiamin retention decreased from 83 to 74% for bread and 93 to 88% for pan rolls as cooking time increased.[177] Chemical leavening of baked products is very destructive to thiamin. Baking powders have been shown to destroy up to 84% of vitamin $B_1$ when incorporated in large amounts of doughs.[19,20] The recovery of thiamin added to self-rise flour doughs is proportional to the acidity of the dough: the lower the pH, the better the recovery.[11] A pH of 6 or lower is desirable for satisfactory stability of thiamin during baking.[67]

Bottomly and Nobile[13] reported an average loss of 29.5% of thiamin when baking white bread. The difference in thiamin retention between the crust and the crumb may be as much as 35%.[115] Riboflavin and niacin are largely stable during baking.[67] Keagy et al.[83] investigated stability of natural folacin during bread processing and home flour storage. They found that yeast fermentation increased folacin content of doughs by about 30%, but this gain was lost during baking. Native flour folacin decreased during early storage and then stabilized.

Rosenberg and Rohdenberg[146] investigated the loss of lysine (microbiological assay) from fortified (DL-lysine·HCl or L-lysine·HCl) and unfortified wheat flour during bread baking. They found that L-lysine loss averaged 11% in unfortified loaves, 15% in DL-lysine·HCl-fortified loaves and 32% in L-lysine·HCl-fortified loaves. Toasting a slice of bread reduced the lysine content an additional 5 to 10%. A similar loss occurred when the bread became stale and dry. Jansen et al.[76,77] attributed losses of supplemented L-lysine·HCl during baking to the level of nonfat dry milk in dough. They estimated that 15% of the supplement was lost during baking of "water" bread. Increasing baking time or level of nonfat dry milk decreased both native and supplemented lysine. When 6 to 14% nonfat dry milk was added before baking, the nutritive loss of lysine was estimated to be 36%, presumably because of the high content of the reducing sugar D-lactose. L-Lysine loss is extremely detrimental to the protein quality of baked products, since lysine is already the limiting amino acid of wheat.

*Microwave*

There are not many reports in the literature investigating the nutrient retention of plant substances during microwave cooking. Most deal only with vitamin C retention in vegetables. Gordon and Noble[63] cooked cauliflower, broccoli, and cabbage in an electronic range with a small amount of water, pressure saucepan, or boiling water and found the best retention of ascorbic acid (80 to 90%) with microwave, medium (70 to 82%) with the pressure saucepan, and least (38 to 73%) with boiling. Kylen et al.[89] found no statistical differences in ascorbic acid retention in seven fresh and three frozen vegetables that were boiled or cooked with microwave. In comparison to the work of Gordon and Noble,[63] Kylen and her co-workers used less water and longer cooking time for microwave. Since Gordon and Noble's work reported much lower retentions of ascorbic acid after conventional boiling and slightly higher retentions after microwave cooking, one could assume that the different results were in part due to the quantity of water used.

This issue was taken up with Eheart and Gott[47] when they cooked five vegetables by boiling or microwave cooking with the same amount of water as boiling or without added water. Frozen spinach retained more ascorbic acid (about 66%) when cooked by microwave than by the conventional method (about 50%), but no differences in retention of ascorbic acid were found for peas (65%), potatoes (67%), or broccoli (77%). They found no effect of water use in microwave cooking on vitamin C retention. Carotene was completely retained by all cooking methods.

As mentioned previously, Eheart and Gott[48] compared cooking broccoli and green beans by stir-fry, microwave, and boiling in a large (4:1) or small (1:2) water to vegetable ratio. With broccoli, ascorbic acid retention with microwave cooking was superior to large water-to-food ratio boiling but less than stir-fry or small water-to-food ratio. With green beans the small water-to-food boiling method resulted in significantly better retention of vitamin C than all other methods.

It would appear from the literature that microwave cooking is equivalent to boiling in moderate amounts of water. However, the nutrient retention issue is far from closed. Nutrient retention of other vitamins should be investigated along with a conclusive study on the effects of water-to-food ratio in microwave heating.

*Summary: Nutrient Stability During Cooking*

Many of the same statements found in the summary on cooking of animals products also apply here. Since most plant products are cooked for a very short time period, however, more losses occur due to leaching than heat destruction. In many cases short-time, waterless heating, such as steaming of vegetables, can lead to almost full recovery of nutrients.

The most labile nutrient of concern in plant products is ascorbic acid. Vitamin C is very labile to moisture, air, heat, and any oxidizing agents. Ascorbic acid is lost in greater amounts than other vitamins in most cooking procedures and can therefore be used as an indicator of quality of total nutrient retention in plant foods.

Thiamin and folacin are possibly the next most labile vitamins in plant products. Thiamin is unstable at alkaline pH and to prolonged heating. Bicarbonate and sulfite treatment are extremely destructive to this nutrient and should be avoided at the home. High losses of both free and total folic acid can occur in foods during short cooking periods.[42]

Riboflavin and niacin are relatively stable to cooking, but more than 50% of these two vitamins along with ascorbic acid, thiamin, folacin, and many minerals can be leached into soaking and/or cooking waters. Natural carotenoids in vegetables and fruits are usually fairly stable during heating and freezing.[42]

Much more research is needed to quantify the stability of nutrients other than ascorbic acid during the various types of cooking. For example, almost no literature reports on vitamin $B_6$, folic acid, and pantothenic acid utilizing proper methodology are available. Some publications are appearing concerned with the stability of nutrients that are added (fortified) to foods.[2,31,42]

### Effect of Holding and Reheating Plant Products

Extensive losses of nutritional value occur when heated plant foods are stored refrigerated for days prior to reheating. Reheated leftovers of plant origin may be a far cry nutritionally from fresh or once-cooked products.

The ascorbic acid content of eight vegetables was determined (1) when raw, (2) after boiling until done with half their weight in water, (3) after holding for 24 hr refrigerated (39 to 48°F), and (4) after 24 hr refrigeration and reheating.[29] Cooked broccoli, brussels sprouts, shredded cabbage, sliced cabbage, cauliflower, peas, and snap beans lost significant amounts of ascorbic acid during 24 hr of refrigerated storage (about 22%), whereas asparagus and spinach lost only 4% each. Reheating resulted in significant losses in all vegetables investigated when compared to the freshly cooked nonrefrigerated products. (average loss equal to 32%.) Five vegetables were subjected to an extended refrigeration of 2 or 3 days. Extended storage resulted in greater losses of ascorbic acid in all vegetables tested (an average additional 9% after 2 days and 14% after 3 days). Of particular interest Charles and Van Duyne's[29] study was their observation that the ascorbic acid in the cooking liquids was stable during refrigeration holding and during reheating, indicating that the vitamin in the vegetable was being specifically destroyed. In another study from the same laboratory, Van Duyne et al.[167] showed that peeled, halved potatoes retained 87% of their ascorbic acid content during boiling. After refrigerated storage for 24 hr, however, they retained only 47% of the original ascorbic acid content, while after 70 hr of refrigerated storage only 18% was retained.

In one study investigating retention of ascorbic acid, thiamin, and riboflavin in large scale preparation of cabbage,[175] drained, cooked cabbage was held in refrigeration for 24 hr and then reheated. A definite loss of ascorbic acid occurred, but no statistically significant loss of vitamin $B_1$ or $B_2$ was observed. Bisset and Berry[12] simulated home storage conditions for studying the ascorbic acid content of orange juice (reconstituted from concentrate) stored at 4.4, 10, or 21.1°F for 7 days. Single-strength orange juice retained 80 to 85% of its ascorbic acid regardless of temperature. They found the differences between plastic and glass refrigerator containers were less than 1%.

These and most other studies concentrate on retention of a single nutrient, ascorbic acid, during refrigeration and reheating. Lack of published research prevents a conclusion of vitamins other than vitamin C. At least with this extremely labile nutrient, refrigerated storage is very damaging.

## Closing Remarks

It is advantageous to nutritionists, physicians, and homemakers alike to be able to check a handbook and determine the average amount of a nutrient that is present in food as consumed. One can simply consult the *Nutritive Value of American Foods.*[1] It would be far better if the same type of handbook would contain a listing of "expected nutrient retentions" resulting from specific common household practices. A quick inspection, for example, could tell us that braising meats reduces nutritive contents as compared to broiling.

Such a handbook would be almost impossible to develop today due to the lack of sufficient nutrient retention data. Many of the results reported in this chapter could not be included because they were obtained using outdated methodologies, improper sampling techniques, or did not provide enough information about cooking conditions. What is required is carefully controlled systematic research to investigate individual preparation practices in various food systems. Nutrients in addition to the classically measured ascorbic acid and thiamin must be investigated. Perhaps a list of "index nutrients" such as vitamin A, $B_6$, folacin, pantothenic acid, magnesium, iron, and calcium, as developed by Pennington[136] for measuring dietary adequacy, could be considered. The index has been selected on the basis of data on the co-occurrence of nutrients in food. Pennington's list contains at least one nutrient that is unstable to oxygen, light, or heat, or neutral, acidic, or alkaline pH.[66] This list could serve as an indicator for nutrient stability of the 50 or so nutrients of potential interest.

Just as Lund[100] pointed out the need to design industrial thermal processes for maximizing nutrient retentions, it is this author's desire to provide the consumer with adequate information to optimize home processes to assure maximum nutrient intake. Since the major loss of vitamins and minerals often occurs during home preparation,[5] the nutrient-conscious consumer deserves to be provided with the necessary data to choose the best food preparation procedure.

# REFERENCES

1. **Adams, C. F.,** *Nutritive Value of American Foods in Common Units,* Agric. Handb. No. 456, U.S. Department of Agriculture, Washington, D.C., 1975.
2. **Anderson, R. H., Maxwell, D. L., Mulley, A. E., and Fritsch, C. W.,** Effects of processing and storage on micronutrients in breakfast cereals, *Food Technol. (Chicago),* 30, 110, 1976.
3. **Andross, M.,** Losses of nutrients in the preparation of foodstuffs, *Proc. Nutr. Soc.,* 4, 155, 1946.
4. **Anon.,** *Recommendations for the Processing and Handling of Frozen Foods,* 2nd ed., International Institute of Refrigeration, Paris, 1972, 144.
5. **Anon.,** The Effects of Food Processing on Nutritional Values, Institute of Food Technologist's Expert Panel on Food Safety and Nutrition and the Committee on Public Information, *Food Technol. (Chicago),* 28, 77, 1974.
6. **Anon.,** Home Canning, Institute of Food Technologist's Expert Panel on Food Safety and Nutrition and the Committee on Public Information, *Food Technol. (Chicago),* 31, 43, 1977.
7. **Anon.,** Food Composition Data, Agricultural Research Service Form No. 200, May 1973.
8. **Aughey, E. and Daniel, E. P.,** Effect of cooking upon the thiamin content of foods, *J. Nutr.,* 19, 285, 1940.
9. **Baldwin, R. E., Korschgen, B. M., Russell, M. S., and Mabesa, L.,** Proximate analysis, free amino acid, vitamin and mineral content of microwave cooked meat, *J. Food Sci.,* 41, 762, 1976.

10. **Bankhead, R. R., Weingartner, K. E., Kuntz, D. A., and Erdman, J. W., Jr.,** The effects of sodium bicarbonate blanch on the retention of micronutrients in soy beverage, *J. Food Sci.,* 43, 345, 1978.
11. **Barockman, R. A.,** Thiamin retention in self-rising flour biscuits, *Cereal Chem.,* 19, 121, 1942.
12. **Bissett, O. W. and Berry, R. E.,** Ascorbic acid retention in orange juice as related to container type, *J. Food Sci.,* 40, 178, 1975.
13. **Bottomley, R. A. and Nobile, S.,** A collaborative study of the determination of thiamine in white flour and bread, *J. Sci. Food Agric.,* 13, 546, 1962.
14. **Bowers, J. A. and Fryer, B. A.,** Thiamin and riboflavin in cooked and frozen, reheated turkey, *J. Am. Diet. Assoc.,* 60, 399, 1972.
15. **Bowers, J. A., Fryer, B. A., and Engler, P. P.,** Vitamin $B_6$ in turkey breast muscle cooked in microwave and conventional ovens, *Poult. Sci.,* 53, 844, 1974.
16. **Bowers, J. A., Fryer, B. A., and Engler, P. P.,** Vitamin $B_6$ in pork muscle cooked in microwave and conventional ovens, *J. Food Sci.,* 39, 426, 1974.
17. **Boyle, M. A. and Funk, K.,** Thiamine in roast beef held by three methods, *J. Am. Diet. Assoc.,* 60, 398, 1972.
18. **Branion, H. D., Roberts, J. S., Cameron, C. R., and McCready, A. M.,** The loss of ascorbic acid in the preparation of old and freshly harvested potatoes, *J. Am. Diet. Assoc.,* 23, 414, 1947.
19. **Briant, A. M. and Hutchins, M. R.,** Influence of ingredients on thiamine retention and quality in baking powder biscuits, *Cereal Chem.,* 23, 512, 1946.
20. **Briant, A. M. and Klosterman, A. M.,** Influence of ingredients on thiamin and riboflavin retention and quality of plain muffins, *Trans. Am. Assoc. Cereal Chem.,* 8, 69, 1950.
21. **Brown, E. J. and Fenton, F.,** Losses of vitamin C during cooking of parsnips, *Food Res.,* 7, 218, 1942.
22. **Burrell, R. C. and Ebright, V. R.,** The vitamin C content of fruits and vegetables, *J. Chem. Educ.,* 17, 180, 1940.
23. **Cameron, E. J., et al.,** *Retention of Nutrients During Canning,* National Canners Association, Washington, D.C., 1955.
24. **Causey, K., Andreasseu, E. G., Hausrath, M. E., Along, C., Ramstad, P. E., and Fenton, F.,** Effect of thawing and cooking methods on palatability and nutritive value of frozen ground meat. I. Pork, *Food Res.,* 15, 237, 1950.
25. **Causey, K., Hansrath, M. E., Ramstad, P. E., and Fenton, F.,** Effect of thawing and cooking methods on palatability and nutritive value of frozen ground meat. II. Beef, *Food Res.,* 15, 249, 1950.
26. **Causey, K., Hansrath, M. E., Ramstad, P. E., and Fenton, F.,** Effect of thawing and cooking methods on palatability and nutritive value of frozen ground meat. III. Lamb, *Food Res.,* 15, 256, 1950.
27. **Causey, K. and Fenton, F.,** Effect of reheating on palatability, nutritive value, and bacterial count of frozen cooked foods. II. Meat dishes, *J. Am. Diet. Assoc.,* 27, 491, 1951.
28. **Chan, C. Y. A. W., Wheeler, E. F., and Leppington, I. M.,** Variations in the apparent nutrient content of foods: a study of sampling error, *Br. J. Nutr.,* 34, 391, 1975.
29. **Charles, V. R. and Van Duyne, F. O.,** Effect of holding and reheating on the ascorbic acid content of cooked vegetables, *J. Home Econ.,* 50, 159, 1958.
30. **Cheldelin, V. H., Woods, A. A., and Williams, R. J.,** Losses of B vitamins due to cooking of foods, *J. Nutr.,* 26, 477, 1943.
31. **Cort, W. M., Borenstein, B., Harley, J. H., Osadca, M., and Scheiner, J.,** Nutrient stability of fortified cereal products, *Food Technol. (Chicago),* 30, 52, 1976.
32. **Cover, S., McLaren, B. A., and Pearson, P. B.,** Retention of the B-vitamins in rare and well-done beef, *J. Nutr.,* 27, 363, 1944.
33. **Cover, S., Dilsaver, E. M., and Hays, R. M.,** Retention of the B vitamins in beef and lamb after stewing. I. Experimental design and standardized cooking procedure, *J. Am. Diet. Assoc.,* 23, 501, 1947.
34. **Cover, S., Dilsaver, E. M., and Hays, R. M.,** Retention of the B vitamins in beef and lamb after stewing. II. Thiamine, *J. Am. Diet. Assoc.,* 23, 613, 1947.
35. **Cover, S., Dilsaver, E. M., and Hays, R. M.,** Retention of the B vitamins in beef and lamb after stewing, III. Pantothenic acid, *J. Am. Diet. Assoc.,* 23, 693, 1947.
36. **Cover, S., Dilsaver, E. M., and Hays, R. M.,** Retention of the B vitamins in beef and lamb after stewing, IV. Niacin, *J. Am. Diet. Assoc.,* 23, 769, 1947.
37. **Cover, S., Dilsaver, E. M., and Hays, R. M.,** Retention of the B vitamins in beef and lamb after stewing. V. Riboflavin, *J. Am. Diet. Assoc.,* 23, 865, 1947.
38. **Cover, S., Dilsaver, E. M., and Hays, R. M.,** Retention of the B vitamins in beef and lamb after stewing. VI. Similarities and differences among the four vitamins, *J. Am. Diet. Assoc.,* 23, 962, 1947.
39. **Cover, S., Dilsaver, E. M., Hays, R. M., and Smith, W. H.,** Retention of B vitamins after large-scale cooking of meat. II. Roasting by two methods, *J. Am. Diet. Assoc.,* 25, 949, 1949.

40. **Cover, S., Dilsaver, E. M., and Hays, R. M.,** Retentions of B vitamins in beef and veal after home canning and storage, *Food Res.*, 14, 104, 1949.

41. **Curran, K. M. and Tressler, D. K.,** Losses of Vitamin C during cooking of northern spy apples, *Food Res.*, 2, 549, 1937.

42. **DeRitter, E.,** Stability characteristics of vitamins in processed foods, *Food Technol. (Chicago)*, 30, 48, 1976.

43. **Derse, P. H. and Teply, L. J.,** Effects of storage conditions on nutrients in frozen green beans, peas, orange juice and strawberries, *J. Agric. Food Chem.*, 6, 309, 1958.

44. **Deuel, H. J., Jr., and Greenberg, S. M.,** A comparison of the retention of vitamin A in margarines and in butter based on bioassay, *Food Res.*, 18, 497, 1953.

45. **Deutsch, R. M.,** *Realities of Nutrition,* Bull Publishing, Palo Alto, California, 1976, 19.

46. **Domah, A. A. M. B., Davidek, J., and Velisek, J.,** Changes of L-ascorbic and L-dehydro-ascorbic acids during cooking and frying of potatoes, *Z. Lebensm. Unters. Forsch.*, 154, 272, 1974.

47. **Eheart, M. S. and Gott, C.,** Conventional and microwave cooking of vegetables, *J. Am. Diet. Assoc.*, 44, 116, 1964.

48. **Eheart, M. S. and Gott, C.,** Chlorophyll, ascorbic acid and pH changes in green vegetables cooked by stir-fry, microwave, and conventional methods and a comparison of chlorophyll methods, *Food Technol. (Chicago)*, 19(5), 185, 1965.

49. **Engler, P. P. and Bowers, J. A.,** Vitamin $B_6$ content of turkey cooked from frozen, partially frozen, and thawed states, *J. Food Sci.*, 40, 615, 1975.

50. **Engler, P. P. and Bowers, J. A.,** Vitamin $B_6$ in reheated, held, and freshly cooked turkey breast, *J. Am. Diet. Assoc.*, 67(7), 42, 1975.

51. **Engler, P. P. and Bowers, J. A.,** B-vitamin retention in meat during storage and preparation, *J. Am. Diet. Assoc.*, 69, 253, 1976.

52. **Evans, R. J., Bandemer, S. L., Bauer, D. H., and Davidson, J. A.,** The vitamin $B_1$ content of fresh and stored shell eggs, *Poult. Sci.*, 34, 922, 1955.

53. **Evans, R. J., Butts, H. A., and Davidson, J. A.,** The niacin content of fresh and stored shell eggs, *Poult. Sci.*, 30, 132, 1951.

54. **Evans, R. J., Butts, H. A., and Davidson, J. A.,** The vitamin $B_6$ content of fresh and stored shell eggs, *Poult. Sci.*, 30, 515, 1951.

55. **Evans, R. J., Butts, H. A., and Davidson, J. A.,** The riboflavin content of fresh and stored shell eggs, *Poult Sci.*, 31, 269, 1952.

56. **Evans, R. J., Butts, H. A., and Davidson, J. A.,** The pantothenic acid content of fresh and stored shell eggs, *Poult. Sci.*, 31, 777, 1952.

57. **Evans, R. J., Davidson, J. A., Bauer, D., and Butts, H. A.,** The biotin content of fresh and stored shell eggs, *Poult. Sci.*, 32, 680, 1953.

58. **Evans, R. J., Davidson, J. A., Bauer, D., and Butts, H. A.,** Folic acid content in fresh and stored shell eggs, *J. Agric. Food Chem.*, 1, 170, 1953.

59. **Feaster, J. F., Jackson, J. M., Greenwood, D. A., and Kraybill, H. R.,** Vitamin retention in processed meat, *Ind. Eng. Chem.*, 38, 87, 1946.

60. **Fennema, O.,** Effects of freeze-preservation on nutrients, in *Nutritional Evaluation of Food Processing,* 2nd ed., Harris, R. S. and Karmas, E., Eds., AVI Publishing, Westport Conn., 1975, 244.

61. **Goldblith, S. A., Tannenbaum, S. R., and Wang, D. I. C.,** Thermal and 2450 MHz microwave energy effect on the destruction of thiamine, *Food Technol. (Chicago)*, 22, 1266, 1968.

62. **Gordon, J. and Noble, I.,** Effect of cooking method on vegetables, *J. Am. Diet. Assoc.*, 35, 578, 1959.

63. **Gordon, J. and Noble, I.,** Comparison of electronic vs. conventional cooking of vegetables, *J. Am. Diet. Assoc.*, 35, 241, 1959.

64. **Gordon, J. and Noble, I.,** "Waterless" vs. boiling water cooking of vegetables, *J. Am. Diet. Assoc.*, 44, 378, 1964.

65. **Harris, R. S.,** Effects of large-scale preparation on nutrients of foods of plant origin, in *Nutritional Evaluation of Food Processing,* Harris, R. S. and Von Loesecke, H., Eds., John Wiley & Sons, New York, 1960, 418.

66. **Harris, R. S.,** General discussion of the stability of nutrients, in *Nutritional Evaluation of Food Processing,* 2nd ed., Harris, R. S. and Karmas, E., Eds., AVI Publishing, Westport, Conn., 1975, 1.

67. **Harris, R. S. and Levenberg, R. K.,** Effects of home preparation on nutrient content of foods of plant origin, in *Nutritional Evaluation of Food Processing,* Harris, R. S. and Von Loesecke, H., Eds., John Wiley & Sons, New York, 1960, 462.

68. **Harris, P. L. and Poland, G. L.,** Variations in ascorbic acid content of bananas, *Food Res.*, 4, 317, 1939.

69. **Hellstrom, V.,** The durability of vitamin C in raw vegetables after mashing, *Z. Vitam. Horm. Fermentforsch.*, 5, 98, 1952.

70. **Henderson, L. M., Waisman, H. A., and Elvehjem, C. A.,** The distribution of pyridoxine (Vitamin B₆) in meats and meat products, *J. Nutr.*, 21, 589, 1941.

71. **Hertzler, A. A. and Hoover, L. W.,** Development of food tables and use with computers, *J. Am. Diet. Assoc.*, 70, 20, 1977.

72. **Hewston, E. M., Dawson, E. H., Alexander, L. M., and Orentkeiles, E.,** Vitamin and Mineral Content of Certain Foods as Affected by Home Preparation, Misc. Publ. 628, U.S. Department of Ag-

73. **Hurdle, A. D. F., Barton, D., and Searles, I. H.,** A method for measuring folate in food and its application to a hospital diet, *Am. J. Clin. Nutr.*, 21, 1202, 1968.

74. **Janicki, L. J. and Appledorf, H.,** Effect of broiling, grill frying and microwave cooking on moisture. Some lipid components and total fatty acids of ground beef, *J. Food Sci.*, 39, 715, 1974.

75. **Jansen, E. F.,** Quality-related chemical and physical changes in frozen foods, in *Quality and Stability of Frozen Foods,* Van Arsdel, W. B., Copley, M. J., and Olson, R. L., Eds., Wiley Interscience, New York, 1969, 19—43.

76. **Jansen, G. R., Ehle, S. R., and Hause, N. L.,** Studies of the nutritive loss of supplemental lysine in baking. I. Loss in a standard white bread containing 4% nonfat dry milk, *Food Technol. (Chicago)*, 18, 367, 1964.

77. **Jansen, G. R., Ehle, S. R., and Hause, N. L.,** Studies of the nutritive loss of supplemental lysine in baking. II. Loss in water bread and in breads supplemented with moderate amounts of nonfat dry milk, *Food Technol. (Chicago)*, 18, 372, 1964.

78. **Jul, M.,** Quality and stability of frozen meats, in *Quality and Stability of Frozen Foods,* Van Arsdel, W. B., Copley, M. J., and Olson, R. L., Eds., Wiley Interscience, New York, 1969, 191—217.

79. **Kahn, L. N. and Livingston, G. E.,** Effect of heating methods on thiamin retention in fresh or frozen prepared foods, *J. Food Sci.*, 35, 349, 1970.

80. **Kahn, R. M. and Halliday, E. G.,** Ascorbic acid content of white potatoes as affected by cooking and standing on steam table, *J. Am. Diet. Assoc.*, 20, 220, 1944.

81. **Kamalanathan, G., Giri, J., Jaya, T. V., and Priyadarsani, P.,** The effect of boiling, steaming, pressure cooking and panning on the mineral and vitamin content of three vegetables, *Indian J. Nutr. Diet.*, 11, 10, 1974.

82. **Kauffman, R. G.,** Biochemical Properties of Pork and Their Relationship to Quality, Ph.D. thesis, University of Wisconsin, Madison, 1961.

83. **Keagy, P. M., Stokstad, E. L. R., and Fellers, D. A.,** Folacin stability during bread processing and family flour storage, *Cereal Chem.*, 52, 348, 1975.

84. **Kemp, J. D., Montgomery, R. E., and Fox, J. D.,** Chemical, palatability and cooking characteristics of normal and low quality pork loins and affected by freezer storage, *J. Food Sci.*, 41, 1, 1976.

85. **Kilgore, L. and Bailey, M.,** Degradation of linoleic acid during potato frying, *J. Am. Diet. Assoc.*, 56, 130, 1970.

86. **Kotschevar, L. H., Mosso, A., and Tugwell, T.,** B-vitamin retention in frozen meat, *J. Am. Diet. Assoc.*, 31, 589, 1955.

87. **Kramer, A., King, R. L., and Westhoff, D. C.,** Effects of frozen storage on prepared foods containing protein concentrates, *Food Technol. (Chicago)*, 30(1), 50, 1976.

88. **Krehl, W. A. and Winters, R. W.,** Effect of cooking method on retention of vitamins and minerals in vegetables, *J. Am. Diet. Assoc.*, 26, 966, 1950.

89. **Kylen, A. M., Charles, V. R., McGrath, B. H., Schleter, J. M., West, L. C., and Van Duyne, F. O.,** Microwave cooking vegetables, *J. Am. Diet. Assoc.*, 39, 321, 1961.

90. **Kylen, A. M., McGrath, B. H., Hallmark, E. L., and Van Duyne, F. O.,** Microwave and conventional cooking of meat, *J. Am. Diet. Assoc.*, 45, 139, 1964.

91. **Lachance, P. A.,** Effects of food preparation procedures on nutrient retention with emphasis upon food service practices, in *Nutritional Evaluation of Food Processing,* 2nd ed., Harris, R. S. and Karmas, E., Eds., AVI Publishing, Westport, Conn., 1975, 463.

92. **Lachance, P. A. and Erdman, J. W., Jr.,** Effects of home food preparation practices on nutrient content of foods, in *Nutritional Evaluation of Food Processing,* 2nd ed., Harris, R. S., and Karmas, E., Eds., AVI Publishing, Westport, Conn., 1975, 529.

93. **Lamb, F. C., Lewis, L. D., and White, D. G.,** The nutritive value of canned foods. The effect of storage on the ascorbic acid content of canned tomato juice and tomato paste, *Food Technol. (Chicago)*, 5, 269, 1951.

94. **Lee, F. A., Brooks, R. F., Pearson, A. M., Miller, J. I., and Wanderstock, J. J.,** Effect of rate of freezing on pork quality. Appearance, palatibility, and vitamin content, *J. Am. Diet. Assoc.*, 30, 351, 1954.

95. **Lee, F. A., Brooks, R. F., Pearson, A. M., Miller, J. I., and Volz, F.,** Effect of freezing rate on meat. Appearance, palatibility, and vitamin content of beef, *Food Res.*, 15, 8, 1950.

96. **Leeking, P., Mahon, P., Hogue, D., Lim, E., and Fenton, F.,** The Quality of smoked hams as affected by adding an antibiotic and fat to the diet and phosphate to the cure. III. Moisture, fat, chloride and thiamin content, *Food Technol. (Chicago)*, 10, 274, 1956.

97. **Lehrer, W. P., Jr., Wiese, A. C., Harvey, W. R., and Moore, P. R.,** Effect of frozen storage and subsequent cooking on the thiamine, riboflavin, and nicotinic acid of pork chops, *Food Res.,* 16, 485, 1951.

98. **Lehrer, W. P., Jr., Wiese, A. C., Harvey, W. R., and Moore, P. R.,** The stability of thiamin, riboflavin, and nicotinic acid of lamb chops during frozen storage and subsequent cooking, *Food Res.,* 17, 24, 1952.

99. **Leverton, R. M. and Odell, G. V.,** The Nutritive Value of Cooked Meat, Oklahoma Agric. Exp. Stn. Misc. Publ. MP-49, 1959.

100. **Lund, D. B.,** Maximizing nutrient retention, *Food Technol. (Chicago),* 42, 71, 1977.

101. **Lushbough, C. H., Weichman, J. M. and Schweigert, B. S.,** The retention of vitamin $B_6$ in meat during cooking, *J. Nutr.,* 67, 451, 1959.

102. **Marston, E. V., Davis, E. A., and Gordon, J.,** Mineral retention in vegetables as affected by phosphates in cooking water, *Home Econ. Res. J.,* 2, 147, 1974.

103. **Matz, S. A.,** Effects of baking on nutrients, in *Nutritional Evaluation of Food Processing,* 2nd ed., Harris, R. S., and Karmas, E., Eds., AVI Publishing, Westport, Conn., 1975, 240.

104. **McCance, R. A., Widdowson, E. M., and Shackleton, L.,** The Nutritive Value of Fruits, Vegetables and Nuts, Med. Res. Counc. Spec. Rep. 213, 1936.

105. **McIntire, J. M., Schweigert, B. S., and Elvehjem, C. A.,** The choline and pyridoxine content of meats, *J. Nutr.,* 28, 219, 1944.

106. **Meiners, C. R., Derise, N. L., Lau, H. C., Crews, M. G., Ritchey, S. J., and Murphy, E. W.,** The content of nine mineral elements in raw and cooked mature dry legumes, *J. Agric. Food Chem.,* 24, 1126, 1976.

107. **Meredith, F. I., Gaskins, M. H., and Dull, G. G.,** Amino acid losses in turnip greens (Brassica rapa L.) during handling and processing, *J. Food Sci.,* 39, 689, 1974.

108. **Meyer, B. H., Hinman, W. F., and Halliday, E. G.,** Retention of some vitamins of the B complex in beef during cooking, *Food Res.,* 12, 203, 1947.

109. **Meyer, B. H., Mysinger, M. A., and Wodarski, L. A.,** Pantothenic acid and vitamin $B_6$ in beef, *J. Am. Diet. Assoc.,* 54, 122, 1969.

110. **Meyer, J. A., Briskey, E. J., Hoekstra, W. G., and Weckel, K. G.,** Niacin, thiamin, and riboflavin in fresh and cooked pale, soft, watery versus dark, firm, dry pork muscle, *Food Technol. (Chicago),* 17, 485, 1963.

111. **Millares, R. and Fellers, C. R.,** Vitamin and amino acid content of processed chicken meat products, *Food Res.,* 14, 131, 1949.

112. **Millross, J., Speht, A., Holdsworth, K., and Glew, G.,** The Utilization of the Cook-Freeze Catering System for School Meals, The University of Leeds, W. S. Maney and Son, Leeds, England, 1973.

113. **Moran, T.,** Nutritional significance of recent work on wheat, flour and bread, *Nutr. Abstr. Rev.,* 29, 1, 1959.

114. **Morgan, A. F.,** Losses of nutrients in foods during home preparation. I. Effects of home preparation on nutrient content of foods of animal origin, in *Nutritional Evaluation of Food Processing,* Harris, R. S. and Von Loesecke, H., Eds., John Wiley & Sons, New York, 1960, 442.

115. **Morgan, A. F. and Federick, H.,** Vitamin B($B_1$) in bread as affected by baking, *Cereal Chem.,* 12, 390, 1935.

116. **Morgan, A. F., Kidder, L. E., Hunner, M., Sharokh, B. K., and Chesbro, R. M.,** Thiamine, riboflavin, and niacin content of chicken tissues, as affected by cooking and frozen storage, *Food Res.,* 14, 439, 1949.

117. **Munsell, H. E., Streightoff, F., Bendor, B., Orr, M., Ezekiel, S. R., Leonard, M. H., Richardson, M. E., and Koch, F. G.,** Effect of large-scale methods of preparation on the vitamin content of food. III. Cabbage, *J. Am. Diet. Assoc.,* 25, 420, 1949.

118. **Murphy, E. W., Criner, P. E., and Gray, B. C.,** Comparisons of methods for calculating retentions of nutrients in cooked foods, *J. Agric. Food Chem.,* 23(6), 1153, 1975.

119. **Murphy, E. W., Watt, B. K., and Rizek, R. L.,** Tables of food consumption: availability, uses, and limitations, *Food Technol. (Chicago),* 38(1), 40, 1973.

120. **Nagy, S. and Smoot, J. M.,** Temperature and storage effects on percent retention and percent U.S. recommended dietary allowance of vitamin C in canned single-strength orange juice, *J. Agric. Food Chem.,* 25, 135, 1977.

121. **Anon.,** Meat Buyers Guide to Portion Control Meat Cuts, Prepared by National Association of Meat Purveyors, Chicago, 1972.

122. **Nelson, A. I., Steinberg, M. P., and Wei, L. S.,** Illinois process for preparation of soy milk, *J. Food Sci.,* 41, 57, 1976.

123. **Nielsen, L. M. and Carlin, A. F.,** Frozen, precooked beef and beef-soy loaves, *J. Am. Diet. Assoc.,* 65, 35, 1974.

124. **Noble, I.,** Thiamine and riboflavin retention in broiled meat, *J. Am. Diet. Assoc.,* 45, 447, 1964.

125. **Noble, I.,** Thiamin and riboflavin retention in braised meat, *J. Am. Diet. Assoc.,* 47, 205, 1965.
126. **Noble, I.,** Thiamin and riboflavin retention in cooked variety meats, *J. Am. Diet. Assoc.,* 56, 225, 1970.
127. **Noble, I. and Gomez, L.,** Thiamine and riboflavin in roast lamb, *J. Am. Diet. Assoc.,* 34, 157, 1958.
128. **Noble, I. and Gomez, L.,** Thiamine and riboflavin in roast beef, *J. Am. Diet. Assoc.,* 36, 46, 1960.
129. **Noble, I. and Gomez, L.,** Vitamin retention in meat cooked electronically, *J. Am. Diet. Assoc.,* 41, 217, 1962.
130. **Odland, D. and Eheart, M. S.,** Ascorbic acid, mineral and quality retention in frozen broccoli blanched in water, steam and ammonia-steam, *J. Food Sci.,* 40, 1004, 1975.
131. **Page, E. and Hanning, F. M.,** Vitamin B$_6$ and niacin in potatoes, *J. Am. Diet. Assoc.,* 42, 42, 1963.
132. **Pantos, C. E. and Markakis, P.,** Ascorbic acid content of artificial ripened tomatoes, *J. Food Sci.,* 38, 550, 1973.
133. **Pearson, A. M., Burnside, J. E., Edwards, H. M., Glasscock, R. S., Cunha, T. J. and Novak, A. F.,** Vitamin losses in drip obtained upon defrosting frozen meat, *Food Res.,* 16, 85, 1951.
134. **Pearson, A. M., West, R. G., and Luecke, R. W.,** The vitamin and amino acid content of drip obtained upon defrosting frozen pork, *Food Res.,* 24, 515, 1959.
135. **Pearson, P. B. and Luecke, R. W.,** The B vitamin content of raw and cooked sweet potatoes, *Food Res.,* 10, 325, 1945.
136. **Pennington, J. A.,** *Dietary Nutrient Guide,* AVI Publishing, Westport, Conn., 1976.
137. **Perry, A. K., Peters, C. R., and Van Duyne, F. O.,** Effect of variety and cooking method on cooking times, thiamin content and palatability of soybeans, *J. Food Sci.,* 41, 1330, 1976.
138. **Ranhotra, G. S.,** Hydrolysis during breadmaking of phytic acid in wheat protein concentrate, *J. Food Sci.,* 37, 12, 1972.
139. **Ranhotra, G. S., Loewe, R. J., and Puyat, L. V.,** Phytic acid in soy and its hydrolysis during bread making, *J. Food Sci.,* 39, 1023, 1974.
140. **Ream, E. E., Wilcox, E. B., Taylor, F. G., and Bennett, J. A.,** Tenderness of beef roasts, *J. Am. Diet. Assoc.,* 65, 155, 1974.
141. **Rice, E. E. and Beuk, J. F.,** Reaction rates for decomposition of thiamin in pork at various cooking temperatures, *Food Res.,* 10, 99, 1945.
142. **Rice, E. E., Fried, J. F., and Hess, W. R.,** Storage and microbial action upon vitamins of the B complex in pork, *Food Res.,* 11, 305, 1946.
143. **Rice, E. E., Squires, E. M., and Fried, J. F.,** Effect of storage and microbial action on vitamin content of pork, *Food Res.,* 13, 195, 1948.
144. **Richardson, L. R., Wilkes, S., and Ritchey, S. J.,** Comparative vitamin B$_6$ activity of frozen, irradiated and heat-processed foods, *J. Nutr.,* 73, 363, 1961.
145. **Rockland, L. B., Miller, C. F., and Hahn, D. M.,** Thiamine, pyridoxine, niacin and folacin in quick-cooked beans, *J. Food Sci.,* 42, 25, 1977.
146. **Rosenberg, H. R. and Rohdenburg, E. L.,** The fortification of bread with lysine. I. The loss of lysine during baking, *J. Nutr.,* 45, 593, 1951.
147. **Anon.,** *Food Stability Survey,* Vol. 2, Department of Food Science, Rutgers University, U.S. Government Printing Office, Washington, D.C., 1971.
148. **Schweigert, B. S., Nielsen, E., McIntire, J. M., and Elvehjem, C. A.,** Biotin content of meat and meat products, *J. Nutr.,* 26, 65, 1943.
149. **Schweigert, B. S., Pollard, A. E., and Elvehjem, C. A.,** The folic acid content of meats and the retention of this vitamin during cooking, *Arch. Biochem.,* 10, 107, 1946.
150. **Sheets, O., Leonard, O. A., and Gieger, M.,** Distribution of minerals and vitamins in different parts of leafy vegetables, *Food Res.,* 6, 553, 1941.
151. **Siedler, A. J.,** Effect of Standard Cooking and Processing Methods on the Nutritional Value of Meat Protein, Bull. No. 51, American Meat Institute Foundation, Chicago, 1961.
152. **Singh, R. P., Heldman, D. R., and Kirk, J. R.,** Kinetic analysis of light-induced riboflavin loss in whole milk, *J. Food Sci.,* 40, 164, 1975.
153. **Singh, S. P. and Essary, E. O.,** Influence of thawing methods on the composition of drip from broiler carcasses, *Poult. Sci.,* 50, 364, 1971.
154. **Singh, S. P. and Essary, E. O.,** Vitamin content of broiler meat as affected by age, sex, thawing and cooking, *Poult. Sci.,* 50, 1150, 1971.
155. **Slavin, J. W.,** Freezing and cold storage, in *Industrial Fishery Technology,* Stansby, M. E. and Dassow, J. A., Eds., Reinhold Publishing, New York, 1963, 288.
156. **Swaminathan, M.,** The effect of washing and cooking on the nicotinic acid content of raw and parboiled rice, *Indian J. Med. Res.,* 29, 83, 1941.
157. **Swaminathan, M.,** The effect of washing and cooking on the vitamin B$_1$ content of raw and parboiled rice, *Indian J. Med. Res.,* 30, 409, 1942.

158. Toepfer, E. W., Pritchett, C. A., and Hewston, E. M., Boneless Beef: Raw, Cooked, and Stewed. Results of Analysis for Moisture, Protein, Fat and Ash, Bull. 1137, U.S. Department of Agriculture, 1955.

159. Thomas, M. H., Brenner, S., Eaton, A., and Craig, V., Effect of electronic cooking on nutritive value of foods, *J. Am. Diet. Assoc.*, 25, 39, 1949.

160. Tucker, R. E., Hinman, W. F., and Halliday, E. G., The retention of thiamin and riboflavin in beef cuts during braising, frying, and broiling, *J. Am. Diet. Assoc.*, 22, 877, 1946.

161. Anon., Conserving the Nutritive Values in Foods, Home and Garden Bull. No. 90, U.S. Department of Agriculture, 1963, (revised January 1971).

162. Anon., Nutritive Value of Foods, Home and Garden Bull. No. 72, U.S. Department of Agriculture, 1964, (revised January 1971).

163. U.S. Department of Interior, Compilation of Laboratory Data: Yields and Losses in Preparation of Foods, U.S. Fish and Wild Life Service Mimeo, 1955.

164. Vail, G. E. and Westerman, B. D., B-complex vitamins in meat. I. Thiamin and riboflavin content of raw and cooked pork, *Food Res.*, 11, 425, 1946.

165. van der Laan, P. J. and Van der Mijll Dekker, L. P., *Voeding*, 6, 128, 1945.

166. Van Duyne, F. O., Chase, J. T., and Simpson, J. I., Effects of various home practices on ascorbic acid content of cabbage, *Food Res.*, 9, 164, 1944.

167. Van Duyne, F. O., Chase, J. T., and Simpson, J. I., Effect of various home practices on ascorbic acid content of potatoes, *Food Res.*, 10, 72, 1945.

168. Van Zante, H. J. and Johnson, S. K., Effect of electronic cookery on thiamine and riboflavin in buffered solutions, *J. Am. Diet. Assoc.*, 56, 133, 1970.

169. Wade, L., Microwave energy for industrial processing, in *Varian Spectrum,* Varian Australia Properietory, 1969.

170. Watt, B. K. and Merrill, A. L., Composition of Foods: Raw, Processed, Prepared, Handbook No. 8, U.S. Department of Agriculture, 1950, (revised 1963).

171. West, L. C., Titus, M. C., and Van Duyne, F. O., Effect of freezer storage and variations in preparation on bacterial count, palatability and thiamine content of ham loaf, Italian rice, and chicken, *Food Technol. (Chicago)*, 13, 323, 1959.

172. Westerman, B. D., Vail, G. E., Kalen, J., Stone, M., and MacKintosh, D. L., B-complex vitamins in meat. III. Influence of storage temperature and time on the vitamins in pork muscle, *J. Am. Diet. Assoc.*, 28, 49, 1952.

173. Westerman, B. D., Vail, G. E., Tinklin, G. L., and Smith, J., B-complex vitamins in meat. II. The influence of different methods of thawing frozen steaks upon their palatability and vitamin content, *Food Technol. (Chicago)*, 3, 184, 1949.

174. Wing, R. W. and Alexander, J. C., Effect of microwave heating on vitamin $B_6$ retention in chicken, *J. Am. Diet. Assoc.*, 61, 661, 1972.

175. Wood, M. A., Collings, A. R., Stodola, V., Burgoin, A. M., and Fenton, F., Effect of large-scale food preparation on vitamin retention: cabbage, *J. Am. Diet. Assoc.*, 22, 677, 1946.

176. Yuki, E. and Ishikawa, Y., Tocopherol contents of nine vegetable frying oils, and their changes under simulated deep-fat frying conditions, *J. Am. Oil Chem. Soc.*, 53, 673, 1976.

177. Zaehringer, M. V. and Personius, C. J., Thiamine retention in bread and rolls baked to different degrees of brownness, *Cereal Chem.*, 26, 384, 1949.

178. Ziprin, Y. A. and Carlin, A. F., Microwave and conventional cooking in relation to quality and nutritive value of beef and beef-soy loaves, *J. Food Sci.*, 41, 4, 1976.

# THE FUNCTION OF FOOD PACKAGING IN PRESERVATION OF NUTRIENTS

## Norman D. Heidelbaugh and Marcus Karel

## THE FOOD PACKAGE AS PART OF FOOD PROCESSING OPERATIONS

Food is produced, processed, and consumed for the purpose of providing nutrients. Any degradation of nutritional value that occurs during processing is significant, because it affects the primary purpose for which food is intended. Obviously, a maximum nutrient loss occurs when the food becomes unacceptable to the consumer. Various degrees of degradation of food quality, as perceived by the consumer, are most often accompanied by a comparable degradation in nutritional value. Food processing is performed primarily to retard such degradations, and/or to make food more acceptable, and/or to make nutrients more available. Packaging is an integral part of most of these food processing operations.

All food processing operations may be thought of in terms of factors that change a food's location, temperature, composition, structure, and/or exposure to irradiation energy. These are the principle factors manipulated by the modern food technologist or engineer in order to adapt food to the needs of a food supply system in industrialized and urbanized societies. Any given food processing procedure may require application of one or a combination of these factors. The basic mechanisms and laws of thermodynamics which underlie any given change in foods are the same basic mechanisms that affect every physical-chemical change. The fact that food is often deeply involved with human emotional overtones and perceived differently by various individuals and groups does not in any way alter the physical-chemical laws that constrain our ability to design, develop, and deliver safe and nutritious food.

Foods are extremely complex biological systems. The magnitude of this complexity becomes evident as we examine the technical problems associated with the use of processed foods in a modern technological society. During and after such processing, most foods are either in a state of disequilibrium with their external environment or are susceptible to degradation if exposed to the environment. It is a function of the food package to regulate the exchange between a food and its environment in a manner that enhances, or at least prevents reduction of, the quality (and hence nutritional value) of the food until it reaches the consumer. The relationships of food packaging to other elements of the food supply system are represented diagramatically in Figure 1.

The ideal food package would be beneficial, or at least nondetrimental, in its interactions with the food. At the same time the ideal package optimally regulates exchanges between the food and all the components of its environment in a manner that enhances the quality of the food or at least prevents deterioration. It follows, therefore, that the success of food packages in enhancing or protecting any quality (especially nutritional value) of a food can be judged by the degree to which the package performs the functions of an ideal barrier between the food and its environment.

## CONTEMPORARY PERSPECTIVES OF FOOD PACKAGING

An adequate food supply system is an essential component of any modern, industrialized society. In today's world, food systems are one of the indispensable life support systems of urban cultures. Indeed, the current world's population could not be supported without a modern food supply system based upon the principles of scientific

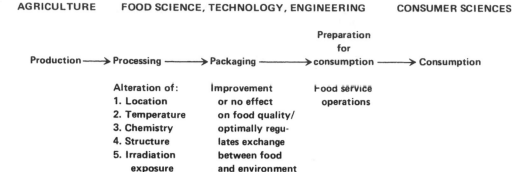

FIGURE 1.    Schematic representation of the food supply system in a modern society.

agriculture, food science, food technology, food engineering, and consumer sciences. Food packaging technology and engineering are essential subcomponents of this modern food supply system. The record of progress in food packaging is, therefore, a part of the excellent record of modern technology in supplying increasing quantities of food with higher quality, improved convenience, and greater acceptability for those populations of the world that are increasing in number and in remoteness from their sources of food production.

In the U.S. today, approximately three out of every four people live in cities, compared to less than 3 out of 100 persons living in cities in 1790. The vast majority of modern-day Americans consume a diet that is composed of a wide variety of foods, many of which are routinely transported hundreds or even thousands of kilometers to reach the consumer. The average U.S. supermarket offers approximately 8000 varieties of food products throughout the year, compared to approximately 100 foods available in urban stores at the turn of the century. Each of these products requires packaging that is individually designed to meet the needs of the food items concerned.

The early settlers coming to America from Europe had a diet while crossing the Atlantic Ocean (Table 1) that, in comparison to the variety available on today's ocean voyages, reveals a great deal about the progress that has been made in our ability to package and transport foodstuffs. In Europe prior to the 19th century, the list of vegetables available throughout the year for the average person was likewise extremely limited (Table 1) compared to today's commonly enjoyed food varieties.

It is important for the consumer in modern urban centers to be aware that the partial degradation in food quality that occurs in modern, packaged foods is only token in magnitude when compared to the greater losses of the food that would have occurred in former times before the advent of modern processing and packaging. Unfortunately, such losses are still experienced today in societies that do not practice modern food technology. The food supply system upon which modern, industrialized societies depend could not exist without modern food packaging. Nevertheless, the demands of modern society continue to expand as the technology of the food distribution system grows in complexity, and/or the relatively uninhibited expectations and entitlements of consumers continue to increase. One of the prices paid by consumers for such expanding services is their increasing dependence upon technologies that are accelerating in complexity and hence in difficulty for the consumer to fully comprehend.

The history of the human food supply is a chronology of change and remarkable variations. Such historic changes in diet probably have been at least equal in biological impact to those resulting from modern food technology and engineering practices. Travelers witness some of the remnants of these changes expressed as changes in cuisine of one locale compared to another.

Table 1
VARIETY OF FOOD AVAILABLE TO
ADVANCED SOCIETIES IN RECENT
HISTORY

| Diet available on Mayflower voyage to America in 1620 | Vegetables typically available to the average person in Europe during an 18th Century winter |
|---|---|
| Biscuits | Beets |
| Bacon | Cabbage |
| Crackers | Carrots |
| Dried/smoked fish | Leeks |
| Dried legumes | Lentils |
| Oatmeal | Onions |
| | Parsnips |
| | Radishes |
| | Turnips |

Prehistoric humans gathered and hunted foods that varied with the seasons. Migrations imposed additional variations on these uncertain food supplies. The introduction of agriculture and animal husbandry was, in its day, a revolution in diet at least equivalent to the changes that have occurred in recent history as the result of application of modern technology. Expansion of trade and the "discovery" by Western man of the "New World", Asia, and the Pacific, touched off a succession of revolutions in the diet of people living in Europe and America. For example, just 500 years ago, only the American Indian consumed such foods as potatoes, corn, tomatoes, lima beans, "French" beans, turkeys, avocados, pineapples, peanuts, red and green peppers, vanilla, and chocolate.[28]

Bread is an example of the change and variability in the processing of human food. Bread is one of man's oldest processed foods. Bread and related bakery-technology products make up a significant amount of the diet throughout many parts of the world. Yet, the variety of bread changes radically from locality to locality. Such variation is a measure of the high degree of tolerance to and actual preference for technological variability in the processing and formulation of the human food supply.

Further insight into changes that have occurred in the ability of a society to provide food can be gained from examination of the foods supplied to expeditions of exploration and in support of military operations. Such food systems characteristically offer the best foods that can be supplied by the state-of-the-art of a given society.

Foods available to 19th and early 20th century explorers were largely limited to canned items supplemented by various dried, shelf-stable items. It becomes evident that a revolution occurred in food technology — especially packaging — when we compare such diets of earlier explorers to the balanced menus provided to America's astronauts who first explored the moon (Table 2).[27] A typical food package used by America's astronauts was a see-through, essentially impermeable, and indestructable pouch (Figure 2). This package was fitted with a one-way, spring-loaded valve for insertion of water to rehydrate the long-life, shelf-stable, freeze-dried food. This package was also designed to form a "bowl" from which, upon cutting open, the astronaut could conveniently consume his rehydrated food by using a standard table fork or spoon. These "spoon-bowl" packages were also fitted with a tablet containing a bacteriostatic agent for insertion into the "bowl" after the food was eaten, so that the package also fulfilled the function of an environmental contamination control device by containing "microbiologically" stabilized food waste.

A comparable revolution can be seen in the foods that are supplied to military forces

**Table 2**
**APOLLO 14 MENUS FOR THE COMMANDER**

Days 1 to 5[b]

| Day | Breakfast Food item | Type[a] | Lunch Food item | Type[a] | Dinner Food item | Type[a] | Calories per day[a] |
|---|---|---|---|---|---|---|---|
| 1 and 5[b] | Peaches | RSB | Chicken and rice | RSB | Cream of tomato soup | RSB | 1748 |
| | Scrambled eggs | RSB | Applesauce | RSB | Spaghetti and meat sauce | RSB | |
| | Bacon squares (8) | IM | Chocolate bar | IM | Peach ambrosia | RSB | |
| | Grapefruit drink | RD | Orange-grapefruit drink | RD | Cheese cracker cubes (4) | D | |
| | Coffee, black | RD | | | Grape drink | RD | |
| 2 | Fruit cocktail | RSB | Turkey and gravy | T | Cream of chicken soup | RSB | 2272 |
| | Sausage patties | RSB | Cranberry-orange | RSB | Frankfurters | T | |
| | Spiced fruit cereal | RSB | sauce | | Banana pudding | RSB | |
| | Orange drink | RD | Pineapple fruitcake | IM | Brownies (4) | IM | |
| | Coffee, black | RD | Grape punch | RD | Pineapple-orange drink | RD | |
| 3 | Peaches | T | Pea soup | RSB | Lobster bisque | RSB | 2157 |
| | Scrambled eggs | RSB | Bread slices (2)[c] | NS | Beef stew | RSB | |
| | Bacon squares (8) | IM | Sandwich spread[d] | T | Beef sandwiches (4) | D | |
| | Grape drink | RD | Butterscotch pudding | RSB | Caramel candy | IM | |
| | Coffee, black | RD | Grapefruit drink | RD | Orange-grapefruit drink | RD | |
| 4 | Mixed fruit | T | Chicken and rice soup | RSB | Beef and gravy | T | 2098 |
| | Canadian bacon and applesauce | RSB | Meatballs with sauce | T | Chicken and vegetables | RSB | |
| | Cornflakes | RSB | Lemon pudding | T | Chocolate pudding | RSB | |
| | Pineapple-grapefruit drink | RD | Graham cracker cubes (4) | D | Sugar cookie cubes (4) | D | |
| | Coffee, black | RD | Grape punch | RD | Grapefruit drink | RD | |

[a]  Definitions: RSB = rehydratable, spoon bowl; RD = rehydratable drink; IM = intermediate moisture; D = dehydrated; T = thermostabilized; NS = natural state.
[b]  Dinner was eaten on day 1; breakfast was eaten on day 5.
[c]  Cheese, rye, or white.
[d]  Chicken, ham, tuna salad, cheddar cheese spread, peanut butter, jelly.

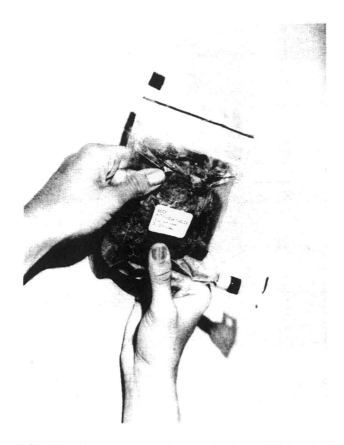

FIGURE 2. Apollo spoon-bowl package for freeze-dried food fitted with one-way spring-loaded valve for insertion of rehydration water and with opening aperture through which food is obtained by using fork or spoon.

on operational duties, patrols, and remote assignments (Table 3).[9,14,18,24] Such impressive advances in our ability to preserve and package foods is a tribute to modern food packaging technology. Without the protective barrier afforded by the package, the natural quality of foods could be lost to the consumer. This quality involves the nutritional value of the food as well as its cosmetic and organoleptic character.

## MATERIALS UTILIZED IN FOOD PACKAGING

There are myriad materials and combinations of materials that may be used in the manufacture of packages for food. The protection afforded by the package is determined principally by the packaging material and the package construction. Materials used in food packaging include glass, metals, paper, wood, and plastics (cellophane, cellulosies, polyolefins, vinyl derivatives, polyesters, rubber hydrochloride, polyfluorocarbons, polyamides, and ionomers).[13] The selection and potential numbers of combinations of these materials is virtually limitless. A single package material may be constructed of six or more layers such as paper, textiles, metals, plastics, waxes, and resins.

## EFFECTS OF PACKAGING ON NUTRIENTS

The losses in food due to inadequate packaging in countries where modern packag-

## Table 3
## EVOLUTION OF COMPONENTS IN U.S. MILITARY
## RATIONS

### Continental Army of 1775

Bread (or flour), 16 oz
Meat, beef, 12 oz, or
pork, 12 oz, or
salted fish, 16 oz

Peas or beans (3 pt/week)
Milk, 1 pt
Rice (½ pt/week) or
Indian meal (1 pt/week)
Beer or cider, 1 qt

### U.S. Army in Southwestern Texas in 1846

Beef, 20 oz (or pork 12 oz)
Bread or flour, 18 oz
Potatoes or dried apples

Coffee (approximately 1 oz)
Sugar (approximately 1 oz)

### U.S. Army Field Ration of 1864

Bread, 22 oz
Meat, 16 oz (beef, fresh or salted, or
saltpork)

Sugar
Coffee
Salt, pepper, vinegar

### U.S. Army Trench Ration of World War I

Canned meats: roast beef, corned beef, salmon, sardines
Salt, sugar, coffee

### Individual Combat Ration (C-4) U.S. Army 1945

Meat in 300×308 size cans
  Pork sausage patties (with gravy)
  Frankfurters and beans
  Chicken and vegetables
  Meat and beans
  Beef stew
  Hamburger (with gravy)

Beans with pork
Ham and lima beans
Corned-beef hash
Meat and noodles
Meat and spaghetti
Ham and eggs (with potatoes)

Fruit in 300×200 size cans
  Cherries
  Peaches
  Pineapple

Pears
Apricots
Fruit cocktail

ing and food technology are not widely practiced is estimated to average between 5 to 10% of the cereal product production with losses frequently as high as 20 to 40%. A 10% loss of cereals represents approximately 50 million tons per year. In tropical African countries, 50% losses of stored corn, beans, and legumes are frequently encountered and losses of 30 to 40% in perishable fruits and vegetables are reported to be not uncommon.[1,2,3,23]

Today's food packages are by no means perfect, because degradations of food quality do occur even when food is packaged by the best techniques now available. Many of these deteriorations are beyond the influence of the package because of chemical and physical degradation reactions that occur even within impermeable containers.

In general, the nutrient value of foods is degraded when the food is subjected to either oxidation, light, heat, and/or a shift of pH. The package is most frequently relied upon to protect the food from changes due to oxidation and light. Specific nutrients that are most sensitive to light include ascorbic acid, thiamin, riboflavin, histidine, tryptophan, tyrosine, phenylalanine, and the sulfur-containing amino acids. Nutrients generally most sensitive to oxidation include unsaturated fatty acids, tocopherols, ascorbic acid, thiamin, and amino acids. A comprehensive review of the literature has recently been published covering the relationship of the package and the stability of nutrients.[13] This review also covers the effect of packaging or preservation of nutrients in specific food products.

The rationale underlying the achievements in food packaging technology has largely been based upon the scientific elucidation of the kinetics and mechanisms of food quality and nutrient deterioration as a function of package barrier characteristics. Some highlights of means to exploit such complex relationships between food degradation and package parameters are outlined below.

## COMPUTER-AIDED PACKAGE DESIGN FOR FOODS

Package-nutrient interactions are exceedingly complex. Until very recently, the prediction of effectiveness of a given package system has been determined by either extended storage testing or predictions based upon empirical knowledge. Such approaches have often resulted in needlessly conservative package protection. Such overprotection imposes unnecessary economic penalties, severely limits package options, and contributes to a wasteful utilization of package resources. This translates into higher costs for the consumer and greater pollution problems for the environment. In addition, these approaches generally rule out the flexibility needed to encourage the implementation of new concepts for food packaging systems.

Empirical long-term storage tests of foods have been conducted since World War II and up to the present time by the U.S. Department of Defense.[4] Unfortunately, much of this work is difficult to relate directly to products and conditions other than those that were specifically tested. Application of these initial findings to other systems is further inhibited by awareness on the part of the technologists, scientists, and engineers of the complexity of factors involved in this problem. This again supports the "conservative" attitude towards food packaging change.

Recent advances in computer-assisted mathematical modeling of such complex systems and their engineering application have given rise to the interest of investigators in the potentials for such techniques in the field of food package design. Several aspects of this subject have recently been published.[6,7,10-13,15-17,25,26] Such data could provide the basis for design of food packages intended for preservation or enhancement of individual nutrients.

A simple example of this mathematical modeling approach may be represented by the predictions of interaction between packaged food and the environment. An approach to this could be taken by assuming five relationships:

First, the properties of a food that determine quality (Q) depend upon the initial condition of the food ($Q_o$) and the reactions that can change these properties over time (t). Such reactions in turn are dependent upon the internal environment of the package, e.g., relative humidity (RH), partial pressure of oxygen ($PO_2$), and temperature (T). Application of this approach rests upon the assumption that the mechanisms of Q change can accurately be expressed by a mathematical function, such that

$$\frac{dQ}{dt} = f(RH, PO_2, t, etc.)$$

Second, a maximum acceptable change in Q can be identified by correlating objective, analytical testing with consumer acceptance, or food safety standards. This is essential to the substitution of discrete, objective, analytical test data and their subsequent relation to consumer desires.

Third, various components of the environment within the package depend upon: (1) the nature of the food, (2) the package's barrier properties, and (3) the external environment. It is then assumed that changes in environmental parameters can be related to food and package properties. For example:

$$a_w = f(a_{wo}, t, RH, k, \ldots k_m, T)$$

when $a_w$ = water activity of the food at any given time, $a_{wo}$ = initial $a_w$, k, ...$k_m$ = constants that characterize sorptive and diffusional properties of the food and the package and T = temperature.

Fourth, the barrier properties of the package can be related to internal and external environments.

Fifth, the various equations accumulated throughout the first four assumptions can be combined and solved such that solutions of predicted storage life can be derived and/or required package properties can be identified for a given storage condition.

As a simplified example, we can cite the application of such assumptions to an analysis of selected changes inside packages of potato chips during storage.[19-22] In this case, the system can be represented by a scheme reduced to just three equations. This example, together with methods for their numerical solution, have been presented in a recent paper.[22] When solved with a computer, these equations predicted changes with time of

1. Oxygen pressure within a package
2. Extent of oxidation (E) expressed as amount of oxygen consumed per unit weight of product and maximum extent of oxidation tolerated (EMAX)
3. Equilibrium relative humidity inside the package (RH) and maximum allowable RH of product RHMAX

These variables are interrelated, because rate of oxidation depends on oxygen pressure and on the equilibrium relative humidity in the package. It has been found more convenient to consider the above variables in their dimensionless form. By this technique, the extent of oxidation can be expressed as a fraction of maximum permissible oxidation level (E/EMAX) and the equilibrium relative humidity (RH) of the chips expressed as a fraction of maximum permissible (RH/RHMAX).

The useful storage life of a package of potato chips was considered at an end when the ratio of oxidation or relative humidities reached unity. The optimum condition (longest possible duration of shelf life) was, therefore, given by that package that had an oxygen and water vapor permeability that enabled both E/EMAX and RH/RHMAX to reach unity at the same time.

Optimization for such assumptions can be calculated only for a specified set of conditions including: initial environment in the package, weight of product, storage conditions, film area, and film thickness. Mathematical methods for optimization are not simple because of the complex interrelationships between variables. A common method of solving this type of problem is the "steepest descent" method,[8] but a more satisfactory method is that of successive corrections.[19] A major advantage of computer simulation is that it allows rapid assessment of the influence of change in product or package conditions without the need to resort to multiple storage studies.

## FUTURE NEEDS IN FOOD PACKAGING

Two advisory groups were established during 1975 in the Office of Science and Technology Policy (OSTP) of the Office of the President of the U.S. for the purpose of preparing an agenda of critical science and technology policy issues for the U.S. These committees were chaired by William O. Baker, President of Bell Laboratories, and Simon Ramo of TRW, Inc. The group consisted of approximately 32 members representing academia, government, and industry.

Eight issues were identified as particularly urgent. Two of these center on food. Briefly, the eight issues have been summarized as:

1. Food, with emphasis on losses that occur in transportation, storage, and processing
2. Nutrition research, with emphasis on adequacy of federal support
3. Effects of government regulation on applications of new technology
4. Energy research, conservation, and environmental impacts
5. Adequacy of oceanographic research support
6. Effective use of new technology to increase productivity
7. Adequacy of support for basic research
8. Role of OSTP in Federal policy making

A recent Massachusetts Institute of Technology workshop sponsored by the National Science Foundation identified critical needs in food science and engineering.[5] The workshop was comprised of approximately 75 leading food scientists and engineers from academia, governments, and industry. The following specific research need was identified as commanding high priority: "Investigate the response of food materials to their protective environment. This research should be instrumental in leading to improved methods of food preservation allowing bulk storage prior to processing and storage in smaller units after processing. Research should include investigation of interactions of food materials with packaging materials."[5]

In recent years, substantial efforts have been undertaken or planned for enhancing our ability to deliver increased food supplies in areas where modern food packaging is not practiced. It should not be overlooked that it is under these very conditions where investments in modern packaging can most often be expected to reap a much higher rate of return on investment than comparable investments in means to increase agricultural productivity.[1-3,23] To put it simply, it is often easier and more efficient to properly package an existing crop than to increase the size of that crop.

As the demands on food packaging increase, the complexity of the technology required to characterize the most desirable package can be expected to continue to accelerate in complexity. The research, development, testing, and engineering that are needed involve such factors as the interrelationship between nutrient stability, cosmetic appearance, organoleptic quality, barrier permeability, head space volume, light spectrum transmission, intentional and unintentional additives, headspace gases, and food-package interactions. The kinetics and mechanisms of such relationships need elucidation and translation to mathematical models for rapid, computerized manipulation so that the most desirable properties of the package can be accurately identified.

## REFERENCES

1. **Anon.**, *Food Losses, the Tragedy and Some Solutions*, Food and Agricultural Organization, Rome, 1969.
2. **Anon.**, *World Food and Nutrition Study — Interim Report of the Steering Committee*, National Research Council, National Academy of Science, Washington, D. C., 1975.

3. Baker, R. C. and Robinsen, W. B., Food Science Research Needs for Improving the Utilization Processing and Nutritive Value of Food Products, Grant Report, National Science Foundation Grant STP 75-225 33, Cornell University, Ithaca, N.Y., 1975.

4. Cecil, S. R. and Woodroof, J. G., *Long-term Storage of Military Rations*, Army Quartermaster Food and Container Institute for the Armed Forces, Chicago, 1962.

5. Heidelbaugh, N. D. and Mudgett, R. E., Material Science of Foods, in *A Workshop on Critical Needs in Food Science and Engineering*, Vol. 1, Massachusetts Institute of Technology, National Technical Information Service, U.S. Department of Commerce, Springfield, Virginia, 1975, 18—25.

6. Herlitze, W., Becker, K., and Heiss, R., Berechnung einer Kunststoffverpackung fuer sauerstofftempfindliche Lebensmittel, *Verpack. Rundsch.*, 24(7), 51, 1973.

7. Herrman, J., Die Haltbarkeit von Lebensmitteln als Wechselbeziehung zwischen Ausgangsqualitaet, Berpackung, Transport und Lagerbedingungen, *Nahrung*, 4, 409, 1974.

8. Himmelblau, D. M., *Process Analysis by Statistical Methods*, John Wiley & Sons, New York, 1970.

9. Horsford, E. N., *The Army Ration*, Van Nostrand, New York, 1864.

10. Karel, M., Quantitative analysis of food packaging and storage stability problems, *Am. Inst. Chem. Eng. Symp. Ser.*, 69(132), 107, 1973.

11. Karel, M., Packaging protection for oxygen-sensitive products, *Food Technol.*, Chicago, 28(8), 50, 1974.

12. Karel, M., Protective packaging of foods, in *Physical Principles of Food Preservation*, Karel, M., Fennema, O. R., and Lund, D. B., Eds., Marcel Dekker, New York, 1975, 399.

13. Karel, M. and Heidelbaugh, N. D., Effects of packaging on nutrients, in *Nutritional Evaluation of Food Processing*, 2nd ed., Harris, R. S. and Karmas, E., Eds., AVI Publishing, Westport, Conn., 1975, 412.

14. Koehler, F. A., *Special Rations for the Armed Forces*, Office of the Quartermaster General, U.S. Army, Washington, D.C., 1958.

15. Labuza, T. P., Nutrient losses during drying and storage of dehydrated foods, *CRC Crit. Rev. Food Technol.*, 3(2), 217, 1972.

16. Labuza, T. P., Effects of dehydration and storage, *Food Technol. (Chicago)*, 27, 21, 1973.

17. Makinde, M. A., Gilbert, S. G., and LaChance, P. A., Nutritional implications of packaging systems, *Food Prod. Dev.*, 10(7), 112—119, 1976.

18. Prescott, Samuel C., *Troop Feeding Program. A Survey of Rationing and Subsistence in the United States Army 1775 to 1940*, National Defense Research Committee of the Office of Scientific Research and Development, Washington, D.C., 1944.

19. Quast, D. G., Computer Simulation of Storage Stability and Package Optimization for Food Products, S.M. thesis, Massachusetts Institute of Technology, Cambridge, 1972.

20. Quast, D. G. and Karel, M., Effects of environmental factors on the oxidation of potato chips, *J. Food Sci.*, 37, 584, 1972.

21. Quast, D. G. and Karel, M., Simulating shelf life, *Mod. Packag.*, 46(3), 50, 1973.

22. Quast, D. G. and Karel, M., Computer simulation of the storage life of food undergoing spoilage by two interacting mechanisms, *J. Food Sci.*, 37, 679, 1972.

23. Schumacher, A., Investment Technology in Food Delivery, presented at National Packaging Week Assembly, New York, N.Y., November 2, 1975 and at World Bank, Washington, D.C., January 1976.

24. Rison, Erna, *Quartermaster Support of the Army. A History of the Corps 1775—1939*, Quartermaster Historian's Office. Office of the Quartermaster General, Washington, D.C., 1962.

25. Singh, R. P. and Heldman, D. R., Simulation of liquid food quality during storage, *Trans. ASAE*, 19, 178, 1976.

26. Singh, R. P., Heldman, D. R., and Kirk, J. R., Kinetic analysis of light-induced riboflavin loss in whole milk, *J. Food Sci.*, 40, 164, 1975.

27. Smith, M. C., Huber, C. S. and Heidelbaugh, N. D., Apollo 14 food system, *Aerosp. Med.*, 42, 1185—1192, 1971.

28. Tannahill, R., *Food in History*, Stein & Day Publishers, New York, 1973.

# EFFECT OF STORAGE ON NUTRITIVE VALUE OF FOOD

## Amihud Kramer

In contrast to the vast literature on nutritive value of fresh and processed foods, it is only in recent years that special attention has been directed to the effect of storage. Thus, the value of foodstuffs has been determined on the basis of their sensory quality retention and freedom from microbial or insect infestation rather than nutrient retention. Yet the same conditions that determine sensory acceptability also affect nutrient retention. The most important of these conditions for determining sensory or nutritional "shelf life" is temperature, but other factors such as packaging, atmosphere within and without the package, and exposure to light, may all be important for specific foods.[1]

As with other quality attributes, the stored or processed product is rarely nutritionally superior to the raw ingredients from which it is produced. Nutrients are destroyed during food processing because of sensitivity to pH, oxygen, light, heat, or a combination of these factors. Trace elements and enzymes catalyze these effects. Where certain nutrients are included as additives they may have an antagonistic effect upon one another (e.g., effect of added iron on vitamin E in milk) or their retention levels may be reduced by other components in the foods (e.g., effect of the anthocyanins on retention of vitamin C added to prune juice).

These changes, usually resulting in lower nutritional levels, may occur during all stages of processing, in the channels of trade, and continue in the home. There is good reason to believe that the maximum damage to nutrient levels in foods occurs during handling and preparation of the foods in the home,[2] to a lesser extent in the retail and distribution channels, to a still lesser extent during storage (particularly if held at low temperatures), and to a relatively minor extent during the actual commercial processing of the foods.

In sensory quality the specific attributes can be weighed in relation to their effect on total quality, and a single overall quality score can be provided. This is next to impossible in considering nutritional quality, although many valiant efforts have been made to provide such a score. For example, a particular product can be given a certain number of "points" for each quantity of each nutrient that it contains. In fact, however, such an exercise is largely meaningless and we must resort to listing the quantity of each of 40 plus nutrients that may be present in a food. The current usual procedure that follows Food and Drug guidelines[3] is to list the actual quantity per serving of protein, calories and fats, and the percentage of the recommended daily dietary allowance (RDA) of protein, vitamins A, $B_1$, $B_2$, niacin, C, and minerals calcium and iron. Other essential vitamins and minerals are usually not listed nor is much attention given to the availability of any of these nutrients, particularly protein, or the nutritionally essential amino acids that must be present and available in the proteins for them to be nutritionally effective.

From the standpoint of temperature control, the situation is not quite so complicated. Although there is eventually some loss in bioavailability if not in actual content of all nutrients during extended storage, and the rate of this loss is attenuated with reduction of storage temperature, all nutrients may be classified into one of three categories:

1. Those that are practically unaffected by temperature of storage
2. Those nutrients that are thermally stable in some foods but not in others
3. Those nutrients that are highly sensitive to storage temperature

We shall consider largely the third category.

The most temperature-sensitive nutrient is undoubtedly ascorbic acid or vitamin C, particularly in nonacid foods and in the presence of air or oxygen. Thus vitamin C in frozen orange concentrate is maintained quite well. During preparation and freezing of nonacid greens, however, vitamin C content is reduced to one quarter (to one tenth when canned). When stored for 6 months at +5°F, vitamin C content is reduced in half again, but when stored at −5°F there is little further loss in vitamin C.[4] Vitamin C loss in storage has been found frequently to parallel sensory quality loss; often vitamin C analysis is used to indicate sensory quality,[5] but this is not always the case. Frozen peaches, for example, maintain sensory quality satisfactorily for 6 months or longer if stored at −5°F. To maintain vitamin C content at the original level, storage temperature must be reduced to −35°F. Since there are quite a few fruits and particularly vegetables that are not acid and are good sources of vitamin C, there is good reason to store them at low temperatures even if they had been thermally stabilized, i.e., sterilized or canned. There is no good argument, for instance, against the refrigerated storage of canned green beans to prevent vitamin C loss except that the vitamin C that is lost may not be considered essential; if the container is labeled for a given vitamin C content, sufficient synthetic vitamin can be added to retain the level declared even at the end of a storage period at high temperature.

The other thermally sensitive vitamin is thiamin or vitamin $B_1$. Where vitamin C is an important nutrient in fruits and vegetables, thiamin, like other B vitamins, is found in greater quantities in animal products, although it is found in vegetable products as well, particularly legumes. Practically everything that has been said about vitamin C applies also to vitamin $B_1$. In this case the only possible argument against use of refrigerated storage to maintain $B_1$ levels is that the standard bread in this country and other countries is fortified with thiamin; so there is little if any thiamin deficiency in the general population. This argument, however, does not prevent a packer from misbranding if he declares his product to contain a certain level of $B_1$ that might very well have been the case when packed but is below this level when stored at ambient temperatures.

Other heat-labile vitamins that may be affected by extended storage are riboflavin, folic acid, pantothenic acid, and biotin. Pyridoxine, niacin, and vitamin $B_{12}$ are reportedly thermally stable.[5]

The vitamin A story is a confused one. Apparently it is not only fully retained in such products as carrots and sweet potatoes, but it seems to increase somewhat during storage. In other products such as leafy greens, it is rapidly lost unless stored at low temperatures.

In contrast to most if not all the other nutrients, there is a real iron deficiency in certain population groups even in the U.S. This is probably due to both an insufficient intake of iron and the unavailability of iron that is consumed. Thus, iron fortification is needed. There is little information on the effect of storage temperature on the bioavailability of iron. Extended storage at any temperature certainly should not cause iron to disappear from the food.

Perhaps the most important and intriguing relationship of nutritional quality and storage temperatures is that of protein. As with iron, there is no reason to believe that protein content as such is reduced with increasing time and temperature of storage. There is, however, mounting evidence to the effect that bioavailability of protein is reduced with increased time and temperature. It has been shown, for example, that the protein in dried milk, when stored at above 70°F and 70% relative humidity, will lose half its nutritional effectiveness (bioavailability) in 6 months. Apparently this is due in part to a change in availability of the amino acid lysine. But this seems to be only part of the story. If the same milk powder is held in refrigerated storage, most of the protein nutritive value is retained for a full year. When stored at 0°F there appears to be little change in nutritive value for 2 years and longer.

Apparently these losses in protein bioavilability are accelerated in the presence of oxygen and water vapor. Thus packaging in vapor and oxygen-tight containers aids in retention of bioavailability. It remains to be seen if products such as milk powder can retain protein nutritive value even at high temperatures of storage if packed in near-total absence of oxygen and water. Recent studies with textured vegetable proteins indicate similar losses in protein bioavailability that were practically eliminated by storage at or below 0°C.

# FRESH FOODS

By definition, fresh foods have not undergone a "stabilizing" processing treatment and are therefore most susceptible to nutritional changes during storage. It is common-place to include as fresh, foods that have been superficially treated chemically, coated, packaged, and/or placed in modified atmospheres. This is because life processes, particularly respiration, have not been arrested but only attenuated, and the main effect is extension of shelf-life through protection of the food from infection or infestation.

## Energy

Practically all fresh foods lose weight after harvest, collection, or storage as a result of transpiration and respiration. This weight loss is generally most rapid in high-moisture foods of plant origin. While transpirational (i.e., moisture) losses may be of major economic importance, no nutrients are affected; respirational losses, however, represent direct loss of carbohydrates and other digestible carbon-containing nutrients, mainly sugar. Thus, respiration losses are generally low in animal products, where the small quantities of glycogen are frequently completely utilized during the slaughtering operation, so that further respiration during storage proceeds at such a slow rate that heat of respiration is not considered a factor in refrigerated storage.

For high-moisture plant foods, however, respiration rates are so rapid that they must be taken into account when calculating refrigeration requirements. As shown in Table 1,[6] heat of respiration increases with storage temperature. It is also substantially lower for "hardware" items such as apples, onions, or potatoes, which are known to have relatively long shelf-life, than for short shelf-life commodities such as green beans, sweet corn, or strawberries.

Moisture percentage is not a good indication of energy loss since under proper conditions moisture loss through transpiration may be proportional to solids' loss through respiration. Thus, for example, green beans stored at 5°C, 60% RH for 10 days lost 20% weight but maintained 88% of initial moisture, indicating that approximately 20% (2.4 of the 12% solids) of the most digestible solids were lost, leaving a higher level of undigestible solids in the stored product.

Sweet corn, harvested at 72% moisture and 4% sugar, lost 50% of the sugar within 12 hr at 30°C and 90% within 3 days. At the same time, moisture content was reduced to 65%, and the indigestible pericarp content increased from 1.8 to 2.8%. When stored at 2°C for 5 days, moisture was reduced by 2%, sugar by 1%, and pericarp increased by 0.2%.[7]

Many "aids" to refrigeration such as controlled atmosphere or hypobaric storage are primarily means of reducing rates of respiration, thereby improving retention of energy value of the products so treated.[8]

Table 1
APPROXIMATE AMOUNT OF RESPIRATION
HEAT PRODUCED BY CERTAIN FRUITS AND
VEGETABLES AT THE TEMPERATURES
INDICATED[b]

| Commodity | Btu per ton per 24 hr | | | |
|---|---|---|---|---|
| | 32°F | 40°F | 60°F | 70°F |
| Apples | 700 | 1,350 | 4,900 | 5,700 |
| Apricots | — | 5,050 | 11,700 | 20,350 |
| Artichokes | 7,700 | 10,450 | 26,400 | 40,700 |
| Asparagus | 9,700 | 18,050 | 38,500 | 48,750 |
| Avocados | — | 5,500 | 24,050 | 46,250 |
| Bananas (green) | — | — | 4,850 | 7,400 |
| Beans | | | | |
|   Green snap | 7,250 | 10,300 | 38,100 | 49,200 |
|   Lima (in pod) | 4,450 | 6,100 | 24,700 | 34,300 |
| Beets | 2,700 | 4,100 | 7,200 | — |
| Blackberries | 4,100 | 7,950 | — | 38,350 |
| Blueberries | 1,400 | 2,350 | 10,550 | 15,300 |
| Broccoli, sprouting | 4,400 | 21,400 | 56,500 | 68,100 |
| Brussels sprouts | 4,400 | 7,700 | 22,000 | 28,350 |
| Cabbage | 1,200 | 2,200 | 4,900 | 8,450 |
| Carrots | 3,300 | 4,300 | 8,750 | 15,500 |
| Cauliflower (trimmed) | 3,900 | 4,500 | 10,100 | 17,700 |
| Celery | 1,600 | 2,400 | 8,200 | 14,200 |
| Cherries | | | | |
|   Sour | 2,100 | 2,850 | 8,500 | 9,800 |
|   Sweet | 1,050 | 2,600 | 7,700 | — |
| Corn (sweet) | 8,950 | 13,850 | 35,850 | 63,700 |
| Cranberries | 650 | 950 | — | 3,200 |
| Cucumbers | — | — | 5,300 | 6,850 |
| Endive and escarole | | | | |
|   (see leaf lettuce) | | | | |
| Figs (fresh) | — | 2,650 | 12,350 | 16,700 |
| Gooseberries | 1,700 | 2,850 | 5,950 | — |
| Grapefruit | — | 1,000 | 3,100 | 4,250 |
| Grapes | | | | |
|   American | 600 | 1,200 | 3,500 | 7,200 |
|   European | 400 | 1,000 | 2,400 | — |
| Kale[1] (whole leaves) | 4,700 | 8,900 | 30,250 | 49,600 |
| Leeks | 2,900 | 5,350 | 21,950 | — |
| Lemons | 700 | 1,250 | 3,650 | 4,850 |
| Lettuce | | | | |
|   Head | 2,500 | 3,650 | 8,450 | 12,200 |
|   Leaf | 5,100 | 6,450 | 13,800 | 22,100 |
| Limes | — | 800 | 1,800 | 2,800 |
| Mangos | — | 3,500 | 9,900 | 24,900 |
| Melons | | | | |
|   Cantaloups | 1,200 | 2,050 | 7,950 | 12,000 |
|   Honeydew | — | 900 | 3,050 | 5,150 |
|   Watermelons | — | 800 | — | 4,650 |
| Mushrooms | 7,900 | 15,600 | 46,000 | 63,800 |
| Nectarines (see peaches) | | | | |
| Okra | — | 12,250 | 32,050 | 57,400 |
| Onions | | | | |
|   Dry | 650 | 750 | 2,400 | 3,650 |
|   Green | 3,600 | 9,400 | 17,950 | 25,800 |
| Oranges | 750 | 1,200 | 4,000 | 6,200 |

Table 1 (continued)
APPROXIMATE AMOUNT OF RESPIRATION
HEAT PRODUCED BY CERTAIN FRUITS AND
VEGETABLES AT THE TEMPERATURES
INDICATED[b]

| Commodity | Btu per ton per 24 hr | | | |
|---|---|---|---|---|
| | 32°F | 40°F | 60°F | 70°F |
| Parsnips | 3,000 | 2,900 | 8,250 | — |
| Peaches | 1,150 | 1,700 | 8,300 | 17,750 |
| Pears | | | | |
| Bartlett | 1,100 | 1,650 | 8,250 | 11,000 |
| Kieffer | 450 | — | 850 | 4,750 |
| Peas (green, in the pod) | 8,500 | 14,450 | 41,900 | 66,750 |
| Peppers (sweet) | — | 2,900 | 8,500 | 9,650 |
| Pineapples | — | 400 | 3,450 | 7,050 |
| Plums (including fresh prunes) | 500 | 1,450 | 2,700 | 4,700 |
| Potatoes | | | | |
| Uncured | — | 2,600 | 4,850 | 6,950 |
| Cured | — | 1,250 | 1,950 | 2,650 |
| Prunes (see plums) | | | | |
| Radishes (topped) | 1,400 | 2,100 | 7,100 | 11,250 |
| Raspberries | 4,700 | 7,650 | 20,200 | — |
| Rhubarb (without leaves) | 2,350 | 3,200 | 8,700 | 10,650 |
| Romaine | — | 4,550 | 9,750 | 15,100 |
| Spinach | 4,550 | 10,150 | 39,350 | 50,550 |
| Squash | | | | |
| Butternut | — | — | — | — |
| Yellow straight-neck | 2,700 | 3,600 | 18,250 | 20,050 |
| Strawberries | 3,300 | 5,450 | 17,950 | 32,800 |
| Sweet potatoes | | | | |
| Cured | — | — | 4,800 | — |
| Uncured | — | — | 6,300 | — |
| Tomatoes | | | | |
| Mature-green | — | 1,450 | 4,900 | 7,650 |
| Pink | — | 1,300 | 5,850 | 7,500 |
| Turnips | 1,900 | 2,150 | 5,000 | 5,400 |
| Watercress | 5,050 | 10,150 | 40,700 | — |

While energy losses in storage for more mature seed crops are not as severe, they can be substantial, particularly if moisture content is above the optimum. Heidman and Lund[9] reported a respiration loss of approximately 2%/day in immature wild rice, about 1% in fully mature rice, and practically no respiration loss in either immature or mature rice when stored in near 100% nitrogen atmosphere.

Studies from Czechoslovakia,[10] Israel,[11] and the U.S.[12] report beneficial effects in using chilled air to cool wheat and soy beans to 20°C. Without such cooling, heat of respiration increases temperatures of stored grain to 40 to 50°C, causing not only losses in carbohydrates and other nutrients, but inducing spoilage and affecting germination. Reports from Japan indicate that to prevent nutritional losses and maintain desirable functional properties, storage temperature of rice should be limited to 15°C.

Feed grains harvested at somewhat higher moisture levels (18 to 20%) than optimal for storage (12 to 14%), have been found to have about a 10% higher feed value. When stored, they must be chilled to ca 5°C to prevent nutrient loss and development of mycotoxins. The alternate control method is treatment with propionic acid or other fungicide, which will also prevent loss of nutrients but will affect germination.[13]

### Vitamin C

Heinze[14] states that ascorbic acid is one of the more important nutrients supplied by fresh fruit and vegetables and is also one of the most sensitive to destruction when subjected to adverse handling and storage conditions. Loss of ascorbic acid is associated with degree of wilting in practically all leafy vegetables such as kale, spinach, and turnip greens, where the degree of wilting and reduction in ascorbic acid is much higher at 10° and certainly at 20°C than at 0°C. Cabbage, which is also a leafy vegetable, loses ascorbic acid more slowly. Seed vegetables, such as peas and beans, should be stored at as low a temperature as possible (slightly under 0°C), not only to prevent multiplication of microorganisms, but also to retard vitamin C loss. Heinze also points out that shelled peas and lima beans lose ascorbic acid at twice the rate of unshelled beans at the same temperature.

Freshly dug potatoes contain 20 + mg/100 g(mg%) ascorbic acid, so that a 5-oz serving of freshly dug potatoes will provide about half the recommended daily dietary allowance (RDA). Potatoes rapidly lose vitamin C in storage however, so that within several weeks ascorbic levels are little more than 5 to 6 mg%. Cooling the freshly dug potatoes rapidly and holding them at close to 0°C not only does not retard vitamin C loss, but accelerates the rate of loss. Thus potatoes at 5°C have been found to lose as much ascorbic acid in 2 months as comparable lots stored at 10 or 15°C lose in 5 months.

Many fruits, particularly citrus, are good sources of vitamin C. It is generally agreed that lemons retain nearly 100% of their ascorbic acid during storage and grapefruit lose very little ascorbic acid. Reports differ for oranges and tangerines, but it has been concluded that loss of vitamin C in fresh citrus is not likely to exceed 10% under reasonable conditions of storage. Temperature of storage may vary depending on the species and variety from as low as 2°C to 15°C.

Green asparagus stalks stored at near 0°C and high relative humidity retain over 80% ascorbic acid after 7 to 10 days and may at the same time reduce fiber content. At 20°C, ascorbic acid content is reduced to 20%.[15]

Tomatoes harvested in the pink stage contain more ascorbic acid than mature green or fully ripe tomatoes. Unripe tomatoes may show an increase in ascorbic acid during the first few days of storage, but will not equal vine-ripened fruit. After 10 days storage at the appropriate temperatures (15 to 20°C for unripe, 5 to 10°C for ripe), all tomatoes retained about 80% of their original ascorbic acid.[16]

Mature, dry seeds of vegetables, grains, and legumes contain practically no ascorbic acid but do contain substantial quantities of other iodine-reducing substances. Upon germination there is a rapid reduction in glutathione and a corresponding increase in ascorbic acid, so that pea and bean sprouts may contain 20 to 30 mg% ascorbic acid.[17]

### Folic Acid

Folic acid or folacin is a vitamin essential to man. Yet, like vitamins E or K, it is difficult to demonstrate deficiency in the human diet. For these reasons it is not usually involved in nutrition labeling. However, with the increasing use of single-cell protein such as yeast as a supplement for protein enrichment, folacin level may become important, since some of these materials are rich in this nutrient. Heinze[14] reports that folic acid is lost rapidly if storage conditions are unfavorable. Leguminous seed vegetables, asparagus, spinach, turnip greens, and other leafy vegetables supply significant quantities of folic acid to the diet. These vegetables, stored for 2 weeks at refrigerated temperatures or in crushed ice, were found to lose little if any of the folic acid content. Storage at room temperature for 3 days, however, resulted in losses of more than 50% of the vitamin.

## Thiamin and Riboflavin

Fruits and vegetables are not considered important sources of thiamin ($B_1$) and riboflavin ($B_2$), but some of the leguminous seed vegetables such as peas and lima beans may supply significant amounts of thiamin. If stored for not more than 2 to 4 days even at ambient temperatures, they should retain about 90% of these nutrients. If stored for longer periods, however, they should be refrigerated. There is some indication that thiamin and riboflavin may initially increase during storage or processing but will decline upon further storage at ambient temperatures.[5,18]

Gas treatments had a profound effect on changes in thiamin content of mushrooms in storage.[19] Controls at both storage temperatures showed little change in thiamin content throughout the 2-month storage period. When stored in nitrogen, thiamin content appeared to increase by about 25% after 1 month's storage, then gradually decreased to original levels during the second month's storage. A similar tendency was noted for the carbon monoxide-treated mushrooms, but to a much more substantial degree with the increase at the end of the first month's storage being practically 100%. For all treatments at all storage periods, thiamin content was higher at the lower storage temperature.

Similar atmospheric modifications of fresh beef patties affected thiamin content differently. The control and carbon monoxide treatments remained fairly stable throughout the storage period. The nitrogen-flushed patties, on the other hand, showed a sharp increase in thiamin content (well over 100%) during the first month's storage; thiamin content tended to drop, but was not reduced to the original levels even after 2-½ month's storage at both the high and low temperatures.

## Vitamin A

There is little if any vitamin A as such in fruits and vegetables; however, many fruits and vegetables, particularly the green and yellow vegetables, contain substantial amounts of carotene, some forms of which are precursors of vitamin A.

Carotene is generally rather stable, so that there have been reports that, in some vegetables such as sweet potatoes, carotene content may actually increase during storage. On the other hand, leafy vegetables subjected to wilting conditions may lose more than half of their carotene when held at or near room temperature for 4 days. Thus to preserve the carotene (or vitamin A) of vegetables such as spinach, which are quite rich in this vitamin when first harvested, they should be held at storage temperatures as low as possible without freezing.[14]

## Hypobaric Storage

The benefits of low-pressure storage in rooms or by means of vacuum packaging for extending storage life of some fresh foods are evident. Some recent data show some beneficial effects on nutrient retention as well. Delaporte[20] found that apples stored at low oxygen tension retained 60% of their original ascorbic acid after 3 months storage at 15°C, as compared to 20% for air-stored apples. Hypobaric storage was reported to reduce rate of ascorbic acid loss in cherries and blueberries, aid retention of sugar in sweet corn, and reduce fiber in asparagus.[21] Vacuum packaging of primal and sub-primal cuts of beef indirectly aided nutrient retention by reducing drip loss.[22]

## FROZEN FOODS

Storage temperature has special significance with frozen foods because they are defined as foods stored at temperatures below −18°C. At such temperatures, although microbial growth is completely arrested, certain enzymatic and non-enzymatic changes continue to limit storage life of frozen foods, but at a much slower rate. Even when

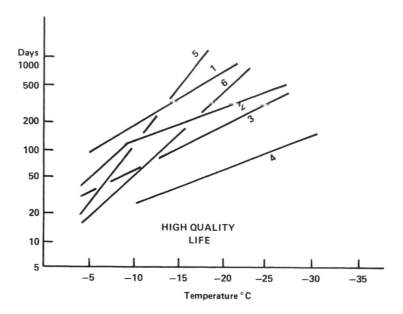

FIGURE 1.    TTT characteristics (HQL-data) for different foods systemized in groups.[24] The groups are (1) Raw, lean meat, and precooked dishes or lean meat in gravy, (2) Raw, fat meat, and precooked dishes of fat meat in gravy, (3) Precooked foods without gravy; lean fish, (4) Fat fish without any qualified protective measures in treatment or packaging, (5) Fruit and berries, and (6) Vegetables.

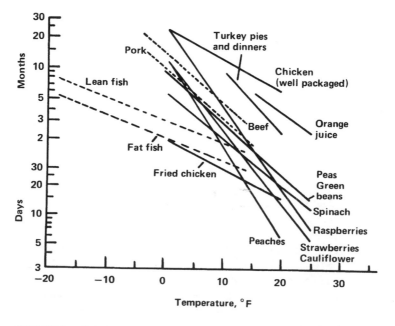

FIGURE 2.    Relation of time and temperature of storage to high quality shelf life of various frozen foods, summarized from U.S. Department of Agriculture T-T-T studies.[23,28]

frozen, the lower the storage temperature, the longer the storage life. As shown in Figure 1, which summarizes much of the information developed in the classic time-temperature-tolerance studies of the U.S. Department of Agriculture,[23] quality losses

Table 2
## MAXIMUM STORAGE TEMPERATURES (°C) FOR FROZEN FRUITS AND VEGETABLES FOR GENERAL QUALITY RETENTION COMPARED TO VITAMIN C LOSSES

| | Months in storage | | | |
|---|---|---|---|---|
| | 6 | 12 | 18 | 24 |
| **Asparagus** | | | | |
| Quality[a] | −18 | −21 | −23 | −25 |
| Vitamin C loss[b] | | | | |
| 10% | −15 | −18 | −19 | −20 |
| 25% | −14 | −15 | −18 | −19 |
| 50% | −13 | −16 | −17 | −18 |
| **Broccoli** | | | | |
| Quality[a] | −18 | −21 | −23 | −25 |
| Vitamin C loss[b] | | | | |
| 10% | −26 | −40 | −46 | — |
| 25% | −17 | −19 | −21 | −22 |
| 50% | −13 | −14 | −16 | −18 |
| **Lima Beans** | | | | |
| Quality[a] | −16 | −20 | −22 | −23 |
| Vitamin C loss[b] | | | | |
| 10% | −16 | −17 | −18 | −19 |
| 25% | −12 | −15 | −17 | −18 |
| 50% | −8 | −13 | −15 | −17 |
| **Green Beans** | | | | |
| Quality[a] | −16 | −19 | −21 | −22 |
| Vitamin C loss[b] | | | | |
| 10% | −20 | −21 | −22 | −23 |
| 25% | −16 | −18 | −19 | −20 |
| 50% | −14 | −16 | −18 | −17 |
| **Cauliflower** | | | | |
| Quality[a] | −16 | −19 | −20 | −21 |
| Vitamin C loss[b] | | | | |
| 10% | −17 | −25 | −37 | — |
| 25% | −16 | −22 | −29 | — |
| 50% | −13 | −18 | −23 | — |
| **Peas** | | | | |
| Quality[a] | −16 | −19 | −21 | −23 |
| Vitamin C loss[b] | | | | |
| 10% | −16 | −19 | −20 | −22 |
| 25% | −13 | −16 | −17 | −18 |
| 50% | −12 | −13 | −14 | −15 |
| **Spinach** | | | | |
| Quality[a] | −19 | −22 | −24 | −25 |
| Vitamin C loss[b] | | | | |
| 10% | −20 | −26 | −28 | −30 |
| 25% | −11 | −20 | −23 | −24 |
| 50% | −14 | −18 | −19 | −20 |

Table 2 (continued)
MAXIMUM STORAGE TEMPERATURES
(°C) FOR FROZEN FRUITS AND
VEGETABLES FOR GENERAL QUALITY
RETENTION COMPARED TO VITAMIN
C LOSSES

| | Months in storage | | | |
|---|---|---|---|---|
| | 6 | 12 | 18 | 24 |
| O. J. and Grapefruit Conc. | | | | |
| Quality[a] | −10 | −14 | −16 | −17 |
| Vitamin C loss[c] | | | | |
| 10% | 5 | 5 | 5 | 5 |
| | | | | |
| Peaches | | | | |
| Quality[a] | −15 | −18 | −16 | −15 |
| Vitamin C loss[d] | | | | |
| 10% | −39 | — | — | — |
| 25% | −18 | −37 | — | — |
| 50% | −12 | −18 | — | — |

[a]   Adapted from WRRL-TTT studies.[23]
[b]   Adapted from Davis.[30]
[c]   Adapted from Haggart et al.[31]
[d]   Adapted from Dubois and Kew.[32]

increase log-linearly with temperature increase, but the slopes of the curves differ for different commodities. Bengtsson et al.,[24] extended this work, and classified all frozen foods into six categories exhibiting different slopes. They found that all categories except No. 2 (Raw fat meat, and precooked dishes of fat meat in gravy) exhibited log-linear curves, and quality losses could therefore be assumed to follow first-order reactions (Figure 2). Since percentage of a nutrient remaining after a given time-temperature of processing or storage is also assumed to be a first-order reaction,[25] and in a few instances has actually been demonstrated to be so,[26] it might be assumed that nutritional losses in storage proceed in much the same manner as previously-reported quality losses (Figures 1, 2). Unfortunately, the above studies provide little data on nutrient losses in frozen storage, and more data on actual rates of nutrient losses are needed before predictions can be made.[25,27]

The nutrient that has been most throughly researched is ascorbic acid, with the finding that kinetics of ascorbic acid destruction during storage are influenced by amount of blanching (to inactivate enzymes), rate of freezing and packaging, as well as time and temperature of storage.[28] A most important finding is that for some frozen foods, such as strawberries, while total and biologically active ascorbic acid remains at essentially the same level for a year or longer, if stored below −18°C; conversion to the partially active dehydroascorbic, and the totally inactive 2, 3-diketogulonic acid increases with increasing storage temperatures, so that practically complete conversion occurs in 8 months at a storage temperature of −10°C, and in less than 2 months at −2°C.[29] Such findings were instrumental in establishing 0°F (−18°C) as the upper limit for frozen food storage, and for using biologically active ascorbic acid as a general indicator of quality deterioration in storage. While this may be appropriate in some instances, it certainly is not in others.

As shown in Table 2,[23,30-32] storage temperature of −20°C will not only maintain quality of asparagus, green beans, lima beans, and peas, but also will retain at least 90% of the original vitamin C content for 12 months. As stated above, this is the reason for using vitamin C determinations as indicators of quality retention. There are, however, many exceptions to this relationship. Although −20°C is adequate to maintain sensory quality of broccoli, cauliflower, spinach, and peaches for 12 months or longer, these products may lose 20 to 50% of their vitamin C under these storage conditions. The reverse may also be true, i.e., sensory quality may deteriorate more rapidly than the vitamin content. An excellent example of this is citrus fruit, particularly orange juice concentrate which will retain quality for over 2 years at −18°C but will lose less than 10% vitamin C even at temperatures as high as + 5°.

Such data may be used for labeling purposes. Freshly frozen asparagus and broccoli both containing 30 mg% ascorbic acid may be held in storage for 12 to 18 months at −18°C to −24°C. It could be safe to label the asparagus as containing 90% of 30, or 27 mg% vitamin C. The broccoli however, stored under the same conditions, could be labeled as containing only 75% of 30, or 22 mg%.

While it is generally assumed that vitamin A (including biologically active carotene precursors) remains quite stable in storage, there are occasional reports that in certain foods stored at above freezing temperatures, vitamin A may be lost rapidly.[14] Such losses are apparently caused by oxidation as demonstrated with two prepared frozen foods. Frozen meat patties and macaroni and cheese were blended in a Waring® blender. The blended samples were stored in a refrigerator at 5°C, and aliquots were removed for various analyses. When the vitamin A analyses were performed immediately after blending, the patties and the macaroni and cheese had 1840 and 1025 IU/100 g, respectively. After 4 days storage, A values were found to increase to 2295 and 1665 IU. With further storage at 5°C, A values began to decrease, so that after 11 days storage, both foods contained less than 800 IU/100 g.

In Table 3, effects of frozen storage are shown for Salisbury steak in tomato sauce, a popular prepared frozen food containing both animal and vegetable ingredients, so that changes in a variety of nutrients could be observed. While quality of product was fully maintained for 6 months when stored at constant −20°C or lower, ascorbic acid content was reduced significantly after 3 months, and to less than 50% after 6 months storage, even at −30°C. Thiamin reduction followed more closely changes in quality. In general, however, losses in both vitamins and sensory quality increased with increasing time-temperature of storage, and were greater under fluctuating (±5°C) temperature conditions than under constant (±1°C) temperatures.

Storage conditions had little or no effect on the macronutrients and minerals or on vitamin A, riboflavin, and niacin. The produce was well-packaged in gas-tight aluminum and the increased "in-package" dessication caused by fluctuating temperatures did not affect the composition of this prepared food, since the ice formed in the package was reabsorbed upon preparation for consumption. Even if the ice were discarded, it is not likely that it would result in a nutritional loss. Other prepared frozen foods behaved similarly.[33]

Although there was no indication of loss of total protein, it is known that heat has a deleterious effect due to either the outright destruction of amino acids, such as lysine in cereal and bread manufacture, or a combination destruction of part of one or more of the amino acids in a linkage that is not hydrolyzed during digestion. This is seen in the Maillard reaction — an amino group from an essential amino acid such as lysine reacting with the carbonyl group of a reducing sugar either during processing or prolonged storage at high temperatures. Obviously, such reactions do take place in the manufacture of precooked foods, but storage of these at 0°F reduces or stops the degree of further deterioration.[28] The data in Table 4 demonstrate not only the beneficial effect of below 0°F on retaining nutritive value of protein in terms of protein efficiency ratio (PER), but indicate that storage at any temperature below 0°C would be practically as effective.

Table 3

CHANGES IN SENSORY, MICROBIAL, AND NUTRITIONAL QUALITY OF SALISBURY
STEAK IN TOMATO SAUCE STORED AT CONSTANT AND FLUCTUATING
TEMPERATURES[33]

| Storage conditions | Quality scores[b] | | Total plate counts[c] | | Ascorbic acid[d] | | Thiamin[d] | |
|---|---|---|---|---|---|---|---|---|
| | Constant[a] | Fluctuating | Constant | Fluctuating | Constant | Fluctuating | Constant | Fluctuating |
| Initial | 4.1 | | 18.0 | | 3.6 | | 3.0 | |
| 3 months | | | | | | | | |
| −10°C | 3.0 | 2.8 | 0.3 | 0.3 | 1.8 | 1.0 | 2.8 | 1.8 |
| −20°C | 3.8 | 3.7 | 17.0 | 14.0 | 2.8 | 2.0 | 2.9 | 2.1 |
| −30°C | 3.8 | 3.7 | 73.0 | 0.3 | 2.8 | 2.5 | 3.2 | 2.6 |
| 6 months | | | | | | | | |
| −10°C | 3.3 | 2.8 | 0.3 | — | 1.2 | 1.1 | 1.9 | 1.8 |
| −20°C | 4.0 | 3.6 | 0.5 | — | 1.6 | 1.1 | 2.7 | 1.7 |
| −30°C | 4.2 | 3.7 | 0.8 | — | 1.8 | 1.1 | 2.7 | 2.6 |

[a]   Constant = ±1°C, fluctuating = ±5°C.
[b]   5 = practically perfect, 2 = poor but acceptable, less than 2 = unacceptable.
[c]   1000s/g.
[d]   mg/100 g.

Table 4
PROTEIN EFFICIENCY RATIOS

| | Storage Temperature | | |
|---|---|---|---|
| Storage duration, months | −30°C | −20°C | −10°C |
| Beef patties + 8.5% TVP | | | |
| 3 | 2.45 | 2.54 | 2.72 |
| 6 | 3.08 | 2.70 | 2.55 |
| 12 | 3.01 | 2.72 | 3.00 |
| 18 | 2.74 | 2.75 | 2.58 |
| Beef patties + 8% TVP + 2.5% SCP | | | |
| 3 | 3.01 | 2.84 | 2.60 |
| 6 | 2.72 | 2.76 | 2.51 |
| 12 | 3.40 | 2.62 | 2.88 |
| 18 | 2.95 | 2.61 | 2.63 |
| TVP, rehydrated, canned | | | |
| 3 | 2.45 | 2.23 | 2.46 |
| 6 | 2.06 | 1.95 | 2.09 |
| 12 | 2.51 | 2.41 | 2.29 |
| 18 | 2.14 | 2.30 | 2.52 |

| | −18°C | +10°C | +23°C |
|---|---|---|---|
| TVP, dry stored at 6 months | 1.95 | 1.89 | 1.51 |

*Note:* All data adjusted to casein control = 2.7.

## CANNED FOODS

Low temperature storage of canned foods may be beneficial to nutrient retention in several ways. The most direct benefit is in the usual improvement in nutrient retention. Canned foods packed in less nutritive media such as water, sugar syrup, or starch gravies gradually suffer a leaching effect of the nutrients from the "meat" into the liquor. This leaching process can be delayed by low-temperature storage. For example, Gangal and Magar[34] demonstrated that canned crab meat packed in brine and stored at 80°F lost about 10% of its protein, 50% of its niacin, and 75% of its riboflavin. In all probability much if not all of the protein and niacin losses and a substantial portion of the riboflavin were not actually destroyed, but leached out of the meat into the brine. Thus, if the consumer utilized the crab meat only, these nutrients would be lost to him, as indicated. If, on the other hand, he had utilized the total can contents, a substantial part of the apparently lost nutrients would have been available.

From the refrigeration standpoint, the important information presented was that these very substantial quantities of soluble nutrients were leached out from canned crab meat during even 3 months of storage when stored at ambient temperatures. Even the relatively heat-stable niacin content of crab meat dropped from 0.98 mg% immediately after canning to 0.82 mg% after 3 months of storage, to 0.65 mg% after 6 months and to 0.57 mg% after 9 months storage. It appears that some equilibrium may have been reached between the niacin retained in the meat and that leached out into the liquor in the can after about 1 year of storage. If, however, the meat had been held in refrigerated storage, this leaching process could have been slowed down considerably, and almost completely arrested at freezer temperatures.

### Canned Juices

The major nutritional contribution of fruit and vegetable juices is vitamin C. Citrus and tomato juice are important sources of vitamin C for human nutrition. Other fruit

Table 5

FRUIT AND VEGETABLE JUICES, MAXIMUM STORAGE TEMPERATURES (°C) FOR 90% RETENTION OF VITAMINS, FOR 12 TO 24 MONTHS[35]

| Canned Juice | Ascorbic acid (vitamin C) | | | Thiamin (vitamin B$_1$) | | | Carotene (vitamin A precursor) | | | Niacin | | |
|---|---|---|---|---|---|---|---|---|---|---|---|---|
| | 12 months | 18 months | 24 months | 12 months | 18 months | 24 months | 12 months | 18 months | 24 months | 12 months | 18 months | 24 months |
| Carrot | — | — | — | — | — | — | 27+ | 27+ | 27+ | — | — | — |
| Grapefruit | 18 | 11 | 7 | — | — | — | — | — | — | — | — | — |
| Orange | 20 | 14 | 8 | — | — | — | — | — | — | — | — | — |
| Pineapple | 28 | 25 | 21 | 27 | 27 | 27 | 27+ | 27+ | 27+ | — | — | — |
| Tomato | 24 | 22 | 20 | 23 | 19 | 16 | 27+ | 27+ | 27+ | — | — | — |

$^a$   10% loss in 24 months, no temperature effect.

and vegetable juices also provide some vitamin C as a natural component. In addition, they may be fortified with vitamin C, i.e., ascorbic acid may be added to the juice drink. At storage temperatures of 5°C or less, there are very small losses of vitamin C from fruit juices, not only after 12 months of storage, but even if the canned juices are "held over" from the previous season. When held at 25 to 30°C for periods up to 12 months however, these canned fruit juices lose approximately one quarter of their vitamin C content. When held over for a second year, the loss is approximately 50%. If held at higher temperatures, such as 98°F, which is unusual except in some tropical regions and central continental areas during the summer months, vitamin C content may be reduced to less than half within a 4-month storage period.

The other nutrient present in substantial amounts in fruit and vegetable juices, particularly the orange-colored juices, is vitamin A (actually its precursor, carotene). Carotene in canned fruit and vegetable juices is more stable than is vitamin C so that in general, refrigerated storage for the purpose of preserving vitamin A is not necessary except for extended storage of several years. Although there may be substantial loss of some of the B vitamins, their presence in the juices is so small that they are not major sources of these nutrients. The same can be said for protein. Niacin is particularly stable with little or no loss during storage at 25 to 30°C even for periods longer than 1 year.

The maximum storage temperatures permitting 90% retention of vitamins in a number of juices are summarized in Table 5. The data indicate that canned citrus juices intended for storage up to 2 years should be stored at not higher than 8°C, if 90% of their vitamin C is to be retained. Pineapple and tomato juice, on the other hand, may be stored at 21°C and 16°C, respectively, while carrot juice may be stored at ambient temperatures with no appreciable loss in its most valuable contribution to nutrition — vitamin A.[35]

## Canned Fruits and Vegetables

The same general comments made for fruit juices apply equally to the fruits and those vegetables such as tomatoes that are essentially fruits. Exceptions are the leguminous vegetables such as peas and beans which, particularly in the immature stage, are good sources of vitamin C, as well as vitamins and protein. Canned peas, green beans, and lima beans, for example, lose just a few percent of their vitamin C content when stored at temperatures below 5°C, but lose about 15% when stored at 25 to 30°C for 1 year, and about 25% when stored for longer than 1 year.

Vitamin B₁ (thiamin) losses are more serious, averaging about 25% when stored up to 12 months at ambient temperatures and about 35% when stored longer than 1 year at 27°C. Losses of vitamin B₁ from canned products such as baked beans are practically nonexistent when stored at 0°C or less for as long as 12 months, and only 8% when stored for over 2 years. At 21°C, on the other hand, there is a 16% loss within one year and a 40% loss at the end of the second year of storage. At 38°C there is more than a 50% loss within 1 year and a 75% loss after 2 years of storage.

The maximum storage temperatures for seasonally produced canned food to assure not more than 10% loss of the vitamins that may be declared are summarized in Table 6. Since practically all these products are packed only during a short period of time each year, there is a certain amount of carryover from year of production to the next year. Storage times are therefore shown for 12, 18, and 24 months. These data illustrate clearly that while there may be increasing losses of niacin with time of storage, these losses are not temperature dependent. For some canned products, but by no means for all, this is also true for carotene.

Vitamin C, B₁, B₂ losses, on the other hand, are both time and temperature dependent. It may be concluded that to protect canned asparagus, green and lima beans,

Table 6

MAXIMUM STORAGE TEMPERATURES (°C) FOR CANNED FOODS TO ASSURE NOT MORE THAN 10% LOSS OF VITAMIN C, B₁, CAROTENE, NIACIN, OR RIBOFLAVIN[35,36]

| Canned product | Ascorbic acid (vitamin C) | | | Thiamin (vitamin B₁) | | | Carotene (vitamin A precursor) | | | Niacin | | | Riboflavin (vitamin B₂) | | |
|---|---|---|---|---|---|---|---|---|---|---|---|---|---|---|---|
| | 12 months | 18 months | 24 months | 12 months | 18 months | 24 months | 12 months | 18 months | 24 months | 12 months | 18 months | 24 months | 12 months | 18 months | 24 months |
| Apricots | 25 | 20 | 16 | >0 | — | — | 21 | 17 | 12 | — | — | — | — | — | — |
| Asparagus | 23 | 18 | 15 | 8 | 3 | 0 | 22 | 15 | 8 | — | — | — | 14 | 10 | 8 |
| Beans, green | 16 | 8 | 0 | 14 | 8 | 0 | — | — | — | — | — | — | 14 | 10 | 8 |
| Beans, lima | 22 | 16 | 8 | >0 | — | — | — | — | — | — | — | — | 18 | 5 | 0 |
| Carrots | — | — | — | — | — | — | 27+ | 27+ | 27+ | — | — | — | — | — | — |
| Corn, sweet | 22 | 16 | 10 | 18 | 14 | 12 | 14 | 19 | 24 | — | — | — | 21 | 13 | 8 |
| Frankfurters and beans | — | — | — | 13 | 9 | 6 | — | — | — | — | — | — | — | — | — |
| Grapefruit segments | 16 | 8 | 0 | — | — | — | — | — | — | — | — | — | — | — | — |
| Peaches | 18 | 10 | 5 | 25 | 27 | 29 | 21 | 5 | 0 | — | — | — | — | — | — |
| Peas | 23 | 19 | 11 | 17 | 13 | 10 | 27 | 14 | 8 | — | — | — | 13 | 10 | 8 |
| Plums | — | — | — | — | — | — | 27+ | 27+ | 27+ | — | — | — | — | — | — |
| Pineapple slices | 20 | 12 | 0 | 27 | 27 | 27 | — | — | — | — | — | — | — | — | — |
| Spinach | 20 | 16 | 11 | 17 | 14 | 9 | 8 | 6 | 3 | — | — | — | 17 | 8 | 0 |
| Tomatoes | 20 | 16 | 8 | 21 | 16 | 10 | — | — | — | — | — | — | — | — | — |

* 10% loss in 17 months — no temperature effect.

ᵇ 20% loss in 12 months, 15% in 24 months, no temperature effect.

ᶜ No loss.

ᵈ 10% loss — no time or temperature effect.

ᵉ 8% loss in 12 months, 13% in 24 months, no temperature effect.

ᶠ 20% loss, no time or temperature effect.

grapefruit segments, and peaches from sustaining more than 10% loss of one or more of the important vitamins during a 1- to 2-year storage period, they should be held at 0°C. Apricots, sweet corn, peas, spinach, and tomatoes, may be stored at 7°C to afford the same protection; whole carrots and plums appear to do very well even at relatively high (25 to 30°C) ambient storage, strictly from the nutrient retention standpoint.[35,36]

In addition to improvement in nutrient retention, benefits of cold temperature storage can be demonstrated for canned fruit and vegetable products from the standpoint of aesthetic quality, particularly eye appeal. It is common knowledge that canned green asparagus retains an attractive green color for a year or more when held in cold storage. In ambient storage, however, canned asparagus color changes to a faded yellow within 1 year and is entirely unsalable when held much longer than 1 year in common storage. Canned cherries are an example of canned fruit that benefits greatly in improved retention of "eye appeal" when stored in cold storage. Unsightly browning of ketchup bottle necks can be reduced by low-temperature storage. While destruction of chlorophyll and anthocyanin pigments may be involved in color changes in canned asparagus and cherries, respectively, no nutrients are inactivated. Ketchup browning, however, is probably the result of a Maillard-reaction, which would result in reducing the bioavailability of the ketchup protein.[27,28]

### Canned Meat and Fish

Much of the above discussion applies to canned foods other than fruits and vegetables, except that different nutrients require protection. As stated above, nutrients such as protein, niacin, and riboflavin may not only be destroyed less rapidly if the canned meat is refrigerated, but the rate of leaching of the nutrients from the meat into the liquor is reduced.

Cecil and Woodroof[37] showed that thiamin loss in canned frankfurters and beans is only 10% when stored for 6 months, but increases to 25% in 1 year and to 50% in 3 years. To retain 90% of the thiamin for a full year, storage temperature should be <13°C, <6°C for 2 years, and not higher than 0°C for 3 years.

The same authors[36] demonstrated that canned meat products generally lost about 50% of their thiamin during 6 months of storage and practically 100% after 2 years at 38°C. At 21°C, thiamin loss was about 15% and 45% after 6 and 24 months storage, respectively. When stored at 0°C, however, 10% loss was recorded only after 3 years while at 18°C there was practically no loss of thiamin. Canned salmon stored for 12 months lost 10% of thiamin at 2°C, 25% at 13°C, and 50% at 28°C.

## DRY AND DEHYDRATED FOODS

The beneficial effect of low-temperature storage on retention of sensory as well as nutritional quality of dry and dehydrated foods has been neglected even to a greater extent than for canned foods. Pretreatments such as thorough scalding, reduction of moisture content to less than 3%, packaging in airtight containers and even addition of oxygen scavengers and desiccants into the package have been proposed. Although some of these measures have been shown to be effective in improving protein availability and retention during ambient storage of nutrients, particularly of vitamins A, $B_1$, C, low water activity equivalent to such low moisture contents was found to accelerate lipid oxidation, thereby increasing the rate of development of rancidity and discoloration. It is for such reasons that acceptable fish protein concentrate must contain not more than 0.5% fat. The only way of maintaining both sensory and nutritional quality in dried foods for extended time periods, therefore, is to store them at appropriately low temperatures and low relative humidities, particularly if the dried products

Table 7

MAXIMUM TEMPERATURE (°C) STORAGE TO
RETAIN VITAMIN C LEVELS IN DEHYDRATED
FOODS PACKED IN VACUUM[37]

| Product | Vitamin C loss (%) | Months in storage | | | | | |
|---|---|---|---|---|---|---|---|
| | | 1 | 3 | 6 | 12 | 18 | 24 |
| Onions | 10 | 21 | 13 | 8 | 3 | 0 | − 2 |
| | 25 | 33 | 26 | 21 | 13 | 10 | 17 |
| | 50 | 38 | 38 | 37 | 25 | 22 | 19 |
| Tomato flakes | 10 | — | 38 | 25 | − 4 | −12 | −17 |
| | 25 | — | — | 38 | 8 | − 4 | −12 |
| | 50 | — | — | — | 23 | 10 | 0 |
| Cabbage | 10 | — | 35 | 27 | 13 | − 4 | −10 |
| | 25 | — | — | 35 | 24 | 10 | 2 |
| | 50 | — | — | 38 | 30 | 20 | 10 |
| White potatoes | 10 | 21 | 8 | 0 | − 5 | − 7 | − 8 |
| | 25 | 27 | 16 | 6 | 0 | − 2 | − 3 |
| | 50 | — | 32 | 24 | 16 | −10 | − 8 |
| Rutabagas | 10 | 21 | 13 | 9 | 3 | 0 | − 3 |
| | 25 | 33 | 26 | 21 | 13 | 10 | 7 |
| | 50 | — | 38 | 32 | 26 | 22 | 19 |

are not packed in airtight containers. Tressler,[38] for example, demonstrated practically no loss in vitamin C in tomato flakes stored at 5°C at moisture levels of 1 to 5%. At 21°C storage, however, vitamin C loss in 1%-moisture flakes was 10% and increased to 30% in 5%-moisture flakes. At a storage temperature of 30°C, a 30% loss in vitamin C was obtained within a 32-week storage period even in tomato flakes having only 1% moisture. In 5% moisture flakes the loss was over 80%.

As shown in Table 7, even some dehydrated vegetables that were packaged in airtight containers that were evacuated and/or the air in the container was replaced with an inert gas, showed substantial losses in vitamin C after ambient storage at 3 to 6 months. To retain vitamin C content of onions, tomato flakes, cabbage, white potatoes, and rutabagas, for as long as 1 year, storage temperatures of −5 to +5°C were found necessary. Sweet potatoes and carrots, on the other hand, showed no appreciable losses when stored at ambient temperatures but in fact seemed to gain in vitamins A, B₁ and/or B₂.

Some dehydrated products such as dried citrus powders are highly hygroscopic and must therefore be stored in airtight containers that automatically help preserve nutrients. Other products such as carrot flakes[39] may be stored in vacuum, in inert atmospheres such as nitrogen, or simply in air. Under the former circumstances, vitamin C is retained quite well at a temperature of about 21°C for as long as 2 years. The same product, if stored in air, will lose about 20% of its vitamin C and 70% of its carotene in 2 months at ambient temperatures.

### Effect of Packaging on Flour Protein Quality

Flours, essentially comminuted dry or dehydrated products, respond to low temperature storage and other environmental conditions and treatments in a manner similar to other products as described above. In addition to storage losses of vitamins, particularly vitamin C, such flours are subject not so much to actual losses in total protein content but to the nutritive value of the proteins, unless stored at low temperatures. Thus, CSM, a blend of corn, soy, and milk flour, has been shipped in great quantities, particularly to developing countries, to improve the nutritional quality of a primarily protein-deficient population. In such a mixture where cereal protein predominates, the

Table 8
MAXIMUM STORAGE TEMPERATURE (°C) FOR
LIMITING % LOSS OF PROTEIN NUTRITIVE
VALUE IN DEHYDRATED PRODUCTS

| | Months in storage | | | |
|---|---|---|---|---|
| | 6 | 12 | 18 | 24 |
| Wheat flour[a] | | | | |
| < 10% loss | | | | |
| In sealed jars | 10 | 33 | 0 | − 2 |
| In bags | 3 | − 3 | − 7 | − 9 |
| < 20% loss | | | | |
| In sealed jars | 38 + | 38 + | 38 | 38 |
| In bags | 38 + | — | 21 | 7 |
| Nonfat milk solids[b] | | | | |
| < 10% loss | | | | |
| In bags, 60°RH | − 1 | −22 | — | — |
| In bags, 40°RH | 11 | 3 | — | — |
| < 25% loss | | | | |
| In bags, 60°RH | 24 | − 1 | −18 | −22 |
| In bags, 40°RH | 36 | 8 | − 7 | −14 |
| In vacuum cans | 38 + | 35 | 20 | 11 |
| < 50% loss | | | | |
| In bags, 60°RH | 27 | 17 | 8 | 3 |
| In bags, 40°RH | 38 + | 33 | 30 | 8 |
| In vacuum cans | 38 + | 38 + | 38 | 35 |

[a]   True protein nitrogen, adapted from Jones and Gersdorff.[41]
[b]   Protein efficiency ratio, adapted from Ben-Gera.[42]

amino acid that usually determines the nutritional quality of the protein is lysine. It has been demonstrated by Bookwalter et al.[40] that at a storage temperature of −18°C there is practically no loss in available lysine. At 25°C there is a loss of over 20% of available lysine when stored for about 1 year. At temperatures of 40°C the loss is about 75% in less than 2 months.

Such losses in nutritional protein quality are demonstrated in Table 8 for wheat flour and nonfat milk solids. It appears that for wheat flour that is not sealed in an airtight bag, a storage temperature of 3°C is required to retain 90% of the protein value for 6 months, and still lower temperatures if the flour will be held longer. When stored in sealed jars, 90% protein value retention is maintained at 3°C storage for 12 months.[41]

If the protein value of nonfat milk solids should not be reduced by more than 10% in 6 months, storage temperature must be maintained at −2°C if the milk solids are not in sealed containers and relative humidity is at 60%. For 90% retention of protein quality for 12 months, milk solids must be held in the freezer. Even if relative humidity is lowered to 40%, storage temperature must still be maintained at about 10°C for 6 months of storage and little over −18°C for 12 month's storage. If stored in vacuum in hermetically-sealed containers, however, protein quality loss can be held to 10% for 1 year at +14°C, but even under these conditions freezer temperature storage of −15°C is needed to retain 90% of the protein quality for 2 years. In fact, cooler storage of 4°C is required to prevent more than 50% loss of protein quality of milk solids if they are not adequately packaged or stored at low humidity for longer than 1 year.[42] Similar results were obtained with storage of protein concentrates, including fat-free milk solids, casein, textured protein, and single-cell protein, even when packaged in four-ply paper bags with one 2-mil ply of polyethylene, as shown in Table 9.

Table 9
EFFECT OF STORAGE
TEMPERATURE ON
BIOAVAILABILITY OF PROTEIN
(P.E.R.) IN SOME PROTEIN
CONCENTRATES

| | | Protein efficiency ratio | | |
| | | After 6 months | | Storage at |
| Product | Initial | 22°C | 0°C | −20°C |
|---|---|---|---|---|
| TVP[a] | 2.27 | 2.12 | 2.24 | 2.25 |
| SCP[b] | 2.23 | 1.79 | 2.12 | 2.23 |
| Milk[c] | 2.37 | 1.75 | 2.35 | 2.36 |

*Note:* Reference casein adjusted to 2.7.

[a]   Textured vegetable protein packed in carton with inner liner.
[b]   Single cell protein, produced from alcohol-yeast fermentation, packed in carton with inner liner.
[c]   Defatted milk solids packed in four-ply paper bag with one 2-mil polyethylene ply.

Daoud and Luh[43] found excellent retention of lysine in dehydrated bell peppers packed in aluminum-film combination pouches when stored at 0°C for 12 months, and there was only a 10% loss after 12 months of storage at 20°C. At 30°C, however, the retention of lysine dropped to not more than 13%. Retention of methionine at 0°C was very good, but there was a 12% loss at 20°C and a 75% loss at 30°C after 12 months of storage.

Loss of vitamins A and C in dehydrated vegetable products packed in various containers is also quite serious if not greater than that of amino acids, and the extent of the loss depends on the gas permeability of the packaging film. For a storage life of 12 months, there is rarely more than 10% loss of these vitamins if they are stored in good, tight film pouches at 0°C. At 20°C, however, there is frequently a loss of as much as half of the vitamin content in 6 months and at a temperature of 30°C in 3 to 4 months.[43]

**Dehydrated Meats**

As with canned meats, the serious nutritional losses that might be expected are in protein availability and the B vitamins. Thiamin retention in stored dehydrated pork may serve as an example. To maintain 90% of the thiamin for just 1 month, storage temperature may not exceed 13°C — substantially higher than for the canned pork. For 12 months of storage, however, a cooler temperature of 0 to 5°C is adequate for 90% retention of the thiamin for both dehydrated and canned pork. At ambient temperatures of 21°C, dehydrated pork will lose over 25% within just 1 month, while a similar loss will not occur in canned pork until after 6 months storage. It appears, therefore, that while cooler storage is desirable for canned meats held for 6 months or longer, it is practically a necessity for dehydrated meats, even if they are to be held in storage for only 2 to 3 months (Table 10).[44]

## Table 10
## A COMPARISON OF CANNED
## AND DEHYDRATED PORK[44]

Maximum Storage Temperatures
(°C) for Limiting % Loss of
Thiamin[a]

|  | %<br>Loss | Months in storage | | | |
|---|---|---|---|---|---|
|  |  | 1 | 3 | 6 | 12 |
| Canned | 10 | 30 | 9 | 3 | 0 |
|  | 25 | — | 27 | 25 | 17 |
|  | 50 | — | 38 | 34 | 21 |
| Dehydrated | 10 | 13 | 11 | 9 | 8 |
|  | 25 | 20 | 16 | 14 | 13 |
|  | 50 | 31 | 24 | 22 | 20 |

**Dehydrated Eggs**

Highly nutritious dehydrated eggs should be held in freezer storage if satisfactory levels of nutrients, particularly vitamin A, are to be maintained for longer than 1 month. As shown in Table 11, maximum temperature of storage for dehydrated eggs packed in barrels is 27°C if there is to be 90% retention of vitamin A over a 1-month storage period. If 90% retention is required for a 12-month period, freezer temperatures should be maintained at −24°C. If freezer temperature is at −18°C, vitamin A loss during 1 year of storage will exceed 25% and will reach 50% if storage temperature is about −12°C.

Requirements for thiamin retention in dehydrated eggs are not quite as rigid, but −18°C storage is required for 90% thiamin retention for a full year. If 25% loss of thiamin is permissible, then storage can be maintained at 0°C. At this temperature, however, there will be a 50% loss in vitamin A.

For other vitamins such as B₂, niacin, pantothenic acid, and D, there is little change as a result of time or temperature of storage up to 9 months. Beyond that time period, there is also a rapidly increasing loss of some of these vitamins.[45]

## CONCENTRATED FOODS

Concentrated foods generally behave in an intermediate manner between the single-strength and dehydrated products. Tomato paste, for example, loses vitamin C three times as rapidly as canned peeled tomatoes or tomato juice; however, it should be pointed out that the vitamin C concentration in the tomato paste is much higher than in the single-strength products.[46]

Canned cheese, a concentrated milk product, retains vitamin A very well for up to 2 years at 21°C. If, however, it is to be maintained for longer than 2 years, it should be stored at 10°C. Riboflavin losses in the canned cheese reach about 15% at 21°C in 2 years, increasing rather sharply beyond that time. It appears, therefore, that for canned cheeses, ambient-temperature storage is adequate for 1 year or more but if the cheese is to be stored for 2 years or longer, it should be held in the refrigerator even if it is processed and hermetically sealed in a can. Condensed milk, another concentrated milk product that is usually canned, shows no appreciable losses of vitamins except for thiamin, which may be maintained at reasonably high levels in prolonged storage only at refrigerator temperatures.

Vitamin C retention in marmalade[47] and thiamin retention in peanut butter[36] are

### Table 11
### MAXIMUM STORAGE
### TEMPERATURES (°C) FOR
### LIMITING LOSSES OF THIAMIN
### AND VITAMIN A IN DEHYDRATED
### EGGS[45]

|  | %<br>Loss | Months in storage | | | |
|---|---|---|---|---|---|
|  |  | 1 | 3 | 6 | 12 |
| Thiamin | 10 | — | 33 | 5 | −18 |
|  | 25 | — | 37 | 31 | 0 |
|  | 50 | — | — | 37 | 31 |
| Vitamin A | 10 | 27 | −15 | −18 | −24 |
|  | 25 | 34 | −12 | −16 | −19 |
|  | 50 | — | 18 | 2 | −12 |

### Table 12
### MAXIMUM STORAGE TEMPERATURES (°C)
### FOR LIMITING CERTAIN NUTRIENT LOSSES
### OF SOME CONCENTRATED FOODS

| Concentrated food | %<br>Loss | Months in storage | | | | | |
|---|---|---|---|---|---|---|---|
|  |  | 1 | 3 | 6 | 12 | 18 | 24 |
| Marmalade, citrus |  |  |  |  |  |  |  |
| Vitamin C | 10 | 22 | 11 | 8 | 6 | — | — |
|  | 25 | 38 | 23 | 18 | 12 | — | — |
|  | 50 | — | 34 | 27 | 18 | — | — |
| Peanut butter |  |  |  |  |  |  |  |
| Thiamin | 10 | — | — | 38 | 30 | 21 | 18 |
|  | 25 | — | — | — | — | 38 | 32 |
| Condensed milk | 10 | 21 | 10 | 5 | 1 | — | — |
|  | 25 | 33 | 22 | 13 | 9 | — | — |
|  | 50 | — | 34 | 26 | 16 | — | — |

[a]  Lincoln and McCay.[47]
[b]  Cecil and Woodroof.[36]
[c]  Cecil and Woodroof.[37]

shown in Table 12. It may be seen that from the standpoint of thiamin retention, at least, cold storage is not required for peanut butter unless it is to be held for well over 1 year. Rapid losses of vitamin C in citrus marmalade, on the other hand, indicate the need for refrigeration of this product, which is a very good source of vitamin C, even if it is to be stored for just a few months. At ambient temperatures of 21 to 27°C, there is a 10% loss of vitamin C within 1 month, a 25% loss with 3 months, and 50% loss in little more than 6 months.

## SOME GENERAL PRINCIPLES

With the possible exception of ascorbic acid, there are insufficient data to predict the fate of the various nutrients during storage, although there is good reason to believe that, with more than a few notable exceptions, nutrient losses in storage follow a first-order reaction. Heat is undoubtedly the prime cause of nutrient losses, particularly ascorbic acid, thiamin, folic acid, and the amino acid lysine. Riboflavin and vitamin

A are similarly influenced in some instances but not in others, while niacin, carotene, and gross protein content, in most cases are time-temperature independent.

Long-term effects of temperature may be attenuated by prompt, short, high-temperature treatment which inactivates enzymes in the fresh foods and in the microorganisms in the food environment. While the heat treatment may cause an immediate moderate reduction in nutrients, remaining nutrients may be stabilized so that their subsequent rate of destruction during prolonged storage is reduced.

The most direct method of preventing nutrient losses in storage is low temperature. Although benefits of low temperature storage are frequently assumed to follow $Q_{10}$ = 2, i.e., reduction in nutrient loss rate by half with every reduction of 10°C, $Q_{10}$ is rarely equal to two or even three. While it is frequently four, it may be as high as 50.[48,49] Thus, fresh foods which do not suffer frost damage, should be stored at or slightly above their freezing point. Foods containing low moisture levels rarely suffer appreciable nutrient losses, even in prolonged storage at or below −10°C. Some high-moisture foods may sustain nutrient losses even at −10°C, or lower.

Moisture content and presence of oxygen in the environment (within the package) are also important in nutrient retention, particularly with low-moisture foods. Variable effects on different nutrients in different food media, are created by the pH level.

# REFERENCES

1. **Richardson, K. C.**, Shelf life of packaged foods, *CSIRO Food Res. Q.*, 36(1), 1—9, 1976.
2. **Lachance, P. A., Ranadive, A. S., and Matas, J.**, Effects of reheating convenience foods, *Food Technol.*, (Chicago), 27(1), 36-38, 1973.
3. **Edwards, C. C.**, Nutrition labeling, *Fed. Regist.*, 38(13), Part III, 2125—2130, 1973.
4. **Kramer, A. and Smith, J.**, Palatability and nutritive value of fresh, canned, and frozen collard greens, *J. Am. Soc. Hortic. Sci.*, 97(2), 161-163, 1972.
5. **Cain, R. F.**, Water soluble vitamins — changes during processing and storage of fruits and vegetables, *Food Technol.*, (Chicago), 21(7), 60-69, 1967.
6. ASHRAE Guide and Data Book, Applications, p. 464, 1971.
7. **Kramer, A., Guyer, R. B., Ide, L. E.**, Factors affecting the objective and organoleptic evaluation of quality in sweet corn, *J. Am. Soc. Hortic. Sci.*, 54, 342-356, 1949.
8. **Dewey, D. H., Herner, R. C., and Dilley, D. R., Eds.** *Controlled Atmospheres for the Storage and Transport of Horticultural Crops*, Horticultural Report, No. 9, Michigan State University, 1969.
9. **Heideman, R. and Lund, D. B.**, Influence of Respiration of Wild Rice Kernels on Yield Losses During Storage, Paper No. 426, Proc., 36th Meeting, Instit. Food Technol., Anaheim, Calif., June 9, 1976.
10. **Urban, B.**, Application of Refrigeration Technology in Deep Silo Storage of Grains, Paper No. D 1.32., in Proc. XIV Int. Congr. Refrigeration, Moscow, September 1975.
11. Institute for Technology and Storage, Scientific Activities, Volcani Cent. Agric. Res., Bet Dagan, Israel, Annual Report, 1974-1975.
12. U.S. Department of Agriculture Northern Regional Res. Lab., Proc. Collaborators Conf., Philadelphia, July 1975.
13. **Berg, G. L., Ed.**, Master manual on molds and mycotomins, *Farm Technol.*, (Chicago), 28(5), 19-49, 1972.
14. **Heinze, P. H.**, Effects of Storage, Transportation, and Marketing Conditions on the Composition and Nutritional Values of Fresh Fruit and Vegetables, U.S. Department of Agriculture Eastern Regional Res. Lab. Publ. No. 3786, Philadelphia, 1973, 29-34.
15. **Scott, L. E. and Kramer, A.**, Physiological changes in asparagus after harvest, *Proc. Am. Soc. Hortic. Sci.*, 54, 357-366, 1949.
16. **Scott, L. E. and Kramer, A.**, Effect of storage upon ascorbic acid content of tomatoes harvested at different stages of maturity, *Proc. Am. Soc. Hortic. Sci.*, 54, 277—280, 1949.
17. **Siegel, T.**, Relation of the Curve of Growth to Ascorbic Acid and Glutathione Production in the Pea, M. Sci. thesis, University of Maryland, College Park, Maryland, 1947.

18. **Underdal, B., Nordal, J., Lunde, G., and Eggum, B.,** The effect of ionizing radiation on the nutritional value of mackerel, *Lebensm. Wiss. Technol.* 9, 2, 72—74, 1976.
19. **Besser, T. and Kramer, A.,** Changes in quality and nutritional composition of foods preserved by gas exchange, *J. Food Sci.,* 37, 820-823, 1972.
20. **Delaporte, N.,** Influence de la teneur en oxygen des atmospheres sur le taux d'acide ascorbique des pommes au cours de leur conservation, *Lebensm. Wiss Technol.* 4, 106-112, 1971.
21. Proc. Northeastern Regional Fruit Marketing Comm., Rutgers University, New Brunswick, New Jersey, 1975.
22. **Seideman, S. C., Carpenter, Z. L., Smith, G. C., and Hoke, K. E.,** Effect of degree of vacuum and length of storage on the physical characteristics of vacuum packed beef wholesale cuts, *J. Food Sci.,* 41(4), 732-737, 1976.
23. **Van Arsdel, W. B., Copley, M. J., and Olson, R. L.,** *Quality and Stability of Frozen Foods,* Wiley-Interscience, 1969.
24. **Bengtsson, M., Liljemark, A., Olsson, P., and Nilsson, B.,** An attempt to systemize time-temperature-tolerance (T.T.T.) data as a basis for the development of time-temperature indicators, *Bull. Inst. Int. Froid,* Annexe 2, 303-311, 1972.
25. **Labuza, T. P.,** Effects of dehydration and storage, *Food Technol., (Chicago),* 27(1), 20-26, 1973.
26. **Lee, Y. C., Kirk, J. R., Heldman, D. R., and Medford, C. L.,** Kinetics and computer simulation of nutritional quality degradation in canned tomato juice during storage, Paper No. 421, in Proc. 36th Meet. Inst. Food Technol., June 9, 1976.
27. **Kramer, A.,** Storage retention of nutrients, *Food Technol., (Chicago),* 28(1), 50-60, 1974.
28. **Goldblith, S. A.,** Food processing, nutrition and the feeding of man during the next 25 years, *Proc. Frigoscandia Symp. World Food Supply and Refrigeration,* Frigoscandia AB, Halsinborg, Sweden, May 23, 1975, 17-38.
29. **Guadagni, D. C. and Kelly, S. H.,** Time-temperature tolerance of frozen foods. XIV. Ascorbic acid and its oxidation products as a measure of temperature history in frozen strawberries, *Food Technol. (Chicago)* 12(12), 645-647, 1958.
30. **Davis, L. G.,** Below zero temperature important for vitamin retention in frozen foods, *Food Can.,* 16(4), 24-30, 1956.
31. **Haggart, R. L., Harman, D. A., and Moore, E. L.,** *J. Am. Diet. Assoc.,* 39, 682, 1954.
32. **DuBois, C. W. and Kew, T. S.,** *Refrig. Eng.,* 59, 772, 1954.
33. **Kramer, A., King, R. L., and Westhoff, D. C.,** Effects of frozen storage on prepared foods containing protein concentrates, *Food Technol. (Chicago),* 30(1), 46—62, 1976.
34. **Gangal, S. and Magar, N. G.,** Canning and storage of crabmeat, *Food Technol., (Chicago),* 21(3A), 397-400, 1967.
35. **Feaster, J. F.,** *Nutritional Evaluation of Food Processing,* Harris, R. S. and Von Loesecke, H., Eds., John Wiley & Sons, New York, 1960, 337-358.
36. **Cecil, S. R. and Woodroof, J. G.,** The stability of canned foods in long-term storage, *Food Technol., (Chicago),* 17(5), 131-138, 1963.
37. **Cecil, S. R. and Woodroof, J. G.,** Long-term storage of military rations, *Georgia Exp. Stn. Tech. Bull.,* 25, 1962.
38. **Tressler, D. T.,** New developments in the dehydration of fruits and vegetables, *Food Technol., (Chicago),* 10, 119-124, 1956.
39. **Stephens, T. S. and McLemore, T. A.,** Preparation and storages of dehydrated carrot flakes, *Food Technol., (Chicago),* 23(12), 104-109, 1969.
40. **Bookwalter, G. N., Moser, H. A., Kwolek, W. F., Pfeifer, V. F., and Griffin, E. L., Jr.,** Storage stability of CSM: alternate formulations for corn-soy-milk, *J. Food Sci.,* 36(5), 732, 1971.
41. **Jones, D. and Gersdorff, J.,** The effect of storage on the protein of wheat, white flour and whole wheat, *Cereal Chem. Bull.,* 18, 417-423, 1941.
42. **Ben-Gera, I.,** Changes in the Nitrogenous Constituents of Staple Foods and Feeds Under Storage Conditions, Ph.D. thesis, Technion, Haifa, Israel, 1965.
43. **Daoud, H. N. and Luh, B. S.,** Packaging of foods in laminate and aluminum-combination pouches. IV. Freeze dried red bell peppers, *Food Technol., (Chicago),* 21(3A), 339-343, 1967.
44. **Rice, E. E. and Robinson, H. E.,** Nutritive value of canned and dehydrated meat products, *Am. J. Public Health,* 34, 587, 1944.
45. **Klose, A. H., Jones, G. I., and Fevold, H. L.,** Vitamin content of spray dried whole egg, *Ind. Eng. Chem.* 35, 1203-1206, 1943.
46. **Hummel, M. and Okey, R.,** Relation of concentration of canned tomato products to storage losses of ascorbic acid, *Food Res.,* 15, 405, 1950.
47. **Lincoln, R. and McCay, C. M.,** Retention of ascorbic acid in marmalade during preparation and storage, *Food Res.,* 10, 357-359, 1945.

48. **Kramer, A. and Farquhar, J. W.,** Testing of time-temperature indicating and defrost devices, *Food Technol. (Chicago)*, 30(2), 50-56, 1976.
49. **Labuza, T. P.,** Should specify reaction order, *Food Technol., (Chicago)*, 30(5), 34, 1976.

*Specific Foods*

# EFFECT OF PROCESSING ON NUTRIENT COMPOSITION OF FOODS: FRUITS AND FRUIT PRODUCTS

## Harold R. Bolin*

## INTRODUCTION

Fruits have traditionally played an important part in man's diet. In the earlier years it was strictly a seasonal item which could only be consumed in the fresh state. The earliest science of food preservation began to develop with the discovery that foods would not support microbial growth and decomposition if most of the water was removed. By sun-drying foods, man began to enjoy a greater variety of food products in his regular diet. With the advent of modern processing methods, an even larger variety of flavorful and healthful products became available to the consumer throughout the year. This is especially noticed in fruits and fruit-related products. This has resulted in a steady increase in the consumption of processed fruits. From 1940 to 1970, the per capita consumption of fresh fruits dropped from 110 lb to 24 lb. However, during the same time, the total consumption of process fruits increased from 30 lb to 56 lb per person, and there is every indication that this trend will continue.

Fruits are consumed for their flavor and nutritional properties. Fruits are a good source of vitamin C, providing about 35% of this vitamin to the diet (Table 1).[1] In addition they are an aid in regulating the body's elimination processes.

The nutrient composition of foods is not static, but changes even during the growing cycle. The goal of food preservation is to provide a flavorful, nutritious, and attractive product that will retain these qualities during extended storage. We experience a better standard of living today because of our year-round availability of high quality nutritious foods. Processing can destroy some food nutrients, as can also cold storage. The amount of change depends upon many factors, such as the maturity, variety, and condition of the fruit, as well as the particular processing conditions used. Table 2 indicates the relative stability of some of the vitamins and amino acids under various conditions.[2] Vitamin A is sensitive to heat in the presence of oxygen and to ultraviolet light. Ascorbic acid decomposes rapidly in the presence of copper, iron, oxygen, or alkalies. Biotin is susceptible to oxidation in the presence of strong acids or bases. Vitamin D is slowly destroyed in an alkaline medium or in the presence of light and air. Folic acid decomposes if held at high temperatures in either an acid or alkaline solution, especially in the presence of oxygen and light. Some essential fatty acid losses occur when they are heated in an alkaline solution and subjected to light, oxygen, and high temperature. Riboflavin is sensitive to light, especially at higher pH and temperature. Thiamin is unstable in air at higher temperatures and is destroyed when it is exposed to sulfites, alkaline conditions, or autoclaving. The tocopherols oxidize easily, even at room temperature, and they are also sensitive to alkalies, ferric salts, and ultraviolet light. Therefore, the degree that a particular processing method violates the stability requirements of these individual nutrients determines the nutrient loss in the final product.

## PRESERVATION METHOD

### Canning

Canned fruits can be divided into two categories, those canned without peeling and

---

* Figures and tables appear at end of text.

those peeled before canning. This preparatory treatment influences the nutrient retention during processing because of the larger surface of cut tissue that is available for oxidation reactions and loss of soluble solids.

Unpeeled fruit is exposed to a minimum of handling before being placed in the can for processing. For most fruits, this pretreatment consists mainly of washing; however, it may sometimes include a pit-removal operation, such as with cherries. Guerrant et al.[3] found that Montmorency cherries retained 96% of their ascorbic acid during processing and that their retention of carotenoids was essentially complete. With cranberries, canning the whole fruit product results in about a 25% loss of vitamin C, but if the product is strained to produce a smooth sauce, over 80% of this vitamin is lost.[4,5] The pumping and straining operation evidently causes a rapid degradation of this vitamin. In preparing cranberry juice, the freshly expressed product does not lose any of its vitamin C. However, upon pasteurization and bottling it is essentially all lost. When guava is canned, it also loses most of its vitamin C, especially if the fruit is very mature.[6] Strawberries were found to lose about 50% of their ascorbic acid upon canning; however, when they were made into jam this loss was reduced.[7] With canned, unpeeled apricots, an ascorbic acid retention of about 85% and a carotenoid retention of 89% is usually realized[8] (Table 3). Maturity influences final quality, with the riper fruit being higher in total solids, ascorbic acid, and vitamin A.

In studying the nutrient losses of peeled peaches during processing, Lamb et al.[9] found essentially no loss of β-carotene. If the peeled fruit was exposed to air for 30, 60, or 120 min, there was a loss of 29, 34, and 45% ascorbic acid, respectively. Slices exposed for similar times lost 42, 52, and 58%, respectively. There was also a distinct drop in ascorbic acid and thiamin after lye peeling, and a further drop if the fruit was held for very long before being processed (Figure 1). Ascorbic acid did show a slight increase after processing, with thiamin continuing to decrease. Niacin was relatively stable through all operations. Mitchell et al.[10] did notice that the canning process caused the carotenoids of peaches to be degraded, with only about 50% remaining in the final product.

The lye-peeling step is the most severe on ascorbic acid and thiamin degradation in peaches. The least destruction of these vitamins is obtained when the peaches are held in the peeling bath for a minimum time. In addition, the time lapse between preparation and processing needs to be limited. With freestone peaches, steam is sometimes used to loosen the peel, after which it is removed by hand. In studying an operation at a commercial cannery, Lamb et al.[9] found a 72 to 86% ascorbic acid retention after steam peeling and 59 to 70% after processing. This would indicate that steam peeling is more destructive to ascorbic acid than lye peeling. They found also that there was a carotenoid retention of 100%, a thiamin retention of 71 to 93%, and a niacin retention of 82 to 86%.

Elkins et al.[11] studied vitamin degradation in clingstone peaches canned and retorted by two different procedures, with the emphasis on ascorbic acid and thiamin (Table 4). Retorting did not have any significant effect on vitamin losses or on carotene stereoisomer changes in clingstone peaches (Table 5). Also, the processing method did not markedly affect mineral loss, which would be expected, since the fruit is not blanched (Table 6). Retorting method did not have any effect. They also found that the total solids and the protein and carbohydrate contents were slightly higher in the solid portion of canned peaches, as compared to the liquid (Table 7). The differences, which are about 0.6% (0.3% of the total carbohydrates) are accounted for by this loss being the approximate amount of insoluble carbohydrates in canned peaches. There is no significant difference between the liquid and solid phases in the water-soluble vitamins; however, the water-insoluble carotene is all in the fruit. Calcium, magnesium and phosphorous are higher in the solid portion by 17, 26, and 42%, respectively. Copper is also higher in the solids. Brush et al.[12] studied this relationship with respect to other canned fruits (Table 8).

Apples have an active ascorbic acid oxidase system which can accelerate the degradation of this vitamin during processing. For example, in the preparation of apple juice, most of the vitamin C is thought to be lost during the disintegrating step. However, if the process could be modified to where the apples were rapidly disintegrated in the absence of oxygen and quickly pasteurized, the juice should contain almost all of its original ascorbic acid.

Citrus fruits are recognized as a good source of vitamin C. The stability of this vitamin in grapefruit juice was studied by determining the average ascorbic acid retention in juice processed by different commercial canneries from Florida to California (Table 9). There was an average retention of 97%, with greater losses occurring in plants where the hot, freshly expressed juice came into direct contact with copper alloys, or if the hot juice was held for any length of time before cooling.

The effect of processing on biotin, folic acid, pyridoxine, and inositol in canned grapefruit juice was studied by Krehl and Cowgill.[13] They found little change in these vitamins as a result of the canning operation or storage. This same stability was found with orange juice, where there was an ascorbic acid retention of over 98% (Table 9). With orange juice, aeration and length of holding time did not have as great an influence on ascorbic acid loss as it did with grapefruit juice. However, here again the juice should not come in direct contact with copper.

Prune juice production differs from other juice manufacturing methods in that it is made by a water extraction of the soluble solids from dried prunes. Because of this extraction method, the final canned juice does not contain any of the fat-soluble components of the whole prunes. Prunes are high in vitamin A, but prune juice does not contain any since this fat-soluble vitamin is held up on the fruit fiber. Bolin et al.[14] developed a rapid procedure for making prune juice, where a portion of the finer fiber is incorporated into the final juice. By using this procedure, prune juice that contained 260 IU vitamin A per 100 g was produced (Table 10).

Overall, nutrient loss from the canning operation is minimal if the products are processed properly. This preservation method has the advantage of producing a product that is ready to eat, and also a product that can be stored at room temperature. With the recent advent of flexible pouches capable of being retorted, these products will continue to command a definite place in the consumer's kitchen.

## Drying

Drying method has an influence on nutrient retention in some fruits. With apricot halves, the drying method affects significantly carotenoid retention.[15] If the halves were sulfured and then hot air dehydrated, no noticeable carotenoid degradation occurred. However, if they were sun dried, there was a 10% loss (Figure 2). A loss was also noticed in producing leather, where the sun-dried, sulfured product had a 20% greater loss of carotene than the sulfured dehydrated or shade-dried products (Table 11). Similar effects were observed in unsulfured samples.

Sulfuring also affects carotenoid loss during drying, where only a slight difference was noticed in dried halves, but a more pronounced effect was observed from drum drying. Apricot sheets prepared by drum drying the sulfur-free concentrate lost 12% of the $\beta$-carotene during drying, compared to a 5% loss in the sample prepared from the 0.3% sulfured puree (Table 12).

Processing and drying method did not have as great an effect on ascorbic acid as it did on $\beta$-carotene. Halves dried without sulfuring lost 95% of their ascorbic acid during drying, compared to a 75% loss from the sulfured samples (Figure 2). Drum-dried sulfured puree also retained more ascorbic acid than the unsulfured product. Drying methods did have some effect, which was noticed in apricot leather production where sun-dried, shade-dried, and dehydrated samples lost 29, 19, and 12%, respectively.

Other drum-dried products have been found to lose nutrients during processing. Escher and Neukom,[16] in their production of apple flakes, found that there was an 8% loss of ascorbic acid during the slicing operation, 62% during blanching, 10% from pureeing, and 5% during the drum-drying step.

Dried fruits tend to lose some vitamins during their drying process. For example, dried figs contain 42% less riboflavin, 48% less thiamin, 37% less niacin, and 33% less pantothenic acid than the fresh fruit.[17] Also, drying unsulfured fruits in the sun accelerates vitamin C loss. Raisins dried in the sun lose almost all of the vitamin C during drying; however, this is not serious since the fresh grapes are not high in this vitamin originally. Dried prunes also contain almost no ascorbic acid; however, the fresh fruit does contain some. When the prunes are dried by hot air dehydration, they have a higher vitamin content, especially A, $B_1$, and riboflavin.[18] If the fruit is sulfured, most of the vitamin C is retained, but most of the $B_1$ is destroyed.

Another fruit that loses vitamin C during drying is cranberries. The drying procedure consists of pricking the berry skin with steel needles and dehydrating for 8 to 12 hr at 49 to 65°C. The resultant product, which contains about 5% moisture, loses about 55% of its ascorbic acid during the drying.[4,5] Also, because of the large surface area exposed, the remaining ascorbic acid is rapidly lost during storage.

Orange juice powder can be prepared by freeze drying or vacuum puff-drying. Foda et al.[19] observed that when a freeze-dried product was produced, there was only a slight ascorbic acid or $\beta$-carotene loss (Table 13). In preparing vacuum puff-dried orange juice powder from concentrate, Curl and Bailey[20] found that the carotenoid distribution was not altered (Table 14), nor was there any loss in the provitamin A (cryptoxanthin and $\alpha$- and $\beta$-carotene) during concentration. The frozen sixfold concentrated Florida valencia orange juice contained 39 ppm total carotenoids, as did the powder, indicating that drying the product to a 3% moisture powder was not detrimental to the carotenoids.

Niacin and riboflavin are water-soluble, but they are fairly stable to heat, oxidation, and sulfiting. Hollingsworth[21] found that neither of these vitamins, nor $B_{12}$, were lost to any degree during dehydration. Ascorbic acid is easily oxidized, especially at higher temperatures, but it is stabilized to a degree by sulfite addition.

The main loss of the fat-soluble vitamins that occur during dehydration, and also storage, is thought to be due to their interaction with the peroxides of free radicals.[22] The peroxides and radicals are produced from the oxidation of the lipids in the product; therefore, anything that would prevent lipid oxidation should increase the retention of the fat-soluble vitamins, like vitamin A and tocopherol.

Fruits are not recognized as a protein source, but they do contain an average of about 3%. Proteins are fairly stable to food preservation procedures. However, hot air dehydration in general causes a slight reduction in protein quality that does not occur in products that are freeze-dried;[23] also biological availability continues to decrease if the product is subjected to higher temperatures. This emphasizes that with drying, as with other preservation methods, the product should not be subjected to a higher temperature than is absolutely necessary, and only for a minimum time.

### Freezing

There is a limited amount of information available on the effect of freezing on nutrient loss. Some workers compiled a table using information from the United States Department of Agriculture Handbook 8 and indicated that there was an appreciable vitamin loss from freezing fruits[2] (Table 15). However, some of these losses could be from the trimming and peeling operation. Specifically an average of 15% of vitamin B₆ and 7% of pantothenic acid was lost from fruits in general during the freezing operation.[24] Loeffler[25] found that there was no loss of ascorbic acid during freezing of raspberries, as did Wolfe et al.[26] with grapefruit sections. However, there was a loss of about 70% of reduced vitamin C in frozen muskmelons.

## Fermentation

Wine, which is the naturally fermented juice of fresh grapes, is not known for its vitamin or mineral content. Fresh grapes contain up to 18 mg ascorbic acid per 100 g. However, finished wines never have more than about 8 mg/100 g and in many there is none.[27] A large percentage of the ascorbic acid is probably lost during the grape-crushing step. Thiamin ranges from 0.1 to 1.2 mg per liter in must, but is markedly degraded by the sulfiting treatment that is used in some wines. Up to 50% of the riboflavin is lost. Also, sugar content is greatly reduced in the fermentation step, with ethanol and carbon dioxide being produced.

## Gamma Radiation

Gamma radiation is not used to a significant degree in commercial food preparation. Experimentally, Salunkhe et al.[28] studied the effect of doses of up to $3.7 \times 10^6$ rads on various fruits and fruit products. They found that radiation at this level did not have any apparent effect on the carotenoids of canned apricot nectar, peach nectar, or peach halves. The radiation did affect anthocyanin pigment and texture, especially at higher radiation levels. The texture effect can be caused by the degradation of intercellular pectin and cellulose.[29,30]

## SUMMARY

As a greater percentage of our fruits continue to be processed by some method of food preservation, there will continue to remain the challenge to the food processor to produce a product that will retain an ever increasing amount of the original nutrients of the food. This challenge is being met today by developing processing procedures that are faster and less damaging, such as in the heat processing of products in flexible pouches, where the heating and cooling time are greatly reduced. Also, process modifications will continue to be made as more basic information is obtained on factors that contribute to nutrient degradation. This information, coupled with our computer technology, will enable the food processor in the near future to readily predetermine the optimum parameters for a given processing operation to insure a retention of the greatest amount of nutrients.

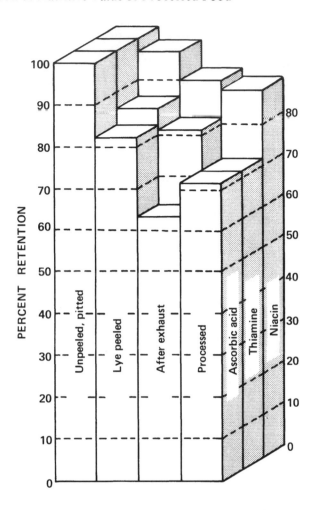

FIGURE 1.   Retention of ascorbic acid, thiamin, and niacin during the commercial canning of clingstone peaches. (From Lamb, F. C., *Retention of Nutrients During Canning*, National Canners Association, Berkeley, Calif., 1955, 15. With permission.)

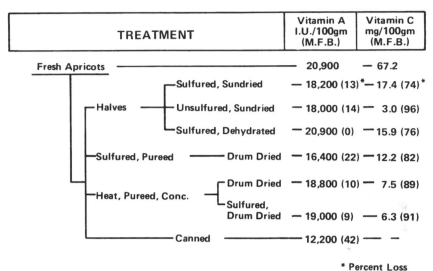

FIGURE 2.    Vitamin A and C content of processed apricots.

### Table 1
### VITAMINS: PERCENTAGE OF TOTAL CONTRIBUTION BY FOOD GROUPS — 1968

| Food Group | Vitamin A | Thiamin | Riboflavin | Niacin | Ascorbic acid |
|---|---|---|---|---|---|
| Meat, poultry, fish | 22.9 | 29.4 | 24.6 | 46.0 | 1.1 |
| Eggs | 6.8 | 2.5 | 5.9 | 0.1 | 0 |
| Dairy products | 11.8 | 9.9 | 43.1 | 1.7 | 4.7 |
| Fats and oils | 8.6 | 0.0 | 0.0 | 0.0 | 0.0 |
| Fruits | 7.3 | 4.3 | 2.0 | 2.5 | 35.0 |
| Potatoes (inc. sweet) | 5.7 | 6.7 | 1.9 | 7.6 | 20.9 |
| Vegetables | 36.4 | 8.0 | 5.6 | 6.8 | 38.3 |
| Dry beans and peas | TR | 5.5 | 1.8 | 7.0 | Tr |
| Flour (cereal prod.) | 0.4 | 33.6 | 14.2 | 22.7 | 0.0 |
| Sugar and sweeteners | 0.0 | Tr | 0.1 | Tr | 0.0 |
| Total | 100% | 100% | 100% | 100% | 100% |
| | 7700 IU | 1.82 mg | 2.24 mg | 22.1 mg | 107 mg |

*Note:* Quantities available for consumption per capita per day, 1968.

From Hein, R. E. and Hutchings, I. J., *Nutrients in Processed Foods — Vitamins, Minerals,* American Medical Association, Publishing Sciences Group, Acton, Mass., 1974, 67. With permission.

## Table 2
## STABILITY OF NUTRIENTS

| Vitamins | | Essential amino acids | |
|---|---|---|---|
| Vitamin A | 2, 3 | Isoleucine | 1—6 |
| Ascorbic acid | 1 | Leucine | 1—6 |
| Biotin | 1—5 | Lysine | 1—5 |
| Choline | 1—3, 5, 6 | Methionine | 1—6 |
| Cobalamine | 1—3, 6 | Phenylalanine | 1—6 |
| Vitamin D | 2 | Threonine | 2, 4, 5 |
| Folic acid | 3 | Tryptophan | 2—4, 6 |
| Inositol | 1—5 | Valine | 1—6 |
| Vitamin K | 2, 4, 6 | | |
| Niacin | — | | |
| Pantothenic acid | 2, 4, 5 | | |
| p-Amino benzoic acid | 1—3, 5, 6 | | |
| Pyridoxine | 1—4 | | |
| Riboflavin | 1, 2, 4 | | |
| Thiamin | 1, 5 | | |
| Tocopherol | 1—3 | | |

*    Stable to: 1-low pH, 2-mid pH, 3-high pH, 4-oxygen, 5-light, 6-heat.

## Table 3
## ASCORBIC ACID AND CAROTENE CONTENT OF RAW AND CANNED APRICOTS OF DIFFERENT DEGREES OF MATURITY AND THE RETENTION OF ASCORBIC ACID AND CAROTENE AFTER CANNING

| Code variety | Growing district | Maturity | Total solids raw fruit (%) | Apricot solids canned fruit (%) | Ascorbic Acid Actual values (mg/100g) Raw | Canned | Retention[a] (%) | Carotene Actual values (mg/100g) Raw | Canned | Retention[a] (%) |
|---|---|---|---|---|---|---|---|---|---|---|
| A 1 Blenheim | Santa Clara | Soft-ripe | 16.4 | 10.3 | 12.6 | 7.4 | 94 | 2.02 | 1.24 | 98 |
| 2 | | Ripe | 15.2 | 9.6 | 11.1 | 5.7 | 81 | 1.61 | 0.85 | 84 |
| 3 | | Firm-ripe | 13.6 | 8.6 | 10.8 | 5.5 | 81 | 1.08 | 0.56 | 82 |
| 4 | | Immature | 13.1 | — | 10.2 | — | — | 0.85 | — | — |
| B 1 Blenheim | Hollister | Soft-ripe | 17.8 | 10.6 | 12.0 | 6.0 | 84 | 2.04 | 1.16 | 96 |
| 2 | | Ripe | 15.1 | 9.6 | 10.1 | 6.1 | 95 | 1.67 | 1.01 | 95 |
| 3 | | Firm-ripe | 13.4 | 8.2 | 9.2 | 4.3 | 76 | 1.32 | 0.63 | 78 |
| C 1 Tilton | San Joaquin | Soft-ripe | 14.8 | 9.4 | 9.2 | 5.3 | 91 | 2.14 | 1.07 | 79 |
| 2 | | Ripe | 13.1 | 8.4 | 9.0 | 5.6 | 97 | 1.58 | 0.95 | 94 |
| 3 | | Firm-ripe | 11.7 | 7.7 | 8.2 | 4.4 | 82 | 0.81 | 0.49 | 92 |
| 4 | | Immature | 10.5 | 5.8 | 6.5 | 3.0 | 84 | 0.34 | 0.18 | 96 |

[a] Retentions calculated on the basis of apricot solids which corrects for dilution factor of packing medium.

From Cameron, E. J., Clifcorn, L. E., Esty, J. R., Feaster, J. F., Lamb, F. C., Monroe, K. H., and Royce, H., *Retention of Nutrients During Canning*, Research Laboratories National Canners Association, Berkeley, Calif., 1955, 14. With permission.

Table 4
## SUMMARY OF THE EFFECT OF HEAT PROCESSING AND STORAGE ON VITAMIN CONTENT OF CLINGSTONE PEACHES

Retorting Method

| Vitamin | Stationary (% retained) | Continuous (% retained) |
|---|---|---|
| Thiamin | 79 | 91 |
| Riboflavin | 103 | 101 |
| Niacin | 94 | 96 |
| Ascorbic acid | 76 | 83 |
| Total carotene AOAC | 40 | 41 |
| Total carotene stereoisomers | 97 | 104 |
| Total carotene effective | 96 | 101 |

From Elkins, E. R., Jr., Kemper, K., and Lamb, F. C., *Investigations to Determine the Nutrient Content of Canned Fruits and Vegetables,* National Canners Association Research Foundation, Washington, D.C., 1976, 75. With permission.


Table 5
## AVERAGE CAROTENE AND CAROTENE STEREOISOMERS IN THREE PACKS OF CLINGSTONE PEACHES

Zero Month

| Process | μg/100g solid | Entire contents | % of isomers | % activity[b] | Effective carotene |
|---|---|---|---|---|---|
| | | **Raw** | | | |
| All-*trans*-α | 2 | | 0.4 | 53 | 1 |
| Neo-β-D | T | | | 53 | |
| Neo-β-B | 51 | | 11.2 | 53 | 27 |
| All-*trans*-β | 185 | | 40.5 | 100 | 185 |
| Neo-β-U | 18 | | 3.9 | 38 | 7 |
| Cryptoxanthin | 201 | | 44.0 | 50 | 101 |
| Total isomers[a] | 457 | | 100 | 70[c] | |
| Total effective[d] | | | | | 321 |
| Total carotene AOAC | 1790 | | | | |
| | | **Stationary** | | | |
| All-*trans*-α | 3 | | 1.1 | 53 | 2 |
| Neo-β-D | T | | | 53 | |
| Neo-β-B | 23 | | 8.3 | 53 | 12 |
| All-*trans*-β | 107 | | 38.8 | 100 | 107 |
| Neo-β-U | 22 | | 8.0 | 38 | 8 |
| Cryptoxanthin | 121 | | 43.8 | 50 | 61 |
| Total isomers | 276 | | 100 | 69 | |
| Total effective | | | | | 190 |
| Total carotene AOAC | | 441 | | | |

## Table 5 (continued)
## AVERAGE CAROTENE AND CAROTENE STEREOISOMERS IN THREE PACKS OF CLINGSTONE PEACHES

### Zero Month

| Process | µg/100g solid | Entire contents | % of isomers | % activity[b] | Effective carotene |
|---|---|---|---|---|---|
| | | Continuous | | | |
| All-*trans*-α | | T | | 53 | |
| Neo-β-D | | T | | 53 | |
| Neo-β-B | | 23 | 7.7 | 53 | 12 |
| All-*trans*-β | | 109 | 36.5 | 100 | 109 |
| Neo-β-U | | 19 | 6.4 | 38 | 7 |
| Cryptoxanthin | | 148 | 49.5 | 50 | 74 |
| Total isomers | | 299 | 100 | 68 | |
| Total effective | | | | | 202 |
| Total carotene AOAC | | 459 | | | |

[a]  Total carotene isomers assumes that all carotene is all-trans-β-carotene.
[b]  Percent activity of each isomer.
[c]  Percentage of value if all carotene were assumed to be all-trans-β-carotene.
[d]  Total effective carotene is corrected for isomers having vitamin A activity less than all-trans-β-carotene.

From Elkins, E. R., Jr., Kemper, K., and Lamb, F. G., *Investigations to Determine the Nutrient Content of Canned Fruits and Vegetables,* National Canning Association Research Foundation, Washington, D.C., 1976, 75. With permission.

## Table 6
## SUMMARY OF THE EFFECT OF HEAT PROCESSING AND STORAGE ON MINERAL CONTENT OF CLINGSTONE PEACHES

| | Retort Method | |
|---|---|---|
| Mineral | Stationary (% retained) | Continuous (% retained) |
| Calcium | 109 | 100 |
| Phosphorus | 105 | 109 |
| Magnesium | 103 | 93 |
| Potassium | 103 | 101 |
| Iron | 76 | 92 |
| Copper | 71 | 66 |
| Manganese | 118 | 109 |
| Zinc | 110 | 99 |

From Elkins, E. R., Jr., Kemper, K., and Lamb, F. C., *Investigations to Determine the Nutrient Content of Canned Fruits and Vegetables,* National Canners Association, Research Foundation, Washington, D.C., 1976, 75. With permission.

Table 7

## COMPARISON OF THE COMPOSITION OF SOLIDS AND LIQUID IN CLINGSTONE PEACHES

| | Pack 1 | | Pack 2 | | Pack 3 | | Average | |
|---|---|---|---|---|---|---|---|---|
| | Solid | Liquid | Solid | Liquid | Solid | Liquid | Solid | Liquid |
| **Proximate Constituents** | | | | | | | | |
| °Brix | 19.4 | 19.4 | 20.7 | 20.3 | 17.6 | 17.5 | 19.3 | 19.1 |
| % Solids | 20.2 | 19.5 | 21.3 | 20.5 | 18.6 | 17.6 | 20.1 | 19.2 |
| % Protein | 0.4 | 0.3 | 0.6 | 0.4 | 0.6 | 0.4 | 0.6 | 0.4 |
| % Ash | 0.2 | 0.2 | 0.2 | 0.2 | 0.3 | 0.3 | 0.2 | 0.3 |
| % Carbohydrate | 19.5 | 19.0 | 20.4 | 19.9 | 17.6 | 17.0 | 19.2 | 18.7 |
| Calories/100g | 76.3 | 74.3 | 79.8 | 78.5 | 69.2 | 66.9 | 75.1 | 73.2 |
| **Vitamins** | | | | | | | | |
| Thiamin | 0.006 | 0.006 | 0.005 | 0.005 | 0.008 | 0.007 | 0.007 | 0.006 |
| Riboflavin | 0.18 | 0.019 | 0.025 | 0.021 | 0.024 | 0.022 | 0.023 | 0.021 |
| Niacin | 0.54 | 0.53 | 0.63 | 0.61 | 0.57 | 0.54 | 0.58 | 0.56 |
| Ascorbic acid | 1.2 | 1.2 | 3.4 | 3.6 | 3.7 | 4.0 | 2.8 | 2.9 |
| Total carotene AOAC | 431 | 0 | 409 | 0 | 588 | 0 | 478 | 0 |
| **Minerals** | | | | | | | | |
| Calcium | 4.16 | 3.58 | 4.34 | 3.63 | 4.25 | 3.69 | 4.25 | 3.64 |
| Phosphorus | 11.0 | 7.1 | 10.0 | 7.8 | 12.2 | 8.6 | 11.1 | 7.8 |
| Magnesium | 5.27 | 4.07 | 6.50 | 4.75 | 5.68 | 5.07 | 5.82 | 4.63 |
| Sodium | 5.3 | 5.1 | 7.9 | 8.1 | 7.8 | 7.7 | 7.0 | 7.0 |
| Potassium | 106 | 98 | 111 | 109 | 114 | 86 | 110 | 98 |
| Iron | 0.34 | 0.41 | 0.29 | 0.32 | 0.35 | 0.31 | 0.33 | 0.35 |
| Copper | 0.064 | 0.047 | 0.044 | 0.029 | 0.058 | 0.020 | 0.055 | 0.032 |
| Manganese | 0.046 | 0.049 | 0.048 | 0.049 | 0.057 | 0.057 | 0.050 | 0.052 |
| Zinc | 0.074 | 0.078 | 0.070 | 0.073 | 0.086 | 0.084 | 0.077 | 0.078 |

From Elkins, E. R., Jr., Kemper, K., and Lamb, F. C., *Investigations to Determine the Nutrient Content of Canned Fruits and Vegetables,* National Canners Association Research Foundation, Washington, D.C., 1976, 75. With permission.

Table 8

## DISTRIBUTION OF WATER-SOLUBLE VITAMINS IN CONSUMER SIZE CANS OF FRUITS. [a]

| Fruit | | Weight | | Ascorbic acid | | Thiamin | | Riboflavin | |
|---|---|---|---|---|---|---|---|---|---|
| | | Total per can (g) | Distribution (%) | Concentration (mg/100 g) | Distribution (%) | Concentration (mg/100 g) | Distribution (%) | Concentration (mg/100 g) | Distribution (%) |
| Apricots, unpeeled | Solid | 467 | 53 | 3.25 | 53 | 0.020 | 50 | 0.012 | 65 |
| halves (ripe) | Liquid | 419 | 47 | 3.21 | 47 | 0.022 | 50 | 0.011 | 45 |
| Grapefruit segments | Solid | 347 | 57 | 23.0 | 56 | 0.034 | 58 | 0.006 | 67 |
| | Liquid | 262 | 43 | 24.0 | 44 | 0.032 | 42 | 0.004 | 33 |
| Peaches, clingstone | Solid | 567 | 67 | 4.81 | 67 | 0.007 | 70 | 0.012 | 61 |
| | Liquid | 284 | 33 | 4.68 | 33 | 0.006 | 30 | 0.015 | 39 |
| Peaches, freestone | Solid | 431 | 51 | 2.42 | 49 | 0.006 | 61 | 0.011 | 56 |
| | Liquid | 417 | 49 | 2.64 | 51 | 0.004 | 39 | 0.009 | 44 |
| Pears | Solid | 518 | 61 | 1.18 | 68 | 0.006 | 57 | 0.011 | 69 |
| | Liquid | 329 | 39 | 0.86 | 32 | 0.007 | 43 | 0.008 | 31 |
| Pineapple, sliced | Solid | 523 | 60 | 4.76 | 59 | 0.077 | 60 | 0.004 | 66 |
| | Liquid | 352 | 40 | 4.89 | 41 | 0.078 | 40 | 0.003 | 34 |
| Prunes, Italian | Solid | 383 | 46 | 0.96 | 49 | 0.022 | 51 | 0.012 | 53 |
| | Liquid | 456 | 54 | 0.85 | 51 | 0.018 | 49 | 0.009 | 47 |

*Note:* Six no. 2½ cans were mixed for all fruits except grapefruit for which six no. 2 cans were used. Each value is from a single experiment.

From Brush, M. K., Hinman, W. F., and Halliday, E. G., *J. Nutr.*, 28, 138, 1944. With permission.

## Table 9
## ASCORBIC ACID RETENTION DURING CANNING OF GRAPEFRUIT JUICE AND ORANGE JUICE

| Plant[a] | Freshly extracted | After screening | From holding tank | From filler | After processing and cooling | Retention ascorbic acid (%) |
|---|---|---|---|---|---|---|
| | | | mg/100 ml | | | |
| | | | **Grapefruit Juice** | | | |
| | | | Florida[b] | | | |
| A | 37.6 | | 38.7 | 37.3 | 37.5 | 99.7 |
| B | 38.5 | | 38.3 | 37.4 | 37.7 | 97.9 |
| C | 36.6 | 36.0 | 37.3 | 37.2 | 37.0 | 101.1 |
| D | 38.4 | | 37.8 | 37.0 | 36.6 | 95.3 |
| E | 38.8 | 38.5 | 38.3 | 35.4 | 34.4 | 88.7 |
| F | 39.1 | 38.4 | 39.1 | 37.6 | 38.3 | 98.0 |
| G | 40.6 | 40.9 | 41.1 | 40.4 | 40.6 | 100.0 |
| H | 38.9 | 39.6 | 38.6 | 38.4 | 38.0 | 97.7 |
| I | 37.9 | — | 39.1 | 37.5 | 37.6 | 99.2 |
| J | 38.9 | 38.8 | 37.1 | 36.7 | 36.4 | 93.6 |
| K | 41.1 | 41.2 | | 39.4 | 38.8 | 94.4 |
| L | 41.2 | 41.3 | 41.3 | 40.8 | 40.7 | 98.8 |
| | | | Texas[c] | | | |
| I | 42.2 | 41.4 | 41.7 | 42.4 | 41.1 | 99.3 |
| II | 48.7 | 51.3 | 50.5 | 47.2 | 49.7 | 96.9 |
| III | 42.8 | 44.8 | 41.6 | 41.1 | 41.3 | 92.2 |
| IV | 42.6 | 43.1 | 42.4 | 41.4 | 40.4 | 93.7 |
| V | 37.7 | 38.7 | 38.7 | 36.5 | 36.7 | 94.8 |
| VI | 38.5 | 38.4 | | 38.0 | 37.6 | 97.9 |
| VII | 39.7 | 39.5 | 39.7 | 38.4 | 38.3 | 97.0 |
| VIII | 39.5 | 41.5 | 41.0 | 39.0 | 40.1 | 96.6 |
| IX | 37.6 | 38.4 | | 37.0 | 37.6 | 97.9 |
| X | 42.1 | 41.8 | 41.2 | 40.1 | 40.2 | 96.2 |
| XI | 39.6 | 39.9 | | 38.9 | 39.0 | 97.7 |
| XII | 40.8 | 43.1 | 41.7 | 40.2 | 41.2 | 95.6 |
| | | | California[d] | | | |
| A | — | 46.3 | | 47.1 | 46.9 | 101.3 |
| B | 44.7 | 41.5 | 43.3 | 41.8 | 42.1 | 96.6 |
| C | 44.3 | | 44.4 | | 44.1 | 99.5 |
| | | | Arizona[d] | | | |
| D | — | 42.3 | 43.6 | | 43.2 | 102.1 |
| E | — | 43.4 | 41.4 | | 40.8 | 94.0 |
| F | — | 41.1 | | | 39.7 | 96.6 |
| G | 42.7 | 41.5 | | | 41.8 | 97.9 |
| | | | **Orange Juice** | | | |
| | | | California[d] | | | |
| A | | 43.4 | | 43.5 | 43.2 | 99.5 |
| B | | 40.9 | | 41.7 | 40.9 | 100.0 |
| C | | 48.4 | 48.2 | | 47.3 | 97.8 |
| D | 38.8 | 38.5 | 38.8 | | 38.0 | 97.9 |
| E | 41.7 | 41.7 | 41.0 | | 39.6 | 95.1 |
| | | | Florida[b] | | | |
| A | 49.2 | 49.2 | 49.5 | 49.0 | 48.7 | 99.0 |

**Table 9 (continued)**
## ASCORBIC ACID RETENTION DURING CANNING OF GRAPEFRUIT JUICE AND ORANGE JUICE

[a] Values for individual plants represent averages for all the surveys made at the plant.
[b] Retentions based on freshly extracted juice.
[c] Retentions based on juice after screening.
[d] Retentions based on freshly extracted juice whenever this was tested, otherwise on juice after screening.

From Cameron, E. J., Clifcorn, L. E., Esty, J. R., Feaster, J. F., Lamb, F. C., Monroe, K. H., and Royce, Handle, *Retention of Nutrients During Canning,* Research Laboratories National Canners Association, Berkeley, Calif., 1955, 14. With permission.

**Table 10**
## ANALYSIS OF ENZYMATIC PRUNE JUICE PROCESSING PRODUCTS

| Product | Soluble solids, degrees brix | Insoluble solids, (%) | Vitamin A (IU/100 g) | Moisture (%) |
|---|---|---|---|---|
| Prunes | — | — | 1170 | 18 |
| Slurry from press | 22.0 | 35 | 560 | — |
| Sludge from press | 22.0 | — | 1620 | 75 |
| Finished prune juice | 19.9 | 10 | 260 | — |
| Commercial prune juice | 19.0 | 0.5 | 0 | — |

**Table 11**
## $\beta$-CAROTENE LOST DURING SULFURED APRICOT LEATHER DRYING

| Drying method | Moisture | $\beta$-carotene IU/100 g (MFB)[a] | $\beta$-carotene lost % |
|---|---|---|---|
| None | 68.8 | 19,000 | — |
| Dehydrated | 12.6 | 17,390 | 9.2 |
| Shade dried | 17.1 | 17,080 | 10.1 |
| Sun dried | 16.0 | 13,300 | 30.0 |

[a] Moisture-free basis.

**Table 12**
## $\beta$-CAROTENE IN APRICOT CONCENTRATE AND DRIED SHEETS

(IU/100 g  Moisture-free basis)

| Sulfur dioxide level | Concentrate | Sheets Time 0 | Sheets 13 wk at 32°C |
|---|---|---|---|
| 0 | 15,100 | 13,300 | 9,100 |
| 0.03 | 15,100 | — | 10,100 |
| 0.10 | 15,100 | — | 10,800 |
| 0.30 | 15,100 | 14,400 | 11,800 |

## Table 13

## EFFECT OF FREEZE DRYING ON SOME CHEMICAL PROPERTIES OF ORANGE AND GUAVA JUICES

(Calculated on Dry Weight Basis)

| Components | Raw material of orange juice | | | | | | Raw material of guava juice | | | |
| | Single strength 13% T.S.S. | | Concentrated | | | | Pasteurized | | Nonpasteurized | |
| | | | 20% T.S.S. | | 36% T.S.S. | | | | | |
| | Before f.d.ᵃ | After f.d. | Before f.d. | After f.d. | Before f.d. | After f.d. | Before f.d. | After f.d. | Before f.d. | After f.d. |
|---|---|---|---|---|---|---|---|---|---|---|
| Ascorbic acid, mg/100 g | 452.01 | 439.98 | 451.01 | 436.88 | 440.51 | 433.64 | 586.36 | 678.04 | 567.49 | 559.62 |
| Carotene, mg/100 g | 1.69 | 1.63 | 1.60 | 1.56 | 1.58 | 1.50 | — | — | — | — |
| Pectin as calcium pectate, % | 3.32 | 3.29 | 3.35 | 3.32 | 3.78 | 3.75 | 6.01 | 5.98 | 5.66 | 5.64 |
| Pectin-methylesterase as mg $CH_3O$/100 g | 41.69 | 41.83 | 42.02 | 42.02 | 41.65 | 41.89 | 52.57 | 52.26 | 101.73 | 101.55 |
| Reducing sugars, % | 35.55 | 35.91 | 41.11 | 41.08 | 43.18 | 43.26 | 30.11 | 29.91 | 29.26 | 29.23 |
| Nonreducing sugars, % | 31.80 | 31.35 | 26.86 | 26.78 | 21.65 | 24.58 | 15.83 | 16.07 | 16.60 | 16.61 |
| Total sugars, % | 67.35 | 67.26 | 67.97 | 67.86 | 67.83 | 67.84 | 45.94 | 45.98 | 45.86 | 45.84 |
| Acidity as citric acid, % | 6.01 | 5.86 | 5.57 | 5.68 | 5.61 | 5.57 | 3.12 | 3.08 | 3.26 | 3.17 |
| pH value | 3.45 | 3.50 | 3.45 | 3.51 | 3.45 | 3.48 | 4.24 | 4.20 | 4.20 | 4.25 |

ᵃ f.d. = Freeze drying.

Reprinted from Foda, Y. C., Hamed, M. G. E., and Abd-Allah, M. A., *Food Technol.*, 24, 1394, 1970. Copyright© by Institute of Food Technologists. With permission.

**Table 14**
**CAROTENOID COMPOSITION OF FLORIDA VALENCIA ORANGE JUICES**

| Constituent | Approximate percent of carotenoid mixture[a] | | | | | Ratio to amount found in freshly prepared powder | |
|---|---|---|---|---|---|---|---|
| | Single strength | Concentrate | Fresh powder | Conditioned powder | Aged powder | Conditioned | Aged |
| Phytoene | 1.4 | —[b] | 2.1 | 2.5 | 3.2 | 1.02 | 1.00 |
| Phytofluene | 0.6 | 0.6 | 0.6 | 0.8 | 0.9 | 1.08 | 0.98 |
| Alpha-carotene | 1.0 | 1.4 | 1.1 | 1.5 | 1.7 | 1.09 | 1.01 |
| Beta-carotene | 1.2 | 1.8 | 1.6 | 2.1 | 2.4 | 1.11 | 0.98 |
| Zeta-carotene | 1.1 | 1.5 | 1.7 | 2.2 | 2.4 | 1.07 | 0.91 |
| Gamma-carotene-like | 0 | 0.2 | 0.2 | 0.2 | 0.5[c] | 0.88 | — |
| Hydroxy-alpha-carotene | 2.9 | 2.8 | 2.5 | 2.5 | 2.8 | 0.85 | 0.73 |
| Cryptoxanthin | 5.4 | 5.6 | 4.4 | 4.9 | 6.6 | 0.93 | 0.98 |
| Lutein | 7.1 | 7.1 | 7.2 | 8.7 | 9.2 | 1.03 | 0.85 |
| Zeaxanthin | 9.2 | 9.0 | 8.3 | 9.9 | 11.3 | 1.01 | 0.90 |
| Lutein 5.6-epoxide | 0.3 | 0.3 | 0.3 | 0 | 0.04 | 0 | 0.10 |
| Antheraxanthin | 11.6 | 13.4 | 12.2 | 5.4 | 0.7 | 0.38 | 0.007 |
| Flavoxanthin | 0.14 | 0.3 | 0 | 0.3 | 0.4 | — | — |
| Mutatoxanthins | 7.3 | 8.0 | 9.4 | 16.7 | 22.9 | 1.50 | 1.63 |
| Violaxanthin | 14.7 | 18.8 | 13.6 | 1.5 | 0 | 0.09 | 0 |
| Luteoxanthins | 12.7 | 11.5 | 15.0 | 10.6 | 0.7 | 0.60 | 0.03 |
| Auroxanthins | 3.9 | 2.8 | 5.0 | 14.8 | 19.7 | 2.50 | 2.63 |
| Valenciaxanthin | 1.8 | 1.5 | 1.5 | 1.3 | 0.14 | 0.73 | 0.06 |
| Sinensiaxanthin | 1.6 | 1.6 | 1.5 | 0.4 | 0 | 0.24 | 0 |
| Trollixanthin-like | 10.4 | 7.6 | 7.1 | 6.1 | 0 | 0.73 | 0 |
| Trollein | —[d] | —[d] | —[d] | —[d] | 4.4 | — | — |
| Valenciachromes | 0.5 | 0.2 | 0.9 | 1.6 | 3.1 | 1.46 | 2.20 |
| Trollichrome-like | 3.4 | 1.7 | 2.1 | 4.5 | 6.4 | 1.87 | 1.99 |
| Sinensiachrome | 0.8 | 0.5 | 0.4 | 0.8 | 0 | 1.72 | 0.72 |
| | | | | | Entire sample | 0.91 | 0.72 |

[a] Calculated from sum of adsorbances at principal maximum on Cary spectrophotometer curve for each constituent.

[b] Probably present but obscured by impurity.

[c] Spectrophotometer curve indicated band was quite impure.

[d] Probably present but obscured by trollixanthin-like pigment.

Reprinted from Curl, A. L. and Bailey, G. F., *Food Technol.*, 13, 394, 1959. Copyright© Institute Food Technologists. With permission.

## Table 15
## COMPARATIVE LOSSES OF VITAMINS
## FROM APPLE, APRICOT, PEACH, AND
## PRUNE FROM PROCESSING

| Preservation method | Mean loss from fresh fruit (%) | | | | |
|---|---|---|---|---|---|
| | A | B-1 | B-2 | Niacin | C |
| Frozen, not thawed[a] | 36 | 39 | 0 | 10 | 4 |
| Canned | 23 | 46 | 38 | 16 | 58 |
| Dried | 6 | 55 | 0 | 10 | 56 |

*Note:* Source — USDA Handbbok 8 (Watt and Merrill 1963). Values based on edible portions of fruits "as purchased".

[a]    No prune included.

# REFERENCES

1. **Hein, R. E. and Hutchings, I. J.,** Influence of processing on vitamin-mineral content and biological availability in processed foods, in *Nutrients in Processed Foods — Vitamins, Minerals,* American Medical Association, Publishing Sciences Group, Acton, Mass., 1974, 67.
2. **Harris, R. S. and Karmas, E.,** *Nutritional Evaluation of Food Processing,* AVI Publishing, Westport, Conn., 1975, 3.
3. **Guerrant, N. B., Vavich, M. G., Fardig, O. B., Dutcher, R. A., and Stern, R. M.,** The nutritive value of canned foods, *J. Nutr.,* 32, 449—450, 1946.
4. **Fellers, C. R. and Esselen, W. B.,** Cranberries and cranberry products, *Mass. Agric. Exp. Stn. Bull.* 481, 40—56, 1955.
5. **Licciardello, J. J., Esselen, W. B., Jr., and Fellers, C. R.,** Stability of ascorbic acid during the preparation of cranberry products, *Food Res.,* 17, 338—342, 1952.
6. **Golberg, L. and Levy, L.,** Vitamin C content of fresh, canned, and dried guavas, *Nature (London),* 148, 286, 1941.
7. **Mayfield, H. L. and Richardson, J. E.,** Ascorbic acid content of strawberries and their products, *Mont. State Coll. Agric. Exp. Stn. Bull.,* 412, 11, 1943.
8. **Cameron, E. J., Clifcorn, L. E., Esty, J. R., Feaster, J. F., Lamb, F. C., Monroe, K. H., and Royce, H.,** *Retention of Nutrients During Canning,* Research Laboratories National Canners Association, Berkeley, Calif., 1955, 14—19.
9. **Lamb, F. C.,** *Studies of Factors Affecting the Retention of Nutrients During Canning Operations,* National Canners Association, Berkeley, Calif., 1946, 1—50.
10. **Mitchell, J. H., Van Blaricom, L. O., and Roderick, D. B.,** The effect of canning and freezing on the carotenoids and ascorbic acid content of peaches, *S. C. Agric. Stn. Bull.,* 372, 7, 1948.
11. **Elkins, E. R., Jr., Kemper, K., and Lamb, F. C.,** Investigations to Determine the Nutrient Content of Canned Fruits and Vegetables, Report USDA-ARS-12-14-11, 054(62), National Canners Association Research Foundation, Washington, D. C., 1976, 75—93.
12. **Brush, M. K., Hinman, W. F., and Halliday, E. G.,** The nutritive value of canned foods. V. Distribution of water soluble vitamins between solid and liquid portions of canned vegetables and fruits, *J. Nutr.,* 28, 138, 1944.
13. **Krehl, W. A. and Cowgill, G. R.,** Vitamin content of citrus products, *Food Res.,* 15, 179—191, 1950.
14. **Bolin, H. R., Stafford, A. E., and Fuller, G.,** Rapid enzymatic process yields nutritious, mild-flavored prune juice, *Food Prod. Dev.,* 9, 92—94, 1975.

15. **Bolin, H. R. and Stafford, A. E.**, Effect of processing and storage on provitamin A and vitamin C in apricots, *J. Food Sci.*, 39, 1034—1035, 1974.
16. **Escher, F. and Neukom, H.**, Studies on drum-drying apple flakes, *Trav. Chim. Ailment Hyg.*, 61, 339—348, 1970 (German).
17. **Hall, A. P., Morgan, A. F., and Wheeler, P.**, The amounts of six B-vitamins in fresh and dried figs, *Food Res.*, 18, 206—216, 1953.
18. **Mrak, E. M.**, Retention of vitamins by dried fruits and vegetables, *Fruit Products J.*, 21, 13—15, 1941.
19. **Foda, Y. H., Hamed, M. G. E., and Abd-Allah, M. A.**, Preservation of orange and guava juice by freeze-drying, *Food Technol. (Chicago)*, 24, 1394, 1970.
20. **Curl, A. L. and Bailey, G. F.**, Changes in the carotenoid pigments in preparation and storage of Valencia orange juice powder, *Food Technol. (Chicago)*, 13, 394—398, 1959.
21. **Hollingsworth, D. F.**, Effects of some new production and processing methods on nutritive values, *J. Am. Diet. Assoc.*, 57, 246—249, 1970.
22. **Labuza, T. P.**, Nutrient losses during drying and storage of dehydrated foods, *CRC Crit. Rev. Food Technol.*, 3(2), 217—240, 1972.
23. **de Groot, A. P.**, The influence of dehydration of foods on digestibility and the biological value of the protein, *Food Technol. (Chicago)*, 17, 339—341, 1963.
24. **Schroeder, H. A.**, Losses of vitamins and trace minerals resulting from processing and preservation of foods, *Am. J. Clin. Nutr.*, 24, 562—573, 1971.
25. **Loeffler, H. J.**, Retention of ascorbic acid in raspberries during freezing, frozen storage, pureeing, and manufacture into velva fruit, *Food Res.*, 11, 507—515, 1946.
26. **Wolfe, J. C., Owen, R. F., Charles, V. R., and Van Duyne, F. O.**, Effect of freezing and freezer storage on the ascorbic acid content of muskmelon, grapefruit sections, and strawberry puree, *Food Res.*, 14, 243—251, 1949.
27. **Amerine, M. A., Berg, M. S., and Cruess, W. V.**, *The Technology of Wine Making*, 3rd ed., Avi Publishing, Westport, Conn., 1972, Ch. 10.
28. **Salunkhe, D. K., Gerber, R. K., and Pollard, L. H.**, Physiological and chemical effects of gamma radiation on certain fruits, vegetables, and their products, *Proc. Am. Soc. Hortic. Sci.*, 74, 423, 1959.
29. **Massey, L. M., Jr. and Bourke, J. B.**, Radiative Preservation of Foods, Advances in Chemistry Series No. 65, American Chemical Society, Washington, D. C., 1967, 1—11.
30. **Kertesz, Z. I., Glegg, R. E., Boyle, F. P., Parsons, G. F., and Massey, L. M., Jr.**, Effect of ionizing radiations on plant tissues. III. Softening and changes in pectins and cellulose of apples, carrots, and beets, *J. Food Sci.*, 29, 47, 1964.

# EFFECT OF PROCESSING ON NUTRITIVE VALUE OF FOOD: MEAT AND MEAT PRODUCTS

## I. H. Burger

## INTRODUCTION

Meat and meat products are generally considered to be foods of high nutritional value and are probably regarded as one of the most palatable and appetizing food commodities. The nutritional value of any food is, however, a composite of many factors, and it is important to consider the contribution made by any food group to the nutrient intake of the population to appreciate fully the significance of nutrient losses during processing. In Great Britain, meat and meat products contribute a large proportion of protein, fat, iron, and vitamins of the B complex[1] (Table 1). If processing leads to destruction of these nutrients, this will represent important losses with regard to human nutrition.

In general, vitamins are the most unstable nutrients with protein less so, although some individual amino acids (e.g., lysine) are sensitive to processing. Fats and mineral salts are fairly stable under most processing conditions.[2] The effects of processing on meat products follow this pattern, and it will be seen that the most significant losses are those of the B vitamins (especially thiamin) and protein.

Although some discussion of the practical techniques of meat processing will inevitably appear in the text, a comprehensive consideration of these procedures is beyond the scope of this review and the reader is referred elsewhere for this information.[3]

## EFFECTS OF PROCESSING

### Curing and Smoking

Curing consists of the addition of salt, sodium nitrate, sodium nitrite and other components to meat, both as a preservation technique and to promote or improve the organoleptic properties of the food. Smoking has a similar function. The degree of salting and smoking vary considerably throughout the world, but current procedures are generally mild and have little effect on nutritional quality.

Early studies in this area[4] showed that only small losses (1 to 5%) of thiamin, riboflavin, and nicotinic acid resulted from the curing of meat. An increased thiamin loss (15 to 20%) occurred if the product was smoked, and this is probably attributable to the heat lability of this vitamin, as the losses of riboflavin and nicotinic acid remained low. In fact, thiamin appears to be the only vitamin consistently lost in the preparation of several types of processed meats and sausages (2 to 26% loss),[5] although losses of riboflavin (11 to 43%), thiamin (16 to 26%), and nicotinic acid (4 to 19%) have been reported in smoked bacon.[6]

It is generally assumed that the protein quality of cured meat is close to that of the raw material. Schweigert and Payne[7] showed that the amino acid compositions of several processed meats were virtually the same as unprocessed samples. However, amino acid analysis of protein is not necessarily a good indicator of protein quality,[8] and reductions in the *available* lysine content of smoked meat and meat products have been reported. These losses appear to be temperature dependent: cold smoking at 30°C for 1 to 2 days resulted in an available lysine reduction of 12%,[9] whereas smoking at 65°C for only 10 hr increased the loss to 44%. Protein quality may also be affected by the interaction of nitrite and meat. It is known that several gases are formed when nitrite

Table 1

CONTRIBUTION OF MEAT PRODUCTS TO NUTRIENT INTAKE OF GREAT BRITAIN POPULATION IN 1973

| | Protein | Fatty Acids | | | Carbohydrate | Calcium | Iron | Thiamin* | Riboflavin | Niacin | Vitamin C | Vitamin A (as retinol equivalent) | Vitamin D |
|---|---|---|---|---|---|---|---|---|---|---|---|---|---|
| | | Saturated | Monounsaturated | Polyunsaturated | | | | | | | | | |
| Beef and veal | | 4.5 | 5.3 | 1.4 | — | 0.3 | 7.8 | 0.7 | 2.8 | 7.4 | — | 0.3 | — |
| Mutton and lamb | | 4.1 | 4.1 | 1.9 | — | 0.2 | 2.5 | 1.1 | 2.2 | 4.7 | — | 0.2 | — |
| Pork | | 3.2 | 4.7 | 2.8 | — | 0.1 | 0.9 | 5.0 | 1.2 | 3.2 | — | — | — |
| Bacon and ham (uncooked) | | 5.1 | 7.4 | 8.2 | — | 0.2 | 1.4 | 4.0 | 1.4 | 1.7 | — | — | — |
| Liver | | 0.2 | 0.2 | 0.5 | — | — | 3.3 | 0.5 | 5.0 | 2.4 | 0.9 | 23.3 | 0.8 |
| Poultry (uncooked) | | 0.7 | 1.2 | 2.6 | — | 0.2 | 2.2 | 0.5 | 1.5 | 6.0 | — | — | — |
| Sausages | | 2.8 | 3.8 | 1.9 | 0.7 | 0.3 | 1.4 | — | 0.6 | 1.6 | — | — | — |
| Other meat | | 5.7 | 7.7 | 6.2 | 1.2 | 0.8 | 8.6 | 5.5 | 4.0 | 7.2 | 0.3 | 0.6 | 0.2 |
| Total | | 26.3 | 34.4 | 25.6 | 2.0 | 2.1 | 28.1 | 17.5 | 18.7 | 34.2 | 1.2 | 24.4 | 0.9 |

*Note:* Figures show percentage contribution of each product to the nutrient intake.

*   Thiamin percentages allow for some losses in cooking unless otherwise stated.

From Ministry of Agriculture, Fisheries, and Food, *Household Food Consumption and Expenditure in 1973*, Her Majesty's Stationery Office, London, 1975, 105. With permission.

Table 2
LOSSES OF B VITAMINS IN CANNED MEAT
PRODUCTS[17]

| | | Percentage lost during processing | | |
|---|---|---|---|---|
| Food | Type | Thiamin | Riboflavin | Niacin |
| Beef | Corned | 76 | 6 | 0 |
| | Diced | 67 | 0 | 0 |
| Veal | Diced | 79 | 0 | 0 |
| | Loaf | 81 | 24 | 44 |
| Pork | Chopped | 55 | 0 | 16 |
| | Diced | 66 | 0 | 0 |
| | Pork and Gravy | 67 | 0 | 23 |
| | Ham, chopped | 45 | 0 | 0 |
| | Bacon | 59 | 29 | 52 |
| Lamb | Strained | 84 | 0 | 13 |
| Poultry | Light meat | 67 | — | — |
| | Dark meat | 77 | — | — |

*Note:* Figures show percentage vitamin loss in relation to raw
meat.

interacts with meat under curing conditions,[11,12] and there are indications that nitrite nitrogen is incorporated into meat. Nitrites have also been reported to interact with SH-groups[13] and mitochondrial enzymes.[14]

There is little information on the fate of minerals and trace elements in curing. It is unlikely, however, that substantial losses will occur, and a recent Canadian study[15] suggests that the trace metal content of cured meats is comparable to the level found in meat groups of the total diet.

A review of nutritional changes resulting from curing and smoking would be incomplete without some reference to a possible hazard associated with this type of meat preservation, namely the formation of N-nitrosamines. The nitrosamines are a group of carcinogenic chemicals which have been detected in cured and smoked meat products, although generally at very low concentrations. It is thought that nitrosamines may be generated during the curing process, but concern has also been expressed that they may be formed in the body by the interaction of secondary and tertiary amines (supplied in the food) and nitrite in the stomach. The whole question of nitrosamines in food is the subject of a recent, comprehensive review.[16] Much research is currently being conducted to evaluate the degree of hazard presented by nitrosamine formation and to balance this against the beneficial preservative action of nitrite in meat products.

## Heat Processing

The heat processing (canning) of meat products is the harshest form of preservation to which these foods are likely to be subjected, but it produces a bacteriologically stable food which does not require sophisticated storage conditions. Some loss of nutritional quality can occur during storage at ambient temperatures; this is discussed later in this chapter.

The losses of some B-vitamins on canning are presented in Table 2. As expected, the losses for thiamin are higher than those reported for the milder process of curing. Although information on other vitamins is scarce, it appears that thiamin is generally the only vitamin lost in appreciable amounts during the canning of meats. Nevertheless, it has been reported that 30 to 40% of panthothenic acid[18] and a substantial proportion of folic acid[19] can be lost during commercial heat processing. A more recent study[20] involving ten samples of canned meats (veal, pork, chicken, and beef) showed losses of only 19, 7, and 22% for thiamin, riboflavin, and niacin, respectively. Separate analysis of the meat and gelatin in the finished product suggested that there was some transfer of the vitamins into the gelatin and that the overall content of the three vitamins was little different from raw meat when considered for the whole product.

The range of vitamin losses (especially thiamin) reported for heat processing of meat products is very wide as a result of variations in raw material, severity of heat treatment, type of product, and so on.

However, it has been demonstrated that vitamin losses can be reduced if a high-temperature, short-time (HTST) method of processing is used. In this procedure the food is handled mechanically to reduce bacterial contamination, and as yet it is only practicable for meat products in the form of a liquid. Large-particle foods present technical problems with regard to handling and heat penetration. It has been shown in a pilot study[21] that beef stew or puree given a conventional heat treatment (115°C for 42 min) showed a 22% reduction in thiamin content compared with a loss of only 7% in an HTST process (149°C for 79 sec). Pyridoxine has been reported to be similarly affected.[22] Thiamin has been used as a reference nutrient in a computer-oriented study[23] of the optimum heat processing procedure for nutrient retention that confirmed the HTST process as the best for minimizing nutrient loss.

Although thiamin destruction is probably the most notable effect of heat processing, protein quality can also be influenced by this preservation method as a result of destruction or unavailability of the constituent amino acids. Broadly speaking, three types of reactions are responsible for changes in nutritional value.[24]

1.  Maillard reactions in which amino groups, notably the ε-amino group of lysine, react with aldehyde groups of reducing sugars or carbonyls from oxidized fat rendering lysine metabolically unavailable to the body
2.  Protein-protein interactions resulting in the formation of chemical links that are resistant to hydrolysis by gut enzymes
3.  Oxidation or desulfydration of sulfur amino acids

Mayfield and Hedrick[25] reported only small decreases in the digestibility (98 reduced to 94%) and biological value (BV) (86 reduced to 79%) of beef protein processed at 121°C for 85 min. In another study, pork subjected to longer processing (110°C for 24 hr) lost 44% cystine, 34% available lysine, and up to 20% of other amino acids.[24] In addition, the net protein utilization (NPU) was seriously lowered (by 49%) and it was suggested that the losses of amino acids underestimated the true degree of nutritional damage. Pork processed at 112°C, also for 24 hr, had losses of 70% cystine and 50 to 65% of other essential amino acids as assayed by enzymic hydrolysis.[26]

It is important to appreciate that, although prolonged heating at high temperatures can cause extensive damage to the protein of meat foods, these particular conditions are often inapplicable to normal commercial processing where the most severe conditions involve heating for 4 to 5 hr at 115°C. For example, Rubin[27] has reported that luncheon meat has a protein efficiency ratio (PER) of 2.66 to 2.76, which is similar to that of fresh pork (approximately 3.0). In contrast, the processing of corned beef reduces NPU from 75 to 55,[28] and these observations reflect the degree of heat processing used for these products: luncheon meat is processed for 1.5 hr, whereas corned beef undergoes a 4 to 5-hr heat treatment. In commercially canned meat products, losses of amino acids have been reported to be small, of the order of 10 to 20%.[29] In the same study lysine was found to increase, an observation explained by the gelatinization of collagen.

A great deal of research has been devoted to the effects of processing on the available lysine in meat products, and it is likely that any reductions in nutritional quality are in large measure the result of interactions of lysine with oxidized fat in Maillard-type reactions.[30] This type of reaction can also occur if carbohydrate is present. Reductions in peptic digestibility and free amino acid content have been reported in pork and beef processed at 110°C for 50 min or 130°C for 30 min in the presence of 3% starch.[31] Maillard browning on heating has also been reported in meats containing small amounts of ribose.[32] Nevertheless, it is generally considered that under normal canning procedures meat products show little reduction in available lysine and are the foods showing the greatest resistance to the Maillard reaction and subsequent protein degradation.[33]

Heller et al.[34] showed that from 74 to 92% of the available lysine was retained in pork, beef, and lamb muscle after standard cooking procedures. Only after 16 hr of autoclaving was the amount substantially reduced. It has recently been reported[35] that the destruction of trypsin inhibitors in meat products containing soya bean is accelerated and that this may be due to a factor in meat that decreases the thermostability of the inhibitors. This does not seem to be present in other foods tested. Heat processing is likely, therefore, to improve the nutritional value of meat/soya products and is an interesting development in view of the increasing use of this type of food product.

## Freezing

It is generally accepted that the nutritional losses during freezing are minimal and that freezing is probably the best method for preserving meat.[36] The losses of B-vitamins (thiamin, riboflavin, niacin, pyridoxine, and pantothenic acid) from various animal tissues have been reported to be insignificant during the freezing process per se.[37,38] Precooking and freezing of pork chops did not have any great adverse effect on the content of thiamin, riboflavin, and vitamin $B_{12}$.[39] Nutritional losses can occur during subsequent storage, thawing, and cooking of meat products, but these will be discussed later in this chapter.

The rate of freezing does not have a significant effect on the levels of thiamin, riboflavin, niacin, pyridoxine, and pantothenic acid in bovine,[40] ovine,[41] or porcine[42] muscle tissues. In contrast, oxidative changes in beef and pork have been reported to be influenced by freezing rate.[43] Slow freezing inhibited oxidation more than rapid freezing, and the absence of air circulation during freezing aided this inhibition. If confirmed, this finding could have wide nutritional significance in terms of protein quality and vitamin retention in frozen meats.

## Freeze-Drying

As regards meat and meat products, freeze-drying has a similar effect on nutritional quality to freezing in that few losses have been reported as a result of the freeze-drying process as such, but changes can occur on subsequent storage. The latter are discussed later in this review. In a study of certain B-vitamins in chicken muscle, Rowe et al.[44] showed that the thiamin and riboflavin losses in a product which had been freeze-dried in the raw state, rehydrated, and then cooked were not substantially greater than those in a freshly cooked sample. In a complementary study, De Groot[45] reported that freeze-drying did not significantly alter the BV or digestibility of a variety of meat products, including beef and chicken. Thomas and Calloway[46] found only small (5%) losses of thiamin in freeze-dried pork, chicken, and beef, and complete retention of thiamin and riboflavin has been reported in meat after freeze-drying to a moisture content of below 2%.[47]

## Irradiation

Irradiation is not used routinely for meat preservation in the United Kingdom, but research conducted mainly in the U.S. suggests that, in general, irradiation causes less nutritional damage to meat products than heat processing. There are basically two levels of radiation used in food processing: radappertization, which involves doses in excess of one megarad (Mrad), and radicidation, which involves doses less than this. The former is analogous to heat sterilization (canning), the latter to pasteurization. [60]Co appears to be the most frequently used radiation source.

Even large doses of radiation (4.5 Mrad) result in only small losses of the B-vitamins thiamin, riboflavin, niacin, and pyridoxine from pork[48] with retentions of 85, 78, 78, and 98%, respectively, compared with an unirradiated control. These figures compare favorably with those for heat processing, particularly in the case of thiamin, where heat treatment can result in only 20 to 25% retention. In this study very low temperatures (−80°C) were used, and this seems important to ensure nutrient retention. A thiamin loss of 60% was reported when a similar radiation level (4.7 to 7.1 Mrad) was used at −40°C on beef,[49] although the loss was still no greater than for conventional thermal processing. Smaller radiation treatments have also been reported to cause thiamin loss. A 14% loss was caused by 100 Krad in minced pig meat after 3 days storage,[50] and 600 Krad caused a 36% loss in pig muscle which had previously been fried, cooled, and hermetically packaged.[51] The loss increased to 50% after five months storage at 18 to 23°C.

There is little information on the effect of irradiation on the protein quality of meat products, but the amino acid content of beef irradiated at 4.7 to 7.1 Mrad and stored for 15 months was little different from that of a frozen control sample.[49] Lipids also seem to be relatively unaffected by these levels of irradiation.[49] Goldblith[52] has reviewed the effect of irradiation on food including meat products, concluding that it generally produces only small changes in nutritive value.

## EFFECTS OF STORAGE

Although the nutrient losses resulting from processing may be quite small, they can increase during storage of food. This is an important subject for all types of meat products, but it is particularly relevant to frozen foods in view of the extensive use of commercial frozen storage and the growth of domestic freezer usage.

Information on the losses of B-vitamins in a variety of frozen meat products is summarized in Table 3, and it appears that at temperatures typical of domestic deep freezers, nutrient retention over a 6 month period is good. It is generally considered that the overall freezing process comprising freezing, storage, and thawing results in relatively small decreases in the nutritional quality of meat products.[37]

The same is not true for canned or dehydrated meats stored at ambient temperatures for long periods. Dvorak[55] found that freeze-dried beef stored in bottles at room temperature for 4 years lost about 32% lysine, 40% tryptophan, 12% leucine, and 12% methionine as assessed by enzyme availability tests. Long-term storage of canned meats has been reported to decrease the content of the amino acids lysine, methionine, and threonine.[29] The reductions in biological values of proteins during storage have been ascribed to the Maillard reaction and possibly lipid oxidation.[56] Oxidative deterioration has been found to be a problem in freeze-dried and dehydrated foods where the large relative surface area and low moisture content make foods susceptible to lipid oxidation; the primary lipid contributing to these changes is reported to be linoleic acid.[57] The use of antioxidants and the rigorous exclusion of oxygen have been found to be useful in preventing or reducing oxidative deterioration, and it is interesting that

Table 3
EFFECT OF FROZEN STORAGE ON B VITAMINS

| Product | Conditions of storage | Percentage loss of vitamins | | | | | Ref. |
|---|---|---|---|---|---|---|---|
| | | Thiamin | Riboflavin | Niacin | Pyridoxine | Pantothenic acid | |
| Beef steaks | −18°C, 6 months | 0 | < 1 | + | < 10 | 22 | 37 |
| Pork loins | −16°C, 120 d | 21 | — | — | — | — | 53 |
| Pork chops and roasts | −18°C, 6 months | + to 18 | 0—37 | + to 5 | 0—8 | 18 | 37 |
| Lamb chops | −18°C, 6 months | + | — | + | — | — | 37 |
| Meat meals goulash German sausage | −25°C, 6 months | + to 24 | + to 18 | — | — | — | 54 |

*Note:* + indicates an apparent increase in vitamin content.

Table 4
EFFECT OF STORAGE
TEMPERATURE ON THIAMIN
LOSS IN CANNED AND
DEHYDRATED PORK

| | % Loss | Months in storage | | | |
|---|---|---|---|---|---|
| | | 1 | 3 | 6 | 12 |
| Canned | 10 | 30 | 9 | 3 | 0 |
| | 25 | — | 27 | 23 | 17 |
| | 50 | — | 38 | 34 | 31 |
| Dehydrated | 10 | 13 | 11 | 9 | 8 |
| | 25 | 20 | 16 | 14 | 13 |
| | 50 | 31 | 24 | 22 | 20 |

*Note:* Figures show maximum temperatures
(°C) for limiting the percentage loss of
thiamin to the values indicated in the
left hand column.

From Kramer, A., *Food Technol. (Chicago)*,
28(1), 50, 1974. With permission.

freeze-dried meat products stored under nitrogen showed no decrease in PER after 30 days of storage.[58]

As far as vitamin losses are concerned, Kramer[59] has pointed out the desirability of storing dehydrated and canned meats at low temperatures. Using thiamin as the reference nutrient, it has been demonstrated that 10% loss occurred in canned meat products stored at 0°C over 3 years whereas storage at 20°C caused a 43% loss after only 2 years.[60] Table 4 summarizes the effect of various storage temperatures on thiamin retention in canned and dehydrated pork and shows that, for effective nutrient retention over storage periods of up to 1 year, the temperature should be no higher than

8°C. At temperatures of 20°C or above losses can be considerable, particularly in the dehydrated product.

In a comprehensive study of nutrient retention in canned meals containing meat stored at room temperature (22°C), Hellendoorn et al.[61] showed that the levels of vitamin A, thiamin, niacin, and pantothenic acid decreased during storage of up to 5 years but the other vitamins investigated (i.e., pyridoxine, $B_{12}$, folic acid, riboflavin, and choline chloride) showed only small losses. Vitamin E decreased only after prolonged storage. Protein quality was only slightly affected during storage, and this was attributed mainly to small (10%) losses of methionine and cystine. The lysine content decreased only 3 to 5% on storage. The NPU of corned beef has been reported to be unaffected by a 9-year storage period, but two rather antique samples of canned meat (veal 110-years-old and mutton 136-years-old) had NPU values of 29 and 27, respectively,[28] which represent considerable reductions in nutritive value compared with fresh and canned meat.

It seems that some nutrient loss can occur during prolonged storage of canned and dehydrated meat products at ambient temperatures. In the case of a labile nutrient such as thiamin, these losses, when added to those occurring in processing, represent large overall losses of nutritional quality. In general, storage at low temperatures offers the best way of reducing nutrient loss over long periods, although oxidative deterioration is most effectively prevented by the exclusion of oxygen and/or the use of antioxidants. Very low temperatures (−30°C) have also been reported to be useful in this respect.[36] Of the various nutritional parameters, protein quality seems the least affected by storage in the major proportion of meat products.

## EFFECTS OF FOOD PREPARATION PROCEDURES

As might be expected, the cooking and general preparation of meat products can markedly alter their nutritional quality. These alterations very much reflect the changes observed in commercial processing in that the principal reduction in nutrient value is the loss of B-vitamins, particularly heat-labile thiamin.

### Thawing

Some vitamin loss can occur during thawing of frozen meats, and Pearson et al.[62] have reported losses of thiamin (12%), riboflavin (10%), niacin (14%), pyridoxine (32%), and folic acid (8%) in the thaw juice of a beef carcass. Larson[63] noted defrosting losses of up to 50% of the thiamin, riboflavin, and niacin content of frozen poultry. Nevertheless, comparisons of the vitamin retention of meats cooked from the frozen state with those cooked after thawing show little difference in the content of thiamin, riboflavin,[64] or pyridoxine.[65] The losses of protein and fat in thaw juices are reported to be very low.[66]

### Cooking

The losses of vitamins increase when food is cooked and, as with commercial processing, it is thiamin retention which has attracted the most attention. Table 5 summarizes the losses of thiamin in some meat and meat products during various cooking procedures.

There is clearly a large amount of variation in the thiamin lost in different types of meat for a given cooking process, but in general, braising seems to cause the greatest nutrient loss (60%) with other procedures showing about half this. Tilgner[70] has reported that braising of beef destroys most of the thiamin. Losses of other B-vitamins occur during cooking, but these are usually less than that of thiamin, and it is the

## Table 5
## LOSS OF THIAMIN IN MEAT AND MEAT PRODUCTS
## DURING VARIOUS COOKING PROCESSES

| Food | Percentage loss of thiamin | | | | | |
|---|---|---|---|---|---|---|
| | Frying | Roasting | Broiling (grilling) | Braising | Boiling | Ref. |
| Chicken | 35 | — | 22 | — | 42 | 67 |
| Beef | | | | | | |
| Patties | 8 | 17 | 28 | — | — | 68, 69 |
| Steak | 15 | 10 | 31 | — | — | 68, 69 |
| Various cuts | — | 40 | — | 68 | — | 69 |
| Pork | | | | | | |
| Chops | 40 | 28 | — | — | — | 68 |
| Ham | — | — | 35 | — | — | 69 |
| Bacon | — | — | 21 | — | — | 69 |
| Various cuts | — | — | — | 58 | — | 69 |
| Lamb | | | | | | |
| Chops | 32 | 30 | 34 | — | — | 68, 69 |
| Patties | — | — | 39 | — | — | 69 |
| Various cuts | — | 36 | — | — | — | 69 |
| Veal | | | | | | |
| Chops | — | — | — | 62 | — | 69 |
| Steak | — | — | — | 52 | — | 69 |
| Mean | 26 | 27 | 30 | 60 | 42 | |

latter which is the best indicator of the overall nutrient damage. Losses of vitamin A have been reported during the cooking of liver,[71] but these were generally of the same level as other vitamins and varied between 0 and 29% with an average of 12%. Individual livers differed markedly in vitamin A loss.

A good proportion of the cooking losses of B-vitamins from meat products is probably due to passage into the meat juices. Thomas et al.[72] recovered appreciable amounts (around 20%) of thiamin, riboflavin, and niacin in the juice from beef patties, and Wing and Alexander[73] found 5% pyridoxine in the drip from roasting chicken breast. During the boiling of several meat products, up to 33% of the vitamin $B_{12}$ was lost in the cooking liquid.[74] These studies stress the desirability of using meat juices in gravies, etc., to improve the overall nutritional value of the food.

Protein losses on cooking are generally less than those of B-vitamins unless meat is cooked at very high temperatures. Dvorak and Vognarova[9] reported increasing reductions in the available lysine content of beef as the cooking temperature was raised, ranging from 8% loss at 70°C to 50% at 160°C. Beef cooked at 100 to 120°C suffered only minor changes in its amino acid content apart from cystine and methionine. Cooking in liquid increased the amino acid losses.[75] Choi et al.[76] measured the peptic digestibility of beef round subjected to various cooking processes and found that it was highest for beef autoclaved at 104°C for 30 min and lowest for dry heating at 160°C for 2 hr.

There is little information on the losses of fat on cooking, but fat does not appear to suffer much deterioration during normal cooking procedures. It has been reported that there is little destruction of fatty acids in pork during roasting at 169°C to an internal temperature of 82°C, although roasting resulted in decreased quantities of several phospholipid fatty acids from ham, picnic, and loin.[77] Reductions in the unsaturated-to-saturated fatty acid ratio[78] and in linoleic acid content[79] have been reported for cooked beef steaks compared with the raw material.

## Microwave Cooking

At this stage it is appropriate to compare briefly the relative merits of conventional and electronic (microwave) cooking on nutrient retention, as this has received much attention in recent years. It is conceivable that the rapid heat penetration in microwave cooking might be less destructive of vitamins than the slower rise in temperature in conventional ovens. Goldblith et al.[80] showed that microwave radiation per se had no destructive effect on thiamin and that loss of the vitamin was the result only of heat. However, the bulk of the available evidence suggests that microwave cooking does not significantly increase the retention of B-vitamins in meat and meat products. Kylen et al.[81] found very little difference in the retention of thiamin in beef roast, pork, and beef and ham loaves cooked by microwave or conventional methods. Losses of thiamin and riboflavin[82] and pyridoxine[83] in turkey breast muscle were not significantly different between the two cooking methods. Differences were generally greater between tissue samples than cooking methods. Similar results were obtained for pyridoxine in pork,[84] for thiamin in beef-soy loaves,[85] and for thiamin and riboflavin in retail cuts of turkey, beef, and pork.[86] In addition, conventional methods are reported to score higher on palatability.[87] Nevertheless, Kahn and Livingston[88] showed that thiamin retention was better in frozen meals (including beef and chicken dishes) reheated in a microwave oven than in freshly prepared food held at 82°C. The difference in thiamin availability could be equivalent to as much as 18% of the recommended daily intake of certain age groups. Swiderski[89] has also reported that thiamin is lost in meat dishes held hot, with reductions of up to 23% after 3 hr and 40% after 6 hr.

There is very little information on the effect of infrared radiation on nutritional quality, but Bolshakow et al.[90] have reported that chicken meat grilled using this procedure is superior in BV to a conventionally-cooked product.

## Lysinoalanine Formation

Although the main effects of cooking on nutritional quality in meat products are loss of vitamins, reduction in protein value, and so on, it is important to consider other factors which may influence the overall "goodness value" of the food. It is in this context that lysinoalanine (LAL) is worthy of brief mention. LAL is a nephrotoxic amino acid which is reported to be widely distributed in cooked, high-protein foods. For example, it has been shown[91] that concentrations of up to 200 and 170 ppm can occur in cooked chicken and in heated frankfurters, respectively, whereas none was detected in the raw state or, in the case of the frankfurters, as purchased before cooking.

However, it now appears that the danger to the consumer from LAL formation is much less than was first feared. Although synthetic LAL has caused kidney lesions in rats, it is ineffective when fed combined in food protein.[92] The hypothesis has been advanced that LAL is not released from protein by normal digestive processes. In addition, the rat may be particularly susceptible to this substance, as other species tested including the dog, mouse, hamster, Japanese quail, and monkey, do not develop lesions, even with free LAL. A recent review[93] suggests that LAL presents only a very small risk as a toxic component in the food of man.

## CONCLUDING REMARKS

In the 3 to 4 years since a previous review,[94] there has been a significant amount of new research into the nutritional effects of meat processing. There remain, however, few causes for serious concern about the nutritional damage to meat resulting from processing. This generalization should not obscure the fact that there are specific instances where the loss of B-vitamins, particularly thiamin, can be appreciable — for example, if a product was submitted to heat processing, stored at a high ambient temperature, and then harshly cooked. The losses of nutrients under this set of circumstances would be nutritionally important because meat and meat products are significant sources of these vitamins to the majority of the population.

The best method of preserving meat seems to be deep freezing at very low temperatures, which minimizes vitamin loss and has a negligible deleterious effect on protein and fat quality. Some loss of vitamins can occur in thaw juices, but these are not significant compared with normal losses occurring on cooking. This raises an important point: that virtually all meat products are cooked in one way or another, and nutrient losses during domestic or institutional cooking can be as high as or higher than those resulting from industrial processing, particularly if meat dishes are held hot for long periods.

Barratt[95] and the Institute of Food Technologists[96] have reviewed the overall effect of processing on the nutritive value of food and conclude that, in general, commercial processing does not result in major losses of nutritional quality. Nevertheless, there is no room for complacency, and it will be important to investigate the nutritional impact of more recent methods of meat processing, e.g., fermentation technology, and to improve existing procedures where possible. Several areas such as fat deterioration on storage and the effect of processing on mineral retention are worthy of further research. In addition, it will be important to monitor the effects of processing and cooking on the possible formation of toxic compounds (e.g., nitrosamines) in meat products. In the future it will be necessary to consider the home preparation and institutional handling of meat products as well as industrial processing to guarantee the best possible nutritional quality of the food on the plate.

# REFERENCES

1. **Ministry of Agriculture, Fisheries and Food,** *Household Food Consumption and Expenditure in 1973,* Her Majesty's Stationery Office, London, 1975, 105—108.
2. **Harris, R. S.,** General discussion on the stability of nutrients, in *Nutritional Evaluation of Food Processing,* 2nd ed., Harris, R. S. and Karmas, E., Eds., AVI Publishing, Westport, Conn., 1975, 3.
3. **Hill, M. H.,** Commercial methods of preserving meat and meat products, *Process Biochem.,* 10(10), 23—30, 1975.
4. **Rice, E. E., Beuk, J. F., and Fried, J. F.,** Effect of commercial curing, smoking, storage, and cooking operations upon vitamin content of pork hams, *Food Res.,* 12, 239—246, 1947.
5. **Beuk, J. F., Fried, J. F., and Rice, E. E.,** Nutritive values of sausage and other table-ready meats as affected by processing, *Food Res.,* 15, 302—307, 1950.
6. **Jackson, S. H., Crook, A., Malone, V., and Drake, T. G. H.,** The retention of thiamin, riboflavin and niacin in cooking pork and in processing bacon, *J. Nutr.,* 29, 391, 1945.
7. **Schweigert, B. S. and Payne, B. Y.,** A summary of the nutrient content of meat, *Am. Meat Inst. Found. Bull.,* No. 30, 1956.
8. **Miller, E. L., Hartley, A. W., and Thomas, D. C.,** Availability of sulphur amino acids in protein foods. IV. Effect of heat treatment upon the total amino acid content of cod muscle, *Br. J. Nutr.,* 19, 565, 1965.
9. **Dvorak, Z. and Vognarova, I.,** Available lysine in meat and meat products, *J. Sci. Food Agric.,* 16, 305—312, 1965.

10. Chen, L. and Issenberg, P., Interactions of some wood smoke components with amino groups in proteins, *J. Agric. Food Chem.*, 20, 1113—1115, 1972.

11. Walters, C. L. and Casselden, R. J., The gaseous products of nitrite incubation with skeletal muscle, *Z. Lebensm. Unters. Forsch.*, 150, 335, 1972.

12. Woolford, G., Casselden, R. J., Walters, C. L., Parke, D. V., and Gould, B. J., Gaseous products of the interaction of sodium nitrite with porcine skeletal muscle, *Biochem. J.*, 130, 82P, 1972.

13. Mirna, E. and Hofmann, K., The behaviour of nitrite in meat products, *Fleischwirtschaft*, 49, 1361—1363 and 1366, 1969.

14. Walters, C. L., Burger, I. H., Jewell, G. G., Lewis, D. F., and Parke, D. V., Mitochondrial enzyme pathways and their possible role during curing, *Z. Lebensm. Unters. Forsch.*, 158, 193—203, 1975.

15. Kirkpatrick, D. C. and Coffin, D. E., Trace metal content of various cured meats, *J. Sci. Food. Agric.*, 26, 43—46, 1975.

16. Scanlan, R. A., N-nitrosamines in foods, *CRC Crit. Rev. Food Technol.*, 5, 357—402, 1975.

17. Schweigert, B. S. and Lushbough, C. H., Effects of processing on meat products, in *Nutritional Evaluation of Food Processing*, Harris, R. S. and von Loesecke, H., Eds., John Wiley & Sons, New York, 1960, 98 and 270.

18. Waisman, H. A., Henderson, L. M., McIntire, J. M., and Elvehjem, C. A., The effect of enzymatic digestion on the pantothenic acid content of meats determined by the microbiological method, *J. Nutr.*, 23, 239, 1942.

19. Neilands, J. B., Strong, F. M., and Elvehjem, C. A., The nutritive value of canned foods. XXV. Vitamin content of canned fish products, *J. Nutr.*, 34, 633, 1947.

20. Cantoni, C. and Minoccheri, F., Distribution of vitamins $B_1$, $B_2$ and PP (nicotinic acid) in canned meats, *Indust. Alim. Prod. Anim.*, 12, 107—108, 1973.

21. Everson, G. J., Chang, J., Leonard, S., Luh, B. S., and Simone, M., Aseptic canning of foods, *Food Technol. (Chicago)*, 18, 84—88, 1964.

22. Chichester, C. O., Nutrition in food processing, *World Rev. Nutr. Diet.*, 16, 318—333, 1973.

23. Texeira, A. A., Dixon, J. R., Zahradnik, J. W., and Zinsmeister, G. E., Computer optimization of nutrient retention in the thermal processing of conduction-heating foods, *Food Technol. (Chicago)*, 23, 845—850, 1969.

24. Donoso, G., Lewis, O. A. M., Miller, D. S., and Payne, P. R., Effect of heat treatment on the nutritive value of proteins: chemical and balance studies, *J. Sci. Food Agric.*, 13, 192—196, 1962.

25. Mayfield, H. L. and Hedrick, M. T., The effect of canning, roasting and corning on the biological value of the proteins of Western beef, finished on either grass or grain, *J. Nutr.*, 37, 487, 1949.

26. Beuk, J. F., Chornock, F. W., and Rice, E. E., The effect of severe heat treatment upon the amino acids of fresh and cured pork, *J. Biol. Chem.*, 175, 291, 1948.

27. Rubin, L. J., Nutrition — a new dimension in food processing, *Food Can.*, 32, 23—27, 1972.

28. Bender, A. E., Loss of nutritive value of proteins through processing and storage, *Proc. 1st Int. Congr. Food Sci. Technol.*, III, Leitch, J. M., Ed., Gordon and Breach, New York, 1962, 449.

29. Svabova-Stronova, M., Changes in the biological value of proteins in canned foods, *Cesk. Hyg.*, 13, 449—452, 1968; *Chem. Abstr.*, 70, 18981a, 1969.

30. Osner, R. C. and Johnson, R. M., Nutritional changes in proteins during heat processing, *J. Food Technol.*, 3, 81—86, 1968.

31. Karakas, R., Dinic, J., and Bem, Z., Influence of heat treatment on the biological value of canned meat products, *Proc. Eur. Mtg. Meat Res. Workers*, Institute of Meat Technology, University of Helsinki, 1969. 15, 413, (Summary III, 107).

32. Tarr, H. L. A., The Maillard reaction in flesh foods, *Food Technol. (Chicago)*, 8, 15, 1954.

33. Adrian, J., Nutritional aspects of the Maillard reaction. II. Behaviour of individual foods, *Ind. Alim. Prod. Veg.*, 89, 1713—1720, 1972.

34. Heller, B. S., Chutkow, M. R., Lushbough, C. H., Siedler, A. J., and Schweigert, B. S., Utilization of amino acids from foods by the rat. V. Effects of heat treatment on lysine in meat, *J. Nutr.*, 73, 113—116, 1961.

35. Nordal, J. and Fossum, K., The heat stability of some trypsin inhibitors in meat products with special reference to added soybean protein, *Z. Lebensm. Unters. Forsch.*, 154, 144—150, 1974.

36. Ingram, M., Meat preservation — past, present and future, *R. Soc. Health J.*, 92, 121—130 and 150, 1972.

37. Fennema, O., Effects of freeze-preservation on nutrients, in *Nutritional Evaluation of Food Processing*, 2nd ed., Harris, R. S. and Karmas, E., Eds., AVI Publishing, Westport, Conn., 1975, 244—288.

38. Cutting, C. L. and Hollingsworth, D., Effect of freezing on the nutritive value of meat, *Meat Res. Inst. Symp.*, Cutting, C. L., Ed., Meat Research Institute, Bristol, England, 1974, 3, 12.1—12.5.

39. Cantoni, C., Busolo, C., Minoccheri, F. and Merlino, M., Behaviour of peroxides, free fatty acids and vitamins $B_1$, $B_2$ and $B_{12}$ during preparation, preservation and reheating of precooked frozen foods, *Indust. Alim.*, 11, 80—82, 1972.

40. Lee, F. A., Brooks, R. F., Pearson, A. M., Miller, J. J., and Volz, F., Effect of freezing rate on meat. Appearance, palatability and vitamin content of beef, *Food Res.*, 15, 8—15, 1950.
41. Lehrer, W. P., Jr., Wiese, A. C., Harvey, W. R., and Moore, P. R., The stability of thiamin, riboflavin and nicotinic acid of lamb chops during frozen storage and subsequent cooking, *Food Res.*, 17, 24—30, 1952.
42. Lee, F. A., Brooks, R. F., Pearson, A. M., Miller, J. J., and Wanderstock, J. J., Effect of rate of freezing on pork quality, *J. Am. Diet. Assoc.*, 30, 351—354, 1954.
43. Nestorov, N., Vasilyev, T., Lilov, L., Tyutyundgiyev, N., Ivanov, L., Dgevisov, S., and Miteva, K., Oxidative processes in beef and pork fat as affected with the temperature conditions of freezing and cold storage, *Proc. Eur. Mtg. Meat Res. Workers*, Institute of Meat Technology, University of Helsinki, 1969, 15, II, 110, (Summary III, 129).
44. Rowe, D. M., Mountney, G. J., and Prudent, I., Effect of freeze-drying on the thiamin, riboflavin and niacin content of chicken muscle, *Food Technol. (Chicago)*, 17, 1449—1450, 1963.
45. De Groot, A. P., The influence of dehydration of foods on the digestibility and the biological value of protein, *Food Technol. (Chicago)*, 17, 339—343, 1963.
46. Thomas, M. and Calloway, D., Nutritional value of dehydrated food, *J. Am. Diet. Assoc.*, 39, 105—116, 1961.
47. Svabensky, O., Pickova, J., and Martinovska, M., Stability of thiamin and riboflavin in meat after freeze-drying, *Prum. Potravin*, 18, 378—380, 1967; *Chem. Abstr.*, 67, 72575x, 1967.
48. Thomas, M. H. and Josephson, E. S., Radiation preservation of foods and its effect on nutrients, *Sci. Teacher*, 37, 59—63, 1970.
49. Josephson, E. S., Thomas, M. H., and Calhoun, W. K., Effects of treatment of foods with ionizing radiation, in *Nutritional Evaluation of Food Processing*, 2nd ed., Harris, R. S. and Karmas, E., Eds., AVI Publishing, Westport, Conn., 1975, 393—411.
50. Diehl, J. F., Thiamin in irradiated foodstuffs. I. Influence of different irradiation conditions and of time after irradiation, *Z. Lebensm. Unters. Forsch.*, 157, 317—321, 1975.
51. Krylova, N. N., Piulskaya, V. I., and Krasilnikova, T. F., Effect of gamma-radiation on thiamin stability in fried pork, *Vopr. Pitan.*, No. 2, 83—84, 1973; *Food Sci. Technol. Abstr.*, 5, 7 S 829, 1973.
52. Goldblith, S. A., Radiation preservation of food. The current status, *J. Food Technol.*, 5, 103—110, 1970.
53. Kemp, J. D., Montgomery, R. E., and Fox, J. D., Chemical, palatability and cooking characteristics of normal and low quality pork loins as affected by freezer storage, *J. Food Sci.*, 41, 1—3, 1976.
54. Rogowski, B., The effect of storing and heating frozen ready-to-eat meals on vitamins $B_1$ and $B_2$ in the meat, *Fleischwirtschaft*, 56, 250—252, 1976.
55. Dvorak, Z., Availability of essential amino acids from proteins. II. Food proteins, *J. Sci. Food Agric.*, 19, 77, 1968.
56. Labuza, T. P., Nutrient losses during drying and storage of dehydrated foods, *CRC Crit. Rev. Food Technol.*, 3, 217—240, 1972.
57. Ammu, K. and Sharma, T. R., Changes in the nutritional value of accelerated freeze-dried (AFD) foodstuffs during processing and storage, *Indian Food Packer*, 29(2), 5—10, 1975.
58. Regier, L. W. and Tappel, A. L., Freeze-dried meat. III. Nonoxidative deterioration of freeze-dried meat, *Food Res.*, 21, 630, 1956.
59. Kramer, A., Storage retention of nutrients, *Food Technol. (Chicago)*, 28(1), 50—60, 1974.
60. Cecil, S. R. and Woodroof, J. G., The stability of canned foods in long-term storage, *Food Technol. (Chicago)*, 17(5), 131, 1963.
61. Hellendoorn, E. W., De Groot, A. P., Van der Mijlldekker, L. P., Slump, P., and Willems, J. J. L., Nutritive value of canned meals, *J. Am. Diet. Assoc.*, 58, 434—441, 1971.
62. Pearson, A. M., Burnside, J. E., Edwards, H. M., Glasscock, R. R., Cunha, T. J., and Novak, A. F., Vitamin losses in drip obtained upon defrosting frozen meat, *Food Res.*, 16, 85—87, 1951.
63. Larson, E. R., Vitamin losses in the drip from thawed, frozen poultry, *J. Am. Diet. Assoc.*, 32, 716, 1956.
64. Westerman, B. D., Vail, G. E., Tinklin, G. L., and Smith, J., B complex vitamins in meat. II. The influence of different methods of thawing frozen steaks upon their palatability and vitamin content, *Food Technol. (Chicago)*, 3, 184—187, 1949.
65. Engler, P. P. and Bowers, J. A., Vitamin $B_6$ content of turkey cooked from frozen, partially frozen and thawed states, *J. Food Sci.*, 40, 615—617, 1975.
66. Toepfer, E. W., Pritchett, C. A., and Hewston, E. M., Boneless beef: raw, cooked and stewed. Results of analysis for moisture, protein, fat and ash, *U.S. Dep. Agric. Bull.*, No. 1137, 1955.
67. Rognerud, G., Contents of some nutrients in raw and prepared broiler chickens. I. Thiamin, calcium and iron, *Tidsskr. Hermetikind.*, 58, 125—129, 1972; *Food Sci. Technol. Abstr.*, 5, 1 S 107, 1973.

68. Tronstad, T. and Blegen, E., Thiamin retention in some meat products after pan frying and oven roasting, *Tidsskr. Hermetikind.*, 58, 313—315, 1972; *Food Sci. Technol. Abstr.*, 5, 7 S 721, 1973.

69. LaChance, P. A., Effects of food preparation procedures on nutrient retention with emphasis upon food service practices, in *Nutritional Evaluation of Food Processing*, 2nd ed., Harris, R. S. and Karmas, E., Eds., AVI Publishing, Westport, Conn., 1975, 463—528.

70. Tilgner, D. J., The technology of braising meat, *Fleischwirtschaft*, 52, 853—857, 1972.

71. Hannukainen, F. and Niinivaara, F. P., Destruction of vitamin A in liver during processing, *Fleischwirtschaft*, 54, 1363—1370, 1974.

72. Thomas, M. H., Brenner, S., Eaton, A., and Craig, V., Effect of electronic cooking on nutritive value of foods, *J. Am. Diet Assoc.*, 25, 39, 1949.

73. Wing, R. W. and Alexander, J. C., Effect of microwave heating on vitamin $B_6$ retention in chicken, *J. Am. Diet. Assoc.*, 61, 661, 1972.

74. Yamaguchi, K. and Hayashi, J., Effects of various cooking methods on vitamin $B_{12}$. II. Influence of heating procedures (2), *Jpn. J. Nutr.*, 31, 26—31, 1973.

75. Bognar, A., Effect of thermal treatment on the content of amino acids in beef, *Ernaehr. Umsch.*, 18, 200, 1971.

76. Choi, H. M., Shin, K. S., Youn, J. E., and Lee, B. W., Effect of cooking condition on the enzymic digestibility of meat protein. The digestibility of edible beef and squid, *Korean J. Food Sci. Technol.*, 6, 70—74, 1974.

77. De Lumen, B. O., Witte, V. C., and Bailey, M. E., Effects of processing on the major fatty acids of separable porcine tissues. I. Influence of roasting fresh pork, *J. Anim. Sci.*, 39, 309—316, 1974.

78. Terrell, R. N., Lewis, R. W., Cassens, R. G., and Bray, R. W., Fatty acid compositions of bovine subcutaneous fat depots determined by gas-liquid chromatography, *J. Food Sci.*, 32, 516, 1967.

79. Terrell, R. N., Suess, G. G., Cassens, R. G., and Bray, R. W., Broiling, sex and interrelationships with carcase and growth characteristics and their effect on the neutral and phospholipid fatty acids of the bovine *longissimus dorsi*, *J. Food Sci.*, 33, 562, 1968.

80. Goldblith, S. A., Tannenbaum, S. R., and Wang, D. I. C., Thermal and 2450 MHz microwave energy effect on the destruction of thiamin, *Food Technol. (Chicago)*, 22, 1266, 1968.

81. Kylen, A. M., McGrath, B. H., Hallmark, E. L., and van Duyne, F. O., Microwave and conventional cooking of meat, *J. Am. Diet. Assoc.*, 45, 139, 1964.

82. Bowers, J. A. and Fryer, B. A., Thiamin and riboflavin in cooked and frozen reheated turkey, *J. Am. Diet. Assoc.*, 60, 399—401, 1972.

83. Bowers, J. A., Fryer, B. A., and Engler, P. P., Vitamin $B_6$ in turkey breast muscle cooked in microwave and conventional ovens, *Poult. Sci.*, 53, 844—846, 1974.

84. Bowers, J. A., Fryer, B. A., and Engler, P. P., Vitamin $B_6$ in pork muscle cooked in microwave and conventional ovens, *J. Food Sci.*, 39, 426—427, 1974.

85. Ziprin, Y. A. and Carlin, A. F., Microwave and conventional cooking in relation to quality and nutritive value of beef and beef-soy loaves, *J. Food Sci.*, 41, 4—8, 1976.

86. McMullen, E. A., A comparison of the weight loss, tenderness and nutrient retention of selected meat products cooked uncovered and in oven film, *Diss. Abstr. Int. B*, 35, 1779, 1974.

87. Bender, A. E., Nutritional effects of food processing, *J. Food Technol.*, 1, 261, 1966.

88. Kahn, L. N. and Livingston, G. E., Effect of heating methods on thiamin retention in fresh or frozen prepared foods, *J. Food Sci.*, 35, 349—351, 1970.

89. Swiderski, F., Organoleptic and nutritive changes in prepared dishes during transportation in containers, *Przem. Spozyw.*, 23, 448, 1969.; *Food Sci. Technol. Abstr.*, 2, 4 G 195, 1970.

90. Bolshakow, A. S., Fedorov, N. E., Shablii, V. Ya., and Mitrofanov, N. S., Biological value of chicken meat subjected to heat treatment by infra-red radiation, *Vopr. Pitan.*, 29, 60, 1970; *Food Sci. Technol. Abstr.*, 3, 5 S 617, 1971.

91. Sternberg, M., Kim, C. Y., and Schwende, F. J., Lysinoalanine: presence in foods and food ingredients, *Science*, 190, 992—994, 1974.

92. Van Beek, L., Feron, V. J., and De Groot, A. P., Nutritional effects of alkali-treated soyprotein in rats, *J. Nutr.*, 104, 1630—1636, 1974.

93. Anon., Processed protein foods and lysinoalanine, *Nutr. Rev.*, 34, 120—122, 1976.

94. Burger, I. H. and Walters, C. L., The effect of processing on the nutritive value of flesh foods, *Proc. Nutr. Soc.*, 32, 1—8, 1973.

95. Barratt, B., Nutrition: II. Effects of processing, *Food Can.*, 33, 28—31, 1973.

96. Anon., The effects of food processing on nutritional values, *Food Technol. (Chicago)*, 28(10), 78—81, 1974.

# EFFECT OF PROCESSING ON NUTRIENT CONTENT OF MEATS OF MOLLUSKAN, CRUSTACEAN, AND OTHER INVERTEBRATE ORIGIN

## Bohdan M. Slabyj

## INTRODUCTION

Very few studies have been reported in the literature showing the effect of processing on nutritional content of shellfish. Information published is incidental to other studies, often not giving details needed for proper interpretation. The first and the second table shown have been prepared using primarily review articles to indicate nutritional content of raw and processed edible portions, respectively. The remainder of the tables presented have been selected to show changes in composition due to a given processing of a specific shellfish. It must be pointed out that shellfish exhibit significant seasonal and harvest area variability in nutritional content. Significant differences in composition have also been detected among various body parts of crustacea. Consequently, data of studies paying special attention to these factors are included.

Table 1
NUTRITIONAL CONTENT OF RAW EDIBLE PORTION OF CRUSTACEA AND MOLLUSCS

| | Moisture g/100 g | Protein g/100 g | Lipid g/100 g | Ash g/100 g | Carbohydrate g/100 g | Energy Cal/100 g | Ca mg/100 g | P mg/100 g | Fe mg/100 g | Na mg/100 g | K mg/100 g | Cholesterol mg/100 g | Thiamin mg/100 g | Riboflavin mg/100 g | Niacin mg/100 g | Vitamin $B_6$ mg/100 g | Vitamin $B_{12}$ mg/100 g | Pantothenic Acid mg/100 g | Biotin mg/100 g | Ref. |
|---|---|---|---|---|---|---|---|---|---|---|---|---|---|---|---|---|---|---|---|---|
| **Abalone** | | | | | | | | | | | | | | | | | | | | |
| *Halotis* spp. | 76.9(2.9) | 14.9 (0.2) | 0.5 (0.1) | 1.8 (0.6) | — | — | 27(6) | — | 2.35* | — | — | — | — | — | — | — | — | — | — | 9, 10 |
| **Clam** | | | | | | | | | | | | | | | | | | | | |
| Miscellaneous spp. | 83.0(0.7) | 11.7 (0.4) | 1.4 (0.2) | 1.8 (0.2) | — | — | 99(9) | 156(19) | 6.14 | 190(10) | 137(56) | 50 | 0.09 | 0.18 | 1.3 | 0.04 | — | — | — | 1, 2, 4, 9, 10 |
| Clam, butter — *Saxidomus nuttal* | 83.0 | 13.3 | 1.3 | 1.9 | — | — | — | — | — | — | — | — | — | — | — | — | — | — | — | 1 |
| Clam, hard shell — *Mercenaria mercenaria* | 91.8(0.1) | 4.41(0.17) | 0.21(0.02) | 1.97(0.02) | — | — | 65(3) | 69(3) | — | — | — | — | — | 0.13 | — | — | — | — | — | 4, 8 |
| Clam, short neck — *Venerupis semi decusata* | 84.9 | 12.8 (0.2) | 0.8 (0.4) | — | — | — | — | — | — | — | — | — | — | — | — | — | — | — | — | 9 |
| Clam, soft shell — *Mya arenarea* | 83.3(0.9) | 9.51(0.43) | 1.27(0.16) | 1.19(0.09) | — | — | 53(3) | 152(6) | — | — | — | — | — | — | — | — | — | — | — | 8 |
| | 84.8(1.0) | 11.2 (0.6) | 2.0 | 1.7 | 1.7 | 89 | — | — | — | — | — | — | — | — | — | — | — | — | — | 9 |
| Clam, surf — *Spisula solidissima* | 79.4(0.2) | 15.6 (0.1) | 0.34(0.06) | 2.29(0.10) | — | — | 41(3) | 194(5) | — | — | — | — | — | — | — | — | — | — | — | 8 |
| **Crab** | | | | | | | | | | | | | | | | | | | | |
| Miscellaneous spp. | 76.1(1.8) | 15.8 (1.4) | 3.1 (1.3) | 2.5 (0.5) | — | — | 94(22) | 233(63) | 2.19 | 262(73) | 233(63) | 100 | — | 0.09 | 2.3 | 0.013 | 0.23 | 0.71 | 0.01 | 1, 2, 9, 10 |
| Crab, blue — *Callinectes sapidus* | 81.2(0.6) | 16.1 (0.5) | 1.0 (0.1) | 1.6 (0.1) | 1.25 | 81.5 | 94(11) | 152(30) | — | 188 | — | — | — | — | — | — | — | — | — | 9, 10 |
| | 77.4(0.3) | 19.8 (0.1) | 1.02(0.07) | 2.06(0.04) | — | — | 102(12) | 272(10) | — | — | — | 84 | 0.075 | — | — | — | — | — | — | 3, 8 |
| Crab, Dungeness — *Cancer magister* | 80.5(0.3) | 17.2 (0.7) | 1.4 (0.1) | 1.4 (0.1) | — | 85 (4.6) | — | — | — | — | 57.5 | — | — | — | — | — | — | — | — | 9 |
| Crab, deep sea — *Neptunis* spp. | 78.4(0.6) | 16.5 (0.5) | 0.5 | 1.45 | 1 | — | 174(10) | — | — | — | 134 | — | — | — | — | — | — | — | — | 9, 10 |
| Crab, king — *Paralithodes camchatica* | 80.7(0.6) | 17.2 (0.7) | 0.7 (0.2) | 1.6 (0.2) | — | 160 | — | — | — | 55 | — | — | — | — | — | — | — | — | — | 9, 10 |
| *Paralithodes camchatica* (body) | 79.2(0.3) | 18.3 (0.2) | 0.38(0.02) | 1.60(0.05) | — | — | 42(3) | 212(10) | — | — | — | — | — | — | — | — | — | — | — | 8 |
| *Paralithodes camchatica* (leg) | 76.8(0.7) | 20.1 (0.5) | 0.40(0.03) | 1.81(0.06) | — | — | 55(4) | 228(10) | — | — | — | — | — | — | — | — | — | — | — | 8 |
| Crab, Samoan — *Scylla serrata* | 80.3(0.5) | 14.9 (0.4) | 2.9 (1.1) | 1.8 (0.1) | 0.6 | — | 118(45) | 209(65) | — | — | — | — | — | — | — | — | — | — | — | 9, 10 |
| **Crayfish** | | | | | | | | | | | | | | | | | | | | |
| Miscellaneous spp. | 76.3(0.2) | 18.7 (0.9) | 1.7 | 1.1 | — | — | 39(5) | 239(36) | 4.73 | 121(61) | 392(35) | — | — | 0.06 | 2.4 | 0.003 | 0.21 | 0.41 | 0.004 | 1, 9, 10 |
| **Lobster, spiny** | | | | | | | | | | | | | | | | | | | | |
| *Panulirus argus* | 75.8(0.3) | 23.1 (0.2) | 0.33(0.03) | 1.71(0.02) | — | — | 47(4) | 237(11) | — | — | — | — | — | — | — | — | — | — | — | 8 |
| **Mussel** | | | | | | | | | | | | | | | | | | | | |
| *Mytilus edulis* | 81.2(1.0) | 11.8 (0.1) | 2.87(0.12) | 1.47(0.02) | 2.65(0.02) | 95 | 26.3(5.6) | 197(4) | 3.95(0.38) | 286(6) | 320(17) | 21 | — | 0.13 | — | — | — | — | — | 4, 10, 12, 16 |
| **Octopus** | | | | | | | | | | | | | | | | | | | | |
| Miscellaneous spp. | 82.2 | 15.3 | 0.8 | 1.5 | — | 73 | 28(8) | 109(25) | 1.47 | 363 | 232 | 122 | 0.03 | 0.04 | — | — | 0.36 | — | 0.005 | 1, 6, 10 |
| **Oyster** | | | | | | | | | | | | | | | | | | | | |
| *Ostrea* spp. | 84.8(0.9) | 7.8 (0.5) | 1.5 (0.1) | 1.8 (0.1) | 4.2 (0.3) | 78.5(5.7) | 98(16) | 153(14) | — | 160(78) | 248(111) | 262(53) | 0.12 | 0.18 | 2.0 | 0.2 | 0.22 | 0.34 | 0.009 | 1, 9, 10, 16 |
| **Oyster, American** | | | | | | | | | | | | | | | | | | | | |
| *Crassostrea virginica* | 85.7(0.5) | 6.9 (0.3) | 1.5 (0.1) | 1.5 (0.1) | 3.3 (0.2) | — | — | — | 2.16 | — | — | 47.5 | — | 0.21 | — | — | — | — | — | 4, 9 |
| *Crassostrea virginica* Long Island | 85.4(0.2) | 7.86(0.23) | 1.13(0.07) | 1.11(0.02) | — | — | 52(3) | 145(6) | — | — | — | — | — | — | — | — | — | — | — | 8 |
| *Crassostrea virginica* Maryland and Virginia | 88.3(0.2) | 5.77(0.24) | 1.06(0.08) | 0.65(0.02) | — | — | 36(4) | 121(5) | — | — | — | — | — | — | — | — | — | — | — | 8 |
| **Prawn** | | | | | | | | | | | | | | | | | | | | |
| Miscellaneous spp. | 75.3(1.0) | 16.8 (1.1) | 1.2 (0.2) | 2.7 (0.3) | — | — | — | — | — | — | — | 137 | — | — | — | — | — | — | — | 5, 9 |
| **Scallop** | | | | | | | | | | | | | | | | | | | | |
| Miscellaneous spp. | 79.2(0.8) | 17.2 (0.7) | 0.7 (0.2) | 1.7 (0.1) | — | — | 78(38) | 270(38) | 1.90 | 182(19) | 278(58) | 35 | — | — | — | — | — | — | — | 2, 9 |
| *Pecten* spp. | 78.8(0.7) | 14.1 (0.1) | 0.20(0.03) | 1.42(0.02) | — | — | 32(5) | 207(5) | — | — | — | — | — | — | — | — | — | — | — | 1, 8 |
| **Scallop** | | | | | | | | | | | | | | | | | | | | |
| *Pecten irradians* | 80.7(0.4) | 15.4 (0.2) | 0.5 (0.3) | 1.4 (0.4) | 1.7 (0.2) | — | — | — | — | — | — | 106(35) | — | — | — | — | — | — | — | 9 |

| | | | | | | | | | | | | | | | | | | | | |
|---|---|---|---|---|---|---|---|---|---|---|---|---|---|---|---|---|---|---|---|---|
| Scallop, calico | | | | | | | | | | | | | | | | | | | | |
| *Acquipecten gibbus* | 79.8(0.4) | 15.9(0.2) | 0.6 (0.1) | 1.5 (0.3) | — | — | — | 32(2) | 215(5) | — | — | — | — | — | — | — | — | — | — | 9 |
| Scallop, sea | 77.8(0.4) | 16.9(0.1) | 0.21(0.02) | 1.79(0.01) | — | — | — | — | — | — | — | — | — | — | — | — | — | — | — | 8 |
| *Placopecten magellanicus* | 78.2(0.2) | 18.2(0.1) | 0.17(0.02) | 1.50(0.02) | — | — | — | 22(1) | 234(15) | — | — | — | — | — | — | — | — | — | — | 8 |
| Shrimp | | | | | | | | | | | | | | | | | | | | |
| Miscellaneous spp. | 76.2(0.7) | 20.5(0.7) | 1.1 (0.2) | 2.6 (0.5) | 2.2 | 2.20 | 88.3(9.7) | 142(18) | 239(21) | 132(22) | 248(40) | 160(14) | — | 0.02 | 0.03 | 2.15 | 0.001 | 0.025 | 0.25 | 1, 9, 10, 11 |
| | 77.4(0.3) | 20.1(0.4) | 0.64(0.02) | 2.26(0.14) | — | — | — | 49(4) | 187(4) | — | — | — | — | — | — | — | — | — | — | 8 |
| Shrimp, Asian | | | | | | | | | | | | | | | | | | | | |
| Miscellaneous spp. | 84.0(0.4) | 15.2(0.4) | 0.42(0.17) | 0.77(0.03) | — | — | — | 68(5) | 181(10) | — | — | — | — | — | — | — | — | — | — | 8 |
| Shrimp, brown | | | | | | | | | | | | | | | | | | | | |
| *Penaeus aztecus* | 76.2(0.1) | 21.4(0.2) | 0.14(0.01) | 1.63(0.01) | — | — | — | 59(2) | 248(5) | — | — | — | — | — | — | — | — | — | — | 8 |
| Shrimp, Maine | | | | | | | | | | | | | | | | | | | | |
| *Pandalus borealis* | 81.5(0.5) | 17.1(0.4) | 0.39(0.05) | 1.30(0.06) | — | — | — | 54(4) | 177(9) | — | — | — | 0.05 | 0.05 | 2.0 | 0.005 | 0.12 | 0.23 | 0.003 | 1, 8 |
| Shrimp, Mexican | | | | | | | | | | | | | | | | | | | | |
| Miscellaneous spp. | 80.4(0.3) | 18.1(0.3) | 0.18(0.03) | 1.40(0.04) | — | — | — | 95(2) | 176(4) | — | — | — | — | — | — | — | — | — | — | 8 |
| Shrimp, white | | | | | | | | | | | | | | | | | | | | |
| *Penaeus setiferus* (Gulf) | 77.4(0.2) | 20.6(0.1) | 0.20(0.02) | 1.41(0.02) | — | — | — | 50(1) | 233(9) | — | — | — | — | — | — | — | — | — | — | 8 |
| *Penaeus setiferus* (S. Atlantic) | 76.2(0.02) | 22.0(0.02) | 0.17(0.02) | 1.9(0.05) | — | — | — | 64(3) | 281(11) | — | — | — | — | — | — | — | — | — | — | 8 |
| Squid | | | | | | | | | | | | | | | | | | | | |
| *Loligo* spp. | 79.2(1.6) | 15.3(1.1) | 1.0 (0.2) | 1.8 (0.3) | 3 | 3.2 | 89 | 50(11) | 221(41) | 176 | 275(20) | — | — | — | — | — | — | — | — | 9, 10, 11 |

*Note:* Values in parenthesis indicate standard deviation.

## REFERENCES

1. Braekkan, O. R., *Fish in Nutrition*, Heen, E. and Kreuzer, R., Eds., Fishing News, London, 1962, 132—140.
2. Feeley, R. M., Criner, P. E., and Watt, B. K., *J. Am. Diet. Assoc.* 61, 134—148, 1972.
3. Harris, R. S. and von Loesecke, Eds., *Nutritional Evaluation of Food Processing*, John Wiley & Sons, New York, 1960.
4. Hoar, W. S. and Barberie, M., *Can. J. Res.*, 23, 8—18, 1965.
5. Kanazawa, A., Techima, S., Sakamoto, Y., and Guary, J. B., *Bull. Jpn. Soc. Sci. Fish.*, 42, 1003—1007, 1976.
6. Koga, Y., *Stud. Jpn. Foods*, 23, 412—421, 1970.
7. Pitcher, R. W., Ed., *The Canned Food Reference Manual*, American Can Co., New York, 1949.
8. Sidwell, V. D., Bonnet, J. C., and Zook, E. G., *Mar. Fish. Rev.*, 35(2), 16—19, 1973.
9. Sidwell, V. D., Foncannon, P. R., Moore, N. S., and Bonnet, J. C., *Mar. Fish. Rev.*, 36(3), 21—35, 1974.
10. Sidwell, V. D., Buzzell, D. H., Foncannon, P. R., and Smith, A. L., *Mar. Fish. Rev.*, 39(1), 1—11, 1977.
11. Sidwell, V. D., personal communication.
12. Slabyj, B. M. and Carpenter, P. N., *J. Food Sci.*, 42, 1153—1155, 1977.
13. Slabyj, B. M., Creamer, D. L., and True, R. H., *Mar. Fish Rev.*, 40(8), 18—23, 1980.
14. Stansby, M. E., Proximate composition of fish, in *Fish in Nutrition*, Heen, E. and Kreuzer, R., Eds., Fishing News, London, 1972, 55—60.
15. Teshima, S. and Kanazawa, A., *Comp. Biochem. Physiol.*, 47B, 555—561, 1974.
16. Watt, B. K. and Merrill, A. L., *Composition of Foods. Agric. Handbook 8*, U.S. Department of Agriculture, Washington, D.C., 1965.

**Table 2**

**NUTRITIONAL CONTENT OF PROCESSED EDIBLE PORTION OF CRUSTACEA AND MOLLUSCS**

| | Moisture g/100 g | Protein g/100 g | Lipid g/100 g | Ash g/100 g | Carbohydrate g/100 g | Energy Cal/100 g | Ca mg/100 g | P mg/100 g | Fe mg/100 g | Na mg/100 g | K mg/100 g | Cholesterol mg/100 g | Thiamin mg/100 g | Riboflavin mg/100 g | Niacin mg/100 g | Vitamin $B_{12}$ mg/100 g | Vitamin $B_6$ mg/100 g | Pantothenic acid mg/100 g | Biotin mg/100 g | Ref. |
|---|---|---|---|---|---|---|---|---|---|---|---|---|---|---|---|---|---|---|---|---|
| **Abalone** | | | | | | | | | | | | | | | | | | | | |
| Canned | | | | | | | | | | | | | | | | | | | | |
| Solids and liquid | 80.2 | 16.0 | 0.3 | 1.2 | 2.3 | 80 | 14 | 128 | — | — | — | 41 | 0.12 | — | — | — | — | — | — | 9, 10 |
| Drained solids | 73.2 | 21.7 | 0.1 | 1.3 | 3.7 | 103 | — | — | — | — | — | — | — | — | — | — | — | — | — | 6 |
| **Clam** | | | | | | | | | | | | | | | | | | | | |
| Canned | | | | | | | | | | | | | | | | | | | | |
| Solids and liquid | 85.0 | 8.9 | 0.9 | 2.0 | 2.9 | 56 | 55 | 137 | 41 | — | 140 | 63 | 0.01 | 0.11 | 1.1 | — | 0.08 | — | — | 6, 10 |
| Drained solids | 76.9 | 15.8 | 2.5 | 2.8 | 2.0 | 96 | — | — | — | — | — | 129 | 0.01 | 0.09 | 0.95 | — | — | — | — | 4, 6, 10 |
| Fritters | — | — | — | — | — | — | — | — | — | — | — | — | — | — | — | — | — | — | — | 4 |
| **Crab** | | | | | | | | | | | | | | | | | | | | |
| Steamed | 78.5 | 17.3 | 1.9 | 1.8 | 0.5 | 93 | 43 | 175 | 0.8 | — | — | 100 | 0.16 | 0.08 | 2.8 | — | — | — | — | 4, 12 |
| Canned | | | | | | | | | | | | | | | | | | | | |
| Drained solids | 77.4 | 17.3 | 2.8 | 1.8 | 1.1 | 99 | 45 | 182 | 0.8 | — | 110 | 100 | 0.16 | 0.18 | 2.0 | 0.01 | 0.25 | 0.17 | 0.01 | 1, 4, 6, 10 |
| Imperial | — | — | — | — | — | — | — | — | — | 1000 | — | 140 | — | — | — | — | — | — | — | 4 |
| Paste | 66.7 | 18.8 | 5.2 | 2.6 | 6.8 | — | — | — | — | 236 | — | — | — | — | — | — | — | — | — | 2 |
| **Crab** | | | | | | | | | | | | | | | | | | | | |
| Queen crab | | | | | | | | | | | | | | | | | | | | |
| Cooked (frozen) | 80.6(1.8) | 18.5(2.5) | 14(0.1) | 2.0(0.2) | — | 92 | 26(13) | 133(68) | — | 539(113) | 173(42) | — | — | — | — | — | — | — | — | 3 |
| **Lobster** | | | | | | | | | | | | | | | | | | | | |
| Cooked or canned (solids) | 76.8 | 18.7 | 1.5 | 2.7 | 0.3 | 95 | 65 | 192 | 0.8 | 210 | 180 | 85 | 0.10 | 0.07 | — | — | — | — | — | 4, 5, 10 |
| Frozen in brine (blanched) | 81.2(0.7) | 15.8(1.4) | 1.2(0.2) | 2.4(0.3) | — | 78 | 33(18) | 204(67) | — | 689(164) | 114(25) | — | — | — | — | — | — | — | — | 3 |
| Newburg | — | — | — | — | — | — | — | — | — | — | — | 182 | — | — | — | — | — | — | — | 4 |
| Paste | 68.8 | 15.5 | 9.8 | 3.1 | 3.1 | — | — | — | — | 401 | — | — | — | — | — | — | — | — | — | 2 |
| **Mussel** | | | | | | | | | | | | | | | | | | | | |
| Steamed | | | | | | | | | | | | | | | | | | | | |
| Cultivated stock | 73.0(1.6) | 18.5(2.1) | 3.1(0.3) | 2.3(0.2) | 3.1(1.8) | — | — | — | — | — | — | — | — | — | — | — | — | — | — | 8 |
| Natural stock | 73.2(1.7) | 18.1(1.6) | 3.0(0.3) | 2.3(0.3) | 3.5(1.7) | — | 41(8) | 302(15) | 7.4(1.3) | 269(38) | 325(10) | — | — | — | — | — | — | — | — | 7, 8 |
| Canned | | | | | | | | | | | | | | | | | | | | |
| Drained solids (Natural stock) | 74.6 | 18.2 | 3.3 | 2.4 | 1.5 | 111 | 29(5) | 275(10) | 6.1(0.5) | 440(2) | 231(10) | — | — | 0.13 | — | — | — | — | — | 2, 7, 8 |
| **Prawn** | | | | | | | | | | | | | | | | | | | | |
| Paste | 66.2 | 21.6 | 8.6 | 4.0 | 0 | — | — | — | — | 669 | — | — | — | — | — | — | — | — | — | 2 |
| **Oyster** | | | | | | | | | | | | | | | | | | | | |
| Canned | | | | | | | | | | | | | | | | | | | | |
| Solids and liquid | 84.7 | 7.3 | 1.7 | 0.1 | 4.3 | 63 | 28 | 124 | 5.6 | — | 70 | 45 | — | 0.02 | 0.8 | — | — | — | — | 4, 6, 10 |
| Drained solids | 80.3 | 9.8 | 2.0 | 2.1 | 5.9 | 81 | — | — | — | — | — | — | 0.02 | 0.2 | 1.0 | — | 0.04 | — | — | 1, 6 |
| Stew, homemade | — | — | — | — | — | — | — | — | — | — | — | 25 | — | — | — | — | — | — | — | 4 |
| **Scallop** | | | | | | | | | | | | | | | | | | | | |
| Breaded and frozen | 59.6(6.9) | 13.4(1.6) | 9.2(6.4) | 2.0(0.4) | 15.8 | 204 | 6(3) | 164(48) | — | 512(161) | 264(54) | — | — | — | — | — | — | — | — | 3 |
| Frozen (raw) | 78.5(1.2) | 15.2(1.1) | 1.0(0.2) | 1.60(0.2) | 3.7 | 89 | 4(1) | 191(48) | — | 161(138) | 349(68) | — | — | — | — | — | — | — | — | 3 |
| Steamed | 73.1 | 23.2 | 1.4 | — | — | 112 | 115 | 338 | 3.0 | 265 | 476 | 53 | — | — | — | — | — | — | — | 4, 10 |
| **Shrimp** | | | | | | | | | | | | | | | | | | | | |
| Breaded and frozen (raw) | 60.0(0.6) | 12.6(2.1) | 1.4(0.3) | 2.5(0.1) | 23.5 | 161 | 139(42) | 79(48) | — | 649(18) | 115(7) | — | — | — | — | — | — | — | — | 3 |
| Breaded, fried and frozen | 54.5(3.9) | 10.5(1.1) | 17.0(6.5) | 2.5(0.2) | 15.5 | 261 | 21(1) | 161(72) | — | 733(71) | 93(13) | — | — | — | — | — | — | — | — | 3 |
| Canned | | | | | | | | | | | | | | | | | | | | |
| Solids and liquid | 78.2 | 15.9 | 0.8 | 4.4 | 0.6 | 76 | 59 | 152 | 1.8 | — | — | — | 0.01 | 0.03 | 1.5 | — | — | — | — | 6, 10 |
| Drained solids | 68.6 | 25.3 | 1.2 | 3.8 | 0.6 | 117 | 115 | 263 | 3.1 | — | — | — | 0.03 | 0.25 | 1.5 | — | 0.02 | — | — | 1, 4, 6, 10 |
| French fried | 56.9 | 20.3 | 10.8 | 2.0 | 10.0 | 225 | 72 | 191 | 2.0 | 186 | 122 | 150 | 0.04 | 0.08 | 2.7 | 0.03 | — | 0.25 | — | 10 |
| Frozen (raw) | 81.9(3.1) | 16.9(3.9) | 1.0(0.4) | 1.70(0.7) | 3.0 | 81 | 23(9) | 139(49) | — | 520(268) | 229 | — | — | — | — | — | — | — | — | 3 |
| Paste | 64.7 | 18.4 | 11.5 | 3.0 | 2.5 | — | — | — | — | 716 | 59(47) | — | — | — | — | — | — | — | — | 2 |

*Note:* Values in parenthesis indicate standard deviation.

## REFERENCES

1. **Braekkan, O. R.**, In *Fish in Nutrition*, Heen, E. and Kreuzer, R., Eds., Fishing News, London, 1962, 141—145.
2. **Cox, H. E.**, *Analyst*, 60, 71—76, 1935.
3. **Dyer, W. J., Hiltz, D. F., Hayes, E. R., and Munro, V. G.**, *J. Inst. Can. Sci. Technol. Aliment.*, 10, 185—190, 1977.
4. **Feeley, R. M., Criner, P. E., and Watt, B. K.**, *J. Am. Diet. Assoc.*, 61, 134—148, 1972.
5. **Hoar, W. S. and Barberie, M.**, *Can. J. Res.*, Sec. E, 23, 8—18, 1945.
6. **Pilcher, R. W.**, *The canned food reference manual*, Am. Can Co., New York, 1949.
7. **Slabyj, B. and and Carpenter, P. N.**, *J. Food Sci*, 42, 1153—1155, 1977.
8. **Slabyj, B. M., Creamer, D. L., and True, R. H.**, *Mar. Fish. Rev.*, 40(8), 18—23, 1980.
9. **Standal, B. R., Bassett, D. R., Policar, P. B., and Thom, M.**, *Hawaii Agr. Exp. Station, Univ. Hawaii. Res. Bull.*, 146.
10. **Watt, B. K. and Merrill, A. L.**, *Composition of Foods*, Agriculture Handbook No. 8, U.S. Department of Agriculture, Washington, D.C., 1963.

## Table 3
### THE EFFECT OF REFRIGERATED STORAGE, HEAT PROCESSING (CANNING), AND IRRADIATION ON AMINO ACID AND VITAMIN CONTENT OF SOFT SHELL CLAM (*MYA ARENAREA*)

Amino Acids (% protein)

| | Storage at 0.6°C (days) | | | | | | Fresh | Heat-processed (months at room temperature) | | | Fresh | Irradiated (rads) | | | | | |
| | 0 | | 3 | | 5 | | | | | | | 4,500,000 No storage Air-packed | | 450,000 Air-packed Stored 30 days at 0.6°C | | 350,000 Vac-packed | |
| | Raw | Stm'd | Raw | Stm'd | Raw | Stm'd | Raw | 0 | 6 | 12 | Raw | Raw | Stm'd | Raw | Stm'd | Raw | Stm'd |
|---|---|---|---|---|---|---|---|---|---|---|---|---|---|---|---|---|---|
| Tryptophan | .200 | .040 | .170 | .060 | .180 | .070 | .080 | .049 | .028 | .034 | .200 | .190 | .190 | .170 | .150 | .200 | .200 |
| Lysine | .876 | .143 | .750 | .370 | .540 | .451 | .643 | .427 | .369 | .309 | .148 | .372 | .413 | .555 | .547 | .597 | .609 |
| Histidine | .143 | .037 | .150 | .090 | .210 | .140 | .174 | .059 | .047 | .043 | .058 | .073 | .122 | .161 | .163 | .172 | .166 |
| Threonine | .333 | .062 | .330 | .160 | .270 | .230 | .177 | .094 | .084 | .077 | .091 | .202 | .272 | .338 | .323 | .299 | .356 |
| Valine | .314 | .065 | .280 | .190 | .300 | .220 | .142 | .065 | .069 | .060 | .071 | .226 | .238 | .343 | .348 | .350 | .371 |
| Methionine | .150 | .034 | .160 | .100 | .140 | .120 | .079 | .038 | .028 | .007 | .036 | .094 | .117 | .145 | .136 | .117 | .150 |
| Isoleucine | .194 | .042 | .200 | .100 | .200 | .160 | .131 | .064 | .043 | .012 | .053 | .170 | .252 | .256 | .255 | .296 | .285 |
| Leucine | .328 | .067 | .340 | .170 | .280 | .250 | .151 | .130 | .076 | .060 | .085 | .094 | .102 | .357 | .350 | .403 | .390 |
| Phenyl-alanine | .101 | .037 | .130 | .070 | .130 | .115 | .064 | .053 | .028 | .026 | .092 | .113 | .120 | .162 | .179 | .195 | .204 |

Free Amino Acids

| | Raw | Stm'd | Raw | Stm'd | Raw | Stm'd | Raw | 0 | 6 | 12 | Raw | Raw | Stm'd | Raw | Stm'd | Raw | Stm'd |
|---|---|---|---|---|---|---|---|---|---|---|---|---|---|---|---|---|---|
| ½ Cystine | .150 | .150 | .140 | .140 | .150 | .150 | .040 | .056 | .057 | .026 | .200 | .330 | .280 | .280 | .290 | .260 | .283 |
| Ammonia | .253 | .157 | .190 | .150 | .190 | .180 | .029 | .088 | .179 | .129 | .159 | .172 | .163 | .254 | .253 | .176 | .193 |
| Arginine | .831 | .620 | .870 | .770 | .520 | .780 | .200 | .056 | .417 | .412 | .410 | .615 | .613 | .504 | .626 | .745 | .693 |
| Aspartic acid | .224 | .133 | .180 | .160 | .110 | .260 | .080 | .328 | .294 | .155 | .075 | .150 | .185 | .255 | .273 | .299 | .357 |

| | | | | | | | | | | | | | | | | |
|---|---|---|---|---|---|---|---|---|---|---|---|---|---|---|---|---|
| Serine | .399 | .436 | .323 | .432 | .380 | .369 | .162 | .627 | .368 | .118 | .259 | .380 | .270 | .250 | .540 | .093 | .541 |
| Glutamic acid | 1.160 | 1.237 | 1.136 | 1.199 | .953 | .892 | .454 | .627 | .368 | .876 | .393 | 1.035 | .940 | .920 | 1.310 | .905 | 1.438 |
| Proline | .343 | .325 | .307 | .333 | .226 | .161 | .083 | .051 | .066 | .059 | .137 | .170 | .240 | .090 | .250 | .053 | .250 |
| Glycine | 1.813 | 2.093 | 1.637 | 1.635 | 2.008 | 1.910 | 2.043 | .197 | .218 | .204 | .293 | 2.307 | 2.100 | 2.290 | 2.540 | 1.440 | 2.532 |
| Alanine | 1.921 | 2.492 | 1.991 | 1.932 | 2.678 | 2.569 | 1.849 | .751 | .767 | 1.180 | 1.330 | 2.225 | 2.030 | 2.500 | 1.474 | 1.820 | 2.507 |
| Tyrosine | .204 | .203 | .142 | .179 | .153 | .141 | .041 | .034 | .047 | .054 | .062 | .155 | .160 | .110 | .160 | .037 | 0.140 |
| Total | 10.079 | 10.895 | 9.429 | 9.490 | 9.465 | 8.843 | 6.310 | 3.647 | 3.555 | 3.998 | 4.464 | 9.402 | 8.960 | 8.290 | 10.164 | 5.935 | 11.555 |

## Total Amino Acids

| | | | | | | | | | | | | | | | | |
|---|---|---|---|---|---|---|---|---|---|---|---|---|---|---|---|---|
| Tryptophan | 1.12 | 1.15 | 1.18 | 1.24 | 1.05 | 1.15 | 1.10 | 1.14 | 0.99 | 1.19 | 1.13 | 1.08 | 1.09 | 1.15 | 1.24 | 1.01 | 1.23 |
| Lysine | 6.30 | 7.35 | 6.66 | 6.69 | 6.62 | 6.50 | 6.89 | 8.75 | 8.90 | 8.51 | 8.64 | 7.13 | 6.99 | 7.30 | 7.46 | 7.34 | 7.15 |
| Histidine | 1.22 | 1.35 | 1.67 | 1.74 | 1.33 | 1.35 | 1.31 | 1.66 | 2.06 | 1.69 | 1.84 | 1.89 | 1.74 | 1.97 | 1.99 | 1.72 | 1.85 |
| Threonine | 4.14 | 4.15 | 3.98 | 4.05 | 3.48 | 3.67 | 3.49 | 4.50 | 4.51 | 4.13 | 3.93 | 4.30 | 4.19 | 4.50 | 4.67 | 4.40 | 4.34 |
| Valine | 3.88 | 3.99 | 3.96 | 4.12 | 3.19 | 3.72 | 3.89 | 4.69 | 4.67 | 4.45 | 4.31 | 4.36 | 4.32 | 4.48 | 4.45 | 4.09 | 4.36 |
| Methionine | 2.20 | 2.12 | 2.31 | 2.30 | 1.79 | 2.11 | 2.18 | 2.55 | 2.84 | 2.30 | 2.28 | 2.42 | 2.36 | 2.49 | 2.39 | 2.31 | 2.33 |
| Isoleucine | 3.88 | 3.68 | 3.88 | 4.00 | 3.57 | 3.77 | 3.75 | 4.48 | 4.86 | 5.06 | 5.27 | 3.87 | 3.29 | 4.17 | 4.00 | 4.11 | 4.22 |
| Leucine | 5.65 | 5.89 | 6.67 | 6.50 | 5.24 | 6.45 | 6.27 | 5.89 | 7.61 | 6.58 | 6.43 | 6.83 | 7.01 | 6.77 | 6.70 | 6.58 | 6.40 |
| Phenylalanine | 3.08 | 2.68 | 3.13 | 3.43 | 2.74 | 2.86 | 2.88 | 3.48 | 3.62 | 3.46 | 3.32 | 3.26 | 3.18 | 3.58 | 3.55 | 3.33 | 3.37 |
| ½ Cystine | 1.08 | 1.05 | 1.07 | 1.02 | 0.93 | 1.03 | 1.09 | 0.93 | 0.97 | 1.05 | 1.09 | 1.05 | 0.93 | 1.04 | 1.05 | 0.99 | 1.09 |
| Ammonia | 2.18 | 2.04 | 1.77 | 1.78 | 1.52 | 1.44 | 1.42 | 1.88 | 2.20 | 2.15 | 1.33 | 1.89 | 1.74 | 1.64 | 1.72 | 1.51 | 1.74 |
| Arginine | 7.07 | 6.93 | 6.53 | 6.79 | 5.82 | 5.44 | 6.24 | 8.37 | 8.20 | 6.40 | 6.07 | 7.81 | 7.33 | 7.41 | 6.90 | 7.13 | 7.27 |
| Aspartic acid | 7.66 | 7.75 | 7.50 | 7.60 | 6.97 | 7.01 | 7.46 | 10.49 | 10.32 | 9.39 | 8.98 | 9.32 | 9.20 | 9.79 | 9.70 | 9.81 | 9.03 |
| Serine | 3.86 | 3.81 | 3.89 | 4.08 | 3.49 | 3.71 | 3.47 | 4.50 | 4.77 | 4.36 | 4.80 | 4.60 | 4.64 | 4.59 | 4.44 | 4.32 | 4.14 |
| Glutamic acid | 11.86 | 12.41 | 11.92 | 12.11 | 10.02 | 10.87 | 11.35 | 11.36 | 11.83 | 11.85 | 11.96 | 12.83 | 12.44 | 13.36 | 13.22 | 13.58 | 13.48 |
| Proline | 2.97 | 3.14 | 3.08 | 3.24 | 3.07 | 2.97 | 2.85 | 3.09 | 3.33 | 3.25 | 3.22 | 3.57 | 3.23 | 3.31 | 3.56 | 3.71 | 3.54 |
| Glycine | 6.91 | 7.01 | 7.51 | 6.85 | 6.75 | 7.02 | 6.45 | 4.34 | 4.31 | 4.24 | 4.35 | 7.05 | 6.96 | 7.59 | 7.60 | 7.15 | 7.18 |
| Alanine | 7.89 | 7.97 | 7.99 | 7.76 | 8.00 | 8.07 | 7.62 | 5.36 | 5.74 | 5.57 | 5.90 | 6.26 | 6.29 | 7.01 | 7.29 | 6.36 | 6.56 |
| Tyrosine | 2.83 | 2.51 | 2.89 | 3.11 | 2.67 | 2.55 | 2.88 | 3.10 | 3.08 | 2.97 | 2.91 | 3.11 | 3.00 | 3.46 | 3.34 | 3.32 | 3.36 |
| Protein % | 10.29 | 10.05 | 9.19 | 8.97 | 10.81 | 10.38 | 10.75 | 11.65 | 12.03 | 11.12 | 12.04 | 9.99 | 9.85 | 9.91 | 9.79 | 10.11 | 9.65 |
| Moisture % | 86.20 | 86.30 | 87.83 | 88.28 | 85.07 | 85.28 | 85.50 | | | | | 85.76 | 85.14 | 84.75 | 85.06 | 85.10 | 85.13 |

## Table 3 (continued)
### THE EFFECT OF REFRIGERATED STORAGE, HEAT PROCESSING (CANNING), AND IRRADIATION ON AMINO ACID AND VITAMIN CONTENT OF SOFT SHELL CLAM (*MYA ARENAREA*)

#### Vitamins (μg/g)

| | Storage at 0.6°C (days) | | | | | | Fresh | Heat-processed (months at room temperature) | | | Fresh | Irradiated (rads) | | | | | |
| | 0 | | 3 | | 5 | | | 0 | 6 | 12 | | 4,500,000 No storage | | 450,000 | | 350,000 Stored 30 days at 0.6°C | |
| | | | | | | | | | | | | Air-packed | | Air-packed | | Vac-packed | |
| | Raw | Stm'd | Raw | Stm'd | Raw | Stm'd | Raw | | | | Raw | Raw | Stm'd | Raw | Stm'd | Raw | Stm d |
|---|---|---|---|---|---|---|---|---|---|---|---|---|---|---|---|---|---|
| Riboflavin | 2.33 | 2.10 | 2.23 | 2.10 | 2.22 | 2.18 | 1.91 | 1.97 | 1.95 | 1.92 | 2.14 | 1.83 | 2.17 | 2.12 | 2.07 | 2.37 | 2.13 |
| Thiamin | 0.013 | 0.005 | 0.010 | 0.010 | 0.013 | 0.012 | 0.016 | 0.010 | 0.030 | 0.010 | 0.015 | 0.009 | 0.009 | 0.012 | 0.009 | 0.010 | 0.010 |
| Niacin | 19.8 | 20.0 | 18.8 | 22.5 | 22.8 | 17.5 | 25.3 | 21.3 | 18.4 | 20.2 | 11.6 | 11.3 | 10.0 | 9.8 | 9.1 | 11.2 | 11.3 |
| Pyridoxine | 0.76 | 0.58 | 0.80 | 0.79 | 0.86 | 0.74 | 0.80 | 0.75 | 1.02 | 0.75 | 1.06 | 0.67 | 0.74 | 0.67 | 0.74 | 0.99 | 0.80 |
| Pantothenic acid | 3.6 | 3.1 | 3.3 | 2.8 | 2.6 | 2.6 | 3.10 | 3.27 | 3.12 | 3.10 | 2.60 | 2.90 | 2.20 | 3.00 | 3.40 | 3.00 | 3.00 |
| $B_{12}$ | 1.08 | 1.09 | 1.09 | 1.15 | 1.06 | 1.15 | 1.05 | 0.83 | 0.71 | 0.76 | 0.75 | 0.75 | 0.83 | 0.69 | 0.66 | 0.68 | 0.68 |

Reprinted with permission from Brooke, R. O., Ravesi, E. M., Gadbois, D. F., and Steinberg, M. A., *Food Technol.*, 18, 1060, 1964, copyright © by Institute of Food Technologists.

Table 4

THE EFFECT OF COOKING AND FROZEN STORAGE ON FATTY ACID
CONTENT OF BLUE CRAB (*CALLINECTES SAPIDUS*)

| | Raw | | Cooked | | Cooked and stored 8 months at −29°C | |
|---|---|---|---|---|---|---|
| Total lipid (%) | 1.3 | | 1.2 | | 1.9 | |

Fatty acids[a]

| | Total lipid | Phospholipid fraction | Total lipid | Phospholipid fraction | Total lipid | Phospholipid fraction |
|---|---|---|---|---|---|---|
| 16:0 | 17.0(1.0) | 12.8(2.6) | 16.2(1.8) | 15.1(0.8) | 14.1(1.0) | 13.2(1.8) |
| 16:1 | 7.1(1.1) | 6.9(0.5) | 7.1(1.0) | 7.3(1.3) | 11.6(1.3) | 9.7(0.3) |
| 18:0 | 9.8(2.7) | 7.0(1.3) | 8.3(1.7) | 7.4(2.0) | 3.5(0.8) | 4.5(0.3) |
| 18:1 | 12.5(2.0) | 10.7(1.2) | 13.1(1.6) | 12.3(1.6) | 15.7(0.6) | 14.8(1.1) |
| 18:2 | 1.5(0.4) | 0.8(0.6) | 1.9(0.4) | 1.0(0.1) | 2.1(0.4) | 1.3(0.4) |
| 20:1 | 3.5(2.1) | 1.8(0.4) | 2.1(0.4) | 1.6(0.3) | 3.6(0.5) | 1.6(0.2) |
| 20:4 | 6.6(3.8) | 6.7(3.6) | 8.0(4.7) | 9.1(5.0) | 6.0(0.2) | 7.7(0.2) |
| 20:5 | 20.4(0.6) | 23.5(4.1) | 20.1(1.1) | 22.9(0.8) | 18.3(0.4) | 26.5(0.6) |
| 22:6 | 18.1(2.7) | 20.3(5.8) | 16.6(3.1) | 17.8(3.7) | 15.4(0.4) | 17.3(1.1) |

*Note:* Values in parenthesis indicate standard deviation.

[a] Weight percent of fatty acid methyl esters.

Reprinted with permission from Giddings, G. G. and Hill, L. H., *J. Food Sci.,* 40, 1127, 1975, copyright © by Institute of Food Technolgoists.

Table 5

THE EFFECT OF STORAGE, COOKING, AND
RINSING ON COPPER CONTENT OF DUNGENESS
CRAB (*CANCER MAGISTER*)

| | Days stored at 2 ± 1°C | | |
|---|---|---|---|
| Treatment at sampling | 0 | 2 | 4 |
| | Cu μg/g | | |
| Raw | 21.50 (0.26) | 23.26 (0.28) | 29.06 (2.09) |
| Precooked (60°C for 20 min) | 9.66 (1.29) | 12.04 (0.01) | 21.97 (0.14) |
| Precooked, rinsed and boiled | 14.21 (1.99) | 14.59 (0.33) | 17.42 (0.87) |
| Boiled (12 min) | 20.20 (0.06) | 23.91 (1.61) | 28.57 (0.34) |

*Note:* Values in parenthesis indicate standard deviation.

Reprinted with permission from Babbitt, J. K., Law, D. K., and Crawford, D. L., *J. Food Sci.,* 40, 649, 1975, copyright © by Institute of Food Technologists.

**Table 6**
**SEASONAL FLUCTUATION AND THE**
**EFFECT OF HEAT PROCESSING**
**(CANNING) ON PROXIMATE**
**COMPOSITION OF DUNGENESS**
**CRAB *(CANCER MAGISTER)***

| Time harvested | Moisture | Protein | Lipid | Ash |
|---|---|---|---|---|
| **Raw Body Meat** | | | | |
| January | 80.0 | 17.5 | 1.6 | 1.36 |
| March | 79.0 | 17.8 | 1.5 | 1.43 |
| June | 80.3 | 16.6 | 0.9 | 1.45 |
| August | 79.2 | 17.1 | 0.9 | 1.54 |
| **Raw Claw Meat** | | | | |
| January | 80.3 | 18.5 | 0.8 | 1.32 |
| March | 78.5 | 18.6 | 0.8 | 1.40 |
| June | 82.3 | 15.2 | 1.7 | 1.91 |
| August | 81.5 | 15.6 | 0.7 | 1.71 |
| **Body and Claw Meat (50/50) Canned in Brine** | | | | |
| January | 77.9 | 17.9 | 1.4 | 2.32 |
| March | 76.9 | 18.9 | 1.0 | 2.43 |
| June | 77.7 | 18.9 | 1.2 | 2.78 |
| August | 78.5 | 16.8 | 0.9 | 2.42 |
| **Body and Claw Meat (50/50) Canned Without Brine** | | | | |
| January | 77.7 | 19.6 | 1.1 | 1.18 |
| March | 78.5 | 19.8 | 1.2 | 1.31 |
| June | 76.6 | 21.3 | 1.1 | 1.49 |
| August | 82.9 | 14.7 | 1.1 | 0.97 |

From Farragut, R. N. and Thompson, M. H., *Fish Ind. Res.*, 3(3), 1, 1966.

Table 7
PROXIMATE COMPOSITION AND FATTY ACID CONTENT OF EDIBLE
PARTS OF KING CRAB *(PARALITHODES CAMCHATICA)*

| Fatty acids | Whole meat | Body shoulder | Propodus carpus | Claw and arms | Tails | Merus | Merus without skin | Skin |
|---|---|---|---|---|---|---|---|---|
| | | | Fatty acids[a] | | | | | |
| 10:0 | 0.4 | 0.5 | 0.6 | 0.3 | 0.1 | 0.4 | 0.3 | 0.4 |
| 12:0 | 0.5 | 0.8 | 0.5 | 0.3 | 0.1 | 0.6 | 0.6 | 0.6 |
| 14:0 | 1.4 | 1.6 | 1.4 | 1.2 | 1.6 | 1.4 | 1.3 | 1.5 |
| 15:0 | Tr | Tr | Tr | Tr | Tr | Tr | Tr | Tr |
| 16:0 | 9.2 | 10.0 | 9.5 | 8.7 | 9.6 | 10.1 | 11.7 | 9.5 |
| 18:0 | 4.3 | 3.7 | 4.3 | 4.1 | 4.7 | 4.0 | 3.1 | 4.5 |
| 19:0 | Tr | Tr | Tr | Tr | Tr | Tr | Tr | Tr |
| 20:0 | Tr | Tr | Tr | Tr | Tr | Tr | Tr | Tr |
| 24:0 | Tr | Tr | Tr | Tr | Tr | Tr | Tr | Tr |
| Total | 15.8 | 16.6 | 16.3 | 14.6 | 16.1 | 16.5 | 17.0 | 16.5 |
| 14:1 ω 6 | 0.9 | 1.0 | 0.7 | 0.6 | 0.6 | 0.8 | 1.4 | 1.2 |
| 15:1 ω 6 | 1.5 | 1.5 | 1.4 | 1.1 | 1.0 | 1.2 | 2.5 | 1.6 |
| 16:1 ω 7 | 5.0 | 5.1 | 5.1 | 4.6 | 5.9 | 5.1 | 4.6 | 3.9 |
| 17:1 ω 8 | Tr | Tr | Tr | Tr | Tr | Tr | Tr | Tr |
| 18:1 ω 9 | 15.0 | 15.8 | 15.8 | 15.1 | 15.9 | 16.2 | 17.1 | 15.6 |
| 20:1 ω 9 | 3.5 | 3.8 | 3.7 | 4.2 | 6.0 | 3.5 | 1.7 | 4.3 |
| 22:1 ω 9 | 3.9 | 3.9 | 4.2 | 4.2 | 4.1 | 4.0 | 2.7 | 4.7 |
| Total | 29.8 | 30.1 | 30.9 | 29.8 | 33.5 | 30.8 | 30.0 | 31.3 |
| 15:2 ω 6 | 1.3 | 0.8 | 1.3 | 1.3 | Tr | 1.0 | 1.0 | 1.3 |
| 16:2 ω 4 | 2.9 | 2.1 | 3.3 | 3.1 | 2.9 | 2.4 | 2.6 | 3.4 |
| 18:2 ω 6 | 3.2 | 2.7 | 2.8 | 3.0 | 2.9 | 2.9 | 1.0 | 0.9 |
| 18:3 ω 3 | 3.3 | 2.6 | 2.9 | 3.1 | 1.7 | 2.0 | 1.6 | 1.9 |
| 18:3 ω 6 | 1.3 | 1.0 | 1.5 | 1.4 | 1.7 | 1.6 | 1.2 | Tr |
| 18:4 ω 3 | 2.3 | 1.8 | 1.6 | 2.0 | 2.5 | 1.5 | 0.9 | 1.9 |
| 20:2 ω 6 | 2.4 | 1.8 | 1.5 | 2.0 | 1.3 | 1.3 | 0.7 | 0.9 |
| 20:3 ω 6 | Tr | Tr | Tr | Tr | Tr | Tr | Tr | Tr |
| 20:4 ω 6 | 0.6 | 1.2 | 1.7 | 1.1 | 1.5 | 0.9 | 0.4 | 1.3 |
| 20:4 ω 3 | Tr | Tr | Tr | Tr | Tr | Tr | Tr | Tr |
| 20:5 ω 3 | 21.5 | 22.6 | 21.9 | 22.6 | 20.0 | 23.1 | 29.5 | 23.4 |
| 22:3 ω 6 | 1.6 | 1.5 | 1.4 | 1.5 | 1.4 | 1.3 | 1.1 | 1.5 |
| 22:4 ω 6 | 1.1 | 1.2 | 0.6 | 1.3 | 0.9 | 1.0 | 0.5 | 0.9 |
| 22:5 ω 3 | 1.4 | 1.7 | 1.5 | 1.6 | 1.9 | 1.4 | 0.8 | 1.9 |
| 22:6 ω 3 | 10.2 | 11.1 | 10.8 | 10.9 | 10.2 | 10.9 | 11.2 | 10.6 |
| 23:5 | 0.9 | 0.8 | 0.6 | 0.7 | 0.3 | 0.8 | 1.0 | 1.0 |
| 24:5 | Tr | Tr | Tr | Tr | Tr | Tr | Tr | Tr |
| 24.6 | 1.0 | 0.8 | 0.7 | 0.8 | 1.0 | 1.1 | 1.0 | 1.0 |
| Total | 55.0 | 53.7 | 54.1 | 56.4 | 50.2 | 51.3 | 54.5 | 52.0 |
| | | | Proximate Composition | | | | | |
| Protein (%) | 18.0 | 16.9 | 16.3 | 20.7 | 17.4 | 17.8 | — | — |
| Lipid (%) | 2.0 | 1.5 | 1.9 | 1.6 | 3.3 | 1.3 | — | — |
| Ash (%) | 1.8 | 1.7 | 1.9 | 1.9 | 1.3 | 1.8 | — | — |
| Moisture (%) | 78.6 | 78.5 | 79.6 | 76.5 | 76.2 | 78.2 | — | — |

[a]   Weight percent of fatty acid methyl esters.

Reprinted with permission from Krzeczkowski, R. A., Tenney, R. D., and Kelley, C., *J. Food Sci.*, 36, 604, 1971, copyright © by Institute of Food Technologists.

## Table 8
## THE EFFECT OF PACKAGING AND FROZEN STORAGE AT −18°C ON PROXIMATE COMPOSITION OF SAMOAN CRAB (*SCYLLA SERRATA*)

Crab meat

| | Fresh | Polyethelene bag | | | Bag in carton[a] | | | Dipped[b] + bag in carton | | | Whole crab in bag | | |
|---|---|---|---|---|---|---|---|---|---|---|---|---|---|
| Months stored | 0 | 1.5 | 4 | 7 | 1.5 | 4 | 7 | 1.5 | 4 | 7 | 1.5 | 4 | 7 |
| **Quick Frozen (−40°C)** | | | | | | | | | | | | | |
| Moisture (%) | 80.2 | 77.9 | 75.8 | 74.2 | 77.0 | 75.9 | 75.8 | 76.3 | 74.0 | 73.5 | 77.1 | 76.5 | 76.0 |
| Protein (%) | — | 20.6 | 22.4 | 23.2 | 20.4 | 22.2 | 22.9 | 21.0 | 22.8 | 23.3 | 19.4 | 20.2 | 22.0 |
| Soluble protein (% retention) | 30.0 | 22.0 | 21.1 | 20.0 | 22.3 | 20.5 | 20.1 | 18.8 | 14.9 | 8.4 | 23.4 | 21.7 | 20.9 |
| NPN (%) | 0.53 | 0.51 | 0.57 | 0.51 | 0.50 | 0.65 | 0.52 | 0.32 | 0.30 | 0.15 | 0.50 | 0.56 | 0.51 |
| Total amino nitrogen (%) | 1.92 | 2.16 | 2.45 | 2.43 | 2.2 | 2.38 | 2.37 | 2.67 | 2.94 | 2.83 | 2.04 | 2.17 | 2.12 |
| Thiamin (µg %) | 4.5 | 3.9 | 2.2 | Tr | 4.6 | 2.4 | Tr | 4.0 | 2.3 | Tr | 4.3 | 3.0 | Tr |
| Riboflavin (µg %) | 724 | 573 | 355 | 267 | 552 | 319 | 257 | 570 | 419 | 371 | 555 | 330 | 310 |
| Niacin (mg %) | 1.4 | 1.2 | 1.0 | 1.0 | 1.4 | 1.2 | 1.2 | 1.3 | 1.3 | 1.1 | 1.5 | 1.2 | 1.1 |
| **Slow Frozen (−18°C)** | | | | | | | | | | | | | |
| Moisture (%) | 80.2 | 76.1 | 74.0 | 70.5 | 76.1 | 74.6 | 73.5 | 75.5 | 71.3 | 69.1 | 76.7 | 74.5 | 74.5 |
| Protein (%) | — | 20.8 | 22.8 | 23.7 | 20.9 | 22.4 | 22.9 | 22.6 | 22.9 | 23.8 | 21.4 | 22.0 | 22.6 |
| Soluble protein (% retention) | 30.0 | 21.5 | 18.5 | 17.5 | 22.0 | 18.5 | 15.8 | 17.6 | 12.9 | 9.9 | 24.7 | 19.6 | 19.3 |
| NPN (%) | 0.53 | 0.50 | 0.50 | 0.49 | 0.50 | 0.49 | 0.48 | 0.31 | 0.30 | 0.29 | 0.44 | 0.41 | 0.42 |
| Total amino nitrogen (%) | 1.92 | 2.15 | 2.31 | 2.71 | 2.20 | 2.40 | 2.42 | 2.60 | 2.99 | 3.08 | 2.01 | 2.33 | 2.38 |
| Thiamin (µg %) | 4.5 | 3.7 | 3.2 | Tr | 3.6 | 3.4 | Tr | 3.0 | 3.0 | Tr | 3.0 | 2.7 | Tr |
| Riboflavin (µg %) | 724 | 621 | 345 | 318 | 518 | 377 | 208 | 465 | 382 | 259 | 499 | 420 | 367 |
| Niacin (mg %) | 1.45 | 1.20 | 1.13 | 1.04 | 1.39 | 1.30 | 1.07 | 1.17 | 1.08 | 1.06 | 1.24 | 1.14 | 0.99 |

[a] Polyethelene bags in heavy waxed cartons.

[b] Two minute dip in 1.5% citric acid.

Reprinted with permission from Gangal, S. V. and Magar, N. G., *Food Technol.*, 17, 1573, 1963, Copyright © by Institute of Food Technologists.

Table 9
## PROXIMATE COMPOSITION AND FATTY ACID CONTENT OF EDIBLE PARTS OF HEAT PROCESSED (CANNED) SNOW CRAB *(CHIONECTES BAIRDI)*

| Fatty acids | Whole meat (composite) | Canned[a] | Body-shoulder | Claws | Propodus carpus | Merus | Merus without skin | Skin |
|---|---|---|---|---|---|---|---|---|
| | | | Fatty Acids[b] | | | | | |
| 10:0 | 0.3 | 0.4 | 0.1 | 0.1 | 0.1 | 0.3 | Tr | 0.2 |
| 12:0 | 0.4 | 0.4 | 0.2 | 0.2 | 0.2 | 0.4 | Tr | 0.2 |
| 14:0 | 0.4 | 0.4 | 0.2 | 0.6 | 0.4 | 0.5 | 0.5 | 1.2 |
| 15:0 | 0.7 | 0.7 | 0.9 | 0.9 | 0.5 | 0.5 | 0.5 | 1.5 |
| 16:0 | 13.5 | 12.5 | 13.2 | 12.5 | 13.5 | 13.5 | 13.7 | 11.6 |
| 17:0 | 0.9 | 1.3 | 1.0 | 0.9 | 1.2 | 1.1 | 0.9 | 0.3 |
| 18:0 | 3.1 | 3.4 | 3.5 | 3.8 | 3.6 | 2.9 | 2.8 | 5.8 |
| 19:0 | Tr | Tr | Tr | Tr | Tr | Tr | Tr | Tr |
| 20:0 | Tr | Tr | Tr | Tr | Tr | Tr | Tr | Tr |
| 22:0 | Tr | Tr | Tr | Tr | Tr | Tr | Tr | Tr |
| 24:0 | Tr | Tr | Tr | Tr | Tr | Tr | Tr | Tr |
| Total | 19.3 | 19.1 | 19.1 | 19.0 | 19.5 | 19.2 | 18.4 | 20.8 |
| 14:1 | 0.2 | 0.4 | 0.4 | 0.2 | 0.5 | 0.4 | 0.3 | 0.6 |
| 15:1 | 0.2 | 0.3 | 0.1 | 0.2 | 0.5 | 0.3 | 0.2 | 0.5 |
| 16:1 | 3.0 | 3.3 | 3.4 | 3.8 | 3.2 | 3.3 | 3.5 | 4.5 |
| 17:1 | 0.9 | 0.9 | 0.9 | 0.8 | 0.9 | 0.7 | 0.7 | 1.0 |
| 18:1 | 17.8 | 16.0 | 17.5 | 19.3 | 17.3 | 17.0 | 16.3 | 21.9 |
| 20:1 | 1.4 | 1.2 | 0.5 | 1.5 | 1.6 | 1.0 | 1.4 | 3.0 |
| 22:1 | 0.5 | 0.6 | 0.5 | 0.5 | 0.5 | 0.5 | 0.4 | 0.2 |
| Total | 24.0 | 22.7 | 23.3 | 26.3 | 24.5 | 23.2 | 22.8 | 31.7 |
| 16:2ω4 | 0.7 | 0.4 | 0.6 | 0.8 | 0.6 | 1.0 | 0.5 | 0.8 |
| 18:2ω6 | 1.1 | 3.5 | 2.7 | 1.9 | 1.4 | 1.9 | 1.1 | 1.2 |
| 18:3ω3 | 0.4 | 0.5 | 0.2 | 0.1 | 0.5 | 0.4 | 0.4 | 0.4 |
| 18:4ω3 | 0.5 | 0.6 | 0.5 | 0.1 | 0.5 | 0.3 | 0.1 | 0.2 |
| 20:2ω6 | 0.4 | 0.3 | 0.4 | 0.2 | 0.5 | 0.4 | 0.4 | 0.7 |
| 20:4ω6 | 3.9 | 4.8 | 3.7 | 4.7 | 6.4 | 3.7 | 3.7 | 8.5 |
| 20:4ω3 | Tr | Tr | Tr | Tr | Tr | Tr | Tr | Tr |
| 20:5ω3 | 29.0 | 28.0 | 29.6 | 26.3 | 26.2 | 30.0 | 31.9 | 22.2 |
| 22:3ω6 | 1.8 | 1.4 | 1.2 | 1.1 | 1.1 | 1.1 | 1.0 | 1.1 |
| 22:4ω6 | 0.5 | 0.9 | 0.6 | 1.0 | 0.5 | 0.9 | 0.8 | 0.9 |
| 22:5ω3 | 1.2 | 1.4 | 1.5 | 1.3 | 1.3 | 1.1 | 1.7 | 1.5 |
| 22:6ω3 | 16.3 | 15.0 | 16.6 | 15.7 | 16.5 | 15.6 | 15.1 | 9.4 |
| 23:5? | 0.5 | 0.5 | 0.3 | 0.5 | 0.5 | 0.5 | 1.0 | 0.5 |
| Total | 56.3 | 57.3 | 57.9 | 53.7 | 56.0 | 56.9 | 57.7 | 47.4 |
| | | | Proximate Composition | | | | | |
| Protein % | 18.8 | 19.5 | 18.8 | 18.0 | 16.6 | 19.9 | — | — |
| Lipid % | 1.5 | 1.0 | 1.6 | 1.0 | 1.5 | 1.5 | — | — |
| Ash % | 1.0 | 1.6 | 0.4 | 1.3 | 1.1 | 1.2 | — | — |
| Moisture % | 79.4 | 78.2 | 80.0 | 80.0 | 81.4 | 78.6 | — | — |
| Salt % | 0.3 | 1.3 | 0.2 | 0.7 | 0.3 | 0.3 | — | — |

[a]  Content made up of 28% merus and 72% body-shoulder with claws.
[b]  Weight percent of fatty acid methyl esters.

Reprinted with permission from Krzeczkowski, R. A. and Stone, F. E., *J. Food Sci.*, 39, 386, 1974, copyright © by Institute of Food Technologists.

## Table 10
### THE EFFECT OF BOILING ON CHOLESTEROL CONTENT OF EDIBLE PARTS OF AMERICAN LOBSTER *(HOMARUS AMERICANUS)*

| | Claw | Body | Tail |
|---|---|---|---|
| | | mg/100 g | |
| Raw | 53 | 58 | 79 |
| Boiled | 84 | 87 | 106 |

From Mathes, A. J., The Cholesterol Content of Seafood, Masters thesis, Massachusetts Institute of Technology, Cambridge, 1977.

## Table 11
### THE EFFECT OF STEAMING, FREEZING, AND HEAT PROCESSING (CANNING) ON PROXIMATE COMPOSITION AND MINERAL CONTENT OF BLUE MUSSELS *(MYTILUS EDULIS)*

#### Proximate Composition

| | Raw | Steamed | | |
|---|---|---|---|---|
| | | Fresh | Frozen | Canned |
| Moisture (%) | 81.2 (1.0) | 74.6 (1.6) | 76.8 (0.9) | 75.7 (3.6) |
| Protein (%) | 11.76 (0.06) | 17.65 (0.10) | 16.19 (0.05) | 17.16 (0.10) |
| Crude fat (%) | 2.88 (0.02) | 4.04 (0.03) | 3.74 (0.05) | 4.25 (0.05) |
| Ash (%) | 1.47 (0.02) | 1.57 (0.03) | 1.58 (0.02) | 1.63 (0.02) |
| Carbohydrate (%) | 2.65 (0.02) | 2.08 (0.05) | 1.67 (0.02) | 1.22 (0.02) |

#### Elemental Content (μg/g Wet Weight)

| | Raw | Fresh | Frozen | Canned |
|---|---|---|---|---|
| Al | 17.5 (1.1) | 30.0 (4.3) | 25.5 (2.1) | 22.1 (2.2) |
| As | 0.24 (0.08) | 0.38 (0.10) | 0.44 (0.16) | 0.44 (0.02) |
| B | 2.12 (0.26) | 2.36 (0.15) | 1.97 (0.32) | 2.09 (0.19) |
| Cd | 0.41 (0.02) | 0.66 (0.10) | 0.60 (0.05) | 0.70 (0.02) |
| Ca | 263 (56) | 406 (76) | 278 (46) | 292 (49) |
| Cr | 2.56 (0.34) | 3.66 (0.38) | 3.27 (0.39) | 3.30 (0.44) |
| Co | 0.49 (0.06) | 0.64 (0.05) | 0.51 (0.02) | 0.53 (0.07) |
| Cu | 0.94 (0.15) | 1.47 (0.36) | 1.11 (0.14) | 1.90 (0.24) |
| F | 5.5 (0.8) | 8.9 (1.5) | 8.1 (1.4) | 10.2 (1.7) |
| I | 1.13 (0.11) | 0.38 (0.03) | 0.32 (0.02) | 0.36 (0.02) |
| Fe | 39.5 (3.8) | 73.7 (12.7) | 67.3 (7.0) | 60.8 (4.9) |
| Pb | 0.092 (0.041) | 0.079 (0.030) | 0.111 (0.028) | 0.085 (0.010) |
| Mg | 338 (19) | 432 (25) | 371 (23) | 316 (24) |
| Mn | 30.1 (0.9) | 33.0 (3.8) | 44.1 (2.3) | 41.3 (3.6) |
| Hg | 0.0023 (0.0004) | 0.0036 (0.0008) | 0.0028 (0.0005) | 0.0041 (0.0010) |
| Mo | 0.41 (0.04) | 0.56 (0.08) | 0.42 (0.05) | 0.41 (0.07) |
| Ni | 0.71 (0.08) | 1.22 (0.58) | 0.84 (0.07) | 0.90 (0.07) |
| P | 1974 (38) | 3023 (152) | 2784 (162) | 2746 (97) |
| K | 3196 (169) | 3251 (102) | 2482 (186) | 2309 (97) |
| Se | 0.094 (0.034) | 0.137 (0.038) | 0.077 (0.009) | 0.070 (0.010) |
| Na | 2858 (56) | 2692 (381) | 3967 (70) | 4398 (24) |

### Table 11 (continued)
### THE EFFECT OF STEAMING, FREEZING, AND HEAT PROCESSING (CANNING) ON PROXIMATE COMPOSITION AND MINERAL CONTENT OF BLUE MUSSELS *(MYTILUS EDULIS)*

Proximate Composition

| | Raw | Steamed | | |
| | | Fresh | Frozen | Canned |
| --- | --- | --- | --- | --- |
| V | 0.164 (0.024) | 0.203 (0.008) | 0.151 (0.016) | 0.158 (0.024) |
| Zn | 15.9 (0.8) | 24.1 (1.0) | 25.1 (4.9) | 30.9 (5.1) |

*Note:* Values in parenthesis indicate standard deviation.

Reprinted with permission from Slabyj, B. M. and Carpenter, P. N., *J. Food Sci.*, 42, 1153, 1977, copyright © by Institute of Food Technologists.

### Table 12
### THE EFFECT OF 6 MONTHS OF LIVE-HOLDING AT 1 TO 2°C ON LIPIDS AND FATTY ACIDS OF OYSTERS *(CRASSOSTREA VIRGINICA)*

| Experiment | I | | II | |
| Condition of oysters | Fresh | Stored | Fresh | Stored |
| --- | --- | --- | --- | --- |
| Number of animals | 3 | 9 | 3 | 9 |
| Av. wt. of whole animal (g) | 121.1 | 79.9 | 141 | 101 |
| Av. wt. of dry meat (g) | 10.9 | 8.2 | 13.3 | 8.8 |

Lipids (g/100 g Tissue)

| | Fresh | Stored | Fresh | Stored |
| --- | --- | --- | --- | --- |
| Total lipid | 0.35 | 0.53 | 0.52 | 0.94 |
| Fatty acids | 0.215 | 0.229 | 0.318 | 0.388 |
| Nonsaponifiable | 0.051 | 0.073 | 0.083 | 0.092 |
| Total polar lipids | 0.121 | 0.176 | 0.170 | 0.346 |
| Fatty acids | 0.104 | 0.100 | 0.128 | 0.141 |
| Nonsaponifiable | — | 0.012 | 0.013 | 0.046 |
| Total nonpolar lipids | 0.177 | 0.338 | 0.290 | 0.590 |
| Triglyceride | — | 0.169 | — | 0.407 |
| Sterol ester | — | 0.043 | — | 0.045 |
| Sterol | — | 0.095 | — | 0.079 |
| Fatty acids[a] | 0.111 | 0.129 | 0.198 | 0.247 |

Fatty Acids (mg/100 g Tissue)

Experiment I

| Lipid | Neutral | | Polar | | Total | |
| Condition | Fresh | Stored | Fresh | Stored | Fresh | Stored |
| --- | --- | --- | --- | --- | --- | --- |
| Fatty acid | | | | | | |
| 14:0 | 4.2 | 7.2 | 2.3 | 3.6 | 6.0 | 16.7 |
| 16:0 | 47.5 | 52.1 | 30.7 | 26.2 | 70.7 | 71.2 |
| 18:0 | 4.4 | 4.1 | 9.8 | 7.1 | 14.8 | 11.2 |
| Actual total | 65.5 | 74.6 | 55.1 | 47.8 | 111.4 | 125.0 |

## Table 12 (continued)
## THE EFFECT OF 6 MONTHS OF LIVE-HOLDING AT 1 TO 2°C ON LIPIDS AND FATTY ACIDS OF OYSTERS *(CRASSOSTREA VIRGINICA)*

Fatty Acids (mg/100 g Tissue)

Experiment I

| Lipid | Neutral | | Polar | | Total | |
|---|---|---|---|---|---|---|
| Condition | Fresh | Stored | Fresh | Stored | Fresh | Stored |
| 16:1 | 5.9 | 8.1 | 2.8 | 4.5 | 10.1 | 18.1 |
| 18:1 | 11.3 | 14.8 | 7.4 | 5.1 | 18.5 | 16.7 |
| 20:1 | 5.1 | 4.1 | 11.5 | 4.1 | 18.3 | 4.6 |
| 22:1 | 0.9 | 0.1 | 4.6 | 0.1 | 5.4 | 2.1 |
| Actual total | 24.3 | 27.5 | 26.4 | 14.6 | 52.9 | 43.3 |
| | | | | | | |
| 18:2 ω 6 | 3.2 | 3.1 | 1.0 | 1.4 | 6.0 | 3.9 |
| 18:3 ω 3 | 1.4 | 2.3 | 1.6 | 1.7 | 5.6 | 4.4 |
| 18:4 ω 3 | 1.9 | 2.7 | 1.0 | 0.9 | 6.2 | 7.3 |
| 20:4 ω 6 | 0.7 | 0.9 | 2.0 | 3.5 | 2.6 | 1.8 |
| 20:5 ω 3 | 5.1 | 6.1 | 5.3 | 12.5 | 9.5 | 14.0 |
| 22:5 ω 3 | 0.6 | 0.1 | 0.3 | 0.2 | 0.6 | 0.7 |
| 22:6 ω 3 | 2.3 | 2.6 | 5.7 | 8.3 | 9.0 | 6.2 |
| Actual total | 21.1 | 26.8 | 21.7 | 37.9 | 49.9 | 60.7 |

Experiment II

| Fatty acid | | | | | | |
|---|---|---|---|---|---|---|
| 14:0 | 9.9 | 10.1 | 3.2 | 3.5 | 9.9 | 14.7 |
| 16:0 | 68.5 | 65.2 | 34.3 | 31.3 | 99.5 | 92.0 |
| 18:0 | 7.7 | 7.2 | 7.2 | 5.9 | 21.6 | 7.4 |
| Actual total | 105.3 | 101.3 | 59.1 | 49.4 | 153.6 | 132.3 |
| | | | | | | |
| 16:1 | 11.9 | 15.1 | 3.1 | 7.2 | 15.6 | 22.5 |
| 18:1 | 21.4 | 25.9 | 7.8 | 8.3 | 30.2 | 31.0 |
| 20:1 | 7.1 | 10.4 | 15.2 | 6.1 | 23.2 | 12.8 |
| 22:1 | 5.1 | 2.0 | 3.1 | 1.3 | 4.1 | 1.9 |
| Actual total | 44.9 | 53.8 | 29.2 | 23.1 | 73.1 | 69.1 |
| | | | | | | |
| 18:2 ω 6 | 4.4 | 5.7 | 1.3 | 0.8 | 5.1 | 7.8 |
| 18:3 ω 3 | 3.8 | 6.2 | 1.4 | 2.5 | 3.8 | 10.5 |
| 18:4 ω 3 | 4.8 | 8.6 | 1.3 | 2.1 | 4.1 | 16.7 |
| 20:4 ω 6 | 1.6 | 2.7 | 4.4 | 5.1 | 6.4 | 8.9 |
| 20:5 ω 3 | 10.7 | 21.7 | 7.9 | 18.2 | 16.9 | 48.5 |
| 22:5 ω 3 | 1.8 | 1.0 | 0.5 | 0.6 | 1.9 | 2.7 |
| 22:6 ω 3 | 6.9 | 23.0 | 9.5 | 21.7 | 21.9 | 61.3 |
| Actual total | 47.7 | 91.9 | 39.6 | 68.5 | 90.0 | 167.2 |

[*] Fatty acid weight of nonpolar lipids estimated by subtracting fatty acids of polar lipids from total fatty acids.

Watanabe, T. and Ackman, R. G., *J. Can. Sci. Technol. Aliment*, 10, 40, 1977. With permission.

## Table 13
### THE EFFECT OF CANNING ON ASCORBIC
### ACID CONTENT OF OYSTERS *(OSTREA GIGAS)*

| | | Ascorbic acid | | |
|---|---|---|---|---|
| Product | Free | Bound | Total | Moisture |
| | | mg/100 g | | g/100 g |
| Fresh | 20.0 | 2.3 | 22.3 | 80 |
| Canned meat | 10.5 | 3.3 | 13.8 | 76 |
| Canned liquor | 11.7 | 0.13 | 11.8 | 93 |

From Hastings, W. H. and Spencer, C. F., *J. Mar. Res.*, 11, 241, 1952.

## Table 14
### THE EFFECT OF TWO MONTHS OF LIVE-HOLDING AND AREA OF HARVEST
### ON FATTY ACID CONTENT OF QUAHAUGS *(ARTICA ISLANDICA)*

| | Phospholipids | | | Triglycerides | | | Sterol esters | | |
|---|---|---|---|---|---|---|---|---|---|
| | N.S.[b] | N.B.[c] | | N.S. | N.B. | | N.S. | N.B. | |
| Fatty acid[a] | Fresh | Fresh | 10 wk | Fresh | Fresh | 10 wk | Fresh | Fresh | 10 wk |
| 14:0 | 0.37 | 0.37 | 0.64 | 3.53 | 3.91 | 5.28 | 4.19 | 4.02 | 5.89 |
| 4,8,12-TMTD | 0.18 | 0.16 | 0.10 | 0.64 | ND | 4.47 | 1.64 | 1.26 | 2.89 |
| *Iso* 15:0 | 0.04 | 0.03 | ND | 0.21 | 0.18 | 0.24 | 0.28 | 0.32 | 1.17 |
| *Anteiso* 15:0 | 0.02 | 0.06 | ND | 0.11 | 0.18 | 0.71 | 0.55 | 1.28 | 3.50 |
| 15:0 | 0.41 | 0.52 | 0.63 | 0.54 | 0.52 | 1.19 | 0.83 | 2.07 | 1.75 |
| *Iso* 16:0 | 0.29 | 0.41 | 0.62 | 0.21 | 0.61 | 1.41 | 0.66 | 1.42 | ND |
| Pristanic | 0.18 | 0.53 | 0.40 | ND | ND | ND | 0.43 | 0.61 | ND |
| 16:0 | 12.91 | 9.79 | 12.67 | 32.35 | 27.52 | 29.67 | 18.64 | 11.37 | 21.93 |
| 7-MHD | 0.11 | 0.34 | 0.49 | 0.23 | 0.03 | 0.85 | 0.52 | 0.88 | 1.10 |
| *Iso* 17:0 | 0.44 | 0.19 | 0.51 | 0.84 | 0.48 | 0.93 | 0.81 | 1.56 | 1.14 |
| *Anteiso* 17:0 | 0.29 | 0.37 | 1.13 | 0.84 | 1.57 | 2.56 | 2.71 | 4.38 | 2.86 |
| 17:0 | 1.74 | 1.43 | 2.06 | 1.69 | 1.45 | 1.75 | 0.81 | 0.63 | 0.57 |
| Phytanic | ND | ND | 0.30 | ND | ND | 0.14 | ND | 0.15 | 0.28 |
| *Iso* 18:0 | 0.36 | 0.73 | 0.66 | 0.63 | 0.72 | 0.63 | 1.88 | 1.32 | 0.71 |
| 18:0 | 6.26 | 7.02 | 8.76 | 7.93 | 4.06 | 5.25 | 7.79 | 4.33 | 6.89 |
| 19:0 | 0.21 | ND | ND | 0.41 | 1.06 | 0.63 | 0.53 | 0.15 | 0.28 |
| 20:0 | ND | ND | ND | 0.05 | ND | 0.11 | ND | 0.76 | ND |
| Total saturated | 23.8 | 21.9 | 29.0 | 50.2 | 42.3 | 55.9 | 42.2 | 36.5 | 51.4 |
| 14:1 ω 7 | ND | 0.05 | ND | 0.22 | ND | ND | ND | ND | ND |
| 15:1 | ND | 0.20 | ND | ND | ND | ND | 0.44 | 0.16 | ND |
| 16:1 ω 9 | 0.15 | ND | 0.31 | 0.84 | ND | 0.93 | 2.44 | 1.09 | 2.86 |
| 16:1 ω 7 | 1.74 | 1.99 | 2.47 | 12.64 | 12.78 | 12.71 | 2.71 | 3.13 | 6.29 |
| 16:1 ω 5 | 0.15 | ND | 0.41 | ND | ND | 0.47 | ND | ND | ND |
| 17:1 | 0.14 | 0.74 | 0.15 | ND | 0.48 | 0.35 | ND | 0.15 | 0.28 |
| 18:1 ω 13 | 2.07 | 2.07 | 3.03 | 0.83 | 0.35 | 0.80 | 1.06 | 1.84 | 0.70 |
| 18:1 ω 9 | 1.92 | 1.89 | 2.02 | 3.72 | 3.55 | 4.57 | 6.92 | 5.21 | 6.48 |
| 18:1 ω 7 | 2.85 | 1.95 | 1.61 | 8.26 | 6.85 | 6.28 | 5.32 | 3.22 | 3.05 |
| 18:1 ω 5 | ND | 0.12 | 0.25 | 0.41 | 0.24 | 0.40 | ND | ND | 0.10 |
| 19:1 | 0.14 | ND | 0.15 | 0.10 | 0.30 | 0.34 | ND | 0.08 | 1.40 |
| 20:1 ω 11 | 0.28 | 0.90 | 0.45 | 0.41 | 0.58 | 0.51 | 0.79 | 2.27 | 0.27 |
| 20:1 ω 9 | 1.06 | 0.90 | 0.70 | 1.69 | 0.94 | 1.41 | 3.95 | 5.69 | 0.65 |

**Table 14 (continued)**
## THE EFFECT OF TWO MONTHS OF LIVE-HOLDING AND AREA OF HARVEST ON FATTY ACID CONTENT OF QUAHAUGS *(ARTICA ISLANDICA)*

| Fatty acid[a] | Phospholipids | | | Triglycerides | | | Sterol esters | | |
|---|---|---|---|---|---|---|---|---|---|
| | N.S.[b] | N.B.[c] | | N.S. | N.B. | | N.S. | N.B. | |
| | Fresh | Fresh | 10 wk | Fresh | Fresh | 10 wk | Fresh | Fresh | 10 wk |
| 20:1 ω 7 | 1.47 | 4.18 | 2.77 | 5.31 | 3.13 | 2.80 | 18.77 | 16.14 | 6.45 |
| 20:1 ω 5 | ND | ND | ND | ND | ND | ND | ND | ND | ND |
| 22:1 ω 11 + 13 | ND | ND | ND | 0.10 | 0.14 | 0.11 | 0.65 | 2.40 | 0.82 |
| 22:1 ω 9 | ND | ND | ND | 0.25 | 0.07 | ND | 1.30 | 1.13 | 0.48 |
| 22:1 ω 7 | ND | ND | ND | 0.08 | ND | ND | 0.65 | 0.75 | ND |
| Total monoethylenic | 10.5 | 15.0 | 14.3 | 34.1 | 29.4 | 31.7 | 45.0 | 43.3 | 29.8 |
| 18:2 ω 9 | ND | 0.30 | 2.02 | ND | ND | ND | ND | ND | 0.14 |
| 18:2 ω 6 | 0.32 | 0.18 | 0.46 | 0.36 | 0.59 | 0.46 | 0.93 | 1.00 | 0.96 |
| 20:2 ω 6 | 0.91 | 1.19 | 0.54 | 0.56 | 0.41 | 0.22 | 0.65 | 0.38 | ND |
| (20:2)"a" | 10.64 | 7.24 | 13.48 | 0.92 | 0.29 | 0.28 | 2.63 | 2.27 | ND |
| (20:2) "b" | 0.84 | 2.69 | 0.94 | 1.82 | 1.45 | 1.12 | 5.99 | 3.75 | 2.37 |
| (22:2) "A" | 1.85 | 2.69 | 1.23 | 0.66 | 0.52 | 0.22 | 1.63 | 3.00 | 0.41 |
| (22:2) "B" (?) | ND | ND | ND | ND | ND | 0.11 | ND | ND | 0.14 |
| Total diethylenic | 14.6 | 14.3 | 18.7 | 4.3 | 3.3 | 3.4 | 11.8 | 10.4 | 4.0 |
| 18:3 ω 6 | 0.44 | ND | 0.05 | 0.03 | ND | 0.53 | ND | 0.31 | 0.07 |
| 18:3 ω 3 | 1.32 | 0.43 | 0.36 | 1.27 | 0.30 | 0.29 | 0.27 | 0.79 | 0.60 |
| 20:3 ω 6 | ND | ND | ND | ND | ND | ND | ND | ND | ND |
| 20:3 ω 3 | ND | ND | ND | ND | ND | ND | ND | ND | ND |
| Total triethylenic | 1.8 | 0.4 | 0.4 | 1.3 | 0.3 | 0.8 | 0.3 | 1.1 | 0.7 |
| 18:4 ω 3 | ND | ND | 1.06 | 0.65 | 1.60 | 1.11 | 0.28 | ND | 0.66 |
| 20:4 ω 6 | 2.06 | 2.98 | 2.81 | 0.17 | 0.63 | 0.38 | ND | 0.17 | 1.09 |
| 20:4 ω 3 | 2.88 | 0.64 | 0.72 | ND | 0.14 | ND | ND | 0.45 | 0.62 |
| 22:4 ω 6 | 0.60 | 1.35 | 0.31 | ND | ND | ND | ND | ND | ND |
| Total tetraethylenic | 5.5 | 5.0 | 4.9 | 0.8 | 2.4 | 1.5 | 0.3 | 0.6 | 2.4 |
| 20:5 ω 3 | 15.28 | 15.12 | 15.31 | 5.48 | 16.40 | 6.41 | 0.83 | 1.43 | 1.37 |
| 21:5 ω 2 | 0.61 | 1.05 | 0.53 | 0.14 | 0.96 | ND | ND | ND | 0.92 |
| 22:5 ω 6 | 0.15 | 0.70 | 0.14 | ND | ND | ND | ND | ND | ND |
| 22:5 ω 3 | 2.21 | 2.60 | 1.39 | 0.36 | 0.32 | ND | ND | ND | 0.87 |
| Total pentaethylenic | 18.2 | 19.5 | 17.4 | 6.0 | 17.7 | 6.4 | 0.8 | 1.4 | 3.2 |
| 22:6 ω 3 | 23.91 | 18.85 | 14.55 | 2.75 | 4.71 | 2.00 | ND | 5.24 | 2.55 |
| I.V. (Calc.) | 231.9 | 217.0 | 192.7 | 85.4 | 134.8 | 78.5 | 75.8 | 99.7 | 80.0 |

[a]    4,8,12-TMTD = 4,8,12-trimethyltridecanoic acid; pristanic = 2,6,10,14-tetramethylpentadecanoic acid; phytanic = 3,7,11,15-tetramethylhexadecanoic acid; 7-MHD = 7-methylhexadecanoic acid, the latter measured after hydrogenation of methyl esters.

[b]    Nova Scotia, Canada.

[c]    New Brunswick, Canada.

From Ackman, R. G., Epstein, S., and Kelleher, M., *J. Fish. Res. Board Can.*, 31, 1803, 1974. With permission of the Canadian Journal of Fisheries and Aquatic Sciences.

## Table 15
### THE EFFECT OF BLANCHING AND HEAT PROCESSING (CANNING) ON FATTY ACID CONTENT OF SHRIMP *(PANDALUS BOREALIS)*

| Fatty acids | Whole raw shrimp | Shrimp waste | Shrimp meat | | |
|---|---|---|---|---|---|
| | | | Raw | Blanched | Canned |
| | | Fatty Acids[a] | | | |
| 10:0 | 0.6 | 0.6 | 0.7 | 0.3 | 0.5 |
| 12:0 | 0.3 | 0.6 | 0.5 | 0.4 | 0.4 |
| 14:0 | 4.1 | 2.0 | 2.6 | 2.1 | 2.5 |
| 15:0 | 0.5 | 0.6 | 0.6 | 0.6 | 0.5 |
| 16:0 | 14.3 | 13.9 | 15.7 | 15.1 | 16.0 |
| 17:0 | Tr | Tr | Tr | Tr | Tr |
| 18:0 | 3.0 | 3.0 | 2.3 | 2.7 | 2.6 |
| 19:0 | Tr | Tr | Tr | Tr | Tr |
| 20:0 | Tr | Tr | Tr | Tr | Tr |
| 24:0 | Tr | Tr | Tr | Tr | Tr |
| Total | 22.8 | 20.7 | 22.4 | 21.2 | 22.5 |
| | | | | | |
| 14:1 $\omega$ 6 | Tr | Tr | Tr | Tr | Tr |
| 15:1 $\omega$ 6 | 0.7 | 0.9 | 1.0 | 0.9 | 1.1 |
| 16:1 $\omega$ 7 | 9.6 | 6.7 | 6.0 | 5.4 | 5.8 |
| 17:1 $\omega$ 8 | 1.4 | 1.0 | 1.2 | 1.2 | 1.1 |
| 18:1 $\omega$ 9 | 20.3 | 23.5 | 18.6 | 19.9 | 19.0 |
| 20:1 $\omega$ 9 | 3.6 | 2.4 | 2.7 | 2.1 | 2.4 |
| 22:1 $\omega$ 9 | 3.4 | 2.7 | 1.8 | 1.7 | 1.6 |
| Total | 39.0 | 37.2 | 31.3 | 31.2 | 29.9 |
| | | | | | |
| 18:2 $\omega$ 6 | 1.6 | 0.8 | 1.4 | 1.7 | 1.5 |
| 18:3 $\omega$ 3 | 0.6 | 0.9 | 1.2 | 1.6 | 1.4 |
| 18:4 $\omega$ 3 | 1.6 | Tr | 1.2 | 0.5 | 1.0 |
| 20:2 $\omega$ 6 | 0.7 | 1.4 | 1.5 | 0.8 | 1.0 |
| 20:3 $\omega$ 6 | Tr | Tr | Tr | Tr | Tr |
| 20:4 $\omega$ 6 | 1.0 | 0.5 | 0.4 | 0.4 | 0.4 |
| 20:4 $\omega$ 3 | Tr | Tr | 1.0 | 0.5 | 0.8 |
| 20:5 $\omega$ 3 | 17.9 | 18.4 | 21.1 | 22.5 | 22.0 |
| 22:3 $\omega$ 6 | 1.7 | 4.7 | 2.0 | 1.5 | 1.2 |
| 22:4 $\omega$ 6 | 0.7 | Tr | 1.5 | 1.2 | 0.7 |
| 22:5 $\omega$ 3 | 1.0 | 2.4 | 1.2 | 1.4 | 1.2 |
| 22:6 $\omega$ 3 | 11.2 | 13.4 | 14.9 | 16.0 | 16.0 |
| Total | 38.0 | 42.5 | 47.4 | 48.4 | 47.2 |

[a]   Weight percent of fatty acid methyl ester.

From Krzeczkowski, R. A., *J. Am. Oil Chem. Soc.,* 47, 451, 1970. With permission.

## Table 16
## THE EFFECT OF DEHYDRATING, COOKING, AND IRRADIATING ON PROXIMATE COMPOSITION AND UNSATURATED FATTY ACIDS OF SHRIMP

### Proximate Composition and Vitamin Content

| Sample | Moisture | Protein | Fat | Thiamin | Riboflavin | Niacin | Pyridoxine | Pantothenic | Folic Acid |
|---|---|---|---|---|---|---|---|---|---|
| | g/100 g | | | mg/100 g | | | | | |
| Frozen, raw | 84.8 | 14.1 | 0.6 | 0.018 | 0.019 | 0.91 | 0.080 | 0.200 | 0.003 |
| Processed | | | | | | | | | |
| Dehydrated, raw | 1.8 | 90.6 | 3.4 | 0.045 | 0.107 | 2.35 | 0.610 | 0.180 | 0.024 |
| Dehydrated, pre-cooked | 1.5 | 92.3 | 4.1 | 0.048 | 0.123 | 2.22 | 0.400 | 0.250 | 0.009 |
| Irradiated after enzyme inactivated | 77.5 | 19.8 | 1.0 | 0.008 | 0.018 | 0.44 | 0.010 | 0.060 | 0.002 |
| Irradiated, precooked | 74.0 | 24.1 | 1.0 | 0.007 | 0.020 | 0.57 | 0.015 | 0.070 | 0.002 |
| Canned | 75.9 | 18.2 | 1.1 | 0.005 | 0.034 | 0.25 | 0.040 | 0.350 | 0.002 |
| As eaten, boiled, cold | | | | | | | | | |
| Dehydrated, raw | 77.5 | 21.4 | 1.0 | 0.013 | 0.029 | 0.44 | — | — | — |
| Dehydrated, pre-cooked | 78.2 | 21.1 | 0.9 | 0.013 | 0.032 | 0.41 | — | — | — |
| Irradiated after enzyme inactivation | 77.4 | 21.8 | 0.9 | 0.008 | 0.080 | 0.17 | — | — | — |
| Irradiated, precooked | 77.0 | 22.9 | 1.0 | 0.005 | 0.032 | 0.50 | — | — | — |
| Canned | 76.0 | 21.6 | 0.9 | 0.004 | 0.035 | 0.19 | — | — | — |

### Polyunsaturated Fatty Acids (mg/100 g)

| Sample | Hexane | Pentaene | Tetraene | Triene | Diene | Total |
|---|---|---|---|---|---|---|
| Frozen | 42 | 65 | 31 | 14 | 6 | 159 |
| Processed | | | | | | |
| Dehydrated raw | 199 | 238 | 119 | 55 | 46 | 657 |
| Dehydrated pre-cooked | 179 | 249 | 119 | 58 | 38 | 643 |
| Dehydrated after enzyme inactivation | 29 | 36 | 24 | 16 | 8 | 113 |
| Irradiated, precooked | 22 | 34 | 17 | 9 | 11 | 93 |
| Canned | 18 | 20 | 13 | 6 | 5 | 63 |

From Thomas, M. H. and Calloway, D. H., *J. Am. Diet Assoc.*, 39, 105, 1961. With permission.

### Table 17
### THE EFFECT OF FREEZING AND DIFFERENT HEAT PREPARATIONS ON THIAMIN CONTENT OF SHRIMP NEWBERG

| | Thiamin (μg/100 g) |
|---|---|
| Freshly prepared | 0.93 |
| After −10°F storage (brief) | 0.89 |
| Frozen-microwave heated | 0.86 |
| Frozen-infrared heated | 0.82 |
| Frozen-immersion heated | 0.80 |
| Fresh-held at 180°F 1 hr | 0.71 |
| Fresh-held at 180°F 2 hr | 0.68 |
| Fresh-held at 180°F 3 hr | 0.61 |
| Commercial samples | |
| Frozen | 0.88 |
| Frozen-microwave heated | 0.80 |
| Frozen-infrared heated | 0.76 |

Table 18

THE EFFECT OF CANNING, DRYING, AND IRRADIATING ON PROXIMATE COMPOSITION, AMINO ACID CONTENT, LYSINE AVAILABILITY, ENZYMIC DIGESTS, AND VITAMIN CONTENT OF MIXED SHRIMP CATCH (*METAPANAEUS AFFIRNIS AND PANAEUS INDICUS*)

| | Raw | Freeze dried | Air* dried | Canned | Semi-* dried | Irradiated* | | |
|---|---|---|---|---|---|---|---|---|
| | | | | | | Air pack | Vacuum pack | Nitrogen pack |
| **Proximate Composition** | | | | | | | | |
| Moisture (%) | 86.8 | 2.5 | 2.8 | 75.0 | 40.2 | 41.0 | 40.5 | 40.0 |
| Protein (%) | 11.7 | 87.3 | 86.4 | 20.9 | 49.0 | 48.1 | 48.1 | 49.2 |
| Nonprotein nitrogen (%) | 0.06 | <0.1 | 0.7 | — | 0.2 | 0.3 | 0.3 | 0.3 |
| Lipids (%) | 0.50 | 3.5 | 3.4 | 0.9 | 2.0 | 2.2 | 2.1 | 2.1 |
| Ash (%) | 1.04 | 7.9 | 8.1 | 2.0 | 4.7 | 4.4 | 4.5 | 4.6 |
| **Total Amino Acids (% Protein)** | | | | | | | | |
| Aspartic acid | 11.02 | 11.00 | 10.90 | 11.08 | 11.05 | 11.02 | 11.08 | 11.05 |
| Threonine | 4.00 | 3.98 | 3.98 | 3.94 | 4.02 | 4.00 | 4.02 | 4.06 |
| Serine | 4.04 | 4.02 | 4.00 | 4.05 | 3.98 | 3.88 | 3.82 | 3.88 |
| Glutamic acid | 20.12 | 20.45 | 21.60 | 20.80 | 20.14 | 21.25 | 20.02 | 21.06 |
| Proline | 2.18 | 2.24 | 2.09 | 2.19 | 2.28 | 2.26 | 2.28 | 2.30 |
| Glycine | 4.68 | 4.70 | 4.70 | 4.75 | 4.73 | 4.71 | 4.69 | 4.72 |
| Alanine | 6.04 | 6.01 | 6.05 | 6.02 | 6.02 | 5.88 | 5.86 | 5.79 |
| ½ Cystine | 0.65 | 0.68 | 0.70 | 0.72 | 0.69 | 0.73 | 0.75 | 0.70 |
| Valine | 4.69 | 4.73 | 4.72 | 4.70 | 4.71 | 4.70 | 4.66 | 4.62 |
| Methionine | 2.80 | 2.81 | 2.58 | 2.65 | 2.79 | 2.74 | 2.78 | 2.76 |
| Isoleucine | 4.77 | 4.76 | 4.82 | 4.65 | 4.71 | 4.48 | 4.42 | 4.39 |
| Leucine | 8.55 | 8.53 | 8.32 | 8.38 | 8.23 | 7.97 | 7.88 | 7.85 |
| Tyrosine | 3.24 | 3.19 | 3.11 | 3.10 | 3.27 | 3.12 | 3.12 | 3.16 |
| Phenylalanine | 4.78 | 4.82 | 4.72 | 4.72 | 4.75 | 4.70 | 4.72 | 4.78 |
| Lysine | 8.28 | 8.23 | 7.62 | 7.67 | 8.23 | 8.39 | 8.41 | 8.44 |
| Histidine | 1.82 | 1.85 | 1.82 | 1.78 | 1.89 | 1.85 | 1.88 | 1.86 |
| Arginine | 7.29 | 7.20 | 7.08 | 7.11 | 8.42 | 7.29 | 7.35 | 7.40 |

| | 1.56 | 1.58 | 1.45 | 1.40 | 1.56 | 1.54 | 1.56 | 1.55 |
|---|---|---|---|---|---|---|---|---|
| Tryptophan | | | | | | | | |
| **Free Amino Acids (% Protein)** | | | | | | | | |
| Aspartic acid | Tr | Tr | 0.38 | — | — | Tr | Tr | Tr |
| Threonine | 0.55 | 0.59 | 1.13 | — | 0.09 | 0.14 | 0.13 | 0.15 |
| Serine | 0.35 | 0.38 | 0.80 | — | 0.11 | 0.14 | 0.13 | 0.15 |
| Glutamic acid | 0.79 | 0.88 | 1.80 | — | 0.30 | 0.39 | 0.41 | 0.38 |
| Glycine | 5.95 | 6.12 | 8.85 | — | 2.51 | 2.49 | 2.52 | 2.58 |
| Alanine | 1.81 | 1.94 | 4.10 | — | 1.02 | 1.15 | 1.08 | 1.12 |
| Valine | 0.55 | 0.60 | 1.28 | — | 0.30 | 0.32 | 0.38 | 0.39 |
| Methionine | 0.38 | 0.40 | 0.85 | — | 0.22 | 0.20 | 0.18 | 0.24 |
| Isoleucine | 0.44 | 0.46 | 0.98 | — | 0.21 | 0.25 | 0.26 | 0.21 |
| Leucine | 0.69 | 0.72 | 1.82 | — | 0.40 | 0.38 | 0.42 | 0.45 |
| Tyrosine | 0.68 | 0.63 | 1.10 | — | 0.50 | 0.48 | 0.53 | 0.56 |
| Phenylalanine | 0.49 | 0.41 | 1.18 | — | 0.42 | 0.34 | 0.36 | 0.40 |
| Lysine | 1.85 | 1.74 | 2.92 | — | 1.12 | 1.58 | 1.51 | 1.60 |
| Histidine | Tr | Tr | Tr | — | Tr | Tr | Tr | Tr |
| Arginine | 0.50 | 0.52 | 1.05 | — | 0.30 | 0.35 | 0.37 | 0.39 |
| Total | 15.03 | 15.39 | 28.24 | — | 7.55 | 8.21 | 8.30 | 8.60 |
| **Available Lysine (% Protein)** | | | | | | | | |
| Total lysine | — | 8.23 | 7.62 | 7.67 | 8.23 | 8.39 | 8.41 | 8.44 |
| Days stored at 25 to 28°C | | | | | | | | |
| 0 | — | 7.86 | 6.60 | 7.19 | 7.71 | 8.01 | 7.95 | 8.00 |
| 30 | — | 7.77 | 6.58 | 7.18 | 7.73 | 7.89 | 7.89 | 7.96 |
| 60 | — | 7.71 | 6.62 | 7.09 | — | 7.92 | 7.87 | 7.88 |
| 90 | — | 7.62 | 6.54 | 7.14 | — | 7.80 | 7.82 | 7.80 |
| **Enzymic Digests (% Protein)** | | | | | | | | |
| Pepsin, trypsin, and erepsin (72 hr digest) | | | | | | | | |
| Peptides | — | 33.98 | 42.88 | 37.44 | 35.84 | 27.26 | 25.41 | 25.98 |
| Free amino acids | — | 75.14 | 70.27 | 75.71 | 76.99 | 94.27 | 91.46 | 90.11 |

Table 18 (continued)

## THE EFFECT OF CANNING, DRYING, AND IRRADIATING ON PROXIMATE COMPOSITION, AMINO ACID CONTENT, LYSINE AVAILABILITY, ENZYMIC DIGESTS, AND VITAMIN CONTENT OF MIXED SHRIMP CATCH (*METAPANAEUS AFFIRNIS AND PANAEUS INDICUS*)

| | Raw | Freeze dried | Air dried | Canned | Semi-dried | Irradiated[c] Air pack | Irradiated[c] Vacuum pack | Irradiated[c] Nitrogen pack |
|---|---|---|---|---|---|---|---|---|
| Pepsin and Papain (48 hr digest) | | | | | | | | |
| Peptides | — | 76.80 | 84.67 | 79.23 | 77.25 | 61.82 | 58.37 | 60.35 |
| Free amino acid | — | 36.48 | 32.38 | 35.01 | 35.01 | 41.41 | 44.10 | 44.35 |
| **Vitamin (μg/100 g)** | | | | | | | | |
| Thiamin | 128.6 | — | 54.0 | 50.2 | 52.0 | 33.5 | 42.2 | 40.6 |
| Riboflavin | 250.0 | — | 144.5 | 144.5 | 122.5 | 104.4 | 112.4 | 110.0 |
| Nicotinic acid | 14.7 | — | 12.1 | 10.8 | 9.4 | 8.7 | 8.6 | 8.8 |
| Vitamin B$_{12}$ | 18.4 | — | 12.3 | 11.2 | 11.4 | 10.4 | 10.4 | 10.1 |
| Folic acid | 57.1 | — | 33.9 | 31.9 | 29.3 | 23.9 | 25.9 | 25.5 |

| | Days stored at 25 to 28°C | | | | | | |
|---|---|---|---|---|---|---|---|
| | 30 | 30 | 90 | 30 | 90 | 30 | 90 |
| **Vitamin (μg/100 g)** | | | | | | | |
| Thiamin | 47.8 | 31.3 | 27.0 | 39.5 | 37.0 | 37.4 | 34.9 |
| Riboflavin | 121.6 | 103.8 | 89.3 | 110.6 | 103.6 | 110.7 | 101.8 |
| Nicotinic acid | 9.0 | 8.2 | 8.2 | 8.2 | 8.1 | 8.3 | 8.2 |
| Vitamin B$_{12}$ | 10.4 | 9.5 | 8.9 | 9.6 | 9.0 | 9.1 | 8.8 |
| Folic acid | 26.6 | 21.8 | 19.1 | 23.7 | 21.8 | 23.5 | 21.0 |

<sup>a</sup> Air drier operated at 65 to 70°C for 8 to 10 hr.

<sup>b</sup> Shrimp immersed for 1 hr in 0.5% sorbic acid, blanched 5 min in 10% NaCl at 80°C, and air dried at 65 to 70°C to reduce moisture to 40%.

<sup>c</sup> Semidried shrimp packed in polyethelene pouches, sealed in air, vacuum, or nitrogen, and irradiated in the range of 0.25 to 0.32 Mrad.

Reprinted with permission from Srinivas, H., Vakil, U. K., and Sreenivasan, A., *J. Food Sci.*, 39, 807, 1974, copyright © by Institute of Food Technologists.

# EFFECT OF PROCESSING ON NUTRITIVE VALUE OF FOOD: FISH

## B. E. March

## INTRODUCTION

There has been more study of processing alteration of the nutritive value of fishery products intended for poultry and livestock feeding than of those intended for human consumption. This emphasis is not so odd as might appear at first. There are two reasons why this is so. First, when the products are included in animal feeds, the mixed diet has to supply all of the nutrients for the animal during the time that it is fed. There is no opportunity for nutrient deficiencies in one meal to be offset by nutrients contained in a previous or subsequent meal. Secondly, objectives in animal feeding are well-defined and there are procedures for assessing nutritive value in the physiological and/or economic sense. Although the effects of processing on the nutritive characteristics of fish products have been more thoroughly investigated for those products fed to domestic animals, there has been much research dealing with the chemical changes affecting palatability factors and losses associated with various processing and storage conditions in fish for human consumption. In most cases, these chemical changes will doubtless be associated with some loss of nutritive value, while in other cases, effects in this regard will be insignificant. The following processing effects discussed are those that might be expected to involve alteration of nutritional value.

As a source of nutrients, fish contain protein, lipids, minerals, and vitamins. The proteins, as a whole, supply the essential amino acids in proportions to give a high biological value to the protein and to enable fish protein to be used as a supplement to protein sources of lower biological value. The triglycerides contained in fish are well utilized, and also are high in essential fatty acids. Fish are good sources of trace minerals and, depending on the amount of bone consumed, may contribute significant amounts of calcium and phosphorus to the diet. Fish are rich in many of the vitamins, but vary in the amounts supplied depending on the species and the particular tissues in question.

The effects of processing on the nutritive value may be considered from the aspect of selection of only certain tissues for consumption and also from the standpoint of the processing effecting chemical reactions that alter the nutritive value of the final product. Alteration may be either improvement or deterioration of nutritional quality.

The components of fish constitute a labile system capable of reactions that may proceed in different directions depending upon the conditions imposed. Carbohydrate components such as lactose, glucose, or ribose, which are not present in sufficient quantity to be of nutritional significance, may be important factors in the stability of the system and affect nutritive value indirectly by reacting with, and rendering unavailable, essential amino acids.

Because of the confounding effects of the many reactive components in fish tissue, the model system approach has been followed by a number of investigators in order to isolate the effects of certain reactants. However, observations that have been made on individual compounds, or on compounds in relatively simple systems, may not hold for more complex natural systems. The association of different compounds and the concentration of the system can affect response to different processing or storage conditions.

Fish is primarily consumed or fed as a source of protein. Damage to the nutritional value of this component is accordingly of major concern. Fish muscle — in common with muscle from other species — is of high biological value because it contains a large proportion of essential amino acids. In particular, muscle is rich in those essential amino acids that tend to be limiting in many plant proteins and particularly in cereal proteins. Proteins present in the viscera, the integument, cartilage, and gonads generally contain a less favorable balance of amino acids. The quality of the protein in a fish product will therefore vary, depending upon the proportion of muscle protein contained in it. Keratin — a principal protein in fish scales — is not readily digested, and hence, the presence of the skin in fish products will have lower protein availability. The milt from fish contains large amounts of protamines that contain no tryptophan, sulfur amino acids, or tyrosine. They do, however, contain a high percentage of arginine.

The cooking of fish will cause some solubilization of protein that, depending on the process, may result in loss of protein from the final product. The soluble proteins, however, tend to have a somewhat less favorable balance of amino acids than the remainder of the tissue proteins. Gelatin, for example, which is derived from collagen by boiling, does not contain tryptophan and is low in sulfur-containing amino acids (no cysteine or cystine).

Before the general availability of vitamin supplements, either as synthetic or fermentation products, natural feed ingredients had to supply the full complement of vitamins required in animal mixed feeds. Fish meals and condensed fish solubles were accordingly good sources of many of the vitamins, and fish oils were the important sources of vitamins A and D. Because of the great concern about the effects of processing and storage on the vitamin content, many studies were made. In recent years, however, there has been an increasing tendency for manufacturers of feed for poultry and livestock to use vitamin concentrates of guaranteed potency and pure vitamins to meet the full requirement of the animal for many of the vitamins. As a consequence, the practical importance of fishery products as sources of vitamins has declined, although the products may be included in feeds as sources of an "unidentified nutrient factor." Fish supplies some vitamins to the human diet, although it must be acknowledged that the muscle tissue that is consumed is a poorer source of vitamins than some of the organ tissues, which are discarded or included in the raw material for the production of meal for animal feeding.

Braekkan[10] has tabulated values for thiamin, riboflavin, niacin, vitamin $B_{12}$, vitamin $B_6$, pantothenic acid, and biotin in the uncooked edible part of different species of fish. He summarizes the data on processing effects as follows: weight-by-weight cured fish products usually show higher values than the corresponding fillets. Canned products usually show weight-by-weight values of the same order as the corresponding fresh fish. Smoked and canned products of herring, mackerel, tuna, and salmon are fairly good sources of B vitamins, and usually contain high amounts of niacin. Canned cod and herring roe, and canned cod liver are good sources of B vitamins.

Komata et al.[46] measured the effect of canning on the levels of some B vitamins in mackerel and tuna. After canning, mackerel retained 48, 93, 95, and 102% of thiamin, riboflavin, niacin, and vitamin $B_{12}$, respectively. The corresponding values for tuna were 30, 84, 87, and 96%. After storage at room temperature for 6 months, there was little change in the values for the vitamins with the exception of thiamin, which had declined considerably. The liquid in the cans contained 10 to 20% of the vitamins present. Some tabulations of processing effects on vitamins in a variety of fish products are given in Tables 1 to 3.

Table 1 shows thiamin content and percent retention in raw materials and the frozen fried fish product subjected to various heating treatments.[1] Average retention of thiamin after heating was from 77 to 104% relative to the frozen fried fish product.

Table 2 is a summary of nutritional values and vitamin contents for fish and fish

## Table 1
## VITAMIN CONTENT AND PERCENTAGE RETENTION OF FROZEN FRIED FISH PORTIONS SUBJECTED TO VARIOUS HEATING TREATMENTS

| Number | Treatment | Thiamin (mg/100 g)[a] | Retention[b] (%) |
|--------|-----------|------------------------|------------------|
| Raw materials | | | |
| 1A | Frozen raw fish | 0.299 | — |
| 1B | Batter mix (dry) | 0.118[c] | — |
| 1C | Breading mix | 0.226[c] | — |
| 2 | Frozen breaded raw fish portions | 0.250 | — |
| Conventional institutional handling | | | |
| 3 | Heated in convection oven, no holding | 0.250 ± 0.017[d] | 103.73[a] |
| 4 | Heated in convection oven, held ½ hr | 0.241 ± 0.011 | 100.00[ab] |
| 5 | Heated in convection oven, held 1—½ hr | 0.220 ± 0.020 | 91.29[bc] |
| 6 | Heated in convection oven, held 3 hr | 0.186 ± 0.028 | 77.18 |
| Convenience food system handling | | | |
| 7 | Frozen fried fish portions, thawed | 0.241 ± 0.019 | 100.00[ab] |
| 8 | (Same as No. 4) | — | — |
| 9 | Heated in infrared oven, held ½ hr | 0.231 ± 0.014 | 95.85[abc] |
| 10 | Heated in steamer, held ½ hr | 0.215 ± 0.021 | 89.21[c] |
| 11 | Heated in microwave oven, held ½ hr | 0.231 ± 0.026 | 95.8[abc] |

[a] Fat-free, dry weight basis; average of three determinations for raw materials.
[b] Mean percent retention in relation to frozen fried fish portions (No. 7); means followed by the same letters are not significantly different at the 5% level.
[c] Dry weight basis.
[d] Means and standard deviation of six preparations.

Reprinted from Ang, C. Y. W., Chang, C. M., Frey, A. E., and Livingston, G. E., *J. Food Sci.*, 40, 997, 1975, copyright © by Institute of Food Technologists. With permission.

products prepared by the Norwegian Canning Company Industry and the Norwegian Fisheries Research Institute.[90]

Table 3 summarizes losses in frozen and canned fishery products of vitamin $B_6$ and pantothenic acid.[84]

## N-NITROSAMINES

Discovery of the toxicity and carcinogenicity of N-nitrosodimethylamine caused concern regarding the possibility that nitrates and nitrites, used in curing salt, could react with amines present to form nitroso compounds. In one investigation 18 samples of smoked and five of canned fish were analyzed after cooking with and without sodium nitrite. The results indicated that certain kinds of fish, especially those rich in amines, can form nitrodimethylamine during cooking with nitrite.[87] Herring meals made from nitrite-treated fish have been found to contain toxic quantities of nitrosamines.[82,86] Hurst,[38] on the other hand, analyzed 13 samples of herring meal from fish that had not been treated with nitrate or nitrite, and reported concentrations of dimethylnitrosamine from 0.15 to 1.0 ppm.

Studies by Howard et al.[35] indicated that nitrosodimethylamine is not produced in the flesh of fresh-water fish during smoking, but that in raw and smoked sable, salmon, and shad, trace quantities of 4 to 26 ppb were detected. Fong and Chan[30] found nitrosodimethylamine in samples of Chinese marine salt fish.

## Table 2
## NUTRITIONAL VALUES AND VITAMINS OF NORWEGIAN FISH AND FISH PRODUCTS

Fish and Fish Products, Chemical Composition and Vitamin Content

| Product | Chemical composition | | | | | | | | Vitamins | | | | | |
| | g/100 g | | | | mg/100 g | | | | | | ug/100 g | | mg/100 g | |
| | Water | Protein | Fat | Ash | Ca | P | Fe | I | Thiamin $B_1$ | Riboflavin $B_2$ | Pantothenic acid | $B_{12}$ | Niacin | Cal/100 g |
|---|---|---|---|---|---|---|---|---|---|---|---|---|---|---|
| **Cadidae** | | | | | | | | | | | | | | |
| **Cod** | | | | | | | | | | | | | | |
| Fillet | 80.4 | 18.1 | 0.3 | 1.1 | 20 | 200 | 0.6 | 0.50 | 50 | 110 | 180 | 0.8 | 2.0 | 70 |
| Roe | 74.0 | 20.4 | 2.4 | 1.4 | 30 | 500 | 1.5 | 0.20 | 750 | 700 | 3000 | 10.0 | 1.3 | 105 |
| Liver | 32.0 | 6.2 | 60.3 | 0.8 | 25 | 100 | — | 0.40 | 100 | 580 | 640 | 11.0 | 2.9 | 570 |
| Stockfish | 14.8 | 78.5 | 1.4 | 5.9 | 160 | 950 | 2.5 | 1.20 | — | 240 | 1675 | 10.0 | 7.5 | 325 |
| Klipp-fish | 39.5 | 37.8 | 1.0 | 22.2 | 60 | 300 | 1.6 | — | — | 230 | 340 | 3.6 | 2.4 | 160 |
| Lute-fish | 87.9 | 11.4 | 0.3 | 0.3 | 10 | 90 | 0.5 | 0.05 | — | 50 | 75 | 1.2 | 0.2 | 50 |
| **Scombridae** | | | | | | | | | | | | | | |
| **Mackerel** | | | | | | | | | | | | | | |
| Spring mackerel fillet | 74.3 | 18.6 | 5.4 | 1.5 | 20 | 250 | 1.4 | 0.05 | 105 | 360 | 1030 | 12.0 | 9.4 | 125 |
| Autumn-mackerel fillet | 60.0 | 18.5 | 20.2 | 1.3 | 20 | 240 | 2.4 | 0.05 | 105 | 360 | 1030 | 12.0 | 9.4 | 255 |
| Smoked | 61.1 | 21.5 | 10.6 | 5.8 | — | — | — | — | — | 375 | 520 | 12.0 | 6.6 | 180 |
| Tuna fish, fillet | 66.0 | 24.0 | 9.9 | 1.1 | 40 | 200 | 1.0 | 0.05 | 163 | 160 | 660 | 4.8 | 9.1 | 185 |
| **Other Species** | | | | | | | | | | | | | | |
| Redfish, fillet | 77.1 | 18.3 | 3.5 | 1.5 | 20 | 200 | 0.5 | 0.15 | — | 110 | 360 | 1.0 | 2.0 | 105 |
| Catfish | 78.1 | 16.1 | 2.7 | 1.1 | — | — | — | — | 60 | 80 | 570 | 2.2 | 2.2 | 90 |
| Porbeagle | 76.1 | 18.8 | 0.4 | 1.0 | — | — | — | — | 80 | 100 | 330 | 2.6 | 7.0 | 80 |
| Dogfish | 69.7 | 19.1 | 8.9 | 1.3 | — | — | — | — | — | 140 | 690 | 1.8 | 5.2 | 155 |
| Salmon fillet | 71.0 | 20.5 | 6.2 | 1.6 | 20 | 200 | 0.8 | 0.05 | 140 | 220 | 2080 | 4.0 | 8.8 | 140 |
| Smoked | 63.1 | 21.4 | 8.4 | 7.0 | — | — | — | 0.05 | 110 | 190 | 710 | 7.0 | 5.0 | 160 |
| Trout, fillet | 74.5 | 20.0 | 3.3 | 1.5 | 20 | 290 | 1.2 | 0.05 | 100 | 210 | 1950 | 5.0 | 5.2 | 110 |
| Eel, fillet | 56.2 | 15.3 | 27.7 | 1.0 | 20 | 200 | 0.5 | — | — | 40 | 240 | 2.0 | 3.5 | 310 |
| Shrimp | 68.1 | 23.3 | 0.8 | 6.5 | 60 | 130 | 0.7 | 0.15 | — | 70 | 230 | 4.6 | 2.3 | 100 |
| Crayfish | 72.1 | 24.1 | 0.9 | 3.6 | — | — | — | — | — | 60 | 410 | 2.7 | 2.4 | 105 |

| Product | Water | Protein | Fat | | Ash | Ca | P | Fe | I | Thiamin B₁ | Riboflavin B₂ | Pantothenic acid | B₁₂ | Niacin | Cal/100 g |
|---|---|---|---|---|---|---|---|---|---|---|---|---|---|---|---|
| Fresh herrings in tomato sauce | 66.7 | 15.8 | 14.4 | — | 2.6 | 230 | 330 | 3.5 | 0.10 | — | 285 | 750 | 9.2 | 3.8 | 195 |
| Marinated herrings | 64.1 | 15.8 | 15.9 | 0.8 | 2.5 | 230 | 320 | 3.3 | 0.10 | — | 245 | 820 | 9.5 | 4.7 | 210 |
| Kippered herrings | 62.3 | 21.1 | 13.4 | — | 3.5 | 140 | 380 | 0.7 | 0.10 | — | 370 | 1040 | 1.5 | 4.8 | 205 |
| Soft roes | 82.2 | 15.1 | 3.0 | — | 2.8 | 90 | 620 | 3.0 | 0.15 | — | 750 | 1550 | 10.5 | 2.4 | 85 |
| Hard roes | 65.8 | 24.3 | 2.4 | 1.2 | 1.5 | 50 | 390 | 2.8 | 0.15 | — | 320 | 1730 | 10.7 | 1.4 | 130 |
| Mackerel | | | | | | | | | | | | | | | |
| Mackerel fillets in oil | 52.2 | 18.4 | 28.5 | — | 1.2 | 50 | 220 | 1.1 | 0.10 | 60 | 465 | 685 | 9.8 | 10.6 | 335 |
| Small mackerel in oil | 57.4 | 19.3 | 20.4 | — | 2.1 | 240 | 250 | 2.0 | 0.10 | 100 | 350 | 550 | 8.3 | 8.0 | 260 |
| In tomato sauce | 66.1 | 16.9 | 13.7 | 1.2 | 2.2 | 200 | 280 | 1.4 | 0.10 | 100 | 315 | 590 | 5.4 | 8.8 | 195 |
| Marinated | 70.6 | 20.8 | 4.6 | 0.7 | 2.5 | 270 | 340 | 1.9 | 0.15 | 100 | 400 | 560 | 9.4 | 8.3 | 130 |
| In bouillon | 65.2 | 21.4 | 9.9 | — | 2.9 | 280 | 360 | 2.2 | 0.10 | 100 | 290 | 570 | 5.4 | 10.0 | 175 |
| Tuna fish | | | | | | | | | | | | | | | |
| Tuna in oil | 47.9 | 23.3 | 27.7 | — | 1.7 | 40 | 150 | 2.3 | 0.05 | 25 | 100 | 310 | 2.5 | 9.0 | 345 |
| Tuna in bouillon | 65.8 | 22.2 | .8 | — | 3.3 | 60 | 110 | 2.0 | 0.05 | — | 95 | 230 | 3.0 | 9.8 | 170 |
| Cod | | | | | | | | | | | | | | | |
| Liver natural | 32.3 | 4.6 | 55.1 | — | 3.6 | 30 | 100 | 3.6 | 0.50 | — | 340 | 430 | 10.6 | 1.5 | 515 |
| Liver paste | 49.0 | 6.5 | 40.5 | 1.4 | 2.3 | 20 | 80 | 1.0 | 0.45 | 75 | 430 | 1290 | 9.7 | 1.2 | 415 |
| Roe | 69.7 | 24.3 | 1.7 | 2.5 | 1.8 | 30 | 410 | 1.5 | 0.20 | 250 | 550 | 1965 | 15.0 | 0.8 | 125 |
| Roe-liver paste | 45.8 | 13.6 | 38.3 | — | 2.2 | 30 | 180 | 1.5 | 0.40 | 130 | 440 | 1200 | 13.0 | 1.2 | 400 |
| Milt | 82.0 | 14.5 | 1.1 | — | 1.8 | 40 | 220 | 3.5 | 0.10 | — | 200 | 500 | 5.0 | 1.0 | 70 |

Canned Fish Products, Chemical Composition and Vitamin Content

| | Chemical Composition | | | | | | | | Vitamins | | | | | |
|---|---|---|---|---|---|---|---|---|---|---|---|---|---|---|
| | g/100 g | | | | mg/100 g | | | | µg/100 g | | | | mg/100 g | Cal/100 g |
| Product | Water | Protein | Fat | Ash | Ca | P | Fe | I | Thiamin B₁ | Riboflavin B₂ | Pantothenic acid | B₁₂ | Niacin | |
| Brisling | | | | | | | | | | | | | | |
| Brisling sardines smoked, in oil | 50.2 | 18.6 | 29.6 | 2.6 | 250 | 400 | 1.5 | 0.10 | 30 | 325 | 800 | 10.8 | 6.7 | 340 |
| Brisling sardines smoked, in tomato sauce | 64.5 | 16.8 | 14.3 | 3.0 | 250 | 350 | 2.7 | 0.05 | 30 | 325 | 680 | 11.7 | 5.7 | 195 |
| Herring | | | | | | | | | | | | | | |
| Sild sardines smoked, in oil | 50.3 | 18.3 | 29.2 | 3.3 | 350 | 440 | 1.9 | 0.05 | 45 | 270 | 750 | 9.9 | 4.4 | 355 |

Table 2 (continued)
## NUTRITIONAL VALUES AND VITAMINS OF NORWEGIAN FISH AND FISH PRODUCTS

Canned Fish Products, Chemical Composition and Vitamin Content

| Product | Chemical Composition | | | | | | | | Vitamins | | | | | Cal/100 g |
|---|---|---|---|---|---|---|---|---|---|---|---|---|---|---|
| | g/100 g | | | | mg/100 g | | | | Thiamin ug/100 g | Riboflavin | Pantothenic | mg/100 g | | |
| | Water | Protein | Fat | Ash | Ca | P | Fe | I | B₁ | B₂ | acid | B₁₂ | Niacin | |
| Sild sardines smoked, in tomato sauce | 66.6 | 17.1 | 12.2 | 3.5 | 360 | 380 | 2.9 | 0.05 | 45 | 290 | 710 | 10.9 | 4.1 | 180 |
| Sild sardines unsmoked, in oil | 58.8 | 17.5 | 22.1 | 2.9 | 250 | 350 | 1.0 | 0.10 | 45 | 325 | 960 | 8.0 | 5.7 | 270 |
| Sild sardines unsmoked, in tomato sauce | 67.6 | 17.3 | 12.0 | 3.1 | 240 | 370 | 2.7 | 0.05 | 45 | 300 | 739 | 9.0 | 5.8 | 175 |
| Fresh herrings in bouillon | 65.8 | 18.8 | 12.9 | 3.1 | 260 | 350 | 2.3 | 0.10 | — | 240 | 770 | 10.7 | 3.2 | 190 |
| Coalfish, fillet | 78.4 | 19.4 | 0.7 | 1.2 | 20 | 220 | 0.8 | 0.25 | 45 | 200 | 380 | 3.5 | 3.4 | 80 |
| Haddock, fillet | 78.6 | 19.7 | 0.3 | 1.1 | 20 | 200 | 0.7 | 0.60 | — | 110 | 250 | 1.8 | 4.0 | 80 |
| Pollack, fillet | 77.7 | 19.1 | 0.6 | 1.6 | 20 | 220 | — | — | 45 | 100 | 320 | 1.1 | 1.9 | 80 |
| Ling, fillet | 77.7 | 20.5 | 0.3 | 1.5 | 20 | 200 | 0.7 | 0.30 | — | 80 | 320 | 0.5 | 2.3 | 85 |
| Tusk, fillet | 78.7 | 19.0 | 0.3 | 1.5 | 20 | 220 | — | 0.35 | — | 150 | 310 | 1.2 | 2.8 | 80 |
| Pleuronectiidae | | | | | | | | | | | | | | |
| Flounder, fillet | 78.1 | 17.3 | 2.1 | 1.5 | 30 | 200 | 2.2 | 0.05 | 150 | 90 | 1680 | 10.0 | 3.5 | 90 |
| Halibut, fillet | 74.5 | 18.0 | 6.0 | 1.0 | 30 | 220 | 0.5 | 0.10 | 40 | 60 | 360 | 0.9 | 4.4 | 125 |
| Greenland halibut fillet | 70.2 | 12.4 | 15.6 | 1.1 | — | — | — | — | 60 | 80 | 250 | 1.0 | 1.5 | 190 |
| Greenland halibut smoked | 74.6 | 13.4 | 8.8 | 3.7 | — | — | — | — | — | 170 | 720 | 0.6 | 1.5 | 135 |
| Nupidae | | | | | | | | | | | | | | |
| Sprat, whole fish | 68.4 | 16.8 | 10.5 | 2.5 | 280 | 400 | 0.7 | 0.10 | 40 | 260 | 1090 | 10.6 | 4.8 | 160 |
| Herring | | | | | | | | | | | | | | |
| Winter herring, fillet | 69.4 | 16.9 | 12.4 | 1.6 | 50 | 250 | 1.1 | 0.05 | 40 | 300 | 1000 | 14.0 | 4.0 | 80 |
| Fat herring, fillet | 66.1 | 17.3 | 14.9 | 1.7 | 40 | 320 | 0.6 | 0.05 | 40 | 300 | 1000 | 14.0 | 4.0 | 205 |
| Small herring, whole fish | 76.1 | 16.9 | 4.8 | 2.4 | 280 | 400 | 0.7 | 0.05 | 40 | 300 | 1000 | 14.0 | 4.0 | 110 |
| Small herring, smoked | — | — | — | — | — | — | — | — | — | 280 | 880 | 15.0 | 4.2 | — |
| Small herring hot smoked | — | — | — | — | — | — | — | — | — | 260 | 990 | 14.0 | 4.7 | — |
| Salt herring | — | — | — | — | — | — | — | — | — | 170 | 500 | 8.0 | 2.0 | — |

| | | | | | | | | | | | | | | |
|---|---|---|---|---|---|---|---|---|---|---|---|---|---|---|
| **Crab** | | | | | | | | | | | | | | |
| Meat | 72.4 | 22.9 | 1.8 | — | 1.9 | 120 | 220 | 3.5 | 0.15 | 50 | 395 | 710 | 13.5 | 1.7 | 110 |
| Paste | 69.7 | 15.6 | 8.6 | 2.1 | 3.2 | 70 | 490 | 3.1 | 0.15 | 60 | 185 | 1570 | 43.9 | 1.2 | 150 |
| Dressed | 69.1 | 18.3 | 7.8 | 1.1 | 3.4 | 50 | 450 | 1.6 | 0.15 | 50 | 250 | — | — | — | 150 |
| **Shrimps** | | | | | | | | | | | | | | |
| Peeled | 71.8 | 24.1 | 1.2 | — | 2.8 | 90 | 170 | 3.3 | 0.15 | 60 | 40 | 165 | 2.5 | 0.7 | 110 |
| **Miscellaneous** | | | | | | | | | | | | | | |
| Fish pudding | 81.7 | 10.4 | 1.4 | 4.0 | 1.7 | 70 | 110 | 0.9 | 0.10 | 12 | 130 | 320 | 0.9 | 1.5 | 70 |
| Fishballs in bouillon | 86.5 | 7.4 | 0.6 | 3.8 | 1.9 | 60 | 100 | 0.8 | 0.10 | 10 | 95 | 195 | 0.5 | 1.4 | 50 |
| Fishballs extra quality | 83.8 | 8.8 | 1.5 | 4.0 | 1.4 | 110 | 100 | 0.5 | 0.10 | 10 | 100 | 170 | 0.6 | 1.4 | 65 |
| Fried fish cakes in gravy | 81.1 | 8.8 | 3.3 | 4.0 | 2.0 | 50 | 110 | 1.3 | 0.25 | — | 100 | 250 | 1.0 | 1.1 | 80 |
| Fried fish cakes extra quality | 80.7 | 9.0 | 3.8 | 3.9 | 1.7 | 60 | 110 | 0.9 | 0.25 | — | 100 | 250 | 1.0 | 1.1 | 85 |
| Fried fish cakes in bouillon | 81.1 | 9.3 | 2.6 | 4.1 | 2.1 | 50 | 100 | 2.1 | 0.25 | — | 100 | 250 | 1.0 | 1.1 | 65 |
| Fried fish cakes extra quality | 81.9 | 10.5 | 3.3 | 2.6 | 1.6 | 80 | 120 | 0.5 | 0.25 | — | 100 | 250 | 1.0 | 1.1 | 80 |
| Corned fish | 74.9 | 20.0 | 3.9 | — | 1.5 | 30 | 190 | 0.6 | 0.20 | 50 | 115 | 260 | 2.6 | 2.2 | 115 |
| Cod roe caviar | 53.7 | 17.9 | 11.3 | 9.6 | 6.7 | 30 | 140 | 2.2 | 0.15 | 325 | 455 | 1940 | 9.4 | 0.5 | 210 |
| Salmon substitute in oil | 51.9 | 17.8 | 12.4 | — | 8.6 | 30 | 130 | 1.1 | 0.15 | 10 | 205 | 400 | 2.3 | 2.0 | 265 |
| Sugar salt-cured cod roe | 63.7 | 17.7 | 0.4 | 14.2 | 13.2 | 40 | 160 | 2.0 | 0.20 | — | 425 | 3380 | 12.5 | 0.7 | 130 |

Vitamins A and D in Some of the Most Common Fishes and Fish Products

| | Vitamin A IU/g | Vitamin D IU/g |
|---|---|---|
| Cod roe, fresh and canned | 0—1[a] | 1 |
| Cod liver, fresh and canned | 300—500 | 30—50 |
| Herring, fresh and canned | 0.5—1.5 | 1.5—3 |
| Brisling, fresh and canned | 4—10 | 3—10 |
| Mackerel, fresh and canned | 0.5—2.0 | 1—10 |

[a] The value for roe is probably too low; recent investigations have shown 4 to 5 times as high values measured biologically, resulting from the presence of vitamin A aldehyde.

From Taarland, T., Mathiesen E., Orsthus, O., and Braekken, O. R., *Tids. Hermetikind.*, 44, 405—412, 1958. With permission.

Table 3
LOSSES OF VITAMIN B₆ AND PANTOTHENIC ACID IN
FROZEN AND CANNED FOODS
MICROGRAMS PER GRAM (µg/g)

| Food | Vitamin B₆ | | | Pantothenic acid | | |
|------|-----|--------|--------|------|--------|--------|
| | Raw | Frozen | Canned | Raw | Frozen | Canned |
| Fish and sea food | | | | | | |
| Clams | 0.80 | — | 0.83 | — | — | — |
| Eel | 2.30 | — | 1.23 | 1.50 | — | — |
| Turbot | — | — | 0.38 | 2.50 | — | 7.20 |
| Haddock | 0.82 | | — | 1.30 | — | 1.25 |
| Herring | 3.70 | 3.20 | 1.60 | 9.70 | 9.30 | 7.00 |
| Mackerel | 6.60 | 4.10 | 2.80 | 8.50 | 5.20 | 5.00 |
| Oysters | 0.50 | — | 0.37 | 2.50 | — | — |
| Roe, cod | 1.65 | — | 1.40 | 32.00 | — | 19.65 |
| Salmon | 7.00 | 7.00 | 3.00 | 13.00 | 7.10 | 5.50 |
| Sardines, Atlantic | — | — | — | 10.90 | — | 7.00 |
| Sardines, Pacific | 2.80 | — | 2.20 | 10.00 | — | 6.00 |
| Shrimp | 1.00 | — | 0.60 | 2.80 | — | 2.10 |
| Tuna | 9.00 | — | 4.25 | 5.00 | — | 3.20 |
| Mean | 3.54 | — | 1.81 | 7.98 | 7.20 | 6.39 |
| % Loss | — | 17.3 | 48.9 | — | 20.8 | 19.9 |

From Schroeder, H. A., *Am. J. Clin. Nutr.,* 24, 562, 1971. With permission.

## HISTAMINE

A number of microorganisms that may contaminate fish are capable of decarboxylating histidine. Fatty fishes such as tuna, herring, mackerel, and sardine contain considerable quantities of free histidine in their muscle tissue. In the lean fishes free histidine is either absent or present in very low concentration. According to Hughes,[37] as much as 3% on a wet weight basis of free histidine may be present. When certain diamines such as putrescine and cadaverine are present and consumed with histamine, the rate of absorption of histamine from the digestive tract into the blood stream is enhanced. In this event toxic effects may be observed from the ingestion of smaller amounts of histamine than would otherwise be expected to cause any symptoms of toxicity.[69]

Storage above 0°C induces histamine formation. In the case of mackerel, for example, histamine is produced relatively quickly when the fish are held at ambient temperature.[32] Histamine formation is accompanied by rapid deterioration of the fish and the development of malodors. Conversely, in mackerel held on ice, no histamine could be detected even after 2 weeks, although by this time the fish were unacceptable. High values for histamine are likewise reported in herring, reaching 30 to 40 mg/100 g only 40 to 50 hr after death.[36]

Histamine is heat resistant and has been reported to persist in tuna following domestic cooking. Any amounts remaining in canned tuna after proper commercial retorting are, however, well below the level of toxicity.[70] In a survey conducted by Ramel et al.[76] on the incidence of histamine in canned fish, appreciable amounts were found in certain samples of canned tuna, but far less in sardines and mackerel. The same factories were usually the sources of the samples containing histamine.

The toxicity of some samples of tuna meal for chicks has been identified as due to the presence of histamine.[31,89] Harry et al.[33] attribute the gizzard erosion and proventricular abnormalities in chicks fed certain fishmeals to the presence of histamine. With good sanitary practice the amount of histamine present in fish meals is not of practical significance. Bacterial action can, however, result in toxic levels even when the odor of the raw material is not offensive.

## NUTRIENT LOSSES DUE TO SOLUBILIZATION AND LEACHING

The cut surfaces of fresh fish muscle gradually exude water. The amount of exudate or "drip" varies with the species, and is increased if the fish is frozen and then thawed. Further loss is incurred if the fish is refrozen after it has been thawed.

Drip is partly due to denaturation of the proteins that normally tend to retain the water of the muscle. Since the drip contains protein, it represents nutritional and economic loss. Seagan[85] analyzed the protein composition of drip from thawed fillets and compared it with extracts of low ionic strength from fresh fillets. The electrophoresis patterns were the same.

It was reported in 1942 by Tarr[94] that free drip could be reduced by lightly brining unfrozen fish muscle at its natural pH, and that the effect was due to the ability of sodium chloride to cause the proteins to bind liquid firmly. Love and Abel[49] claim that sodium chloride has an adverse effect in that it diffuses into the tissues. As a result, the freezing point is lowered, causing a greater amount of liquid phase to remain in the muscle. Then oxygen is able to diffuse more easily through the tissue, promoting oxidation of lipids and accelerating protein denaturation.

Boyd and Southcott[9] studied pretreatment of fresh fillets of Dover sole *(Microstomus pacificus)*, Pacific cod *(Gadus macrocephalus)*, halibut *(Hippoglossus stenolepis)*, and red snapper *(Sebastodes ruberrimus)* with sodium tripolyphosphate prior to freezing. It was found to be effective in reducing drip loss during thawing. Sodium chloride, in a few trials, was effective in reducing drip and cooking losses. Tripolyphosphate and sodium citrate dip solutions of corresponding ionic strengths were equally effective in reducing drip loss during thawing from fillets of red snapper. Pretreatment of chinook salmon *(Oncorhynchus tshawytscha)* fillets with sodium tripolyphosphate preceding freezer storage was ineffective in retarding lipid oxidation during storage at $-10°C$; however, unlike sodium chloride, sodium tripolyphosphate did not accelerate the development of oxidative rancidity. It should be noted that, although none of the compounds had an appreciable effect on drip loss from frozen salmon flesh, the compounds did reduce the amount of material lost when the fish was cooked and reduced shear strength of the salmon muscle cooked after storage.

Ellinger[27] has reviewed the literature on the use of polyphosphate and other salt solutions as dips or sprays for fish. There are discrepancies in the results reported from different laboratories. One possible source of variation in response is the condition of the fish at the time of treatment. Polyphosphates have little or no effect on good quality fish, but cause fluid retention and reduce weight loss in poorly processed fish. Fluid escape is prevented by the formation of a film of gelled protein over the surface of the fish. When polyphosphate is used in conjunction with sodium chloride, the film of gelled protein appears to block the entry of sodium chloride into the tissue.

Deboned or minced fish flesh is extensively used for the manufacture of such food items as fish sticks, cakes, and sausage. The flesh may be trimmings from a filleting operation or from whole fish. Because of irregularity of supplies of fresh material, it is convenient to freeze the deboned flesh for later use. This practice means that the fish flesh is subjected to two freezings and thawings. Pottinger et al.[73] demonstrated with sea trout fillets that there is an increase in the drip of fish that has been frozen twice. In cod that has been refrozen, the rate of free fatty acid formation is rapid, as is the decrease in extractable protein.[24] Podeszewski et al.[71] have concluded from their investigations of the quality of double-frozen herring that, when evaluating fish that has been frozen twice, attention should be directed primarily to changes relating to alteration of lipids. They report that the changes in lipids are more dynamic than those in nitrogenous compounds both during freezing and after thawing. Their data showed that after initial freezing of herring tissue, the decomposition of triglycerides was about 6% and of phospholipids about 7%. Secondary freezing increased the decomposition of phospholipids to 16%.

Kolakowski et al.[45] studied changes in the protein nutritive value of frozen fish sausage produced from fresh and frozen minced herring flesh. The results indicated that up to 1 month of storage at −20°C, whether the sausage was made from fresh or frozen minced flesh, had little effect on the nutritive value of the protein. After 3 months storage, however, there was considerable difference in the amount of available lysine present in the protein, depending upon whether fresh or frozen flesh had been used. Lysine loss was 21.8% in the frozen sausages made from frozen flesh and only 7.6% in those made from fresh flesh. The minced flesh itself (not made into sausage) showed 31.0 and 8.5% declines in available lysine, depending upon whether it was fresh or refrozen when it went into storage. The reduced loss of lysine availability in the sausage was attributed to the antioxidant properties of the spices that were added.

When deboned fish is to be produced from headed and gutted fish, the kidney substances, blood and, if it is dark in color, the membrane lining the belly cavity must be removed before the carcass is put through the deboning machine. The final product will otherwise be unattractive. An alternative approach would be to debone without removing the dark-colored materials from the headed and gutted carcass and then to wash and dewater the deboned product. Yamamoto et al.[103] attempted this procedure with deboned fish samples from frozen fish of a wide variety of species with disappointing results. Washing improved the general appearance of the flesh, although this varied with the species. There was loss of flavor following the washing and dewatering. Most serious, however, was the loss of water-soluble protein, which ranged from about 12% for herring and grey cod frames, to 20% for perch, and as high as 30 to 40% for some of the flatfish. On the basis of the data presented, washing of deboned flesh cannot be considered as an acceptable procedure.

## FREEZING AND FROZEN STORAGE

Frozen storage of fishery products prevents microbial spoilage and retards most chemical changes, although some reactions may be accelerated. Denaturation of proteins, oxidation and hydrolysis of lipids, protein-lipid interactions, and protein-carbohydrate interactions can all take place during frozen storage. Some of these changes may be important only because they affect texture, flavor and palatability, while others may reduce amino acid availability and destroy vitamins.

There is a temperature at which the rate of protein denaturation in frozen fish is maximal. Love and Elerian[50] determined this to be approximately −1.5° for cod frozen at −29°C. An explanation that has been offered for denaturation is the concentration of inorganic ions that occurs as the tissue water freezes. A crude parallel has been drawn between the frozen and the dehydrated state with respect to solvent water.[23] However, the phenomenon did not occur when fresh tissue was supercooled to the same temperature. Denaturation of cod fillets is inhibited to some extent by treatment with glycerol solution prior to freezing, with 10% being the optimum concentration.[51] Glycerol may inhibit denaturation at low temperature by maintaining more water in association with the protein rather than by dilution of inorganic ions. The denaturation curves of cod muscle at different temperatures showed that fillets soaked in 10% glycerol for 14 hr and stored at −14°C are denatured at a similar rate to control fillets stored at −20°C. The denaturation of fish muscle at low temperature is linked with the release of free fatty acids from lipids. It is not clear whether the free fatty acids themselves are involved in the denaturation process or whether intact triglyceride or phospholipid in association with the protein is necessary for the normal extractability of the protein. The question is well-reviewed by Connell.[18] Many enzyme-catalyzed reactions are accelerated during freezing (or freezing and thawing) in cellular systems. The explanation may be that the normal compartmentalization of enzymes in subcellular particles is disrupted by freezing.[28] Protein denaturation may occur secondarily to the release of fatty acids from lipids.

In cold-stored mackerel the rate of hydroperoxide formation varied as follows: vacuum-packed fillets < foil-wrapped fillets < ungutted fish < gutted fish.[32] It was noticeable that the boxed, ungutted, and gutted fish dehydrated more rapidly than did the foil-wrapped fillets. The dehydration was probably accompanied by more rapid oxidation. Oxidation is similar in herring kept under these conditions.

Glycolysis is known to proceed in fish muscle at temperatures below 0°. There is an early report by Sharp[88] that significant glycolysis occurs in haddock muscle at −10°C. More recently Tomlinson et al.[98] reported changes in lactate concentrations for ling cod muscle at temperatures down to −30°C. Burt[12] studied changes in sugar phosphate and lactate concentration in cod muscle, frozen pre- and postrigor, and stored at different temperatures. Maximum glycolysis in most samples occurred before or during freezing and in the first 2 weeks of storage. In fish frozen pre-rigor, however, in a plate-freezer and stored at −29°, the lactate concentrations increased markedly during the 4 to 16 week period, and then more slowly during the subsequent 14 week period.

## FISH ENSILAGE AND FERMENTATION PRODUCTS

Fish flesh left in the anaerobic condition is likely to become acidic rather than alkaline. The reduction in pH that occurs in most species of fish is generally much less than that which occurs in mammalian muscle following conventional slaughter and is probably related to the lower concentrations of glycogen in fish muscle. Connell[17] observed that fish myosin is more rapidly digested by trypsin and chymotrypsin than are mammalian, chicken, or frog myosins. Autolysis in whole fish seems to be due mainly to the digestive enzymes present in the gut. If the fish is ground, these enzymes are distributed throughout the mixed tissues and autolytic liquification is rapid. The muscle tissue alone liquifies poorly.

Ensiling of fish as a means of preservation for poultry and livestock feeding is practiced only when there are not drying facilities available for the production of meal and where the product does not have to be transported any distance. There are a number of procedures that may be followed. If oily fish is used, as much oil as possible should be separated at an early stage of manufacture, since there is rapid deterioration in oil quality as measured by free fatty acid content and iodine value.[97] Generally the ground fish is acidified from pH 2.5 to 4 with sulfuric, hydrochloric, or formic acid, or a mixture of acids, and allowed to liquefy as a result of action of the enzymes naturally present and not from bacterial action.[54] An insoluble sediment always remains in fish silage even when commercial enzymes are added, although the amount of insoluble sediment varies according to the conditions of incubation. The amino acid composition of the sediment differs from that of the soluble phase.[75] It lacks hydroxyproline and contains less protein than the soluble phase. Hydroxyproline is quickly released from fish skin that is exposed to the soluble phase of silage, and it is therefore concluded that collagen is rapidly solubilized in silage. A high concentration of cystine in the sediment suggests that the S-S cross-linkage may be essential in a protein structure that resists the action of the proteolytic enzymes in silage. The protein of the sediment is sufficiently similar to that of structural glycoproteins in connective tissue to suggest that much of the sediment consists of glycoproteins.

Feeding trials with "liquid herring" preparations made by an enzymatic, and a high pressure acid process, respectively,[54] indicated that the two preparations were similar in nutritive value for the chick.[59] The growth response was intermediate between that obtained from a sample of herring meal and that obtained from condensed herring solubles.

Fermented fish products in the form of sauces and pastes are nutritional adjuncts to human diets otherwise low in good quality protein in some areas of the world. They are important particularly in that they supply lysine, sulfur amino acids, vitamins, and minerals. The fish tissues, often of the entire fish, are broken down under controlled conditions, autolytically and by enzymes contributed by bacteria or molds.[102] Fermentation of fatty fish with certain microorganisms can result in considerable reduction of the fat content.[11]

## DRIED FISH AND FISHMEAL

The preservation by drying of fish for foods for human and livestock consumption is a traditional practice. The nutritive quality of the product will be affected by both the drying and the storage conditions employed.

In the manufacture of fishmeal, drying at too high temperatures will destroy vitamins and render protein unavailable.[5,6,93] Nutritive losses continue to occur during storage of the product.

The storage stability of the dried product may be affected by the freshness of the product at the time of drying and by the amount of heat applied. The most stable dried herring are those made from fresh fish. Keeping the fish in ice for 2 days prior to drying, or holding them in cold storage, much reduces the stability of the dried product.[3] Herring smoked before drying showed increased stability. Cooking at 115°C produces a more stable dehydrated product than cooking at 104°C. Similarly, fish dried at 80 to 90°C is more stable than fish dried at 50 to 70°C. It is assumed that some substances with antioxidant properties are formed at the higher temperatures. Haem compounds formed during meal oxidation have been credited with antioxidant properties.[4,21,34,41] Haem pigments may, on the other hand, act as catalysts during lipid autooxidation[29,77,92] as evidenced by the tendency to rancidity of the red lateral line muscle in fish.

The drying temperatures to which herring presscake is subjected alters the pattern of oxidative changes during storage of the resultant meal when compared to the pattern observed with freeze-dried meal. When the drying temperature is sufficiently high, the more labile compounds may be oxidized prior to storage. Where intermediate products of labile compounds are prooxidants, their rapid turnover during heat drying could reduce subsequent oxidative deterioration of more stabile meal components during storage.

Some browning reaction in fish probably occurs as a result of interaction between amino acids and sugar.[39,40,93,96] More important are products of lipid oxidation that can react with proteins and likewise cause toughening, darkening, and reduction of digestibility.

Roubal[79,80] and Roubal and Tappel[81] have suggested that, in lipid-protein systems, free radicals derived from lipid oxidation are the principal cause of damage to protein. Amino acid analysis before and after the reaction of myosin with malonaldehyde showed that malonaldehyde reacts preferentially with histidine, arginine, tyrosine, and methionine.[13] Oxidizing lipid in lipid-protein systems reacts with the protein component[19,66,91] and, conversely, the protein accelerates the oxidation of the lipid.[25] Interactions among different components of systems containing oxidizable lipid may vary — depending upon a variety of factors — to give apparently contradictory results.[7,8]

The hydroperoxides formed in lipid oxidation are particularly effective in inactivating the S-amino acids, forming methionine sulfoxide from methionine and probably cysteic acid from cystine. Cuq et al.[20] showed that the formation of methionine sulfoxide in an intact protein leads directly to a loss of methionine availability measured by in vitro digestibility.

Oxidative changes involving the protein and the lipids affect both the biological value of the protein and the digestibility of the lipid. Chemical estimation of available lysine[14] may be a more sensitive test of protein alteration under these conditions than pepsin digestibility tests,[25] although the sensitivity of the latter can be altered by adjusting the concentration of pepsin employed.

The oxidative reactions in fishmeal may be retarded by the addition of antioxidants to the meal.[2,26,47,55,56,58,59] The protective effect of antioxidant against changes in both the lipid and the protein components in herring meal may be apparent as early as 2 weeks after preparation of the meal.

## FISH PROTEIN CONCENTRATE

Fish protein concentrate (FPC) is a modern sophisticated version of dried fish, a product that has been used for human consumption since ancient times in many parts of the world. In its present form, FPC can be added to other foods to improve the quality and level of protein intake. Emphasis in developing processing techniques has been on the production of a bland — or flavorless — stable product with good protein quality. The flavor and stability of the FPC are dependent upon the completeness of extraction of lipids. Lipids in FPC are relatively stable when present at levels of 0.1% or less.[60] Studies by Morrison and McLaughlan[62] and Morrison et al.[64] indicate that the method of extraction can markedly influence the nutritional value of FPC. Fish flours prepared from cod, herring, rosefish, or capelin, by a procedure involving the use of chloroform and isopropyl alcohol, were superior to casein at the 5 and 10% protein levels, but were toxic at the 20% protein level. The toxicity was removed by extraction with ether, but was resistant to removal by heating. Residual chloroform per se was not the cause of the toxicity. Morrison and Munro[63] reported that there was a reduction in the cystine content when freeze-dried cod fillets were refluxed for 16 hr with ethylene dichloride. They suggest the formation of a thioether, 5,5′-ethylenebiscysteine. These authors also identified chlorocholine chloride as a toxic compound present in samples of fish flour that had been extracted with dichloroethane.[65]

Decreases in the availability of lysine and the sulfur amino acids during processing have been of particular concern because of the importance of these essential amino acids in any supplement intended for use with a low protein, high cereal diet. Particular attention has been paid to the sulfur amino acids because the levels in fish proteins are not particularly high.[15,61] To assess the heat damage to protein that might be anticipated during manufacture of FPC, Yanez, Ballester, and Donoso[104] dried hake fillets at different temperatures. The fillets were freeze-dried and oven-dried at 105° and 170°C for 6 hr. Available lysine[14] was similar for the freeze-dried and oven-dried at 105° fish, but that subjected to 170° suffered a 20% loss. Damage to sulfur amino acids seemed to start at 105°. In tests with rats, both net protein utilization and protein efficiency ratio indicated protein damage at 170°.

Dubrow et al.[22] compared the chemical composition and nutritive quality of FPC with that of the raw fish before processing. The amino acid composition of the concentrate was not appreciably different from that of the raw material. Available lysine and protein efficiency ratio (rat feeding trials) were likewise comparable in the original and the processed material. Newberne et al.[68] evaluated an FPC prepared from whole red hake *(Urophycis chuss)* by extraction with isopropyl alcohol. The product was evaluated for lack of toxicity over five generations of rats. Growth, reproduction, and lactation of these groups were compared to control groups fed casein. There was no evidence of any significant difference between the rats fed the FPC and the control rats. Regardless of fish species or method of extraction, all FPCs responded similarly to histidine and methionine supplementation as measured by rat growth response and feed intake in experiments conducted by Makdani et al.[52]

The relative nutritive values were studied of the water-soluble fractions from commercially available sources of FPC extracted with different solvents.[53] The water-soluble fractions of hexane-extracted, dichloroethane-extracted, and isopropanol-extracted FPC represented 16, 15, and 9%, respectively, of the original FPCs. Weanling rats fed diets containing the dehydrated water-insoluble fraction, to provide 10% of protein, gained more weight and ate more feed than did rats fed diets containing the intact FPC. On similar diets prepared with the water-soluble fractions, no growth of the rats was observed, and feed intakes were very low. For each of the FPCs the water-soluble fraction contained the essential amino acids as a smaller percentage of the total nitrogen than did the water-insoluble fraction or the original FPC, irrespective of the solvent used for extraction of the fish. Even though the essential amino acid levels in the water-insoluble fractions of the FPCs were approximately the same, weight gains were much lower for dichloroethane-extracted FPC than for the hexane- or isopropanol-extracted FPCs. The dichloroethane extracted FPC evidently still contained some toxic factors formed during extraction with the solvent.

## RADIATION

Ionizing radiation at low doses can, by killing a large proportion of contaminating microflora, considerably extend the shelf life of fish without significantly altering organoleptic quality. The effects on nutritional quality have been studied in fish of both lean and fatty species.

Underdal et al.[100] studied the effects of gamma radiation of mackerel on protein quality. Irradiation was by a cobalt 60 source with 30,000 Ci activity and a dose rate of 780 krad per hr. The radiation doses ranged from 0.1 to 4.5 Mrad. The protein quality of the irradiated flesh was tested with rats on the basis of true digestibility, biological value, and net protein utilization. On the basis of the results of these tests, radiation had no deleterious effect on protein quality. Kennedy and Ley[43] studied the effects of irradiation and cooking, separately and combined, on the protein quality of cod fillets. Irradiation was by a cobalt 60 source with 10,000 Ci activity and a dose rate of 31 krad per hr and a radiation dose of 0.6 Mrad. Cooking was in a pressure cooker for 4 min at 15 lb psi. All drip was retained. Protein nutritive value was unaffected by irradiation, whereas cooking caused a 9% loss. Dried fishmeals likewise show no effect upon irradiation at a dosage of 1.0 Mrad.[42]

There is little alteration of the overall amino acid composition of fish protein following irradiation. Irradiation may increase the amounts of free amines and free amino acids. The increase in free amino acids would probably be more important organoleptically than nutritionally. Differences in volatile substances between irradiated and non-irradiated fish products are likewise probably not of nutritional significance.[44]

With respect to individual amino acids, Van der Schaff and Mossel[101] found no loss of available lysine from fish meal upon irradiation. Underdal et al.[100] noted an insignificant degradation of sulfur amino acids with mackerel but greater loss when cod was irradiated.[99] They suggest the difference may be due to the presence of greater amounts of antioxidants in mackerel than in cod.

Irradiation can cleave disulfide bonds in proteins, whereas lipid peroxides are effective only in the case of the disulfide bond in cystine. Another difference between the effects of radiation and peroxides was discovered by Schaich.[83] Electron spin resonance signals were observed in all gamma irradiated amino acids, but peroxides of methyl linoleate produced free radicals only in cystine, cysteine, lysine, tryptophan, tyrosine, and histidine. No signals were observed in the other common amino acids.

In the experiments of Kennedy and Ley noted above,[43] the effects of irradiation and cooking on some of the B-complex vitamins in the cod fillets were also observed. Irradiation did not affect niacin, reduced riboflavin by 6%, and reduced thiamin by 47%. Cooking reduced niacin by 4%, riboflavin by 9%, and thiamin by 10%. The total loss of vitamins from irradiation followed by cooking was approximately the sum of the losses produced by the two treatments. The sensitivity of thiamin to radiation has also been observed in halibut[74,105] and in swordfish.[48] Underdal et al.[100] compared the concentrations of thiamin, pyridoxine, and niacin in irradiated and nonirradiated samples of mackerel. There was no effect on niacin from irradiation at the doses used. Both thiamin and pyridoxine were reduced by doses as low as 0.3 Mrad. Thiamin was particularly sensitive to irradiation and was reduced to 15% of its original concentration by 4.5 Mrad. The same dosage reduced pyridoxine to 38% retention of the original concentration.

Tocopherol is very radiosensitive in the presence of oxygen (as is vitamin A). It is also important to note that tocopherol was observed to be destroyed when added to rat diets containing irradiated beef.[72]

Irradiation of fish may induce both oxidative and lytic changes depending upon whether oxygen is present or not. Ionizing radiation in the presence of oxygen is oxidative[16] and would accordingly be expected to reduce amounts of polyunsaturated fatty acids. Nawar[67] irradiated mackerel oil — under vacuum — in comparison with other oils and found the radiolytic pattern to be predictable and dependent upon the fatty acid composition of the oil. Each fatty acid yields two major hydrocarbons; one with one carbon atom less than the fatty acid and the other with two carbon atoms less and an extra double bond. The major aldehydes have the same chain length as those of the major fatty acids. The major hydrocarbons identified in irradiated mackerel oil were similar to those found in irradiated mackerel fillets. Ronsivalli et al.,[78] determined the effects of irradiation of cod and haddock muscle on fatty acid composition. There were decreases in 20:5 ω 3 and 22:6 ω 3 after irradiation.

## REFERENCES

1. **Ang, C. Y. W., Chang, C. M., Frey, A. E., and Livingston, G. E.,** Effects of heating methods on vitamin retention in six fresh or frozen prepared food products, *J. Food Sci.*, 40, 997—1003, 1975.
2. **Aure, L.,** Oxidation-stabilization of herring meal by butylene hydroxytoluol (BHT) on a technical scale, *Arsberet. Vedkomm. Nor. Fisk.*, 3, 17—24, 1957.
3. **Banks, A.,** Some factors affecting the oxidation of the fat of dehydrated herrings, *J. Food Sci. Technol.*, 1, 28—34, 1950.
4. **Banks, A., Eddie, E., and Smith, J. G. M.,** Reactions of cytochrome-c with methyl linoleate hydroperoxide, *Nature (London)*, 190, 908—909, 1961.
5. **Biely, J. and March, B. E.,** The nutritive value of herring meals. III. The effects of heat treatment and storage temperature as related to oil content, *Poult. Sci.*, 34, 1274—1278, 1955.

6. Biely, J., March, B. E., and Tarr, H. L. A., The effect of drying temperature on the folic acid content of herring meal, *Science*, 116, 249—250, 1952.

7. Bishov, S. J. and Henick, A. S., Antioxidant effect of protein hydrolyzates in a freeze-dried model system, *J. Food Sci.*, 37, 873—875, 1972.

8. Bishov, S. J., Henick, A. S., and Koch, L. B., Oxidation of fat in model systems related to dehydrated foods, *Food Res.*, 25, 174—182, 1960.

9. Boyd, J. W. and Southcott B. A., Effect of polyphosphates and other salts on drip loss and oxidative rancidity of frozen fish, *J. Fish. Res. Board Can.*, 22, 53—67, 1965.

10. Braekkan, O. R., B-vitamins in some fish products, in *Fish in Nutrition*, Heen, E. and Kreuzer, R., Eds., Fishing News (Books), 1962.

11. Burkholder L., Burkholder, P. R., Chu, A., Kostyk, N., and Roels, O. A., Fish fermentation, *Food Technol. (Chicago)*, 22, 1278—1284, 1968.

12. Burt, J. R., Changes in sugar, phosphate and lactate concentration in trawled cod (Gadus callarias) muscle during frozen storage, *J. Sci. Food Agric.*, 22, 536—539, 1971.

13. Buttkus, H., The reaction of myosin with malonaldehyde., *J. Food Sci.*, 32, 432—434, 1967.

14. Carpenter, K. J., The estimation of the available lysine in animal-protein foods, *Biochem. J.*, 77, 604—610, 1960.

15. Chalupa, W. and Fisher, H., Comparative protein evaluation studies by carcass retention and nitrogen balance methods, *J. Nutr.*, 81, 139—146, 1963.

16. Chipault, J. R., High energy irradiation, in *Symposium on Foods: Lipids and Their Oxidation*, Schultz, H. W., Ed., AVI Publishing, Westport, Conn., 1962, 151—169.

17. Connell, J. J., The relative stabilities of the skeletal muscle myosins of some animals., *Biochem. J.*, 80, 503—509, 1961.

18. Connell, J. J., The effect of freezing and frozen storage on the proteins of fish muscle, in *Low Temperature Biology of Foodstuffs*, Hawthorn, J. and Rolfe, E. J., Eds., Pergamon Press, Oxford, 1968, 333—358.

19. Crawford, D. L., Yu, T. C., and Sinnhuber, R. O., Reaction of malonaldehyde with protein., *J. Food Sci.*, 32, 332—335, 1967.

20. Cuq, J. L., Provansal, M., Guilliux, F., and Cheftel, C., Oxidation of methionine residues of casein by hydrogen peroxide. Effects on in vitro digestibility, *J. Food Sci.*, 38, 11—13, 1973.

21. Dubouloz, P. J., Laurent, J., and Dumas, J., Metabolism of lipid peroxides. I. Characterization of a hematin pigment which destroys lipid peroxides., *Bull. Soc. Chim. Biol.*, 33, 1740—1744, 1951.

22. Dubrow, D. L., Pariser, E. R., Brown, N. L., and Miller, H., Jr., F.P.C.'s quality virtually the same as its raw material's quality, *Commer. Fish. Rev.*, 32, 25—31, 1970.

23. Duckworth, R. B. and Smith, G. M., The environment for chemical change in dried and frozen foods., *Proc. Nutr. Soc.*, 22, 182—189, 1963.

24. Dyer, W. J., Fraser, D. I., Ellis, D. G., Idler, D. R., MacCallum, W. A., and Laishley, E., *Bull. Inst. Int. Froid Annexe*, 1, 515—552, 1962.

25. El-Lakany, S. and March, B. E., A comparison of chemical changes in freeze-dried herring meals and a lipid-protein model system., *J. Sci. Food Agric.*, 25, 889—897, 1974.

26. El-Lakany, S. and March, B. E., Chemical and nutritive changes in herring meal during storage at different temperatures with and without antioxidant treatment., *J. Sci. Food Agric.*, 25, 899—906, 1974.

27. Ellinger, R. H., Phosphate applications in seafood processing, in *Phosphates as Food Ingredients*, CRC Press, Boca Raton, Fla., 1972, 131—147.

28. Fennema, O., Activity of enzymes in partially frozen aqueous systems, in *Water Relations of Foods*, Duckworth, R. B., Ed., Academic Press, New York, 1975, 397—413.

29. Fishwick, M. J., Freeze-dried turkey muscle. II. Role of haem pigments as catalysts in the autoxidation of lipid constituents, *J. Sci. Food Agric.*, 21, 160—163, 1970.

30. Fong, Y. Y. and Chan, W. C., Dimethylnitrosamine in Chinese marine salt fish, *Food Cosmet. Toxicol.*, 11, 841—845, 1973.

31. Grau, C. R., Barnes, R. N., Karrick, N., and McKee, L. G., The effect of raw material on tuna-meal quality, *Commer. Fish. Rev.*, 18(7), 18—20, 1956.

32. Hardy, R. and Smith, J. G. M., The storage of mackerel (*Scomber scombrus*). Development of histamine and rancidity, *J. Sci. Food Agric.*, 27, 595—599, 1976.

33. Harry, E. G., Tucker, J. F., and Laursen-Jones, A. P., The role of histamine and fish meal in the incidence of gizzard erosion and proventricular abnormalities in the fowl, *Br. J. Poult. Sci.*, 16, 69—78, 1975.

34. Hirano, Y. and Olcott, H. S., Effect of heme compounds on lipid oxidation, *J. Am. Oil Chem. Soc.*, 48, 523—524, 1971.

35. **Howard, J. W., Fazio, T., and Watts, J. O.**, Extraction and gas chromatographic determination of N-nitrosodimethylamine in smoked fish: application to smoked nitrite-treated chub., *J. Assoc. Off. Anal. Chem.*, 53, 269—274, 1970.

36. **Hughes, R. B.**, Chemical studies on the herring *(Clupea harengus)*. II. The free amino acids of herring flesh and their behaviour during post-mortem spoilage., *J. Food Sci.*, 10, 558—564, 1959.

37. **Hughes, R. B.**, Chemical studies on the herring *(Clupea harengus)*. X. Histidine and free sugars in herring flesh., *J. Sci. Food Agric.*, 15, 293—299, 1964.

38. **Hurst, R. E.**, Dimethylnitrosamine levels in untreated herring meals, *J. Sci. Food Agric.*, 27, 600—602, 1976.

39. **Jones, N. R.**, "Browning" reactions and the loss of free amino acid and sugar from lyophilized muscle extractives of fresh and chill-stored codling *(Gadus callarias)*, *Food Res.*, 24, 704, 1959.

40. **Jones, N. R.**, Kinetics of phosphate-buffered, ribose-amino reactions at 40° and 70% relative humidity: systems related to the "browning" of dehydrated and salt cod, *J. Sci. Food Agric.*, 10, 615—624, 1959.

41. **Kendrick, J. and Watts, B. M.**, Acceleration and inhibition of lipid oxidation by heme compounds, *Lipids*, 4, 454—458, 1969.

42. **Kennedy, T. S.**, Studies on the nutritional value of foods treated with gamma-radiation. II. Effects on the protein in some animal feeds, egg, and wheat, *J. Sci. Food Agric.*, 16, 433—437, 1965.

43. **Kennedy, T. S. and Ley, F. J.**, Studies on the combined effect of gamma irradiation and cooking on the nutritional value of fish, *J. Sci. Food Agric.*, 22, 146—148, 1971.

44. **King, F. J., Mendelsohn, J. M., Gadbois, D. F., and Bernsteinas, J. B.**, Some chemical changes in irradiated seafoods, *Radiat. Res. Rev.*, 3, 399—415, 1972.

45. **Kolakowski, E., Fik, M., and Karminska, S.**, Investigations into changes in the protein nutritive value of frozen fish sausages produced from fresh and frozen minced flesh., *Bull. Inst. Int. Froid Annexe*, 1972-2 59—62.

46. **Komata, Y., Hashimoto, Y., and Mori, T.**, B-vitamins in marine products and their changes in processing and storage. I. Canned mackerel and tuna in brine, *Bull. Jpn. Soc. Sci. Fish.*, 21, 1236—1240, 1956.

47. **Lea, C. H., Parr, L. J., and Carpenter, K. J.**, Chemical and nutritional changes in stored herring meal, *Br. J. Nutr.*, 12, 297—312, 1958.

48. **Lopes-Matas, A. and Fellers, C. R.**, Composition and nutritive value of fresh, cooked, and processed swordfish, *Food Res.*, 13, 387—396, 1948.

49. **Love, R. M. and Abel, G.**, The effect of phosphate solution on the denaturation of frozen cod muscle, *J. Food Technol.*, 1, 323—332, 1966.

50. **Love, R. M. and Elerian, M. K.**, Protein denaturation in frozen fish. VIII. The temperature of maximum denaturation in cod, *J. Sci. Food Agric.*, 15, 805—809, 1964.

51. **Love, R. M. and Elerian, M. K.**, Protein denaturation in frozen fish. IX. The inhibitory effect of glycerol in cod muscle, *J. Sci. Food Agric.*, 16, 65—70, 1965.

52. **Makdani, D. D., Huber, J. T., and Bergen, W. G.**, Effect of histidine and methionine supplementation on the nutritional quality of commercially prepared fish protein concentrate in rat diets, *J. Nutr.*, 101, 367—376, 1971.

53. **Makdani, D. D., Huber, J. T., Mickelson, O., and Bergen, W. G.**, The influence of water fractionation on the nutritional value of fish protein concentrate, *Nutr. Rep. Int.*, 9, 309—317, 1974.

54. **McBride, J. R., Idler, D. R., and MacLeod, R. A.**, The liquefaction of British Columbia herring by ensilage, proteolytic enzymes, and acid hydrolysis, *J. Fish. Res. Board Can.*, 18, 93—112, 1961.

55. **March, B. E., Biely, J., Claggett, F., and Tarr, H. L. A.**, Nutritional and chemical changes in the lipid fraction of herring meals with and without anti-oxidant treatment, *Poult. Sci.*, 41, 873—880, 1962.

56. **March, B. E., Biely, J., Goudie, C., Claggett, F., and Tarr, H. L. A.**, The effect of storage temperature and antioxidant treatments on the chemical and nutritive characteristics of herring meal, *J. Am. Oil Chem. Soc.*, 38(2), 80—84, 1961.

57. **March, B. E., Biely, J., McBride, J. R., Idler, D. R., and MacLeod, R. A.**, The protein nutritive value of liquid herring preparation, *J. Fish. Res. Board Can.*, 18, 113—116, 1961.

58. **March, B. E., Biely, J., Tarr H. L. A., and Claggett, F.**, The effect of antioxidant treatment on the metabolizable energy and protein value of herring meal, *Poult. Sci.*, 44, 679—685, 1965.

59. **Meade, T. L.**, A new development in fish meal processing, *Feedstuffs*, 28(20), 15—22, 1956.

60. **Medwadowski, B., Haley, A., Van der Veen, J., and Olcott, H. S.**, Effect of storage on lipids of fish protein concentrate, *J. Am. Oil Chem. Soc.*, 48, 782—783, 1971.

61. **Miller, D. S.**, The nutritive value of fish proteins, *J. Sci. Food Agric.*, 7, 337—343, 1956.

62. **Morrison, A. B. and McLaughlin, J. M.**, Variability in nutritional value of fish flour, *Can. J. Biochem. Physiol.*, 39, 511—517, 1961.

63. **Morrison, A. B. and Munro, I. C.**, Factors influencing the nutritional value of fish flour. IV. Reaction between 1,2-dichloroethane and protein, *Can. J. Biochem.*, 43, 33—40, 1965.

64. **Morrison, A. B., Sabry, Z. I., and Middleton, E. J.**, Factors affecting the nutritional value of fish flour. I. Effects of extraction with chloroform or ethylylene dichloride, *J. Nutr.*, 77, 97—104, 1962.
65. **Munro, I. C. and Morrison, A. B.**, Factors influencing the nutritional value of fish flour. V. Chlorocholine chloride, a toxic material in samples extracted with 1,2-dichloroethane, *Can. J. Biochem.*, 45, 1049—1053, 1967.
66. **Narayan, K. A., Sugai, M., and Kummerow, K. A.**, Complex formation between oxidized lipids and egg albumen, *J. Am. Oil Chem. Soc.*, 41, 254—259, 1964.
67. **Nawar, W. W.**, Radiolytic changes in fats, *Radiat. Res. Rev.*, 3, 327—334, 1972.
68. **Newberne, P. M., Glaser, O., Friedman, L., and Stillings, B.**, Safety evaluation of fish protein concentrate over five generations of rats, *Toxicol. Appl. Pharmacol.*, 24, 133—141, 1973.
69. **Parrot, J. L. and Nicot, G.**, Alimentation et la vie 53; p. 4, 5, 6, and 76, 1965; as cited by Hardy, R. and Smith, J. G. M., *J. Sci. Food Agric.*, 27, 595—599, 1976.
70. **Plagnol, H. and Aldrin, J. F.**, Amount of histamine in tuna from the Gulf of Guinea, *Rev. Conserv.*, 1, 1963, 143; as cited in *World Fish. Abstr.*, 16, 47—48, 1965.
71. **Podeszewski, Z., Otto, B., Stodolnik, L., and Swiniarski, J.**, Technological evaluation of double-frozen meat tissue from Baltic herring, *(Clupea harengus L.)*, *Bull. Inst. Int. Froid Annexe*, 1972-2, 85—91.
72. **Poling, C. E., Warner, W. D., Humburg, F. R., Reber, E. F., Urbain, W. M., and Rice, E. E.**, Growth, reproduction, survival, and histopathology of rats fed beef irradiated with electrons, *Food Res.*, 20, 193—214, 1955.
73. **Pottinger, S. R., Kerr, R. G., and Lanham, W. B.**, Effect of refreezing on quality of sea trout, *Commer. Fish. Rev.*, 11, 14—16, 1949.
74. **Proctor, B. E. and Goldblith, S. A.**, Effects of ionizing radiations on food nutrients, in *Nutritional Evaluation of Food Processing*, Harris, R. S. and Von Loesecke, H., Eds., AVI Publishing, Westport, Conn., 1960, 133—144.
75. **Raa, J. and Gildberg, A.**, Autolysis and proteolytic activity of cod viscera, *J. Food Technol.*, 11, 619—628, 1976.
76. **Ramel, P., Girard, P., and Lanteaume, M. T.**, Histamine in canned fish, *Rev. Hyg. Med. Soc.*, 13, 73—83, 1965; Current and Tech. Lit. 19 (Abstr. 370), 72, February 1966.
77. **Robinson, M. E.**, Hemoglobin and methemoglobin as oxidative catalysts, *Biochem. J.*, 18, 255—264, 1924.
78. **Ronsivalli, L. J., King, F. J., Ampola, V. G., and Holston, J. A.**, Study of irradiated pasteurized fishery products, *Isot. Rad. Technol.*, 8, 321—340, 1971.
79. **Roubal, W. T.**, Trapped radicals in dry lipid-protein systems undergoing oxidation, *J. Am. Oil Chem. Soc.*, 47, 141—144, 1969.
80. **Roubal, W. T.**, Free radicals, malonaldehyde, and protein damage in lipid protein systems, *Lipids*, 6, 62—64, 1971.
81. **Roubal, W. T. and Tappel, A. L.**, Damage to proteins, enzymes and amino acids by peroxidizing lipids, *Arch. Biochem. Biophys.*, 113, 5—8, 1966.
82. **Sakshaug, J., Sögnen, E., Hansen, M. A., and Koppang, N.**, Dimethylnitrosamine: its hepatotoxic effect in sheep and its occurrence in toxic batches of herring meal, *Nature (London)*, 206, 1261—1262, 1965.
83. **Schaich, K.**, Free Radical Formation in Proteins Exposed to Peroxidizing Lipid, Sc.D. thesis, Massachusetts Institute of Technology, Cambridge, 1974; as cited by Karel, M. in Free radicals in low moisture systems, in *Water Relations of Foods*, Duckworth, R. B., Ed., Academic Press, New York, 1975.
84. **Schroeder, H. A.**, Losses of vitamins and trace minerals resulting from processing and preservation of foods, *Am. J. Clin. Nutr.*, 24, 562—573, 1971.
85. **Seagan, H. L.**, Analysis of the protein constituents of drips from thawed fish muscle, *Food Res.*, 23, 143—149, 1958.
86. **Sen, N. P., Schwinghamer, L., Donaldson, B. A., and Miles, W. F.**, N-nitrosodimethylamine in fish meal, *J. Agric. Food Chem.*, 20, 1280—1281, 1972.
87. **Sen, N. P., Smith, D. C., Schwinghamer, L., and Howsam, B.**, Formation of nitrosamines in nitrite treated fish, *J. Can. Inst. Food Technol.*, 3, 66—69, 1970.
88. **Sharp, J. G.**, Post mortem breakdown of glycogen and accumulation of lactic acid in fish muscle at low temperatures, *Biochem. J.*, 29, 850—853, 1935.
89. **Shifrine, M., Ousterhout, L. E., Grau, C. R., and Vaughn, R. H.**, Toxicity to chicks of histamine formed during microbial spoilage of tuna, *Appl. Microbiol.*, 7, 46—50, 1959.
90. **Taarland, T., Mathiesen, E., Ovsthus, O., and Braekken, O. R.**, Nutritional values and vitamins of Norwegian fish and fish products, *Tids. Hermetikkind.*, 44, 405—412, 1958.
91. **Tappel, A. L.**, Studies of the mechanism of vitamin E action. III. In vitro copolymerization of oxidized fats with protein, *Arch. Biochem. Biophys.*, 54, 266—280, 1955.

92. **Tappel, A. L.**, Unsaturated lipid oxidation catalyzed by hematin compounds, *J. Biol. Chem.*, 217, 721—733, 1956.
93. **Tarr, H. L. A., Biely, J., and March, B. E.**, The nutritive value of herring meals. I. The effect of heat, *Poult. Sci.*, 33, 242—250, 1954.
94. **Tarr, H. L. A.**, Effect of pH and NaCl on swelling and drip in fish muscle, *J. Fish. Res. Board Can.*, 5, 411—427, 1942.
95. **Tarr, H. L. A.**, The Maillard reaction in flesh foods, *Food Technol. (Chicago)*, 8, 15—19, 1954.
96. **Tarr, H. L. A.**, The origin and quantitative distribution of sugars and sugar phosphates in fish muscles post mortem and the role of these in Maillard browning, Food Sci. and Technol., Proc. First Int. Congr. Food Sci. and Tech. London, Vol. 1, Gordon & Breach, New York, 1962, 18—21.
97. **Tatterson, I. N. and Windsor, M. L.**, Fish silage, *J. Sci. Food Agric.*, 25, 369—379, 1974.
98. **Tomlinson, N., Jonas, R. E. E., and Geiger, S. E.**, Glycolysis in lingcod muscle during frozen storage, *J. Fish. Res. Board Can.*, 20, 1145—1152, 1963.
99. **Underdal, B., Nordal, J., Lunde, G., and Eggum, B.**, The effect of ionizing radiation on the nutritional value of fish (cod) protein, *Lebensm. Wiss. Technol.*, 6, 90—93, 1973.
100. **Underdal, B., Nordal, J., Lunde, G., and Eggum, B.**, The effect of ionizing radiation on the nutritional value of mackerel, *Lebensm. Wiss. Technol.*, 9, 72—74, 1976.
101. **Van der Schaff, A. and Mossel, D. A. A.**, Gamma radiation sanitation of fish and blood meals, *Int. J. Appl. Radiat. Isot.*, 14, 557—562, 1963.
102. **Van der Veen, A. G.**, Fermented and dried seafood products in southeast Asia, in *Fish as Food*, Vol. III, Borgstrom, G., Ed., Academic Press, New York, 1965, 227—250.
103. **Yamamoto, M., Barnes, A., Lou, Y. C., and Wong, J.**, Consequences of Washing Deboned Fish Flesh Upon Appearance and on Protein Loss, Tech. Rep. 580, Fisheries and Marine Service, Canada, 1975, 1—10.
104. **Yanez, E., Ballester, D., and Donoso, G.**, Effect of drying temperature on quality of fish protein, *J. Sci. Food Agric.*, 21, 426—428, 1970.
105. **Ziporin, Z. Z., Kraybill, H. F., and Thach, H. J.**, Vitamin content of foods exposed to ionizing radiations, *J. Nutr.*, 63, 201—209, 1957.

# EFFECT OF PROCESSING ON NUTRITIVE VALUE OF FOOD: MILK AND MILK PRODUCTS

## B. A. Rolls

## INTRODUCTION

Since earliest historical times, the milk of domesticated herbivores has formed an important part of the diet of many peoples. The cow, buffalo, goat, sheep, mare, ass, camel, yak, llama, and reindeer have been domesticated for this purpose, but this section will deal mainly with cow's milk, partly because of its wider distribution and economic importance, (milk production in 1976, in million metric tons: cow, 394.4; buffalo, 23.8; goat, 6.9; sheep, 7.5;)[1] and partly because insufficient work has been carried out on the milks of other species to present figures with confidence. This is not to dismiss the important contribution to human nutrition made by, e.g., the sheep in Europe or the buffalo in Egypt and India. However, it is reasonable to assume that particular treatments will sequester or destroy equivalent proportions of the labile nutrients in the milk of other milch animals as are removed by the treatment of cow's milk.

Remember that, even within a single species, milk is not a uniform product. It is well-known that the milks of the Friesian and Guernsey cows differ markedly in fat and carotene content and that these are also subject to seasonal variation, as are any products made from the milks.[2-4] Moreover, the composition of milk from normal healthy animals will vary with age, nutrition, stage of yield, and simple individual variation, a factor that tends to be obscured in those countries with advanced dairying industries, where milk is bulked in central dairies. Variations between and within breeds of other milk-yielding species is probably at least as great.

Milk is the most complete single food, although in fact, most milks contain insufficient iron and vitamin D for the needs of the young. Unfortunately, once the natural immediate transfer from teat to young is interrupted, the composition of milk makes it an ideal medium for the growth of microorganisms, including pathogens, that may be originally present or introduced during handling. To produce a safe product liquid milk may be treated to control bacterial contamination, to destroy pathogens, and eliminate certain enzymes that would produce off-flavors, after which the milk is packaged to prevent subsequent contamination. The action of microorganisms harmless to man may also be used to make such products as cheese and yogurt, in which the growth of pathogenic organisms is inhibited. Since microorganisms will not proliferate in the absence of water, dried milks remain safe for long periods provided that moisture is rigorously excluded. Processing may affect the nutrients originally present in raw milk in two ways: certain nutrients may be labile to the treatment used to ensure bacteriological safety, and when the process involves a partition, the nutrients are almost certain to be unequally distributed.

This section deals only with nutrient losses resulting from processing. Prolonged storage, particularly under adverse conditions, may lead to losses as great as or greater than those given here.[5]

## LIQUID AND DRIED MILKS

### Common Treatments for Liquid Milk

In general, it can be said that conservative heat treatments used to produce liquid and dried milks do not affect the fat, fat-soluble vitamins, carbohydrates, and minerals of raw milk. Interest has therefore centered on the protein and water-soluble vitamin content. Tables 1 and 2 outline the common treatments used for liquid milk and their effects.

## Other Treatments of Liquid Milk

**Preservative addition** — It is generally regarded as undesirable, and local legislation may forbid the practice. However, nisin or hydrogen peroxide addition may be acceptable where milk cannot be effectively cooled or transported rapidly for processing. Nutrient losses are thought to be minimal, except for vitamin C.

**Irradiation** — X-Rays or ultraviolet light have been used to reduce microbial contamination. In general, the use of ionizing radiation results in nutrient losses similar to those in pasteurization[6,7] although, depending on the dose, somewhat more riboflavin and vitamin A may be lost.[8,9] The organoleptic qualities are often damaged[6] by this process. Ultraviolet light may enhance vitamin D contents,[10] although there are losses of riboflavin and vitamin C.

**Ultrafiltration and reverse osmosis** — These methods have attracted attention recently as concentrative processes that do not utilize heat. The two processes differ in the effective pore size of the membranes employed, that for reverse osmosis being smaller. Fat and protein are well-retained, and with reverse osmosis there are few vitamin losses. However, ultrafiltration retains only those vitamins that are firmly protein-bound, e.g., vitamin $B_{12}$ and folic acid.[11] This is shown in Table 3.

## Treatment of Human Milk

Breast-fed infants are generally considered less susceptible to infectious disease and to sudden infant death syndrome (cot death, crib death) than their bottle-fed counterparts.[12-14] Thus, not only does human milk have a superior balance of nutrients, but its content of immune antibodies and nonspecific antimicrobial factors confers additional advantages on the infant. For these reasons many hospitals are establishing human milk banks so that milk from donor mothers may be used to nourish small, weak, or premature infants or those whose mothers are temporarily unable to nurse them.

Provided that collections are made under hygienic conditions and the milk is immediately cooled, the bacterial count may be sufficiently low to permit its use raw, with all the desired factors preserved. In practice, the bulked milk is usually pasteurized by the holder process (62.5°, 30 min), although a small-scale laboratory high-temperature, short-time (HTST) process has been used in some tests. Nutrient losses may be estimated by analogy from Table 2. The whey proteins of human milk may be less susceptible to heat damage than those of cow's milk.[15] Recent work[12] has shown that this treatment reduces the immunoglobulin A (IgA) by 20%, destroys the immunoglobulin M (IgM) and lactoferrin, but has less effect on the lysozyme and folic acid and vitamin $B_{12}$ binding capacities. Except for vitamin $B_{12}$ binder, destruction was increased by higher treatment temperatures. So, the practice of boiling the milk is to be deplored both on nutritional (see Table 2) and immunological grounds. Indeed, the minimum treatment to ensure bacteriological safety should be employed. For longer-term preservation, freeze-drying following pasteurization, has been used, although this is too expensive to be used in commercial dairying. Little nutrient loss is reported, except that the reconstituted milk contains little vitamin C, a lack easily remedied.

## CREAM, BUTTER, CHEESE, AND YOGURT

Cream is milk in which the fat content has been increased by skimming or centrifugation. It is essentially a mixture of milk fat and skim milk in proportions that vary

## Table 1
## COMMON TREATMENTS FOR LIQUID MILK

| Product | Pretreatment | Treatment | Temperature (°C) | Period | Containers | Keeping qualities |
|---|---|---|---|---|---|---|
| Skim | — | Mechanical removal of fat[a] | — | — | — | As raw milk |
| Homogenized | — | Forced through small tube at high pressure | 60 | <1 sec | — | Inferior to raw milk[b] |
| **Pasteurized** | | | | | | |
| Holder process[c] | — | Heated in batches in SS tank by steam/hot water | 61—66 | 30 min | Bottles, cartons, plastic bags, etc. | Several days if kept cool |
| HTST process | — | Continuous flow: heat exchange, hot water | 71—73[d] | 15 sec | | |
| **Sterilized** | | | | | | |
| **In bottle** | | | | | | |
| Raw milk[e] | — | Heated in batches, in containers | 110—120 | 20—40 min | Sealed bottles | Several months at room temperature |
| UHT milk | UHT | | 110—112 | 15—20min | | |
| UHT process | Homogenized | Indirect: heat exchanger  Direct: steam injection, evaporation at reduced pressure[f] | 130—150 | 1—4 sec | A1-lined plastic-coated cartons[g] | |
| Evaporated[h] | Heated to 95° for 10 min, evaporated at 50°, reduced pressure | Heated in batches in steam autoclave | 115 | 15 min | Cans | >1 Year at room temperature |
| Condensed[h] | None, or UHT | Heated, then evaporated at reduced pressure | 80 | 15 min | Cans | >1 Year at room temperature |
| Roller-dried[h] | Evaporated at reduced pressure, homogenized | Spread on rollers heated by steam[i]  Spread on steam-heated rollers at reduced pressure | 150  40 | 1—5 sec  1—5 sec | Airtight bags, perhaps under nitrogen | >1 Year if cool and dry[j] |

## Table 1 (continued)
## COMMON TREATMENTS FOR LIQUID MILK

| Product | Pretreatment | Treatment | Temperature (°C) | Period | Containers | Keeping qualities |
|---|---|---|---|---|---|---|
| Spray-dried[h] | Heated at 80—90° for 10—15 sec, homogenized, evaporated at reduced pressure | Sprayed as fine mist into hot air | 90 | 4—6 sec | Airtight bags, perhaps under nitrogen | >1 Year if cool and dry[i] |

*Note:* HTST: high-temperature, short-time; UHT: ultra high temperature.

[a]   Milk may be partially or wholly skimmed. Normally about 0.1% fat is left.
[b]   Homogenization breaks up fat globules and renders them susceptible to attack by lipase.
[c]   Now obsolescent.
[d]   Higher temperatures may be used in countries where the presence of thermoduric pathogens is suspected.
[e]   Marked "cooked" flavor. Not necessarily undesirable for certain purposes.
[f]   The addition of water from condensed steam may be controlled by local legislation.
[g]   This is the preferred type of container. Some manufacturers, however, omit the aluminum lining and fill the milk into oxygen-permeable containers, to the detriment of the keeping qualities of the milk.
[h]   Either whole or skim milk may be so treated.
[i]   Skim milk powder will keep for several years.

Table 2
COMPOSITION OF RAW AND TREATED WHOLE AND SKIM MILKS,
CONCENTRATED AND DRIED MILKS, WITH NUTRIENT LOSSES DUE TO
PROCESSING

| Product | Water (g) | Protein (g) | Fat (g) | Carbohydrate (g) | Energy (kJ) | Vitamin A[a,b] ($\mu$g) | Vitamin A[a,b] Loss (%) | Vitamin D[b] ($\mu$g) | Vitamin D[b] Loss (%) |
|---|---|---|---|---|---|---|---|---|---|
| **Whole milk** | | | | | | | | | |
| Raw[d] | 87.6 | 3.3 | 3.8 | 4.8 | 274 | 34 | — | 0.022 | — |
| Pasteurized[f] | 87.6 | 3.3 | 3.8 | 4.8 | 274 | 34 | 0 | 0.022 | 0 |
| Sterilized | | | | | | | | | |
| 1. In bottle | | | | | | | | | |
| (a) Raw | 87.6 | 3.3 | 3.8 | 4.8 | 274 | 34 | 0 | 0.022 | 0 |
| (b) UHT | 87.6 | 3.3 | 3.8 | 4.8 | 274 | 34 | 0 | 0.022 | 0 |
| 2. UHT | 87.6 | 3.3 | 3.8 | 4.8 | 274 | 34 | 0 | 0.022 | 0 |
| Boiled[j] | 87.6 | 2.7 | 3.0 | 4.8 | 234 | 27 | 20 | 0.017 | 20 |
| Evaporated | 68.6 | 8.4 | 9.2 | 12.0 | 705 | 90 | 0 | 0.1[k] | 0 |
| Sweetened condensed[l] | 25.8 | 8.4 | 9.2 | 55.4 | 1410 | 90 | 0 | 0.1 | 0 |
| Roller-dried[m] | 3.0[n] | 25.0 | 27.5 | 37.5 | 2100 | 290[k] | 0 | 0.15[k] | 0 |
| Spray-dried | 3.0[n] | 25.0 | 27.5 | 37.5 | 2100 | 290[k] | 0 | 0.15[k] | 0 |
| **Skim milk[o]** | | | | | | | | | |
| Raw | 90.9 | 3.4 | 0.1 | 5.0 | 142 | 1 | 98 | 0 | 100 |
| Evaporated | 80.0 | 7.4 | 0.2 | 10.7 | 310 | 2 | 0 | 0 | — |
| Sweetened condensed[l] | 29.0 | 9.6 | 0.3 | 58.8 | 1150 | 3 | 0 | 0 | — |
| Dried[p] | 3.0[n] | 36.0 | 1.0 | 50.5 | 1500 | 10 | 0 | 0 | — |

| Product | Thiamin ($\mu$g) | Thiamin Loss (%) | Riboflavin ($\mu$g) | Riboflavin Loss (%) | Nicotinic acid ($\mu$g) | Nicotinic acid Loss (%) | Vitamin B$_6$ ($\mu$g) | Vitamin B$_6$ Loss (%) | Vitamin B$_{12}$ ($\mu$g) | Vitamin B$_{12}$ Loss (%) |
|---|---|---|---|---|---|---|---|---|---|---|
| **Whole milk** | | | | | | | | | | |
| Raw[d] | 45 | — | 180[r] | — | 80 | — | 40 | — | 0.30 | — |
| Pasteurized[f] | 42 | 10 | 180[r] | 0 | 80 | 0 | 40 | 0 | 0.27 | 10[s] |
| Sterilized | | | | | | | | | | |
| 1. In bottle | | | | | | | | | | |
| (a) Raw | 30 | 35 | 180[r] | 0 | 80 | 0 | 20 | 50 | 0.03 | 90 |
| (b) UHT | 36 | 20 | 180[r] | 0 | 80 | 0 | 32 | 20 | 0.24 | 20 |
| 2. UHT | 42 | 10 | 180[r] | 0 | 80 | 0 | 36[i] | 10 | 0.27[i] | 10 |
| Boiled[j] | 32 | 30 | 162[r] | 10 | 80 | 0 | 36 | 10 | 0.15 | 50 |
| Evaporated | 65 | 40 | 450 | 0 | 250 | 5 | 40 | 40 | 0.01 | 80 |
| Sweetened condensed[l] | 100 | 10 | 450 | 0 | 250 | 0 | 40 | 10 | 0.50 | 30 |
| Roller-dried[m] | 280 | 15 | 1200 | 0 | 700 | 0 | 210 | 0 | 2.0 | 30 |
| Spray-dried | 310 | 10 | 1200 | 0 | 700 | 0 | 210 | 0 | 2.0 | 30 |
| **Skim milk[o]** | | | | | | | | | | |
| Raw | 47 | 0 | 175[r] | 2—3 | 82 | 0 | 42 | 0 | 30 | 0 |
| Evaporated | 65 | 40 | 400 | 0 | 250 | 5 | 40 | 40 | 0.01 | 80 |
| Sweetened condensed[l] | 110 | 10 | 500 | 0 | 260 | 0 | 45 | 10 | 0.50 | 30 |
| Dried[p] | 450 | 10 | 1600 | 0 | 1200 | 0 | 260 | 0 | 3.0 | 30 |

## Table 2 (continued)
## COMPOSITION OF RAW AND TREATED WHOLE AND SKIM MILKS, CONCENTRATED AND DRIED MILKS, WITH NUTRIENT LOSSES DUE TO PROCESSING

| Product | Vitamin C (mg) | Loss (%) | Folic acid[c] (μg) | Loss (%) | Pantothenic acid (μg) | Loss (%) | Biotin (μg) | Loss (%) |
|---|---|---|---|---|---|---|---|---|
| **Whole milk** | | | | | | | | |
| Raw[d] | 2.0[e] | — | 5.5 | — | 350 | — | 2.0 | — |
| Pasteurized[f] | 1.5—1.8[e,h] | 10—25 | 5.0 | 10 | 350 | 0 | 2.0 | 0 |
| Sterilized | | | | | | | | |
| 1. In bottle | | | | | | | | |
| (a) Raw | 0.2[e] | 90 | 2.8 | 50 | 350 | 0 | 2.0 | 0 |
| (b) UHT | 0.8[e] | 60 | 3.9 | 30 | 350 | 0 | 2.0 | 0 |
| 2. UHT | 1.5[i] | 25 | 5.0[i] | 10 | 350 | 0 | 2.0 | 0 |
| Boiled[j] | 0.6—1.4 | 30—70 | 4.4 | 20 | 350 | 0 | 2.0 | 0 |
| Evaporated | 1.5 | 60 | 8.0 | 25 | 850 | 0 | 3.0 | 10 |
| Sweetened condensed[l] | 2.5 | 25 | 10.0 | 25 | 850 | 0 | 3.0 | 10 |
| Roller-dried[m] | 10[k] | 30 | 40 | 10 | 2700 | 0 | 10.0 | 10 |
| Spray-dried | 12[k] | 15 | 40 | 10 | 2700 | 0 | 10.0 | 10 |
| **Skim milk[o]** | | | | | | | | |
| Raw | 2.0 | 0 | 5.5 | 0 | 360 | 0 | 2.0 | 0 |
| Evaporated | 1.5 | 60 | 8.0 | 25 | 750 | 0 | 3.0 | 10 |
| Sweetened condensed[l] | 3.0 | 25 | 10.0 | 25 | 1000 | 0 | 3.5 | 10 |
| Dried[p] | 6—18[q] | 15—70 | 20—60[q] | 15—70 | 3600 | 0 | 15.0 | 10 |

*Note:* The content of each nutrient is in 100 g product. Loss is the percentage loss of that nutrient during processing. The figures given are typical values and individual products may vary markedly due to variations in conditions of manufacture.

[a]   Vitamin A activity is made up of retinol and carotene, a precursor, in proportions dependent on the season. Carotene has an activity about 1/6 of that of the same weight of retinol.

[b]   There is considerable seasonal variation. In summer, concentrations are much higher. These are notional "average" figures. In raw milk mean vitamin A may be 27—41, mean vitamin D, 0.012—0.030, and products will vary accordingly.

[c]   Total folic acid, free and bound.

[d]   These figures are for whole, fresh milk from Friesians. Milk from other breeds may differ, e.g., that of Guernseys has higher fat, vitamins A and D, and energy. Percentage losses may be taken to be the same for other breeds' milks. Poor initial storage conditions may exacerbate treatment losses.

[e]   The action of sunlight, diffuse daylight, or fluorescent light destroys riboflavin and vitamin C. Samples stored unprotected will have lower concentrations. Vitamins A and $B_6$ are affected, only much more slowly.

[f]   Homogenization does not affect the nutrients in milk significantly, thus, pasteurized homogenized milk has the contents listed here.

[g]   Vitamin $B_{12}$ is stable to heat. Losses are caused by products of vitamin C destruction.

[h]   Vitamin C (ascorbic acid) is stable to heat, but the action of dissolved oxygen leads to the formation of the heat-labile dehydroascorbic acid. The action continues and after 24 hr pasteurized milk will contain only about 0.5 mg.

[i]   After 60 days storage UHT milk loses 40% of its vitamin $B_6$ and 25—60% of its vitamin $B_{12}$. Losses of vitamin C and folic acid may be total, but these can be reduced by using the direct process, (Table 1) which eliminates dissolved oxygen, but results in a more "cooked" flavor.

[j]   Losses may be minimized by rapid heating and stirring. There is also a loss of about 18% of the calcium.

[k]   These figures are for unfortified products. Milks intended for, or that may be used for, infant feeding are commonly fortified.

## Table 2 (continued)

*l*   Nutrient losses in the preparation of sweetened condensed milks are less than for evaporated milks, as bacteriological safety is partly assured by the high sucrose content.

*m*   A good quality roller-dried milk. Nutrient losses in milks where the conditions are less well controlled may well be much higher — such milks are often intended for animal feeds.

*n*   The water content of dried milks may be much higher, particularly if storage conditions are poor. In this event deterioration may be rapid.

*o*   In the lower half of the table the losses listed for raw skim milk are those resulting from partition of nutrients during separation. The other losses in this section are for nutrient loss from raw skim milk during processing.

*p*   "Instant" milks are spray-dried (usually skim) products that have been moistened and redried to promote rapid solution. No significant nutrient loss should result.

*q*   There is considerable variation, depending on conditions of manufacture.

with the conditions of separation, and its nutrient content varies correspondingly. Thus, a good estimate of the nutrient content of any cream may be calculated from a knowledge of the composition of the original milk and the fat and skim milk content. Four commonly available varieties are given in Table 4. Cream is usually pasteurized by the high-temperature, short-time (HTST) process or sterilized. Percentage nutrient losses are similar to those in pasteurization or sterilization of milk.

Butter was first churned from milk, but is now churned from cream of about 34% fat. The butter grains are strained from the buttermilk and kneaded into a compact mass. The cream may be fresh or soured ("ripened") by bacteria, and it is generally pasteurized at 95° before churning. There is little nutrient loss in processing: the food value of butter consists largely of fat and the fat-soluble vitamins that are stable to moderate heat. The removal of further water to produce ghee or butterfat gives products whose fat contents reflect their vitamin A and D concentrations. Butter stored at −20 to −30° will keep for a year or more.

Cheese is both historically and quantitatively one of the most important ways of preserving some of the nutrients of milk. Most cheese, like most milk, is from cows, but every available milk is used, and the nutrient content of these cheeses may be assessed by analogy. Something between 400 and 1000 varieties are made throughout the world, but these may be grouped into less than 20 types, and in a brief summary it is not misleading to refer to hard, semihard, soft, and blue-vein cheeses. All may be made with whole, partly-skimmed, or skim milk with corresponding variation in nutrient content.[16,17]

Milk is clotted by rennet or a substitute, and the liquid (whey) is drained off. A typical partition of nutrients is shown in Table 5. It can be seen that cheese preserves nearly all the fat and fat-soluble vitamins, 75% of the protein, some water-soluble vitamins — particularly those associated with protein like riboflavin and thiamin — and also much of the calcium of the original milk. Naturally cottage cheese, made from skim milk, contains little fat or fat-soluble vitamins, and cream cheese, made from cream, contains little or no protein, although the cream cheeses made with cream-milk mixtures will have higher protein levels.

True cheeses are ripened by the action of bacteria or molds. During ripening residual vitamin C is destroyed, but some bacterial cultures synthesize several of the B vitamins, although these are mainly in the outer layers, which are not always eaten.[18,19] In addition, cottage cheese, cream cheese, and whey cheese are made. These are not ripened. Processed cheeses and cheese spreads are made, usually from cheese of inferior quality, with or without additional fat or skim milk and flavoring, and the whole is heated to about 80° and poured into suitable containers (tinfoil or plastic). Their good keeping quality is due to this heat treatment, which probably only marginally affects the nutrient content of the constituents.

Raw milk, HTST-pasteurized or warmed milk (at 65° for a few seconds) may be

## Table 3
## PERCENTAGE LOSS OF NUTRIENTS DURING THE TWOFOLD CONCENTRATION OF WHOLE MILK BY ULTRAFILTRATION AND REVERSE OSMOSIS

| | Protein | Fat | Carbohydrate | Energy | Thiamin | Riboflavin | Nicotinic acid | Vitamin B$_6$ | Vitamin B$_{12}$ | Vitamin C | Folic acid | Pantothenic acid | Biotin |
|---|---|---|---|---|---|---|---|---|---|---|---|---|---|
| Ultra filtration | 5 | 0 | 43 | 13 | 38 | 39 | 41 | 36 | 2 | 87 | 5 | 32 | 37 |
| Reverse osmosis | 0 | 0 | 0 | 0 | 0 | 0 | 8 | 3 | 0 | — | 0 | 0 | 0 |

From Glover, F. A., *J. Dairy Res.*, 38, 373, 1971. With permission.

## Table 4
## TREATMENT OF CREAM

| Product | Pretreatment | Treatment | Temperature °C | Period | Containers | Keeping qualities |
|---|---|---|---|---|---|---|
| Single cream | Homogenization, or none | Pasteurization, HTST | 82—88 | 10 sec | Cartons | Over a week if cool |
| Double cream | None[a] | Pasteurization, HTST | 82—88 | 10 sec | Cartons | Over a week if cool |
| Clotted cream | Stood overnight to separate cream | Scalding milk and cream, skim | 82 | about 1 hr | Cartons | Over a week if cool |
| Sterilized cream | Homogenization | Heating in containers | 115 | 20—30 min | Cans, bottles | Several months |

[a] Homogenization destroys the whipping properties of cream.

**Table 5**
**PARTITION OF NUTRIENTS BETWEEN CURD AND WHEY DURING THE INITIAL STAGES OF CHEESEMAKING WITH WHOLE MILK**

| Fraction | Water[a] | Protein | Casein | Soluble proteins | Fat | Carbohydrate | Energy | Vitamin A | Thiamin | Riboflavin | Vitamin $B_{12}$ | Vitamin C | Folic acid | Calcium |
|---|---|---|---|---|---|---|---|---|---|---|---|---|---|---|
| Curd | 6 | 75 | 96 | 4 | 94 | 6 | 65 | 94 | 15 | 26 | 25 | 6 | 5 | 62 |
| Whey | 94 | 25 | 4 | 96 | 6 | 94 | 35 | 6 | 85 | 74 | 75 | 84 | 95 | 38 |

[a] Figures are percentages of total in the milk.
[b] Vitamin C recovery is less than 100% as some is destroyed by light. There are also variable riboflavin losses due to light. Destruction is greater in whey.

From Kon, S. K., *Milk and Milk Products in Human Nutrition*, 2nd ed., Nutrition Studies No. 27, Food and Agricultural Organization, Rome, 1972. With permission.

used in cheese manufacture. Nutrient losses during this pretreatment are slight. The consumption of true cheeses from raw milk presents no hazard as no pathogen survives the 4 to 6 month ripening period.

Typical values for most of these cheeses and cheese products are given in Table 6.

Yogurt is one of the varieties of sour and fermented milks made in many parts of the world. In Europe and North America they are generally made from fresh milk, in Asia from boiled milk (Nutrient losses may be estimated from Table 2). Streptococci, lactobacilli, and yeasts are used to produce foods such as yogurt, laban, dahi (the traditional sour milk of the Balkans and Near East), and kefir and kumiss (which contain appreciable amounts of alcohol). Cultured buttermilks and yogurts are made using specific bacterial strains, usually from skim or partly-skimmed milk, or concentrated milks that have been pasteurized. These are important products in countries with advanced dairying industries. Fruit or fruit juices, and sometimes sugar, are added to some yogurts.

There is a common belief that the bacterial cultures present confer advantages on these foods beyond their content of milk nutrients, and that their consumption promotes health and longevity. There is no firm evidence for this; however, the methods of preparation are mild, and the nutrient content of these soured milks may be taken to be essentially that of the raw material. Some lactose is destroyed, reducing the energy content by 3 to 4% but some bacteria used synthesize certain vitamins, particularly riboflavin and thiamin. Typical values for cultured yogurts, now important commercially, are given in Table 6.

## OTHER MILK PRODUCTS

Milk, milk products, and milk fractions are incorporated into a wide variety of foods. Here it is possible to mention only some of the more important items in which milk or milk products are a major ingredient.

Whey from cheesemaking contains many valuable nutrients.[20,21] Some are used, particularly in Europe, for the preparation of whey cheeses (e.g., sérac, skuta, mysost) and fermented drinks, and is consumed as such. Dried whey is used extensively in the food industry, especially in baking and the preparation of sauces, soups, and whips. The fat is extracted by centrifugation to make whey butter. Whey is an important source of lactose.

Even in the manufacture of spray-dried whey for human foods there are lysine losses due to the Maillard reaction,[22] and the proteins are denatured, destroying the functional properties that make it such an attractive food ingredient. Recently, reverse osmosis has been used to prepare concentrated undenatured whey.[23] Regrettably, its high water content makes whey an expensive product to dry, and much is used for animal feed (particularly for pigs) or wasted, although even its disposal presents a problem.

Ice cream is a term applied loosely to a wide variety of products, some of which contain little or no milk, and have only the frozen state in common. Strictly, ice cream is a milk product made from cream, milk, sugar, and flavorings. Commercially, the constituents vary widely, and may include whole milk, skim milk, or water; cream, butter, butterfat, or vegetable fat; milk powder or condensed milk; sucrose or glucose and cornflour; apart from emulsifiers, stabilizers, flavorings, and colorings.[24] Composition and descriptive terms may be closely controlled by local legislation.

Due to this wide variation, no summary is possible. Estimates of the nutrient content of any particular product can be made from a knowledge of the composition and the known effects of treatment. The ingredients are dispersed, pasteurized, or UHT-sterilized (at temperatures slightly higher than those used for milk), homogenized, cooled, and frozen. Fat may vary from 8 to 20%, milk solids from 5 to 12%, protein is usually

## Table 6
## COMPOSITION OF CREAMS, BUTTER, CHEESES, AND YOGURT

| Product | Water (g) | Protein (g) | Fat (g) | Carbohydrate (g) | Energy (kJ) | Vitamin A[a,b] (µg) | Vitamin D[b] (µg) | Thiamin (µg) | Riboflavin (µg) |
|---|---|---|---|---|---|---|---|---|---|
| **Cream** | | | | | | | | | |
| Single[d] | 74 | 2.4 | 18 | 3.2 | 790 | 170[e] | 0.123 | 30 | 120 |
| Double | 48 | 1.5 | 48 | 2.0 | 1850 | 430[e] | 0.280 | 20 | 80 |
| Clotted | 30 | 1.3 | 63 | 2.0 | 2450 | 560 | 0.370 | 10 | 50 |
| Canned sterilized | 70 | 2.6 | 23 | 2.7 | 950 | 205 | 0.135 | 10 | 100 |
| Butter, salted[f] | 15.4[g] | 0.4 | 82[g] | 0 | 3040 | 730[e,h] | 0.50 | 0 | 0 |
| **Cheese** | | | | | | | | | |
| Hard cheese, e.g., Cheddar, Emmental[i] | 35 | 26 | 33 | 0 | 1670[i] | 380 | 0.26 | 50[i] | 500[j] |
| Semihard cheese, e.g., Edam, Gouda[i] | 43 | 26 | 24 | 0 | 1330 | 250 | 0.18 | 60 | 350 |
| Soft ripe cheese, e.g., Camembert, Brie | 51 | 19 | 23 | 0 | 1180 | 240 | 0.18 | 50 | 450 |
| Blue vein cheese, e.g., Danish Blue | 40 | 21 | 31 | 0 | 1500 | 300 | 0.23 | 30 | 700 |
| Cream cheese, from double cream | 18 | 3.1 | 72 | 0 | 2700 | 730 | 0.45 | 20 | 140 |
| Processed cheese | 44 | 21 | 25 | 0 | 1290 | 240 | 0.15 | 20 | 290 |
| Cheese spread | 51 | 18 | 23 | 1 | 1170 | 180 | 0.13 | 20 | 240 |
| Cottage cheese[m] | 79 | 17 | 0.4[m] | 1.5 | 340[m] | 3[m] | 0.001[m] | 30 | 280 |
| **Yogurt** | | | | | | | | | |
| Reduced fat, plain | 86 | 5.0 | 1.0 | 6.4 | 225 | 8[n] | 0[n] | 50 | 260 |
| Reduced fat, fruit | 75 | 4.8 | 1.0 | 18.1 | 410 | 8[n] | 0[n] | 50 | 230 |

## Table 6 (continued)
## COMPOSITION OF CREAMS, BUTTER, CHEESES, AND YOGURT

| Product | Nicotinic Acid (µg) | Vitamin B$_6$ (µg) | Vitamin B$_{12}$ (µg) | Vitamin C (mg) | Folic[c] acid (µg) | Pantothenic acid (µg) | Biotin (µg) | Calcium (mg) |
|---|---|---|---|---|---|---|---|---|
| **Cream** | | | | | | | | |
| Single [a] | 70 | 30 | 0.2 | 1.2 | 4 | 300 | 1.4 | 79 |
| Double | 40 | 20 | 0.1 | 0.8 | 2 | 190 | 0.8 | 50 |
| Clotted | 30 | 10 | 0.1 | 0.5 | 1 | 100 | 0.5 | 80 |
| Canned sterilized | 60 | 10 | 0 | 0 | 0 | 280 | 1.3 | 80 |
| Butter, salted [f] | 0 | 0 | 0 | 0 | 0 | 0 | 0 | 15 |
| **Cheese** | | | | | | | | |
| Hard cheese, e.g., Cheddar, Emmental [i] | 100 [j] | 80 [j] | 1.5 [j] | 0 | 20 [k] | 300 [k] | 1.7 [k] | 800 |
| Semihard cheese, e.g., Edam, Gouda [l] | 60 | 80 | 1.4 | 0 | 20 | 300 | 1.5 | 740 |
| Soft ripe cheese, e.g., Camembert, Brie | 800 | 200 | 1.2 | 0 | 60 | 1400 | 6.0 | 380 |
| Blue vein cheese, e.g., Danish Blue | 900 | 150 | 1.2 | 0 | 50 | 2000 | 1.5 | 580 |
| Cream cheese, from double cream | 80 | 10 | 0.3 | 0 | 5 | — | — | 98 |
| Processed cheese | 80 | 10 | 0.3 | 0 | 2 | — | — | 700 |
| Cheese spread | 70 | 10 | 0.3 | 0 | 2 | — | — | 510 |
| Cottage cheese [m] | 80 | 10 | 0.5 | 0 | 9 | — | — | 60 |
| **Yogurt** | | | | | | | | |
| Reduced fat, plain | 120 | 40 | 0 | 0.4 | 2 | — | — | 180 |
| Reduced fat, fruit | 110 | 40 | 0 | 1.8 | 3 | — | — | 160 |

*Note:*  The content of each nutrient is in 100 g product. The figures given are typical and individual products may vary markedly.

<sup>a</sup> Vitamin A activity is made up of retinol and carotene, a precursor, in proportion dependent on the season. Carotene has an activity about 1/6 of that of the same weight of retinol.

<sup>b</sup> There is considerable seasonal variation. In summer, concentrations are much higher. These are notional "average" figures. See note <sup>b</sup>, Table 2.

<sup>c</sup> Total folic acid, free and bound.

<sup>d</sup> Single cream is sometimes homogenized. This does not affect its nutrient content significantly.

<sup>e</sup> Seasonal variations are approximately: single cream 155—220; double cream 350—500; butter 570—1080.

<sup>f</sup> Butter is also made unsalted. Nutrient levels are little different, but keeping qualities are inferior.

<sup>g</sup> Limits to these values may be set by local legislation.

<sup>h</sup> Vitamin A is destroyed by light; thus butter wrapped in parchment, rather than foil, and exposed to light may have lower concentrations.

<sup>i</sup> These are representative values. Thus, Gouda from whole milk will have a higher energy value than Edam from partly-skimmed milk.

<sup>j</sup> Concentrations may be much higher in the outer layers of ripened cheeses.

<sup>k</sup> Considerable variations may be found.

<sup>l</sup> Hard and semihard cheese have higher calcium contents than other cheeses.

<sup>m</sup> Cottage cheese prepared from skim milk. Frequently cottage cheese is made from a mixture of skim milk and cream, and local legislation may set a minimum level for fat. A typical commercial product would contain (per 100 g) fat, 4.0 g; energy 400 kJ; vitamin A, 36 μg; vitamin D, 0.023 μg.

<sup>n</sup> Values for unfortified products. Commercial yogurts are often fortified.

Table 7
## TYPICAL PERCENTAGE COMPOSITIONS OF THE AUSTRALIAN AND NEW ZEALAND MILK BISCUITS

|  | Australian | New Zealand |
|---|---|---|
| Protein (Casein, whey proteins) | 20 | 24 |
| Fat (milk fat) | 20 | 25 |
| Total carbohydrate | 50 | 42 |
| Lactose | 0 | 30 |
| Vitamins and minerals | 7 | 6 |
| Water | 3 | 3 |

about 4%, and levels of water-soluble vitamins are low. High quality ice cream is a readily digested and attractive source of energy and the fat-soluble vitamins, but when vegetable fat that is unfortified with vitamins A and D is used, the product, although a pleasant confection, contributes little other than energy to the diet.

Coprecipitates are made by acidifying, or adding calcium chloride to, heated milk or mixtures of cheese whey and skim milk. They conserve practically all the proteins of milk, both casein and whey, together with the calcium and phosphorus associated with the casein. They have good functional properties as food ingredients and high nutritional value.[25] They are used extensively in a milk biscuit developed in Australia. A biscuit developed in New Zealand is made from dried milk and dried whey. It has a substantial lactose content (see Table 7).[26-28] Trials suggest that the Australian biscuit is more acceptable, both in taste and in avoiding the problem of lactose intolerance, that is common in Africa and Asia.[29-32] The biological value of the original milk proteins is well-preserved (see Table 8).[33-35]

Future developments in milk products are likely to include the development of concentrated foods to reduce the large volumes of water currently transported, and the increasing use of individual milk fractions as raw materials.[36]

## CHANGES IN THE NUTRITIVE VALUE OF MILK PROTEINS

The proteins of raw milk are readily digestible and of high biological value. The whey proteins are superior to casein, as the latter has a slight deficiency of the sulfur amino acids (methionine and cystine).[37] This explains both the difference in the biological value of human and cow's milk, and the rather lower nutritive value of cheese proteins.[38]

The more conservative treatments affect the nutritive value of milk proteins relatively little, but the more severe procedures, such as in-bottle sterilization and the older drying processes, result in a lowering of the biological value.[39] Some values are listed in Table 8. Processes such as membrane concentration, efficient spray-drying, freeze-drying, coprecipitation, gel-formation, souring, and preservative addition, may be assumed to leave the protein essentially unaltered. However, the high levels of hydrogen peroxide added in some countries may result in losses of the sulfur amino acids.

Milk proteins may be affected in two ways. Firstly, whey proteins (particularly β-lactoglobulin) are denatured to some degree by any heating (in pasteurization, 10%; in UHT, 40 to 60%; in in-bottle sterilization, 100%. This does not affect biological value as measured with rats or human infants,[40] but calves and, to a lesser degree, pigs are adversely affected.[41-43] Secondly, the availability of amino acids, particularly of sulfur amino acids, may be reduced by protein-protein interactions. The availability of lysine may be reduced by protein-carbohydrate interactions, involving the formation

Table 8

BIOLOGICAL VALUE (B.V.) OF
THE PROTEINS OF MILK AND
MILK PRODUCTS

| Product | b.v. |
|---|---|
| Whey proteins | 1.00 |
| Casein | 0.80 |
| Human milk (whey casein, 1:1) | 1.00 |
| Cow's milk (whey casein, 1:4) | |
| Raw | 0.90 |
| Pasteurized | 0.91 |
| UHT | 0.91 |
| Spray-dried[a] | 0.90 |
| Roller-dried[a] | 0.89 |
| Condensed | 0.89 |
| Evaporated | 0.88 |
| Sterilized | 0.84 |
| Cheese proteins | 0.76 |
| Milk biscuits (Australian) | 0.88—0.91 |

*Note:* Values are taken from assays with rats,
but may be taken as applying to
human nutrition. Estimates are based
on the assumption that whole egg
protein has a b.v. of 1.00.

[a] Values for a good quality product. Inferior
samples may have lower values.

Table 9

AVAILABLE LYSINE (AS A
PERCENTAGE OF TOTAL
LYSINE) IN THE PROTEINS
OF RAW AND TREATED
MILKS

| Product | Lysine availability (%) |
|---|---|
| Raw | 95—99 |
| Evaporated | 88 |
| Spray-dried | 90—98[a] |
| Roller-dried | 60—95[a,b] |

[a] Values vary with the efficiency of the
process.
[b] There may also be a reduction of methionine availability of up to 10%.

of a Schiff base by the Maillard reaction.[44] The loss of lysine activity is the more extensive.

As the biological value of milk proteins is limited by its sulfur-amino acid content, loss of methionine or cystine is more important if milk is to be used as a sole food.[45] As milk contains an abundance of lysine, a reduction of its availability might seem less important. However, its great value in human nutrition is in complementing cereal and other vegetable proteins that tend to be deficient in lysine, so this is the more serious factor in mixed diets.[46] Some idea of this effect is given in Table 9.

## MINERAL CONTENT OF MILK AND MILK PRODUCTS

Most of the minerals required by the body are distributed widely in foods, but good sources of iron and calcium are fewer. Milk and milk products are poor sources of iron, but they are an important source of calcium — raw milk containing 100 to 150 mg/100 g. As said in the section on liquid and dry milks, the treatments outlined in Tables 1 and 2 and preservative addition and irradiation do not affect mineral compositions, so these products remain excellent calcium sources. Membrane filtration, however, can be expected to result in mineral loss, although reliable figures are not available.

Cheese is usually a good source of calcium, since much of the element is retained in the curd (Table 5). Calcium concentrations are high in hard cheeses, lower in soft, pressed, cheeses, and relatively low in soft cheeses. The calcium in cottage cheese derives from the whey fraction, (Table 6). The reason for the variation is that whereas for hard and semihard cheeses there is little mineral loss after the initial separation, for blue-veined, soft, and cottage cheeses substantial proportions of the calcium are lost when the whey becomes acid and is drained or pressed away.

Cow's milk contains more electrolytes than does human milk. Infants given cow's milk have a higher plasma osmolality.[47] The increased renal solute load for the immature kidney may lead to a decreased margin of safety against dehydration brought about by infection or changes in the environment.[48,49] Hence, some manufacturers feel that in the preparations intended for infant feeding the concentrations of calcium, phosphorus, sodium, potassium, and chloride should be adjusted to resemble more nearly those in human milk. Fortification with iron is general, although much supplementary iron is not absorbed.[50]

## ACKNOWLEDGMENT

I should like to thank my colleagues in the Nutrition Department for their generous help and advice and Mr. F. Sayles of the Library and Scientific Information Service for his valuable assistance with the literature.

## GENERAL REFERENCES

Individual references are listed below. In addition the following articles and books have been drawn upon extensively and may be consulted with advantage on almost every aspect of the subject matter. Articles illuminating particular aspects appear regularly in *Dairy Science Abstracts* and *Proceedings of the Nutrition Society.*

Kon, S. K., *Milk and Milk Products in Human Nutrition,* 2nd ed., Nutrition Studies No. 27, Food and Agricultural Organization, Rome, 1972.

Paul, A. A. and Southgate, D. A. T., *McCance and Widdowson's The Composition of Foods* 4th revised and extended ed., Her Majesty's Stationery Office, London, 1978.

Porter, J. W. G., *Nutritional Studies — Recent Advances,* Rothwell, J., Ed., Society of Dairy Technology, London, 1974, 46-50.

Porter, J. W. G., *Milk and Dairy Foods,* Oxford University Press, Oxford, 1975.

# REFERENCES

1. *FAO (FAOUN) Prod. Yearb.*, 30, 1976.
2. Searles, S. K. and Armstrong, J. G., *J. Dairy Sci.*, 53, 150—154, 1970.
3. Henry, K. M., Hosking, Z. D., Thompson, S. Y., Toothill, J., Edwards-Webb, J. D., and Smith, L. P., *J. Dairy Res.*, 38, 209—216, 1971.
4. Bancher, E., Washuttl, J., and Waginger, H., *Osterreich. Milchwirtsch.*, 28, 37—40, 1973.
5. Erbersdobler, H., *Milchwissenschaft*, 25, 280—284, 1970.
6. Milostic, I., *Bull. Sci. Cons. Acad. RSF Yougosl. Sect. A.*, 12, 334, 1967.
7. Luczak, M., *Rocz. Inst. Przem. Mlecz.*, 12, 71—86, 1970.
8. Martinek, M., Milostic, I., and Zilic, S., *Kem. Ind.*, 15, 269—276, 1966.
9. Wagner, K.-H., *Prot. Vitae*, 16, 170—174, 1971.
10. Werner, M., Janecke, H., and Brendel R., *Milchwissenschaft*, 27, 563—569, 1972.
11. Glover, F. A., *J. Dairy Res.*, 38, 373—379, 1971.
12. Ford, J. E., Law, B. A., Marshall, V. M. E., and Reiter, B., *Pediatrics*, 90, 29-35, 1977.
13. Braun, O. H., *Klin. Paediatr.*, 188, 297—310, 1976.
14. Carpenter, R. G., *Sudden and Unexpected Deaths in Infancy, Report of the Proceedings of the Sir Samuel Bedson Symposium held at Addenbrooke's Hospital, Cambridge*, Camps, F. E. and Carpenter, R. G., Eds., John Wright and Sons, Bristol, 1972, 7—15.
15. Nicola, P. and Ponzone, A., *Minerva Pediatr.*, 17, 785—791, 1965.
16. Steen, K. and Eggum, B., *Maelkeritidende*, 81, 479—491, 1968.
17. Davis, J. G., *Cheese*, Vol. I, J. A. Churchill, London, 1965; Vol. 2, 1967.
18. Gregory, M. E., *J. Dairy Res.*, 34, 169—181, 1967.
19. Bijok, F., *Rocz. Inst. Przem. Mlecz.*, 9, 59—78, 1965.
20. Wingerd, W. H., Saperstein, S., and Lutwak, L., *Food Technol. (Chicago)*, 24, 760—761, 764, 1970.
21. de la Bourdonnaye, A., *Rev. Lait. Fr.*, 541—567, 1974.
22. Ferretti, A. and Flanagan, V. P., *J. Dairy Sci.*, 54, 1764—1768, 1971.
23. McDonough, F. E., Mattingly, W. A., and Vestal, J. H., *J. Dairy Sci.*, 54, 1406—1409, 1971.
24. Hyde, K. A. and Rothwell, J., *Ice Cream*, Churchill Livingstone, New York, 1973.
25. Lohrey, E. E., Marshall, K. R., and Southward, C. R., *Proc. Int. Dairy Congr. XIX New Delhi* IE, 1974, 564—565.
26. Chapman, L. P. J., *Dairy Ind.*, 33, 379—383, 1968.
27. Chapman, L. P. J., *Food Technol. (Aust.)*, 20, 516—518, 1968.
28. Bolin, T. D. and Davis, A. E., *Aust. J. Dairy Technol.*, 25, 119—120, 1970.
29. Bayless, T. M. and Rosensweig, N. S., *JAMA*, 197, 968—972, 1966.
30. Buchanan, R. A., *The Australian Milk Biscuit. Report on the Status of the Project as the 1st July 1969 Prepared at the Request of the FAO; diWHO/UNICEF Protein Advisory Group (PAG)*, Food and Agriculture Organization, Rome, 1969, 1—6.
31. Buchanan, R. A., *Proc. Int. Dairy Congr. XVIII Sydney*, IE, 1970, 452.
32. Simoons, F. J., *Am. J. Dig. Dis.*, 14, 819—836, 1969.
33. Townsend, F. R. and Buchanan, R. A., *Aust. J. Dairy Technol.*, 22, 139—143, 1967.
34. Anon., *The New Zealand Wholemilk Biscuit*, New Zealand Dairy Board, Wellington, 1967.
35. Townsend, F. R. and Buchanan, R. A., *Aust. J. Dairy Technol.*, 22, 139—143, 1967.
36. Mann, E. J., *Dairy Sci. Abstr.*, 33, 1—9, 1971.
37. Henry, K. M. and Kon, S. K., *Br. J. Nutr.*, 7, 29—33, 1953.
38. de Vuyst, A., Vervack, W., Vanbelle, M., and Foulon, M., *Lait*, 53, 625—635, 1973.
39. Ford, J. E., Porter, J. W. G., and Burton, H., *Proc. Int. Dairy Congr. XVII, Munich*, B, 1966, 357—360.
40. Henry, K. M., and Porter, J. W. G., *Proc. Int. Dairy Congr. XV, London*, I, 1959, 425—428.
41. Roy, J. H. B., *Vet. Rec.*, 76, 511—526, 1964.
42. Braude, R., Newport, M. J., and Porter, J. W. G., *Br. J. Nutr.*, 25, 113—125, 1971.
43. Perkin, A. G., Henschel, M. J., and Burton, H., *J. Dairy Res.*, 40, 215—220, 1973.
44. Finot, P. A., *Proteins in Human Nutrition*, Porter, J. W. G. and Rolls, B. A., Eds., Academic Press, London, 1973, 501—514.
45. Kisza, J., Zbikowski, Z., and Przybylowski, P., *Z. Ernaehrungswiss.*, 10, 115—122, 1970.
46. Van den Bruel, A. M. R., Jenneskens, P. J., and Mol, J. J., *Ned. Melk. Zuiveltijdschr.*, 26, 19—30, 1972.
47. Davies, D. P., *Arch. Dis. Child.*, 48, 575—579, 1973.
48. Pratt, E. L. and Snyderman, S. E., *Pediatrics*, 11, 65—69, 1953.
49. Ziegler, E. E. and Fomon, S. J., *J. Pediatr.*, 78, 561—568, 1971.
50. Rios, E., Hunter, R. E., Cook, J. D., Smith, N. J., and Finch, C. A., *Pediatrics*, 55, 686—693, 1975.

# Specific Nutrients and Nonnutrients

# EFFECTS OF PROCESSING ON FOOD LIPIDS

## L. A. Witting and P. S. Dimick

Lipids are a heterogeneous group of organic compounds that make up a large proportion of the diet in man. They are distributed widely in both plant and animal tissue and influence many qualities of the food wc eat, including contributions of essential nutrients, energy, mouth-feel, flavor, and emulsifying and complexing characteristics. The physical and chemical makeup of lipids in foods, whether natural or added, are greatly altered by processing procedures that may be beneficial or detrimental to the product.

## RAW MATERIALS

In considering the effect of food processing on lipids, it seems desirable to consider three additional points related to the lipids in the raw materials to be processed: lipid constituents essential to man, potentially undesirable lipid constituents, and reactions occurring in lipids prior to processing.

### Essential Constituents

Fats are our most concentrated source of energy and supply approximately 40% of the calories in normal mixed diets. Approximately 80 to 95% of the dietary fat is ingested in the form of triglycerides. The fatty acids commonly occurring in these triglycerides are straight-chain molecules with an even number of carbon atoms, frequently 16 or 18, and may contain zero to six methylene-interrupted *cis* double bonds, i.e., $CH_3(CH_2)_x(CH=CHCH_2)_{0-6}(CH_2)_yCO_2H$. These fatty acids may be separated into four groups according to chain length. Short-chain fatty acids ($C_4$ to $C_8$) tend to be rather rare except in milk fats and some palm oils such as babassu, coconut, and palm kernel, while medium-chain fatty acids ($C_{10}$ to $C_{14}$) occur in most seed oils. Long-chain fatty acids, $C_{16}$ to $C_{18}$, are the predominant fatty acids in a great variety of lipids. Very long saturated-chain fatty acids (greater than $C_{20}$) are common to marine oils and are frequently restricted to specialized uses such as wax ester formation, or are found to appear in specific lipid classes such as sphingolipids or glycosphingolipids. Fatty acids containing 18 to 22 carbon atoms usually contain one or more *cis* double bonds.

Serious questions have been raised regarding the caloric value of highly unsaturated fatty acids containing five or six double bonds.[1,2] Kaneda and Ishii[3] have shown that such fatty acids are as nutritious as oleic acid if they are rigorously protected from autoxidation. However, this is not always easy to accomplish since such oxidation may take place in the digestive tract.[4]

The polyunsaturated fatty acids are frequently described in terms of an omega ($\omega$) nomenclature,[5] where the position of the double bonds is designated with regard to the terminal methyl group. The series of fatty acids 9,12-octadecadienoic acid (linoleic), 6,9,12-octadecatrienoic acid (linoleic acid), and 5,8,11,14-eicosatetraneoic acid (arachidonic) are all members of the $\omega 6$ family and are usually abbreviated as $18:2\omega 6$, $18:3\omega 6$, and $20:4\omega 6$, respectively. Arachidonic acid, $20:4\omega 6$, appears to be the true essential fatty acid, but linoleic acid, $18:2\omega 6$, is the biological precursor available in quantity in the normal diet.[6,7] Except in certain rare or special situations, the double bonds in the naturally occurring fatty acids are all in the *cis* configuration.

In the absence of dietary essential fatty acids, growth is retarded and dermal symptoms appear. Generally, such observations are restricted to children[7] since it is extremely difficult to deplete the adult of essential fatty acids stored in the adipose tissue. The exceptions are prolonged malabsorption syndromes or intravenous feeding with fat free preparations, particularly where there has been a gross loss of adipose tissue. The one half depletion rate time of linoleate stored in the adipose tissue of man has been reported to be approximately 26 months.[8]

Monoenoic fatty acids, containing *trans* double bonds in various positions, are found in the tissue and milk of ruminants and are produced by rumen organisms[9,10] or during catalytic hydrogenation. Such *trans* fatty acids are not biochemically equivalent to the corresponding *cis* isomers. They do not pass through the placenta[11,12] and, despite the presence of unsaturation, are esterified to the alpha rather than the beta position of glycerol.[13,14]

One sensitive test of the potential biological activity of various positional and geometric isomers of the essential fatty acids is the manner in which they are enzymatically elongated and desaturated.[15-17] Privett and Blank[15] have shown that the the *trans, trans* isomer of linoleate is not utilized, and that the *cis, trans* isomer of $18:2\omega6$ is poorly utilized for $20:4\omega6$ formation.[18] Of the various positional isomers of odd chain length fatty acids, only those retaining the all-*cis* methylene interrupted sequence corresponding to linoleic acid are utilized.[19]

Fats and oils are important sources of the fat-soluble vitamins A, D, E, and K. Vitamin A, retinol, is required in vision and appears to be involved in glycosaminoglycan synthesis.[20] The recommended daily allowance[21] of 4000 to 5000 IU, or 800 to 1000 retinol equivalents recognizes the production of retinol in the cleavage of various carotenoids.[22] Retinol is stored in the liver,[23] where vitamin E is required to protect this highly unsaturated material.[24]

DeLuca[25] has presented strong arguments that cholecalciferol and its biological activated forms that are involved in calcium and phosphorus metabolism are hormones, since with adequate exposure of the individual to sunlight, a dietary precursor of vitamin D is not required. For infants and children, a recommended daily allowance of 400 IU is advised.[21] The well-known deficiency sign is rickets. Excessive intakes of vitamin D are considered to be dangerous.[26]

Various biochemical reactions involve free-radical intermediates. Leakage of free-radicals, such as the hydroxyl free-radical at the flavin level of electron transport, may adventitiously initiate lipid peroxidation.[27] Lipid peroxidation proceeds via a cyclic chain reaction which alpha-tocopherol, vitamin E, competitively terminates by withdrawing free radicals from the system.[28] Since vitamin E is stored in the tissues, particularly the liver,[29] overt pathological signs of deficiency are rarely observed. The recommended daily allowance[21] is stated as 12 to 15 IU of vitamin E activity. Gamma-tocopherol, which occurs at approximately 2.5 times the level of alpha-tocopherol in a normal mixed diet,[30] is assumed to have about 10% of the biological activity of alpha-tocopherol.[31]

Phylloquinone, of plant origin, is the major source of vitamin K in the human diet,[32] although menaquinones of bacterial origin are directly ingested in ruminant tissues such as beef liver.[33] In man, absorption of bacterial menaquinones produced within his own digestive tract satisfies a major portion of the requirement for vitamin K. The vitamin is well known for its involvement in blood clotting.[34]

Tissue storage is an important factor with all the fat-soluble vitamins and essential fatty acids. The requirements for these factors may safely be met by taking the average over a period of time rather than placing emphasis on the daily intake.[21] Man does not have the storage capacity of certain animals, but several well-known facts may be cited to emphasize the documented extremes. It is possible, for instance, to administer enough vitamin A in one or two massive doses to establish liver stores in the rat sufficient to last the remainder of the animal's life span.[35] Similarly, polar bear liver contains levels of vitamins A and D that are toxic to man.[36]

## Potentially Undesirable Constituents

Undesirable is used here in the sense that the constituent is or is thought to be a potential source of problems under certain conditions. Obviously, almost anything may be thought to be undesirable by someone under some set of conditions. By different criteria, both saturated and polyunsaturated fatty acids may be undesirable or desirable in foods.

Oxygenated fatty acids, in general, are undesirable constituents in raw materials for at least two reasons. Such materials appear to strongly promote the autoxidation of polyunsaturated fatty acids.[37,38] Several of these compounds have been shown to irritate or damage the stomach and intestinal mucosa.[39,40] Ricinoleic acid, for example, makes up 90% of the fatty acids in castor oil (the seed oil of *Ricinus communis*) and is an intestinal irritant producing catharsis in man while being well-digested by rats, rabbits, sheep, and guinea pigs.[41,42] Plants contain an enzyme, lipoxidase, which acts on systems containing a *cis, cis* 1,4-diene to produce a *trans, cis* conjugated fatty acid hydroperoxide.[43] Such compounds may be converted enzymatically to keto[44] and hydroxy-keto[45] fatty acids and ethers.[46] The presence of such oxygenated fatty acids is usually associated with damage to plant or seed tissue.[47,48]

Fatty acids containing a cyclopropane ring are rarely seen in plants.[49] Sterculic acid (9,10-methyleneoctadec-9-enoic acid) is a cyclopropene compound and is the Halphen reactive material in cottonseed oil.[50] A similar fatty acid, malvalic acid (8,9-methyleneheptadec-8-enoic acid) is unusual in having an odd chain length.[51] These fatty acids are toxic to nonruminants.[52] The residual amounts of this lipid in cottonseed meal is sufficient to have an adverse effect on poultry, and ingestion results in pink discoloration of the white in stored chicken eggs.[53] Addition of 1% cyclopropene fatty acid to the diet of the weanling rat results in growth retardation, enlargement of the liver and kidneys with fatty infiltration, focal degeneration of the tubular epithelium and shriveling of the hepatic parenchymal nuclei, and increased saturation of the tissue lipids.[54] Malvalic acid blocks the desaturation of stearic acid to oleic acid in several animal species.[55,56] The various biological effects are obviated by hydrogenation of the cyclopropene ring.[54]

The presence of a ring system is not invariably undesirable since a series of cyclopentenoid fatty acids known to occur in a family of tropical shrubs and trees[57] are of interest in the treatment of Hansen's Disease.

Rape (*Brassica campestris*) seed oil has been a major source of edible fat in Canada and is exported to Europe in very large quantities. High levels of rape seed oil fed to male weanling rats have resulted in transitory fatty infiltration of the heart, adrenals, and skeletal muscle with residual necrotic and fibrotic cardiac lesions.[58,59] These observations were initially attributed to the erucic acid (*cis*-13-docosenoic acid) content of the oil.[60] The level of erucic acid in commercial rape seed oil was subsequently reduced from 45 to 55% to approximately 0.5% by genetic selection.[61] Studies with such oils have suggested that other constituents in the lipid may also be involved.[62]

Partially hydrogenated marine fish oils, a source of long chain monoenoic acids, and cetoleic acid (*cis*-11-docosenoic acid) from herring oil have been shown to produce effects similar to those attributed to erucic acid, while *cis*-11-eicosenoic has little effect.[63,64]

In the early 1950s when very little was known regarding the intermediary metabolism of lipids and the regulation of lipid metabolism, attention was focused on the interrelations between dietary lipid serum cholesterol and the incidence of atherosclerotic heart disease.[65-67] It has been demonstrated that the level of serum cholesterol is mildly influenced by the balance of saturated to polyunsaturated fatty acids in the diet.[68,69] A large-scale, national diet-heart survey failed to document a significant direct correlation to dietary lipid.[70] Hyperlipoproteinemias are not a homogeneous entity and have been resolved into at least five distinct subclassifications requiring different treatments.[71] Several general dietary modifications, particularly those increasing the ratio of polyunsaturated to saturated fatty acids, have received wide attention.

As judged from studies of the fatty acid composition of human adipose tissue, the level of linoleate in the dietary fat has doubled from approximately 10 to 20% between 1959 and 1974, with the prospect of still further increases.[72] There have been several interesting attempts made to increase the linoleate content of raw materials. Hydrogenation of dietary fatty acids by rumen microorganisms tends to limit efforts to modify the polyunsaturated fatty acid content of veal, beef, and milk. Some success has been achieved by use of a complex called "protected fat," prepared by treating lipid and protein with formaldehyde.[73-76]

Oils containing large amounts of linolenic acid, such as linseed oil, are classified as "drying" oils and are suitable for use in oil-based paints. "Drying" is used in the sense that a thin layer of the oil will polymerize to a tough film in a reasonable period of time upon exposure to air. The presence of approximately 2 to 8% linolenic acid in soybean oil, for instance, has tended to restrict the potential uses of this oil. Some progress has been reported in the development of a copper catalyst to selectively hydrogenate the linolenic acid in fats.[77,78] It is extremely difficult to protect fats containing highly unsaturated fatty acids against autoxidation. The oxidized material then promotes further oxidation in the product or breaks down to small molecules with undesirable flavors and odors.[79-85]

The normal human diet contains approximately 300 to 700 mg of cholesterol per day, and the normal adult synthesizes approximately 1.7 to 2.4 g of cholesterol *de novo* from acetate. In some animals such as the rat, there is a homeostatic balance between the dietary intake of cholesterol and the biosynthesis[86] and catabolism[87] of this sterol. Since this homeostatic balance in man is poor,[88] the circulating level of cholesterol may be slightly reduced by restricting cholesterol intake. Plant and animal sterols appear to be absorbed at the same intestinal sites. It has been suggested that plant sterols impede the absorption of cholesterol by competing for these absorptive sites.[89] This may be of some importance in selecting dietary items for individuals with a high risk of atherosclerotic heart disease.

Other potentially undesirable constituents besides those defined as lipids may be present due to production methods of the various fat and oil sources. It is important to realize that foods may become contaminated with materials prior to processing. Contamination by agricultural chemicals, pesticide residues, environmental pollutants, polychlorinated hydrocarbons, and mycotoxins are potential hazards to any food system.

The foregoing discussion is intended to convey the impression that dietary lipids are complex materials that cannot be considered merely as a source of energy. It is essential to be aware of the fatty acid composition of the fats in the raw materials as it relates to digestibility, product stability, possible untoward physiological responses, and the economic ramifications of current fads.

## SPECIFIC REACTIONS OF LIPIDS

The principal reactive sites in neutral lipids are the fatty acid carboxyl group and the double bonds in the fatty acid chain. Except in hydrolytic rancidity, the reactions occurring at the double bonds are of primary importance. Certain processing steps affect only the position and configuration of the double bonds without otherwise altering the molecule. However, most reactions involving oxidation, heat, or thermal-oxidation modify the double bond by insertion or formation of new functional groups or structures.

Even though oxidative reactions play a major role in the stability of lipid-containing foods, the formation of breakdown products by nonoxidative mechanisms may also occur and are important in milk and animal tissue lipids. These mechanisms involve the hydrolysis of triglycerides, hydroxyacid glycerides, β-keto acid glycerides, and plasmalogens.

### Positional and/or Configurational Changes

Liquid vegetable oils are converted to solid fats commercially by partial hydrogenation, usually in the presence of a nickel catalyst. At the catalyst surface, both hydrogen addition and hydrogen abstraction occur.[90] The residual double bonds are in somewhat random positions although strongly centering around the original position and, depending on the selectivity of the catalyst, may be largely in the *trans* configuration.

Hydrogenation is seldom carried to completion, since a fully hydrogenated fat would have a relatively high melting point and a low coefficient of digestibility. Fatty acids tend to be hydrogenated in order of their degree of unsaturation, i.e., trienoic acids tend to be hydrogenated before dienoic acids, which in turn tend to be hydrogenated before monoenoic acids. Reduction of all the unsaturated fatty acids in soybean oil to *cis* monoenoic acids would produce a liquid fat containing approximately 88% "oleic" acid. If linoleic and linolenic acids are partially or largely converted to the *trans* positional isomers of elaidic acid, however, a solid fat may be produced, since an acyl dielaiden[91] has a melting point approximately 25 to 30°C higher than the corresponding acyl diolein.[92]

Frequently it is necessary to produce a fat which has a wide "plastic range." Such a fat is soft and spreadable upon removal from refrigerated storage at 5°C and will retain these properties without melting when standing at room temperature. Fats of this type are composed of liquid oil suspended in a solid fat matrix. Elaidic acid and other *trans* monoenoic acids contribute to this solid matrix without exceeding the melting point at which the coefficient of digestibility begins to rapidly decrease. By careful control of the degree and selectivity of the hydrogenation, it is possible to adjust the properties of fats for various uses.

Oleomargarines containing linoleic acid are best obtained by blending unhydrogenated triglycerides with a suitable matrix fat, since the position and configuration of the double bonds in the dienoic acids found in a partially hydrogenated oil is quite variable.

### Oxidative Reactions

Autoxidation[93] of lipid-bound polyunsaturated fatty acids (RH) is usually initiated by the catalytic action of trace metals with abstraction of a proton and formation of a fatty acid free-radical (R). This free-radical may exist in a number of resonance forms, but in the predominant structure the double bond moves into conjugation with the next adjacent double bond and is inverted to the *trans* configuration as follows:

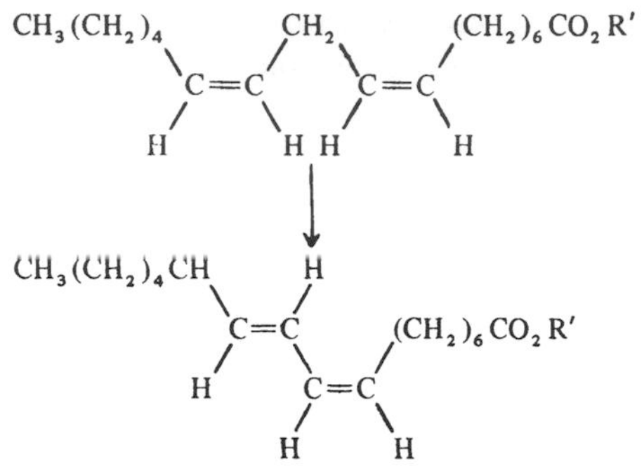

$$CH_3(CH_2)_4 \quad CH_2 \quad (CH_2)_6 CO_2 R'$$

$$CH_3(CH_2)_4 CH \quad H \quad (CH_2)_6 CO_2 R'$$

Autoxidation then proceeds via a cyclic chain reaction process to produce lipid-bound fatty acid hydroperoxides (ROOH).

$$RH \xrightarrow{r_i} R \cdot$$

$$R \cdot + O_2 \xrightarrow{k_2} RO_2 \cdot$$

$$RO_2 \cdot + RH \xrightarrow{k_3} ROOH + R \cdot$$

Chain branching or free-radical multiplication results in an autocatalytic reaction shown below. The presence of even very small quantities

$$ROOH \longrightarrow RO \cdot + OH$$

$$2 ROOH \longrightarrow RO_2 \cdot + RO \cdot + H_2O$$

of hydroperoxides in the lipid is thus a serious threat to the future stability of the product.

Lipid antioxidants (AH) such as the tocopherols do not prevent lipid peroxidation; they do not react directly with hydroperoxide (ROOH) or destroy hydroperoxides.[28] Antioxidants minimize the yield of hydroperoxide per free-radical initiation by competing with the lipid bound fatty acids (RH) for reaction with the peroxy free-radical $(RO_2 \cdot)$[94,95] shown by:

$$RO_2 \cdot + AH \longrightarrow ROOH + (A \cdot)$$

The antioxidant withdraws free-radicals from the system by reactions such as quinone formation or dimerization.[96,97] Some antioxidants do combine directly with the peroxy free-radical, but this is still a competitive reaction, with hydroperoxide formation being minimized but not prevented.[28]

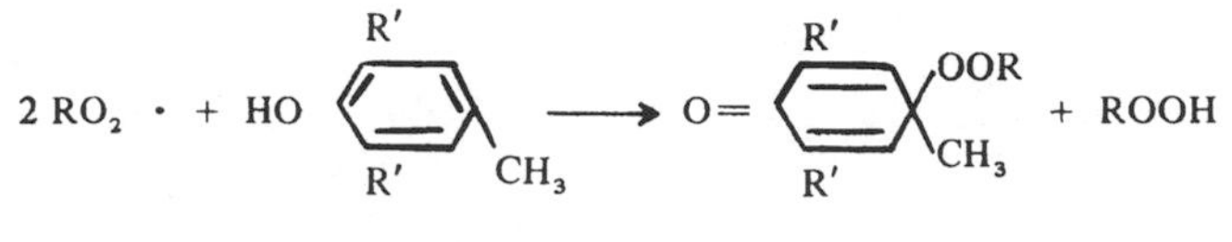

The conjugated diene formed in the original reaction is more reactive than the original fatty acid, and secondary reactions rapidly become important.[98-101] Peroxide concentrates are best prepared at low temperatures. At room temperature, the reaction mixture in pure linoleate reaches a level of approximately 8% simple monohydroperoxide,[102] at which stage secondary reactions and primary reactions proceed at similar rates and there is no further net accumulation of the hydroperoxide. At moderate temperatures, oxygen bonded polymers are formed, probably of a peroxide type R-O-O-R'.[103-106] These polymers may contain a number and variety of functional groups and undergo rearrangements and chain scission on storage, even at low temperatures.

In nonaqueous media, chain scission may occur to produce a variety of products [107-125] including saturated, mono- and diunsaturated aldehydes RCHO, R'CH=CH CHO, and R"CH=CHCH=CHCHO, respectively. Dialdehydes (OHCRCHO) and semialdehydes (OHCR'CO$_2$H) are also produced, although the latter may remain bound to the glyceride. The aldehydes may be oxidized to the corresponding acids and the unsaturated aldehydes may undergo further chain scission.[126,127] When compounds containing free amino groups such as the proteins are present, condensation products are formed.

Various tabulations of volatile products obtained under specified conditions have appeared, and the techniques of gas chromatography and mass spectrometry have been particularly useful in this area.[112-114] In addition to the compounds noted above which are present in homologous series, these lists include alcohols, esters, ketones, and aromatic as well as aliphatic hydrocarbons.

## Thermal Oxidation

The nature and relative proportion of various products formed during thermal oxidation will be dependent on the temperature and the degree of aeration. Many laboratory studies have involved bubbling air through the heated oil, and it is often difficult to compare the composition of various thermally oxidized oils produced by different investigators.

The following observations are reported from a study of thermally oxidized corn oil and are fairly typical.[128] Two reasonably distinct reaction phases were noted. In the first phase, oxygen was taken up and nonconjugated acids were converted to conjugated fatty acids. The carbonyl value increased markedly while the refractive index and viscosity increased only slightly. During the second phase, conjugated acids "disappeared" and the carbonyl value decreased while the refractive index and viscosity increased, indicating polymer formation. Intermittent heating and cooling increased the yield of altered fatty acids formed per hour of heating time.[129] This was attributed to the buildup of peroxides during the cooling period. Foaming of the oil is related to the formation of highly oxygenated polar polymers.[130-132]

As in low-temperature oxidation, chain scission occurs with the production of numerous short chain volatile compounds.[133-139] While the lists of compounds produced are similar, a greater variety of aromatic compounds are noted in thermally oxidized oils. In addition to phenol, toluene, benzaldehyde, and benzoic acid, various aliphatic carbonyl compounds with an aromatic substituent, such as 6-phenyl-3-hexanone, have been characterized. It should be remembered that a portion of the fragmented fatty acid chain usually remains attached to the glycerol.

From the analytical viewpoint it is easier to work with either the oxygenated monomers or the less polar compounds in the nonvolatile fraction. Reported characterizations have, therefore, included a number of nonoxygenated compounds containing cyclohexane, cyclohexene, or aromatic rings.[140-145] The reaction mixture has frequently been subjected to thin-layer chromatography, but more recent fractionations have utilized gel permeation.[146-150] Fatty acids in the polymers are linked by carbon to carbon bonds. While reports of cyclic linkages predominate,[151] there have been reports[152-154] of dimers that could not be aromatized and were, therefore, presumably noncyclic. In a study of the thermal oxidation of trilinolein, the level of cyclic dimer was approximately twice the level of acyclic dimer.[137] The hydroxyl and carbonyl content of the cyclic dimers is dependent on the experimental conditions during the thermal oxidation.

When a heated and/or oxidized oil is converted to methyl or ethyl esters and treated with urea, simple straight-chain molecules form a clathrate; dimers, polymers, and compounds containing a nonterminal ring are excluded. The older literature had frequently considered the material not forming a urea adduct to be polymeric,[155] although cyclic monomers are included in this fraction. A fraction described as a distillable, non-urea adduct-forming material is usually a concentrate of cyclic monomer. The nature of the materials formed in oxidized and thermally oxidized oils will be further considered in a later section dealing with their nutritional and physiological properties.

Foodstuffs are not normally heated to high temperatures in the absence of air. However, extensive literature exists on the deliberate anaerobic thermal polymerization of oils for other purposes. It is usually assumed that some of the same products appear in fats and oils heated in the presence of air at frying temperatures. The mixture of reaction products produced during anaerobic heat treatment is less complex than that produced during aerobic heat treatment, thus facilitating analysis and characterization. In considering thermal reactions a serious controversy arises as to what temperature range should reasonably be considered. Many studies have used temperatures of 250 to 350°C (482 to 662°F). It is somewhat arbitrarily stated that the "nonthermal" oxidation temperature range extends to 100°C, since polymerization by carbon-to-carbon bond formation is noted only at this or higher temperatures.[156-157]

### Nonoxidative Reactions

Even though autoxidation plays a major role in the flavor stability of lipid-containing foods, the formation of breakdown products by nonoxidative mechanisms is by no means less important. The formation of numerous compounds such as free volatile acids, lactones, methyl ketones, and aldehydes may be generated without the presence of oxygen.

Free fatty acids are found naturally in most food systems and, depending on their chain length and concentration, may contribute to the flavor of foods. These trace components may occur in the lipids of foods as products of incomplete biosynthesis of triglycerides (the major class of lipids) or more importantly, from lipolytic enzyme activity and hydrolysis of the glycerides present. The flavor threshold of the fatty acids differ, depending on whether they are present in water or oil.[158] The short-chain acids with less than six carbon atoms have a high degree of water solubility and their flavor is suppressed. The longer-chain fatty acids ($C_8$ to $C_{12}$) have an affinity for the oil phase, resulting in higher flavor thresholds. Therefore, in terms of a complex food, the physical system greatly influences the flavor properties of the free fatty acids.

Lipolytic rancidity, as characterized by the action of lipase, has been a potential source of a variety of off-flavors in fluid milk and is also known to impart characteristic flavors to cheese and other milk fat containing products.[159] The general scheme illustrating the action of lipase (glycerol ester hydrolyase) on glycerides is as follows:

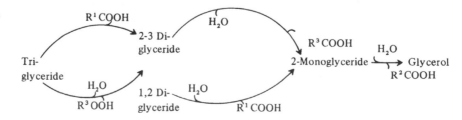

The compositional nature of the milk triglyceride precursors coupled with the specificity of the lipase results in the formation of volatile short chain fatty acids. For example, the flavorful acids butyric and caproic are esterified primarily on the sn-3 position of the glyceride, and due to positional and intermolecular specificity of the enzyme, these acids accumulate following lipolysis. The improved means of milk handling and processing, i.e., rapid cooling, efficient pasteurization, etc., have aided in eliminating lipolytic rancidity in fluid milk.

Other products rely on free fatty acid development in milk fat for their characteristic flavor; for example, cultured cream for butter manufacture, Italian and mold-ripened cheese, chocolate products, confectionery products, and imitation dairy products.

The enzymes involved in the lipolytic activity are found in animals, plants, and microorganisms. An excellent text[160] summarizes the present knowledge of these lipolytic enzymes. An example of lipolytic activity resulting from mold growth in cocoa beans indicates that the free fatty acid content of sound cacao beans from nine geographic origins varied from 2.7 to 4.8 meq/100 g fat, whereas values of 200 meq free acid per 100 g fat were obtained for badly deteriorated samples.[161] These authors point out that even though an increase of free fatty acids was evident in the moldy beans, a significant decrease in the proportion of unsaturated free fatty acids was evident. This decrease may be attributed to the conversion of acids to carbonyls by oxidative mechanisms following lipolysis.

Aliphatic methyl ketones (2-alkanones) have been known to occur in the lipid-soluble phase of many natural systems, i.e., animals, plants, and microorganisms, and in turn may contribute to the flavors of foods.[162] The methyl ketones containing odd-numbered carbon atoms have been observed in a number of dairy products and are apparently not produced by autoxidation through hydroperoxides. The presence of methyl ketones in dairy products, particularly dry whole milk, has been related to the stale-oxidized off-flavor developing during storage. Those products that incorporate milk fat in the formula and where heat is utilized in the process may also develop flavors attributed to the presence of methyl ketones. Milk caramel is an excellent example of where these compounds have been identified in the flavor distillate and were thought to contribute to the flavor.[163]

The methyl ketones in milk fat are formed from β-ketoacids esterified to glycerol.[164] The precursor in the presence of heat (140°C) and trace amount of water liberates the β-ketoacid, which in turn decarboxylates to form a methyl ketone of one less carbon.

$$
\begin{array}{l}
\quad\quad\quad\quad\;\; O \\
\quad\quad\quad\quad\;\; \| \\
CH_2-O-C-R \\
| \quad\quad\quad\;\; O \\
| \quad\quad\quad\;\; \| \\
CH-O-C-R_1 \\
| \quad\quad\quad\;\;\; O \quad\quad\;\; O \\
| \quad\quad\quad\;\;\; \| \quad\quad\;\; \| \\
CH_2-O-C-CH_2-C-(CH_2)_n-CH_3
\end{array}
$$

$+H_2O$

DG    140C

$$
\begin{array}{l}
\quad\; O \quad\quad\quad\;\; O \\
\quad\; \| \quad\quad\quad\;\; \| \\
HO-C-CH_2-C-(CH_2)_n-CH_3
\end{array}
$$

$-CO_2$

$$
\begin{array}{l}
\quad\quad\quad\; O \\
\quad\quad\quad\; \| \\
CH_3-C-(CH_2)_n-CH_3
\end{array}
$$

The origin of the β-ketoacids is the acetate formed during normal fatty acid synthesis in the mammary gland. The free β-ketoacid intermediates are then incorporated into a glyceride without the further reduction as would normally proceed for fatty acid synthesis.[164] Due to the biochemical origin of these flavor precursors, one can expect to see variation in the levels of flavor compounds in milk fat from cows on different feeding regimes and in different stages of lactation.[165]

The methyl ketones also associated with cheese flavor, particularly in mold-ripened cheeses, are derived not only from the β-ketoacid-containing glycerides as previously discussed, but also from the action of fungi during the ripening process.[166] The mechanism involves the abortive β-oxidation of free fatty acids and is illustrated as follows:

$$\text{triglyceride} \xrightarrow{\text{lipase}} \text{free fatty acid} \longrightarrow$$
$$\alpha, \beta\text{-unsaturated fatty acid} \longrightarrow \beta\text{-hydroxy acid} \longrightarrow$$
$$\beta\text{-keto acid} \longrightarrow \text{methyl ketone} + CO_2$$

Methyl ketones have also been identified in several nondairy food systems, i.e., reverted soybean oil, stale potato chips, poultry fat, roasted peanuts, and cocoa.[158] The elaboration of their origin, whether through nonoxidative or oxidative mechanisms, has yet to be determined.

One of the first implications of the aliphatic lactones being important in the flavor of foods was made in 1951 through investigations into the volatile decomposition products of milk fat.[167] This early work on the aliphatic lactones in dairy products stemmed from the unsuitable flavors associated with stored forms of milk, e.g., beverage grade, dry whole milk. These compounds were also thought to play a role in the attractive flavor properties of butter as a cooking and baking additive. Much research has clarified and strengthened the knowledge concerning the occurrence and role of minor but flavorful components in the lipid-soluble phase of both animal and plant systems.[168]

Animal products contain predominately δ-lactones and plant materials contain mainly γ-lactones. Trace levels of numerous unsaturated aliphatic lactones have also been identified in butter, processed vegetable oils, and plant extracts.[158] The flavor potential of any given lipid-containing food system may vary, depending on the amount of lactone precursor present, the level of heating, and the degree of oxidation within the product. Based on the research thus far, milk fat has the greatest potential to form lactones, averaging approximately 90 ppm for cow, 53 ppm for goat, 20 ppm for sheep, 14 ppm for swine, and 5 ppm for human.[169] Lower concentrations of these compounds are associated with meat fats and plant lipids and as yet have not been totally quantified. The ability of bovine milk fat (butter) to produce the γ- and δ-lactones at levels far exceeding the flavor threshold level (<5 ppm) points out the impact these compounds may have on the flavor acceptance of a product where butter is used as an ingredient. For example, they may contribute to the mellowness of milk caramel.[163] It is evident from the data that a doubling of the fat content increases the lactone concentration from 31.97 to 43.49 mg%. An extension of the cooking time lowers the concentration to 19.43 mg%. This suggests that the maximum lactone potential is reached during normal cooking, and extended cooking reduces the lactones through volatilization.

The origin and formation of the lactones in foods is intriguing and very complex. In general, the mechanisms can be classified as being either nonoxidative (occurring primarily in animal and plant systems via a biosynthetic sequence) or oxidative (occurring in highly oxidized vegetable oils).

Freshly secreted milk contains essentially no free lactones, and the formation of these compounds are induced by post-secretion treatments such as the heating and storage of milk fat. Numerous studies mutually confirm that the lactone precursors are monohydroxy alkanoic acid containing glycerides that are secreted in the milk.[170-172] The mechanism of lactone formation from these precursors is as follows:

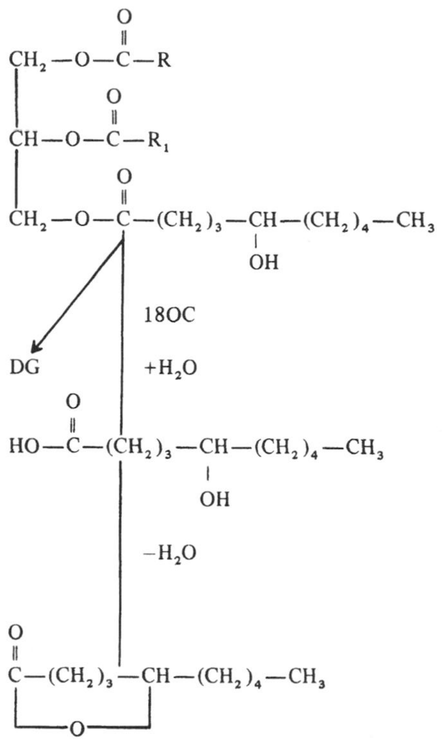

$$
\begin{array}{l}
\overset{\displaystyle O}{\underset{\displaystyle \|}{}} \\
CH_2-O-C-R \\
\quad\quad\quad \overset{\displaystyle O}{\underset{\displaystyle \|}{}} \\
CH-O-C-R_1 \\
\quad\quad\quad \overset{\displaystyle O}{\underset{\displaystyle \|}{}} \\
CH_2-O-C-(CH_2)_3-CH-(CH_2)_4-CH_3 \\
\quad\quad\quad\quad\quad\quad\quad\quad\quad | \\
\quad\quad\quad\quad\quad\quad\quad\quad\quad OH
\end{array}
$$

180C

DG        $+H_2O$

$$
\overset{\displaystyle O}{\underset{\displaystyle \|}{}}\\
HO-C-(CH_2)_3-CH-(CH_2)_4-CH_3 \\
\quad\quad\quad\quad\quad\quad | \\
\quad\quad\quad\quad\quad\quad OH
$$

$-H_2O$

$$
\overset{\displaystyle O}{\underset{\displaystyle \|}{}}\\
C-(CH_2)_3-CH-(CH_2)_4-CH_3 \\
\underline{\quad\quad\quad\quad O \quad\quad\quad\quad}
$$

The formation is the result of heating milk fat to 140°C for 1 hr, liberating a homologous series of lactones from their corresponding hydroxy fatty acids. Investigations on the environmental and physiological factors that influence the production of δ-lactones in bovine milk fat demonstrate a highly significant positive correlation with the esterified short chain fatty acids ($C_4$ to $C_{14}$) synthesized in the mammary gland.[173] Radioisotope studies have shown that acetate, the precursor of saturated fatty acids, is also the precursor for the δ-lactones.[174] This metabolic origin of these flavor precursors points out that the lactone potential may be influenced by the season of the year, stage of lactation, and health of the animals, and in turn may influence the flavor quality of the milk fat and the resulting products where it is utilized.[173]

A postulation on formation of the lactones via a biosynthetic route has been made,[175] demonstrating the presence of these compounds in apricots. This scheme also has been proposed based on studies on goat milk.[176-177]

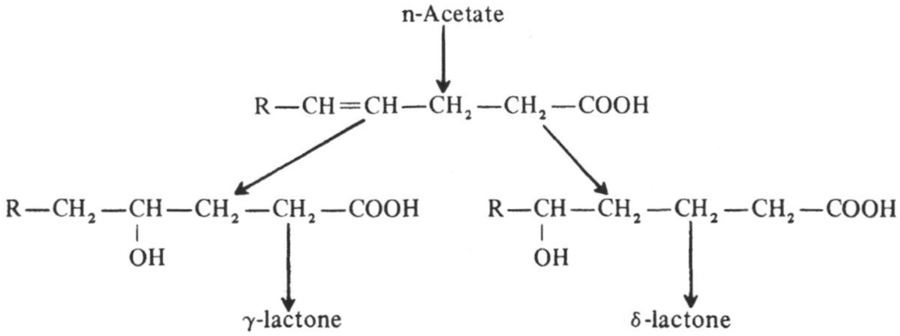

n-Acetate

$$
R-CH=CH-CH_2-CH_2-COOH
$$

$$
R-CH_2-CH-CH_2-CH_2-COOH \quad\quad R-CH-CH_2-CH_2-CH_2-COOH
$$
$$
\quad\quad\quad | \quad\quad\quad\quad\quad\quad\quad\quad\quad\quad\quad\quad | 
$$
$$
\quad\quad\quad OH \quad\quad\quad\quad\quad\quad\quad\quad\quad\quad\quad OH
$$

γ-lactone                    δ-lactone

The 4- and 5-ketoacids have also been proposed as an intermediate in the natural formation of γ- and δ-lactones in animal fats.[178]

Several oxidative mechanisms have been postulated for the occurrence of these same flavorful lactones. Fresh refined cottonseed and soybean oils have been reported to be devoid of δ- and γ-lactones; however, these compounds were present in highly peroxidized samples of cottonseed and soybean oil.[179] The catabolic pathways involve the decomposition of hydroperoxide from unsaturated fatty acids.

In the study of lactone formation in heated meat fats, several precursors were demonstrated in addition to those already discussed.[180] A series of γ- and δ-lactones could be found in the thermal oxidative products of saturated acids, aldehydes, and alcohols that had been heated with pork fat at 180°C for 5 hr with air flow. They suggest that the lactones are secondary products formed by the oxidative degradation of meat fats.

It may be concluded that the presence of lactones in food lipids may originate from many different mechanisms and precursors. Optical activity data of the lactones isolated from both animal and vegetable fats supports this point.[181] Based on the rule that whenever optically active materials are naturally formed only one enantiomer is produced, their data shows that these compounds must be formed via different pathways.

## GENERAL EFFECTS OF PROCESSING ON LIPIDS

### Processing of Foods Other Than by Frying

To a great extent, the effect of various processing techniques on food lipids is easily predicted on the basis of tissue damage, exposure to oxygen, and the temperature range involved.

Simple rapid freezing of raw unblanched plant tissue raises the potential problem of lipoxidase action. The extent of enzymatic action will be a factor of tissue damage, storage temperature, and time. Blanching will inactivate some enzymes, but the reactivation during storage must be considered. Low-temperature storage reduces the rate of lipid autoxidation but does not prevent the reaction.

Both dehydration and freeze-drying have the effect of exposing the food lipid to air while being distributed as a thin film. Autoxidation proceeds most rapidly in the presence of a critical, residual amount of water.[182,183] Excess water protects the lipid from contact with air, but a solution of metal ions catalyzes the autoxidation of the lipid. Again, storage temperature and time are important in determining the extent of oxidative damage. Since dehydration may remove some natural flavor and odor constituents, detection of oxidatively produced off-flavors may be facilitated.

The products of lipid autoxidation in an aqueous emulsion differ from those formed under somewhat anhydrous conditions,[184] with hydroxylated intermediates leaving the lipid phase and being extracted into the aqueous phase. It is interesting to note that these compounds have been reported to inhibit glycolysis and respiration of tumor cells in vitro and to cause morphological changes that quickly lead to their death while not affecting normal cells. Myoglobin, hemoglobin, and other metalloproteins are particularly effective catalysts of lipid autoxidation, although histidine[185,186] has been used in many model system studies.

Distribution of lipids over a large surface area also occurs in many baked products. Such products, however, are usually consumed quite soon after production. The bleaching of wheat flour with strong oxidizing agents also oxidizes the residual lipid, which in turn may combine with the bleaching agent. Other types of fermentations frequently and deliberately produce compounds which would, in other products, be considered undesirable. Consider, for instance, the production of short chain acids and carbonyl compounds in cheeses. Some of the fermented fish and soy products consumed in the Orient are quite rancid by occidental standards.

Ionizing radiation[187-190] has a tendency to destroy essential nutrients and to produce undesirable products. The compounds from gamma-irradiated fat resemble those from oxidized fat. Additional products arise from the interaction of lipid degradation products such as unsaturated carbonyl compounds with protein degradation products such as methyl mercaptan. Sterilizing dosages of radiation fail to inactivate many enzymes, and a heating step prior to irradiation is required with many products.

Lipid antioxidants such as butylated hydroxytoluene or butylated hydroxyanisole and metal chelating agents are routinely added to many foods to stabilize the lipids. Where products are prepared for faddists, the exclusion of these materials shortens the shelf life. Similarly, where the polyunsaturated fatty acid content of a foodstuff is increased, the prevention of autoxidation becomes a greater-than-usual problem.

The introduction of carcinogenic polycyclic hydrocarbons into the food during processing, as may occur in charcoal broiling, is extraneous to this discussion, since this is not a conventional industrial-scale process.

Generally speaking, the processing techniques noted above may, in extreme cases, adversely affect product quality and shelf life and detract from vitamin content without greatly affecting the nutritional or safety aspects of the product. Some controversy exists, however, as to whether or not these statements are equally true regarding the techniques used in the preparation of bulk oils and fats and the processing of foods by frying. The processing of fats and oils as distinguished from the processing of complex foods is discussed later.

### Frying

While discontinuous restaurant batch-type frying operations are quite similar to continuous, commercial frying processing, the former has a much more adverse effect on the fat or oil. In both cases the fried food withdraws oil from the cooking unit that must be replenished periodically or continuously. The critical factors requiring discussion are (1) exclusion of air,[191] (2) removal of volatiles, and (3) attainment of steady state conditions. The first two factors are related to the presence of water in the food. The hot oil is depicted as being blanketed by a layer of steam, which reduces contact with the air, and volatile decomposition products are continuously removed by steam distillation. It should be noted, however, that water increases the extent of oxidation.[192] No mention is usually made of the nonvolatile portion of the scissioned fatty acid chain still attached to the glycerol moiety.

Maintenance of an effective steam blanket requires spraying water on the oil and the presence of a cover over the frying unit,[193] which may consist of a continuous belt carrying the product through a long rectangular tray or trough of heated oil. Such a cover will favor condensation of the volatiles and their reentry into the oil. Some entrained and contained air will, of course, enter the oil with the food to be processed. Factors (1) and (2) are variable and related to the design and operation of the particular frying unit, but the steam blanket is normally not a significant protective factor. Examination of such units quickly reveals that volatiles are, to a great extent, purged out of the oil and that oxidation does indeed take place. Significant oxygen uptake is associated with the first phase of thermal oxidation, while the second phase, polymer formation, does not require a great amount of oxygen.[128]

Attainment of a steady state is most readily discussed in mathematical terms. Continuous addition of fresh oil at the rate of 8% per hr, for instance, results in a "complete" change of oil approximately twice in 24 hr. Obviously, some number of molecules of the original fat placed in the frying unit will remain in the unit no matter how much fresh oil is added. This point is emphasized by a consideration of the addition of fresh oil at discreet intervals. If ⅓ of the total oil is withdrawn by the food in a given time, the original volume is reattained by the addition of this amount of fresh fat at the end of that time period. The origin of the terms in the series thus generated should be readily apparent. If all fat molecules are "equivalent," ⅔ of those present at the start of an interval, *a*, should be present at the end of the interval. With the exception that the final term is always twice the expected term, this is the expansion of ⅓ (⅔)$^{n-1}$ *na*. This series approaches a limiting value, and steady-state or equilibrium conditions are considered to be attained in commercial operations. According to this popular description of the frying operation, the fat is effectively heated for only a short period of time before being removed from the unit by the food product. Thus serious damage cannot occur.

Oil used in the discontinuous batch-type fryer must eventually be discarded because of either high viscosity or excessive foaming. Stable foams are produced by about 9% oxidized polymer.[130] Hydroxyl groups are more effective in contributing to foam production than are carbonyl groups.[131,132] Viscosity, in turn, is closely related to thermal polymer content.[194] Discarded oils are frequently found to contain approximately 25% polymer.[146,195,196] Since the addition of methyl silicone[197] to frying oils to prevent foaming became a standard practice, higher levels of polymer (approximately 35%) are also encountered.

Such badly damaged oils are not usually seen in a well-managed continuous frying operation. An increase in the viscosity of the oil of 1 cs at 100°C was reported to increase the uptake of oil by fry cakes from 10 to 15%.[194] An increase of 2.5 cs substantially reduced product quality. These increases in viscosity appeared to be related to polymer (non-urea adduct-forming materials) levels, of 2 to 4% and 5 to 7%, respectively. An increase of 3.0 cs resulted in a 20% reduction in heat transfer by the oil. Consider that approximately 250,000 tons of oil are used in frying potato chips each year in the U.S., and another 100,000 tons are used in frying doughnuts.[154] Economic considerations would seem to dictate careful preservation of oil quality. It should be noted, however, that the increased oil uptake by the fry cakes with increased oil viscosity suggests that all fat molecules may not indeed be "equivalent" in the frying unit.

## PROCESSING OF EDIBLE FATS AND OILS

### Extraction

The relation of oil or fat quality to the severity of processing techniques has long been recognized and is apparent in the descriptions historically applied to the various grades of lard, tallow, and olive oil. Most vegetable oils are currently obtained by solvent extraction with volatile petroleum hydrocarbons. It has been suggested that such solvents contain undesirable traces of carcinogenic multi-ring aromatic hydrocarbons that are selectively transferred to the oil. Such materials have not yet been detected,[198] but if this contamination did occur, these materials would undoubtedly be removed during the deodorization process that will be discussed below. In studies of the various processing procedures on the polymer content of the oil it was reported that 1 to 2% of polymeric material is present in the raw oil.[199]

The fire and explosion hazard associated with the solvent extraction process cannot be avoided by the use of halogenated hydrocarbons. When this was tried commercially it was found that the solvent reacts with the sulfhydryl groups of the seed protein and attaches to the sulfur atom. This modified protein presents a very serious nutritional and safety hazard.[200]

### Refining

Oils are treated with water and base, usually in a centrifugal apparatus, to remove plant gums, free fatty acids, and the bulk of the phospholipids. Commercial soybean lecithin is a byproduct of this type of operation and the free fatty acids are a source of soap stock. Removal of the various associated materials markedly reduces the stability of the oil.

Fatty acids are also excellent starting materials for the preparation of various industrial chemicals. Frequently this includes a fractional distillation of the fatty acids in the starting material. The still residues or "foots" may be used in animal feeds. It has been found that such foots may occasionally contain levels of polychlorinated hydrocarbons that produce pericardial edema in chicks.[201,202] Actually, the chick is rather unusual in responding to these levels that do not, in fact, bother numerous other species. Such foots are not edible by human standards but they are fed to animals consumed by man.

### Bleaching and Deodorization

Carotenes, chlorophyll, and other plant pigments are removed or reduced in concentration by treatment of the oil with a bleaching clay. This is not a simple adsorptive process and involves oxidation and free-radical production.[203,204] Small quantities of positional and geometric isomers of the fatty acids are formed as are various hydroxy, keto, and epoxy derivatives. This process improves the quality of the oil at the expense of a minor contribution to future instability.

Deodorization, vacuum steam distillation of volatile odoriferous components from the oil,[205-207] may be performed as a batch, semicontinuous, or continuous process. At temperatures of 190 to 230°C (375 to 450°F) approximately 2 to 5 hr are needed for efficient batch deodorization. There has been a trend toward shorter processing times by raising the temperature to 230 to 250°C (445 to 480°F) and/or increasing the vacuum from 6 to 1mm Hg. A byproduct of this process, the deodorizer condensate, is a commercial source of plant sterols and, for practical purposes, is the only source of commercial quantities of the natural tocopherols.[208] Crude corn oil is frequently stated to contain 1 to 2 mg of tocopherols per gram of oil, whereas the oil on the grocery store shelf may contain only 0.5 to 0.7 mg/g. A substantial reduction in the level of an essential nutrient and natural antioxidant occurs in this process.

When the oil is hydrogenated, it is essential to perform the deodorization after the hydrogenation.[209,210] Under somewhat anaerobic conditions, the high temperature in the deodorizer tends to decompose those oxidized materials that would later tend to decompose under aerobic conditions to initiate the cyclic chain reaction of autoxidation. The formation of small quantities of thermal polymers at this stage is clearly preferable to the formation of potentially larger quantities of oxidized material in the product at a later stage. Removal of the volatiles produces a bland oil. The various processing operations tending to remove or produce polymers somewhat balance each other, and the finished oil has been reported to contain slightly less polymer than does the raw oil.[199]

When a stock source of bland unsaturated oil is needed as a reference standard in organoleptic testing, it has been found that despite elaborate precautions changes occur with time.[211] Only the regeneration of fatty acid esters from the urea adduct provided a reproducible, stable standard.[212]

### Hydrogenation

Addition of hydrogen to the double bonds of the fatty acids converts oxidatively unstable liquid oils to stable solid fats. As noted previously, however, the process must be halted at an intermediate stage short of complete saturation. Furthermore, a catalyst is frequently chosen to selectively produce *trans* isomers. A recent advertisement for one such catalyst presented data suggesting an essentially quantitative conversion of the linoleic and linolenic acids in soybean oil to *trans* monoenoic acids.[213] In many ways these *trans* positional isomers of oleic acid, because of their melting point,[91] are the ideal approach to the production of a solid, digestible matrix for the support of lower melting fats or liquid oils.

### Rearrangement

A simple blending of fats and oils does not produce a homogeneous product since the triglycerides of the oil retain their characteristic fatty acids as do the triglycerides of the fat. Introduction of a suitable catalyst such as sodium methoxide results in a rapid ester interchange and produces triglycerides with a random fatty acid composition.[214] This reaction may also be conducted in the directed manner.[215] If the reaction vessel is provided with a low-temperature region, high-melting point triglycerides may be selectively crystallized out as they are formed and withdrawn from the system. The catalyst may be destroyed by addition of a stoichiometric amount of water and the residual methanol removed. This process may have a slight adverse effect on product stability.[216]

A variation of this reaction is used in the laboratory to produce methyl esters from lipids by simply adding a catalyst and a large excess of methanol. Conversely, triglycerides may be synthesized in the laboratory by the ester interchange between glyceryl triacetin and fatty acid methyl esters. Removal of the volatile methyl acetate under vacuum drives the reaction to completion.

## NUTRITIONAL AND SAFETY ASPECTS OF PROCESSING

The literature on oxidized and heated fat must be viewed in historical perspective. During World War II and for a short period thereafter, edible fats and oils were in short supply in some areas and soybeans and soybean oil were relatively novel and minor items in the occidental diet. Deliberate thermal polymerization was seriously considered as an alternative to hydrogenation in some countries.[217,218] The best-known studies in this area are those of Crampton and co-workers with linseed oil.[219-225] They heated this oil to 275°C (550°F) for 12 hr under an atmosphere of carbon dioxide. When fed at the 20% level in the diet of rats, the animals lost weight and mortality rate was high. Toxicity was attributed to products formed from linolenic acid. Subsequent studies indicated that the thermal dimers and higher polymers had low caloric value due to poor intestinal absorption and that their nonabsorption resulted in diarrhea. Subsequent studies involving fractionation of the heated oil attributed the toxicity to the cyclic monomers. A concentrate of these cyclic monomers prepared by distillation of the material not forming an adduct with urea produced weight loss but not death when fed at the 2.5% level in the diet of rats.[226] However, 0.5 m*l* of a comparable concentrate administered by stomach tube for three days to 50 g weanling rats resulted in 40% mortality.[227] This might be equivalent to approximately 10% of the food an animal of this size would eat per day.

In the late 1930s and early 1940s, a series of reports by Roffo[228-234] appeared in Argentinian journals not generally available in the U.S. ascribing carcinogenic activity to heated fats. The starting points for much of the work on thermally oxidized frying fats were these reports of outright toxicity and carcinogenicity in related materials. These topics will be discussed separately below.

### Nutritional Properties of Thermally Oxidized Fats

When considering some of the original experiments in this area, the difficulty of publishing negative reports should be borne in mind. In general, conditions were selected for the production of oxidized, heated, or thermally oxidized materials such that if toxic materials similar to those studied by Crampton and co-workers[219-225] could be produced, they would probably be produced by the conditions used. In the usual scientific experiments, once conditions are established that will produce toxic materials, it becomes feasible to isolate and characterize these materials and to develop techniques for qualitative analysis. At this point it is possible to determine if significant quantities of such materials are produced under "practical" conditions.

In principal, such fats should perhaps have been produced in somewhat the following manner: A relatively highly unsaturated frying fat is used for an excessively prolonged period of time for the actual frying of foods at the highest temperature likely to be encountered in gross misuse that does not ruin the product or involve an actual fire hazard. Heating should be intermittent rather than continuous. Makeup fat is added batchwise after significant removal of fat by the product to increase the ratio of exposed surface to total volume. The equipment should not be covered, and an efficient draft should be provided to minimize steam blanketing of the surface.

Preparation of experimental fats by such a procedure is not economically feasible in most cases. Instead, fats and oils have been heated under vacuum or with air blown through the hot oil.[266-280] Typically, little or no actual product was fried in the oil and therefore the addition of fresh oil was minimal or nonexistent. Fats or oils prepared under such conditions did not reach steady state conditions and "damage" was usually proportional to the treatment time.

Needless to say, reputable scientists in the research laboratories of the major commercial producers of frying fats and oils hastened to point out that data derived from the feeding of such oils were not particularly relevant to the ingestion of fats and oils used in the actual frying of foods. These proved to be quite harmless in their experiments.[235-242] The scientific literature is largely composed of progress reports on various approaches to specific problems, and only to a very limited extent to final solutions to major problems. The professional has the training to read and evaluate such reports in their proper perspective whereas the interested public is usually not aware of the differences between approaches to a problem, the problem itself, nor benefits from these negative reports.

Early in the feeding studies with thermally oxidized fats and oils, confirmation of a rather basic general principal was obtained. In general, the toxicity or carcinogenicity of a material is inversely related to the protein level of the diet furnished to the experimental animal.[243,244] Using a specific heated corn oil, an almost total lack of growth was seen in young rats fed 10% casein. Severe growth depression was noted with 20% casein, and a relatively mild effect was noted when the diets contained 30% or more casein.[245] In adult man the recommended dietary allowance for protein is 56 g or 224 kcal (8.3% of the calories in a 2700 kcal diet). In a rat diet containing 10% fat by weight and usually 4 to 5% minerals, 30% casein corresponds to approximately 28% of the calories. For man this would require approximately 756 kcal of protein or 189 g of protein per day or 2 ¼ lb of roast beef.

Industrially oriented investigators are notably prone to refer to the use of "normal" diets comparable to those eaten by man rather than the customary semisynthetic animal diets; they thus feed a mixture containing 5% casein, 21% nonfat dry milk, 43% ground whole wheat, 3% dried egg white, 3% dried defatted liver, and 0.5% L-lysine.[227] It should be realized that while such an unnatural high-protein diet cannot actually prevent the growth-depressing or toxic effects of a severely treated oil, it may make it difficult or impossible to accurately detect any deleterious effect that might otherwise be produced by a less drastically treated oil. The rat differs from man in its protein requirement, but maximum weight gain and efficiency of food conversion are achieved with 18 to 20% protein.[246]

Although frying oils are described as thermally oxidized there seems to be agreement regarding the absence of nutritionally significant quantities of hydroperoxide per se in these oils. Air blown through fresh corn oil at the rate of 150 ml/min/kg of oil at 120°, 160°, and 200°C (248°, 320°, and 392°F) for 24 hr resulted in peroxide numbers of 81, 6, and 2, respectively.[247] Essentially all of the reported analytical data on heated oils are characterized by quite low peroxide values. More than 20 years ago, Dubouloz[248-253] described the destruction of lipid peroxides in the intestinal lumen by a metalloprotein. In other tissues, enzymes such as glutathione peroxidase[254,255] are now known to efficiently destroy lipid peroxides. Lymph cannulations have shown that oxidized lipids are absorbed but that the absorbed material does not contain the hydroperoxide group.[256-260] Hydroxylated fatty acids such as those prepared from ex-poxidized soybean oil are also well tolerated by the rat.[261] In view of the well-known intolerance of the human gut to a simple hydroxy fatty acid, the relevance of much of these data to the practical problem is questionable.

As little as 0.54% aromatic cyclic monomer from fish oil produced growth depression and was lethal at the 2.15% level.[262] The partially saturated cyclic monomer from linseed oil is not as toxic, since growth depression, but not death, resulted when fed at the 2.5% level.[226] Some fractions of this non-urea adduct-forming type appear to be toxic while others fed at the same level are not. One report[227] appears to state that the level of this fraction does not particularly increase in grossly mistreated oils (1.7 to 2.3%) as compared to fresh oils (1.5 to 2.0%) but nevertheless may result in 20 to 40% mortality when fed as the isolated material.

The cyclic dimers and higher polymers of linseed oil are nontoxic by virtue of poor absorption. The growth depressing effects of polymers from other heated oils are due, in part, to poor absorption; as little as one third of the isolated polymers of some laboratory treated oils are absorbed.[263-265] However, the polymers (nondistillable, non-urea adduct-forming material) from corn oil and cottonseed oil and an isolated dimer from soybean oil all appear to be somewhat toxic. This may be due, in part, to the formation of a definite amount of acyclic polymers[152-154] in oils containing linoleic acid rather than linolenic acid as the predominant polyunsaturated fatty acid. Such a dimer has recently been chromatographically isolated and partially characterized by Japanese investigators.[153]

The laboratory thermal oxidation of oils commonly used for frying purposes definitely produces toxic compounds.[266-280] Even the most sincere advocates of the absolute safety of commercially-used frying oils agree that, qualitatively, essentially the same compounds are produced under actual condition of use. The critical and as yet unresolved problem is the question of the quantitative significance of such compounds in commercially-used oils. In the dog, even the use of a 29.4% protein diet containing 5% casein, 21% nonfat dry milk, 17% toasted soybean meal, 3% blood meal, 30% toasted ground whole wheat, and 2% liver powder would not mask the growth depressing properties of 15% commercially-used oil.[242]

Oils thermally oxidized in the laboratory produce enlarged livers, kidneys, and adrenals in the rat.[281,282] Commercially-used oils have been reported[238] to produce mild enlargement of these organs even when fed in a diet containing 15% lactalbumin, 20.5% ground whole wheat, 15% soybean oil meal, 10% nonfat dry milk solids, 10% meat and bone meal, and 2% alfalfa meal. Laboratory prepared oils produced statistically significant increases in liver weight whereas commercially-used oils did not in a short term, 7-day study. Liver enlargement in these circumstances is viewed, in part, as increased synthesis of the hepatic microsomal mixed-function oxidase system for the metabolism of toxic compounds. It has recently been shown that rats fed heated fat synthesized less hemoglobin and retained more protein in the liver to cope with the metabolic effects of the damaged fat.[283] Modern frying fats contain a minimum level of polyunsaturated fats[284] and therefore are less susceptible to heat damage. However, their nutritional impact is probably more dependent on the protein level of the diet than on the extent of the heat damage.

## Thermally Oxidized Fats and Cancer

All efforts to reproduce the production of gastric cancers as reported by Roffo by feeding heated and/or oxidized fats have failed.[285] Noncancerous lesions of the stomach were produced after 18 to 24 months in Ivy's laboratory using rats of Roffo's strain.[286] One of the critical points in Roffo's studies was the extreme period of time, 27 to 30 months, needed to produce the gastric lesions. Most investigators were unable to maintain their rats for more than two years. The possible exception to these negative results is the study by Sugai and co-workers.[287]

It was considered possible that addition of a low level of a powerful chemical carcinogen such as acetylaminofluorene (AAF) to the diet might sensitize the tissues of the rat to the point where the co-carcinogenic activity of a weak carcinogen could be detected. It was indeed finally possible to carry out an experiment wherein all the rats fed 0.005% AAF and fresh fat survived for 30 months without detectable tumors, whereas none of the rats fed this level of AAF and 2.5% of the non-urea adduct forming material from thermally oxidized corn oil were free of tumors.

At the time these experiments were conducted (1954 to 1961), it was discovered that the N-hydroxylation of AAF enhanced the carcinogenicity of this compound.[288,289] The drug metabolizing capacity of the liver is now known to increase in response to the ingestion of oxidized fats.[290-292] In retrospect, this experiment is now open to the criticism that the inclusion of the thermally oxidized fat in the diet had the side effect[293,294] of increasing the animal's capacity to metabolize the carcinogen AAF to another compound, N-hydroxyl-2-acetylaminofluorene, which is an even more potent carcinogen than its precursor.

## Lipids and Atherosclerosis

The role that dietary fats play in the nutritional perspective, (i.e., their actual role) in atherosclerosis is still not clear. Recommendations are being made and conclusions drawn without knowledge of all the factors involved.

For example, the final report of the National Diet Heart Study stated: "Extensive evidences implicate diet as a key factor in the etiology of atherosclerosis and suggests that the disease can be prevented by changes in diet, particularly by lowering serum cholesterol level."[295]

In addition, a policy statement of the American Medical Association Council on Food and Nutrition[296] and the Food and Nutrition Board of the National Academy of Sciences indicated how changes in diet could be accomplished: "Generally such lowering can be achieved most practically by partial replacement of the dietary sources of saturated fat with sources of unsaturated fat, especially those rich in polyunsaturated fatty acids." This joint statement concluded: "There is abundant evidence that the risk of developing CHD (cardiovascular heart disease) is positively correlated with the cholesterol in the plasma." However, such a nutritional perspective has not fully considered that dietary sources of saturated fat and cholesterol, i.e., meat, eggs, and dairy products, serve as the major source of protein, vitamins, and minerals in the American diet.

Serum cholesterol levels are somewhat responsive to dietary cholesterol level, the relative balance of polyunsaturated and saturated fatty acids in the dietary fat, and certain drugs such as niacin and clofibrate. Either the dietary approach[70] or the drug approach[297] may lower serum cholesterol levels 10%. However, essentially negative results have been obtained with such an approach in two long-term national studies.[70,297]

It has been shown by Van Den Bosch and co-workers[298,299] that the replacement of an unsaturated by a saturated fatty acid influences the physical characteristics of the phospholipid into which it is incorporated and maintains the physical properties of the phospholipid molecule between certain limits. Data on liquid crystals and synthetic membranes support the hypothesis that the properties of membranes are dependent on the physical characteristics of the fatty acid composition of the phospholipids.[300-302] De Kruyff and co-workers[303] incorporated elaidic instead of oleic acid into the phospholipids of *Acholeplasma laidlawii*. They noted a difference in the energy contents of the phase transitions of the isolated lipids, which they believe may have significance to the liquid crystalline state as cholesterol was shown to preferentially interact with lipids that are in the liquid crystalline state. As phospholipids are important components in the cell membranes that make up the myocardium and the intima, the fatty acid composition of these phospholipids may be important to the rate at which lipid infiltration can occur through the cell membrane.

## SUMMARY

Food lipids may suffer loss of nutritional value under conditions that do not differ drastically from normal processing conditions. By occidental standards, however, fats and oils rapidly become unpalatable after relatively mild, adverse treatment. The role of dietary fat in atherosclerosis is still under study.

## REFERENCES

1. Yoshida, M., *J. Agric. Chem. Soc. Jpn.*, 13, 120—147, 1937.
2. Osaki, J., *J. Agric. Chem. Soc. Jpn.*, 8, 1286—1309, 1932.
3. Kaneda, T., and Ishii, S., *Bull. Jpn. Soc. Sci, Fish.*, 19, 171—177, 1953.
4. Green, J., *Ann. N.Y. Acad. Sci.*, 203, 29—44, 1972.
5. Holman, R. T., *Prog. Chem. Fats Other Lipids*, 9, 1—12, 1966.
6. Holman, R. T., *Prog. Chem. Fats Other Lipids*, 9, 611—682, 1970.
7. Soderhjelm, L., Wiese, H. F., and Holman, R. T., *Prog. Chem. Fats Other Lipids*, 9, 557—585, 1970.
8. Witting, L. A., *Prog. Chem. Fats Other Lipids*, 9, 517—553, 1970.
9. Polan, C. E., McNeil, J. J., and Tove, S. B., *J. Bacteriol.*, 88, 1056—1064, 1964.
10. Viviani, R., *Adv. Lipid Res.*, 8, 267—346, 1970.
11. Johnston, P. V., Johnson, O. C., and Kummerow, F. A., *Proc. Soc. Exp. Biol. Med.*, 96, 760—762, 1957.
12. Johnston, P. V., Walton, C. H., and Kummerow, F. A., *Proc. Soc. Exp. Biol. Med.*, 99, 735—736, 1958.
13. Privett, O. S., Nutter, L. J., and Lightly, F. S., *J. Nutr.*, 89, 257—264, 1966.
14. Lands, W. E. M., Blank, M. L., Nutter, L. J., and Privett, O. S., *Lipids*, 1, 224—229, 1966.
15. Privett, O. S., and Blank, M. L., *J. Am. Oil Chem. Soc.*, 41, 292—297, 1964.
16. Sprecher, H. W., Dutton, H. J., Gunstone, F. D., Sykes, P. T., and Holman, R. T., *Lipids*, 2, 122—126, 1967.
17. Schlenk, H., *Prog. Chem. Fats Other Lipids*, 9, 587—605, 1970.
18. Blank, M. L. and Privett, O. S., *J. Lipid Res.*, 4, 470—476, 1963.
19. Schlenk, H., and Sand, D. M., and Sen, N., *Biochim. Biophys. Acta*, 70, 361—364, 1964.
20. DeLuca, L., Little, E. P., Wolf, G., *J. Biol. Chem.*, 244, 701—708, 1969.

21. Food and Nutrition Board, National Research Council, *Recommended Dietary Allowances,* 8th rev. ed., National Academy of Sciences, Washington, D.C., 1974, 1—11.

22. Olson, J. A., and Lakshmanan, M. R., *The Fat Soluble Vitamins,* DeLuca, H. F. and Suttie, J. W., Eds., University of Wisconsin Press, Madison, 1969, 213—226

23. Williams, R. J., *Vitam. Horm.* (N.Y.), 1, 229—247, 1943.

24. Davies, A. W. and Moore, T., *Nature,* 147, 794—796, 1941.

25. DeLuca, H. F., *Am. J. Clin. Nutr.,* 28, 339—345, 1975.

26. Anning, S. T., Dawson, J., Dolby, D. E., and Ingram, J. T., *Q. J. Med.,* 17, 203—228, 1948.

27. Fong, K. L., McCay, P. B., Poyer, J. L., Keele, B. B., and Misra, H., *J. Biol. Chem.,* 248, 7792—7797, 1973.

28. Uri, N., *Autoxidation and Antioxidants,* Lundberg, W. O., Ed., Interscience, New York, 1961, 133—169.

29. Mason, K., *J. Nutr.,* 23, 71—81, 1942.

30. Bieri, J. G. and Evarts, R. P., *J. Am. Diet. Assoc.,* 62, 147—151, 1972.

31. Bieri, J. G. and Evarts, R. P., *J. Nutr.,* 104, 850—857, 1974.

32. Matschiner, J. T. and Taggart, W. V., *Anal. Biochem.,* 18, 88—93, 1967.

33. Matschiner, J. T. and Amelotti, J. M., *J. Lipid Res.,* 9, 176—179, 1968.

34. Suttie, J. W., *The Fat Soluble Vitamins,* DeLuca, H. F. and Suttie, J. W., Eds., University of Wisconsin Press, Madison, 1969, 447—462.

35. Moore, T., *The Fat Soluble Vitamins,* Morton, R. A., Ed., Pergamon, Oxford, 1970, 238—257.

36. Rodahl, K. and Moore, T., *Biochem. J.,* 37, 166—168, 1943.

37. Bhalerao, V. R., Kokatnur, M. G., and Kummerow, F. A., *J. Am. Oil Chem. Soc.,* 39, 28—30, 1962.

38. Anderson, R. H., and Huntley, T. E., *J. Am. Oil Chem. Soc.,* 41, 686—688, 1964.

39. Matsuo, N., *Lipids and Their Oxidation,* Schultz, H. W., Day, E. A., and Sinnhuber, R 0., Eds., AVI Publishing, Westport, Conn., 1962, 321—359.

40. Whipple, D. V., *Proc. Soc. Exp. Biol. Med.,* 30, 319—321, 1932.

41. Paul, H. and McCay, C. M., *Arch. Biochem.,* 1, 247—258, 1942.

42. Stewart, W. C. and Sinclair, R. G., *Arch. Biochem.,* 8, 7—11, 1945.

43. Dolev, A., Rohweddar, W. K., and Dutton, H. J., *Lipids,* 2, 28—32, 1967.

44. Viogue, E. and Holman, R. T., *Arch. Biochem. Biophys,* 99, 522—528, 1962.

45. Zimmerman, D. C., and Vick, B. A., *Plant. Physiol.,* 46, 445—453, 1970.

46. Galliard, T., Wardale, D. A., and Matthew, J. A., *Biochem. J.,* 138, 23—31, 1974.

47. Appelquist, L. A., *J. Am. Oil Chem. Soc.,* 44, 206—208, 1967.

48. Robertson, J. A., Morrison, W. H., III, and Burdick, D., *J. Am. Oil Chem. Soc.,* 50, 443—445, 1973.

49. Kleiman, R., Earle, F. R., and Wolff, I. A., *Lipids,* 4, 317—320, 1969.

50. Faure, P. K., *Nature,* 178, 372—373, 1956.

51. Macfarlane, J. J., Shenstone, F. S., and Vickery, J. R., *Nature,* 179, 830—831, 1957.

52. Phelps, R. A., Shenstone, F. S., Kemmerer, A. R., and Evans, R. J., *Poult. Sci.,* 44, 358—394, 1965.

53. Shenstone, F. S. and Vickery, J. R., *Poult. Sci.,* 38, 1055—1070, 1959.

54. Nixon, J. E., Eisele, T. A., Wales, J. H., and Sinnhuber, R. O., *Lipids,* 9, 314—321, 1974.

55. Allen, E., Johnson, A. R., Fogerty, A. C., Pearson, J. A., and Shenstone, F. S., *Lipids,* 2, 419—423, 1967.

56. Raju, P. K. and Reiser, R., *J. Biol. Chem.,* 242, 379—384, 1967.

57. Shriner, R. L. and Adams, R., *J. Am. Chem. Soc.,* 47, 2727—2739, 1925.

58. Abdellatif, A. M. M. and Vles, R. O., *Nutr. Metab.,* 12, 285—295, 1970.

59. Abdellatif, A. M. M., *Nutr. Rev.,* 30, 2—6, 1972.

60. Abdellatif, A. M. M. and Vles, R. O., *Nutr. Metab.,* 15, 219—231, 1973.

61. Rocquelin, G., Martin, B., and Cluzan, R., *Proc. Int. Conf. Sci. Technol. Marketing of Rapeseed and Rapeseed Products,* (Ste. Adele, Quebec,) Rapeseed Association of Canada in cooperation with the Department of Industry, Trade, and Commerce, Ottawa, 1970, 405—422.

62. Kramer, J. K. G., *Lipids,* 8, 641—648, 1973.

63. Beare-Rogers, J. L., Nera, E. A., and Craig, B. M., *Lipids,* 7, 46—50, 1972.

64. Beare-Rogers, J. L., Near, E. A., and Craig, B. M., *Lipids,* 7, 548—552, 1972.

65. Katz, L. N., Stamler, J., and Pick, R., *Fed. Proc.,* 15, 885—893, 1956.

66. Ahrens, E. A., Jr., Insull, W., Jr., Blomstrand, R., Hirsch, J., Tsaltes, T. T., and Peterson, M. L., *Lancet,* 2, 943—953, 1957.

67. Reiser, R., *Am. J. Clin. Nutr.,* 26, 524—555, 1973.

68. Keys, A., Anderson, J. T., and Grande, F., *Lancet,* 2, 959—966, 1957.

69. Kinsella, L. W., *Am. J. Clin. Nutr.,* 12, 228—229, 1963.

70. Final report, National Diet-Heart Study, *Circulation, 37(Suppl 1)*, 1—208, 1968.
71. Levy, R. I., *Fed. Proc.*, 30, 829—834, 1971.
72. Witting, L. A. and Lee, L., *Am. J. Clin. Nutr.*, 28, 277—283, 1975.
73. Bitman, J., Dryden, L. P., Goering, H. K., Wrenn, T. R., Yoncoskie, R. A., and Edmonson, L. F., *J. Am. Oil Chem. Soc.*, 50, 93—98, 1973.
74. Wong, N. P., Walter, H. E., Vestal, J. H., Lacroix, D. E., and Alford, J. A., *J. Dairy Sci.*, 56, 1271—1275, 1973.
75. Ellis, R., Kimoto, W. I., Bitman, J., and Edmondson, L. F., *J. Am. Oil Chem. Soc.*, 51, 4—7, 1974.
76. Edmondson, L. F., Yoncoskie, R. A., Rainey, N. H., Douglas, F. W., Jr., and Bitman, J., *J. Am. Oil Chem. Soc.*, 51, 72—76, 1974.
77. Moulton, J. J., Beal, R. E., and Griffin, E. L., *J. Am. Oil Chem. Soc.*, 50, 450—454, 1973.
78. List, G. R., Evans, C. D., Beal, R. E., Black, L. T., Moulton, K. J., and Cowan, J. C., *J. Am. Oil Chem. Soc.*, 51, 239—243, 1974.
79. Going, L. H., *J. Am. Oil Chem. Soc.*, 45, 632—634, 1968.
80. Vioque, A., Gutierrez, R., Albi, M. A., and Nosti, N., *J. Am. Oil Chem. Soc.*, 42, 344—345, 1965.
81. Crossley, A. and Thomas, A., *J. Am. Oil Chem. Soc.*, 41, 95—100, 1964.
82. Evans, C. D., Frankel, E. N., Cooney, P. M., and Moser, H. A., *J. Am. Oil Chem. Soc.*, 37, 452—456, 1960.
83. Baumann, L. A., McConnell, D. G., Moser, H. A., and Evans, C. D., *J. Am. Oil Chem. Soc.*, 44, 663—666, 1967.
84. Ackman, R. G., Hooper, S. N., and Hooper, D. L., *J. Am. Oil Chem. Soc.*, 51, 42—49, 1974.
85. Morita, M. and Fujimaki, M., *J. Agric. Food Chem.*, 21, 860—863, 1973.
86. Morris, M. D., Chaikoff, I. L., Felts, J. M., Abraham, S., and Fansah, N. O., *J. Biol. Chem.*, 224, 1039—1045, 1957.
87. Wilson, J. D., *J. Lipid Res.*, 5, 409, 417, 1964.
88. Grundy, S. M., Ahrens, E. H., Jr., and Davignon, J., *J. Lipid Res.*, 10, 304—315, 1969.
89. Ivy, A. C., Lin, T., and Karvnen, E., *Am. J. Physiol.*, 183, 79—85, 1953.
90. Cousins, E. R., *J. Am. Oil Chem. Soc.*, 40, 206—210, 1963.
91. Daubert, B. F., *J. Am. Chem. Soc.*, 66, 290—292, 1944.
92. Daubert, B. F., Spiegel, C. J., and Longnecker, H. E., *J. Am. Chem. Soc.*, 65, 2144—2145, 1943.
93. Uri, N., *Autoxidation and Antioxidants*, Lundberg, W. O., Ed., Interscience, New York, 1961, 55—106.
94. Witting, L. A., *J. Amer. Oil Chem. Soc.*, 52, 64—68, 1975.
95. Mahoney, L. R., *Angew. Chem.*, 81, 555—561, 1969.
96. Boguth, W. and Niemann, H., *Biochim. Biophys. Acta*, 248, 121—130, 1971.
97. Csallany, A. S., *Int. J. Vitam. Nutr. Res.*, 41, 376—384, 1971.
98. Privett, O. S. and Nickell, C., *J. Am. Oil Chem. Soc.*, 33, 156—163, 1956.
99. Privett, O. S., *J. Am. Oil Chem. Soc.*, 36, 507—512, 1959.
100. Johnston, A. E., Zilch, K. T., Selke, E., and Dutton, H. J., *J. Am. Oil Chem. Soc.*, 38, 367—371, 1961.
101. Kokatnur, M. G., Bergman, J. G., and Draper, H. H., *Anal. Biochem.*, 12, 325—331, 1965.
102. Paschke, R. F. and Wheeler, D. H., *J. Am. Oil Chem. Soc.*, 25, 278—283, 1949.
103. Chang, S. S. and Kummerow, F. A., *J. Am. Oil Chem. Soc.*, 30, 251—254, 1953.
104. Chang, S. S. and Kummerow, F. A., *J. Am. Oil Chem. Soc.*, 30, 403—407, 1953.
105. Chang, S. S. and Kummerow, F. A., *J. Am. Oil Chem. Soc.*, 31, 324—327, 1954.
106. Witting, L. A., Chang, S. S., and Kummerow, F. A., *J. Am. Oil Chem. Soc.*, 34, 470—473, 1957.
107. Cobb, W. Y. and Day, E. A., *J. Am. Oil Chem. Soc.*, 42, 420—422, 1965.
108. Cobb, W. Y. and Day, E. A., *J. Am. Oil Chem. Soc.*, 42, 1110—1112, 1965.
109. Chang, S. S., Brobst, K. M., Tai, H., and Ireland, C. E., *J. Am. Oil Chem. Soc.*, 38, 671—674, 1961.
110. Chang, S. S., Krishnamurthy, R. G., and Reddy, B. R., *J. Am. Oil Chem. Soc.*, 44, 159—161, 1967.
111. Gaddis, A. M., Ellis, R., and Currie, G. T., *J. Am. Oil Chem. Soc.*, 38, 371—375, 1961.
112. Horvat, R. J., McFadden, W. H., Ng, H., Lane, W. G., and Shepherd, A. D., *J. Am. Oil Chem. Soc.*, 43, 350—351, 1966.
113. Horvat, R. J., McFadden, W. A., Ng, H., Lee, A., Fuller, G., and Applewhite, T. H., *J. Am. Oil Chem. Soc.*, 46, 273—276, 1969.
114. Horvat, R. J., McFadden, W. H., Ng, H., Black, D. R., Lane, W. G., and Teeter, R. M., *J. Am. Oil Chem. Soc.*, 42, 1112—1115, 1965.
115. Ng, H., Horvat, R. J., Lee, A., McFadden, W. H., Lane, W. G., and Shepherd, A. D., *J. Am. Oil Chem. Soc.*, 45, 708—709, 1968.
116. Keith, R. W. and Day, E. A., *J. Am. Oil Chem. Soc.*, 40, 121—124, 1963.

117. Kawada, T., Krishnamurthy, R. G., Mookherjee, B. D., and Chang, S. S., *J. Am. Oil Chem. Soc.*, 44, 131—315, 1967.
118. Krishnamurthy, R. G. and Chang, S. S., *J. Am. Oil Chem. Soc.*, 44, 136—140, 1967.
119. Meijboom, P. W. and Stroink, J. B. A., *J. Am. Oil Chem. Soc.*, 49, 555—558, 1972.
120. Hoffman, G. and Meijboom, P. W., *J. Am. Oil Chem. Soc.*, 45, 468—470, 1968.
121. Seals, R. G. and Hammond, E. G., *J. Am. Oil Chem. Soc.*, 47, 278—280, 1970.
122. Mookherjee, B. D. and Chang, S. S., *J. Am. Oil Chem. Soc.*, 40, 232—235, 1963.
123. Patton, S., Barnes, I. J., and Evans, L. E., *J. Am. Oil Chem. Soc.*, 36, 280—283, 1959.
124. Scholz, R. G. and Ptak, L. R., *J. Am. Oil Chem. Soc.*, 43, 596—599, 1966.
125. Smouse, T. H. and Chang, S. S., *J. Am. Oil Chem. Soc.*, 44, 509—514, 1967.
126. Lillard, D. A. and Day, E. A., *J. Am. Oil Chem. Soc.*, 41, 549—552, 1964.
127. Matthews, R. F., Scanlan, R. A., and Libbey, L. M., *J. Am. Oil Chem. Soc.*, 48, 745—747, 1971.
128. Johnson, O. C. and Kummerow, F. A., *J. Am. Oil Chem. Soc.*, 34, 407—409, 1957.
129. Perkins, E. G. and Van Akkeren, L. A., *J. Am. Oil Chem. Soc.*, 42, 782—786, 1965.
130. Miyakawa, T., *Fette, Seifen, Anstrichm.*, 66, 1048—1051, 1964.
131. Ota, S., Iwata, N., and Morita, M., *Yukagaku*, 13, 210—216, 1964.
132. Ota, S., Mukai, A., and Yamamoto, I., *Yukagaku*, 13, 264—269, 1964.
133. Endres, J. G., Bhalerao, V. R., and Kummerow, F. A., *J. Am. Oil Chem. Soc.*, 39, 159—162, 1962.
134. Wishner, L. A. and Keeney, M., *J. Am. Oil Chem. Soc.*, 42, 776—781, 1965.
135. Kawada, T., Krishnamurthy, R. G., Mookherjee, B. D., and Chang, S. S., *J. Am. Oil Chem. Soc.*, 44, 131—135, 1967.
136. Krishnamurthy, R. G. and Chang, S. S., *J. Am. Oil Chem. Soc.*, 44, 136—140, 1967.
137. Yasuda, K., Reddy, B. R., and Chang, S. S., *J. Am. Oil Chem. Soc.*, 45, 625—628, 1968.
138. Reddy, B. R., Yasuda, K., Krishnamurthy, R. G., and Chang, S. S., *J. Am. Oil Chem. Soc.*, 45, 629—631, 1968.
139. Chang, S. S. and Hsieh, A., *J. Am. Oil Chem. Soc.*, 51, 526A, 1974.
140. Michael, W. R., *Lipids*, 1, 365—368, 1966.
141. Scharmann, H., Eckert, W. R., and Zeman, A., *Fette, Seifen, Anstrichm.*, 71, 118—122, 1969.
142. Artman, N. R. and Alexander, J. C., *J. Am. Oil Chem. Soc.*, 45, 643—648, 1968.
143. Wantland, L. W. and Perkins, E. G., *Lipids*, 5, 191-200, 1970.
144. Perkins, E. G. and Anfinsen, J. R., *J. Am. Oil Chem. Soc.*, 48, 556—562, 1971.
145. Artman, N. R. and Smith, E. E., *J. Am. Oil Chem. Soc.*, 49, 318—326, 1972.
146. Aitzetmueller, K., *Fette, Seifen, Anstrichm.*, 75, 14—17, 1973.
147. Aitzetmueller, K., *Fette, Seifen, Anstrichm.*, 75, 256—260, 1970.
148. Harris, W. C., Crowell, E. P., and Burnett, B. B., *J. Am. Oil Chem. Soc.*, 50, 537—539, 1973.
149. Inoue, H., Kazuo, K., and Taniguchi, N., *J. Chromatogr.*, 47, 348—354, 1970.
150. Perkins, E. G., Taubold, R., and Heish, A., *J. Am. Oil Chem. Soc.*, 50, 223—225, 1973.
151. Firestone, D., *J. Am. Oil Chem. Soc.*, 40, 247—255, 1963.
152. Perkins, E. G. and Kummerow, F. A., *J. Am. Oil Chem. Soc.*, 36, 371—375, 1959.
153. Ohfuji, T. and Kaneda, T., *Lipids*, 8, 353—359, 1973.
154. Paulose, M. M. and Chang, S. S., *J. Am. Oil Chem. Soc.*, 50, 147—154, 1973.
155. Sahasrabudhe, M. R. and Bhalerao, V. R., *J. Am. Oil Chem. Soc.*, 40, 711—712, 1963.
156. Williamson, L., *J. Appl. Chem.*, 3, 301—307, 1953.
157. Frankel, E. N., Evans, C. D., and Cowan, J. C., *J. Am. Oil Chem. Soc.*, 37, 418—424, 1960.
158. Forss, D. A., *Prog. Chem. Fats Other Lipids*, 13, 204—208, 1972.
159. Jensen, R. G., *Prog. Chem. Fats Other Lipids*, 11, 347—394, 1971.
160. Brockerhoff, H. and Jensen, R. G., *Lipolytic Enzymes*, Academic Press, New York, 1974, 1—330.
161. Kavanagh, T. E., Reineccius, G. A., Keeney, P. G., and Weissberger, W., *J. Am. Oil Chem. Soc.*, 47, 344—346, 1970.
162. Kinsella, J. E., Patton, S., and Dimick, P. S., *J. Am. Oil Chem. Soc.*, 44, 449—454, 1967.
163. Talapatra, K., Studies on the Volatile Compounds in Aroma Fraction of Milk Caramel, Ph.D. thesis, Pennsylvania State University, University Park, 1974.
164. Lawrence, R. C. and Hawke, J. C., *Biochem., J.*, 98, 25—29, 1966.
165. Dimick, P. S. and Walker, H. M., *J. Dairy Sci.*, 51, 478—482, 1968.
166. Forney, F. W. and Markovetz, A. J., *J. Lipid Res.*, 12, 383—395, 1971.
167. Keeney, M. and Doan, F. J., *J. Dairy Sci.*, 34, 728—734, 1951.
168. Dimick, P. S., Walker, N. J., and Patton, S., *J. Agric. Food Chem.*, 17, 649—655, 1969.
169. Dimick, P. S., Patton, S., Kinsella, J. E., and Walker, N. J., *Lipids*, 1, 387—390, 1966.
170. Mattick, L. R., Patton, S., and Keeney, P. G., *J. Dairy Sci.*, 42, 791—798, 1959.
171. Boldingh, J. and Taylor, R. J., *Nature*, 194, 909—913, 1962.
172. Jarriens, G. and Oele, J. M., *Nature*, 207, 864—865, 1965.
173. Dimick, P. S. and Harner, J. L., *J. Dairy Sci.*, 51, 22—27, 1968.

174. Walker, N. J., Patton, S., and Dimick, P. S., *Biochem. Biophys. Acta,* 152, 445—453, 1968.
175. Tang, C. A. and Jennings, W. G., *J. Agric. Food Chem.,* 16, 252—254, 1968.
176. Dimick, P. S., Walker, N. J., and Patton, S., *Biochem. J.,* 111, 395—399, 1969.
177. Swenson, P. E. and Dimick, P. S., *Biochem. J.,* 125, 1139—1140, 1971.
178. Van der Ven, B., *Recl. Trav. Chim. Pays-Bas,* 83, 976—982, 1964.
179. Fioriti, J. A., Krampl, V., and Sims, R. J., *J. Am. Oil Chem. Soc.,* 44, 534—538, 1967.
180. Watanabe, K. and Sato, Y., *Agr. Biol. Chem.,* 34, 464, 472, 1970.
181. Van der Ven, B. and de Jong, K., *J. Am. Oil Chem. Soc.,* 47, 299—302, 1970.
182. Labuza, T. P., Tsuyuki, H., and Karel, M., *J. Am. Oil Chem. Soc.,* 46, 409—416, 1969.
183. Tjhio, K. H., Labuza, T. P., and Karel, M., *J. Am. Oil Chem. Soc.,* 46, 597—600, 1969.
184. Schauenstein, E., *J. Lipid Res.,* 8, 417—428, 1967.
185. Mabrouk, A. F., *J. Am. Oil Chem. Soc.,* 41, 331—334, 1964.
186. Coleman, J. E., Hampson, J. W., and Saunders, D. H., *J. Am. Oil Chem. Soc.,* 41, 347—351, 1964.
187. Dugan, L. R., Jr. and Landis, P. W., *J. Am. Oil Chem. Soc.,* 33, 152—154, 1956.
188. Slover, H. T. and Dugan, L. R., Jr., *J. Am. Oil Chem. Soc.,* 34, 333—335, 1957.
189. Chipault, J. R. and Mizuno, G. R., *J. Am. Oil Chem. Soc.,* 41, 468—473, 1964.
190. Kavalam, J. P. and Nanar, W. W., *J. Am. Oil Chem. Soc.,* 46, 387—390, 1969.
191. Rock, S. P. and Roth, H., *J. Am. Coil Chem. Soc.,* 41, 228—230, 1964.
192. Dornseifer, T. P., Kim, S. C., Keith, E. E., and Powers, J. J., *J. Am. Oil Chem. Soc.,* 42, 1073—1075, 1965.
193. Yuki, E., *Yukagaku,* 16, 654—658, 1967.
194. Rock, S. P. and Roth, H., *J. Am. Oil Chem. Soc.,* 43, 116—118, 1966.
195. Firestone, D., Nesheim, S., and Horowitz, W., *J. Assoc. Off. Agric. Chem.,* 44, 465—474, 1961.
196. Waltking, A. E. and Zmachinski, H., *J. Am. Oil Chem. Soc.,* 47, 530—534, 1970.
197. Freeman, I. P., Padley, F. B., and Shappard, W. L., *J. Am. Oil Chem. Soc.,* 50, 101—103, 1973.
198. Ryder, J. W. and Sullivan, G. P., *J. Am. Oil Chem. Soc.,* 39, 263—266, 1962.
199. Frankel, E. N., Evans, C. D., Moser, H. A., McConnell, D. G., and Cowan, J. C., *J. Am. Oil Chem. Soc.,* 38, 130—134, 1961.
200. McKinney, L. L., Picker, J. C., Jr., Weakly, F. B., Eldridge, A. C., Campbell, R. E., Cowan, J. C., and Biester, H. E., *J. Am. Chem. Soc.,* 81, 909—915, 1959.
201. Firestone, D., Horowitz, W., Friedman, L., and Shue, G. M., *J. Am. Oil Chem. Soc.,* 38, 418—422, 1961.
202. Higginbotham, G. R., Huang, A., Firestone, D., Verrett, J., Ress, J., Campbell, A. D., *Nature,* 220, 702, 1968.
203. Rich, A. D. and Greentree, A., *J. Am. Oil Chem. Soc.,* 35, 284, 287, 1958.
204. Van Den Bosch, G., *J. Am. Oil Chem. Soc.,* 50, 487—493, 1973.
205. White, F. B., *J. Am. Oil Chem. Soc.,* 33, 495—506, 1956.
206. Rini, S. S., *J. Am. Oil Chem. Soc.,* 37, 512—520, 1960.
207. Zehnder, C. T. and McMichael, C. E., *J. Am. Oil Chem. Soc.,* 44, 478A—512A, 1966.
208. Fiala, R. J., *J. Am. Oil Chem. Soc.,* 36, 375—379, 1959.
209. Chang, S. S., Masuda, Y., Mookherjee, B. D., and Silveira, A., Jr., *J. Am. Oil Chem. Soc.,* 40, 721, 724, 1963.
210. Merker, D. R. and Brown, L. C., *J. Am. Oil Chem. Soc.,* 33, 141—143, 1956.
211. Evans, C. D., Moser, H. A., List, G. R., Dutton, H. J., and Cowan, J. C., *J. Am. Oil Chem. Soc.,* 48, 711—714, 1971.
212. List, G. R., Hoffmann, R. L., Moser, H. A., and Evans, C. D., *J. Am. Oil Chem. Soc.,* 44, 485—487, 1967.
213. Sullivan, T. J., *J. Am. Oil Chem. Soc.,* 52, 3A, 1975.
214. Braun, W. Q., *J. Am. Oil Chem. Soc.,* 37, 598—601, 1960.
215. Eckey, E. W., *Ind. Eng. Chem.,* 40, 1138—1139, 1948.
216. Zalewski, S. and Gaddis, A. M., *J. Am. Oil Chem. Soc.,* 44, 576—580, 1967.
217. Jacobson, F., Nergaard, R., and Mathiesen, E., *E. Tids. Hermetikind,* 27, 225—266, 1941.
218. Privett, A. S., Pringle, R. B., and Farlane, W. D., *Oil Soap (Chicago),* 22, 287—289, 1945.
219. Crampton, E. W., Farmer, F. A., and Berryhill, F. M., *J. Nutr.,* 43, 431—440, 1951.
220. Crampton, E. W., Common, R. H., Farmer, F. A., Berryhill, F. M., and Wiseblatt, L., *J. Nutr.,* 43, 533—539, 1951.
221. Crampton, E. W., Common, R. H., Farmer, F. A., Berryhill, F. M., and Wiseblatt, L., *J. Nutr.,* 44, 177—189, 1951.
222. Crampton, E. W., Common, R. H., Farmer, F. A., Wells, A. F., and Crawford, D., *J. Nutr.,* 49, 333—346, 1953.
223. Crampton, E. W., Common, R. H., Pritchard, E. T., and Farmer, F. A., *J. Nutr.,* 60, 13—24, 1956.

224. Common, R. H., Crampton, E. W., Farmer, F. A., and De Freitas, A. S. W., *J. Nutr.*, 62, 341—347, 1957.

225. Wells, A. F., and Common, R. H., *J. Sci. Food Agric.*, 4, 233—237, 1953.

226. McInnes, A. G., Cooper, F. P., and MacDonald, J. A., *Can. J. Chem.*, 39, 1906—1914, 1961.

227. Nolen, G. A., Alexander, J. C., and Artman, N. R., *J. Nutr.*, 93, 337—348, 1967.

228. Roffo, A. H., *Bol. Inst. Med. Exp. Estud. Trat. Cancer Buenos Aires*, 14, 589—592, 1938.

229. Roffo, A. H., *Bol. Inst. Med. Exp. Estud. Trat. Cancer Buenos Aires*, 15, 407—529, 1939.

230. Roffo, A. H., *Prensa Med. Argent.*, 26, 619—648, 1939.

231. Roffo, A. H., *Bol. Inst. Med. Exp. Estud. Trat. Cancer Buenos Aires*, 19, 503—530, 1942.

232. Roffo, A. H., *Bol. Inst. Med. Exp. Estud. Trat. Cancer Buenos Aires*, 20, 471—486, 1943.

233. Roffo, A. H., *Bol. Inst. Med. Exp. Estud. Trat. Cancer Buenos Aires*, 21, 1—41, 1944.

234. Roffo, A. H., *Am. J. Dig. Dis.*, 13, 33—38, 1946.

235. Melnick, D., *J. Am. Oil Chem. Soc.*, 34, 578—582, 1957.

236. Melnick, D., *J. Am. Oil Chem. Soc.*, 34, 351—356, 1957.

237. Melnick, D., Luckman, F. H., and Gooding, C. M., *J. Am. Oil Chem. Soc.*, 35, 271—277, 1958.

238. Poling, C. E., Warner, W. D., Mone, P. E., and Rice, E. E., *J. Nutr.*, 72, 109—120, 1960.

239. Rice, E. E., Poling, C. E., Mone, P. E., and Warner, W. D., *J. Am. Oil Chem. Soc.*, 37, 607—613, 1960.

240. Poling, C. E., Warner, W. D., Mone, P. E., and Rice, E. E., *J. Am. Oil Chem. Soc.*, 39, 315—320, 1962.

241. Poling, C. E., Eagle, E., Rice, E. E., Durand, A. M. A., and Fisher, M., *Lipids*, 5, 128—136, 1970.

242. Nolen, G. A., *J. Nutr.*, 103, 1248—1255, 1973.

243. Wilson, R. H., De Eds, F., and Cox, A. J., *J. Cancer, Res.*, 1, 595—598, 1941.

244. Engel, R. W. and Copeland, D. H., *Cancer Res.*, 12, 905—908, 1952.

245. Witting, L. A., Nishida, T., Johnson, O. C., and Kummerow, F. A., *J. Am. Oil Chem. Soc.*, 34, 421—424, 1957.

246. Bunce, C. E. and King, K. W., *J. Nutr.*, 98, 168—176, 1969.

247. Kummerow, F. A., *Lipids and Their Oxidation*, Schultz, H. W., Day, E. A., Sinnhuber, R. O., Eds., Avi Publ., Westport, Conn., 1962, 294—320.

248. Dubouloz, P., Fondari, J., and Lagarde, C., *Biochim. Biophys. Acta*, 3, 371—377, 1949.

249. Dubouloz, P. and Laurent, J., *C. R. Seances Soc. Biol. Paris*, 144, 1183—1185, 1950.

250. Dubouloz, P., Dumas, J., and Laurent, J., *C. R. Seances Soc. Biol. Paris*, 145, 905—906, 1951.

251. Dubouloz, P., Laurent, J., and Dumas, J., *Bull. Soc. Chim. Biol.*, 33, 1740—1744, 1951.

252. Dubouloz, P. and Fondari, J., *Bull. Soc. Chim. Biol.*, 35, 819—826, 1953.

253. Dubouloz, P. and Laurent, J., *Bull. Soc. Chim. Biol.*, 35, 781—818, 1953.

254. Rotruck, J. T., Pope, A. L., Ganther, H. E., Swanson, A. B., Hafernan, D. G., and Hoekstra, W. G., *Science*, 179, 588—590, 1973.

255. Christopherson, B. O., *Biochim. Biophys. Acta*, 164, 35—46, 1968.

256. Andrews, J. S., Griffith, W. H., Mead, J. F., and Stein, R. S., *J. Nutr.*, 70, 199—210, 1960.

257. Glavind, J. and Tryding, N., *Acta Physiol. Scand.*, 49, 97—102, 1960.

258. Glavind, J., Sondergaard, E., and Dam, H., *Acta Pharmacol. Toxicol.*, 18, 267—277, 1961.

259. Bergan, J. G. and Draper, H. H., *Lipids*, 5, 976—982, 1970.

260. Bhalerao, V. R., Inoue, M., and Kummerow, F. A., *J. Dairy Sci.*, 46, 176—180, 1963.

261. Kaunitz, H. and Johnson, R. E., *J. Am. Oil Chem. Soc.*, 41, 50—52, 1964.

262. Gottenbos, J. J. and Thomasson, H. J., *Bibl. Nutr. Dieta*, 1, 110—129, 1965.

263. Lassen, S., Bacon, E. K., and Dunn, H. J., *Arch. Biochem. Biophys.*, 23, 1—7, 1949.

264. Johnson, O. C., Perkins, E., Sugai, M., and Kummerow, F. A., *J. Am. Oil Chem. Soc.*, 34, 594—597, 1957.

265. Kajimoto, G. and Mukai, K., *Yukagaku*, 19, 66—70, 1970.

266. Johnson, O. C., Sakuragi, T., and Kummerow, F. A., *J. Am. Oil Chem. Soc.*, 33, 433—435, 1956.

267. Perkins, E. G. and Kummerow, F. A., *J. Nutr.*, 68, 101—108, 1959.

268. Friedman, L., Horowitz, W., Shue, G. M., and Firestone, D., *J. Nutr.*, 73, 85—93, 1961.

269. Bottino, N. R., *J. Am. Oil Chem. Soc.*, 39, 25—29, 1962.

270. Czok, G., Griem, W., Kieckebusch, W., Baessler, K. H., and Lang, K., *Z. Ernaehrunsswiss.*, 5, 80—89, 1964.

271. Raju, N. B., Narayan, Rao, M., and Rajagopolan, R., *J. Am. Oil Chem. Soc.*, 42, 774—776, 1965.

272. Bottino, N. R., Anderson, R. E., and Reiser, R., *J. Am. Oil Chem. Soc.*, 42, 1124—1129, 1965.

273. Shue, G. M., Douglass, C. D., Firestone, D., Friedman, L., Friedman, L., and Sage, J. S., *J. Nutr.*, 94, 171—177, 1968.

274. Perkins, E. G., Vaccha, S. M., and Kummerow, F. A., *J. Nutr.*, 100, 725—731, 1970.

275. Van Tilborg, H., De Bruijn, J., Gottenbos, J., and Koch, G. K., *J. Am. Oil Chem. Soc.*, 47, 430—437, 1970.

276. Ohfuji, T., Iwamoto, S., and Kaneda, T., *Yukagaku*, 19, 887—890, 1970.

277. Ohfuki, T. and Kaneda, T., *Yukagaku*, 19, 486—489, 1970.

278. Matsuo, N., *Eiyo To Shokuryo*, 25, 579—589, 1972.

279. Govind Rao, M. K., Hemans, C., and Perkins, E. G., *Lipids*, 8, 342—347, 1973.

280. Hemans, C., Kummerow, F. A., and Perkins, E. G., *J. Nutr.*, 103, 1665—1672, 1973.

281. Kaunitz, H., Slanetz, C. A., Johnson, R. E., Knight, H. B., Saunders, D. H., and Swern, D., *J. Am. Oil Chem. Soc.*, 33, 630—634, 1956.

282. Kaunitz, H., Slanetz, C. A., Johnson, R. E., Knight, H. B., Koos, R. E., and Swern, D., *J. Am. Oil Chem. Soc.*, 36, 611—615, 1959.

283. Miller, J. and Landes, D. R., *J. Food Sci.*, 40, 545—548, 1975.

284. Kummerow, F. A., *J. Food Sci.*, 40, 12—17, 1975.

285. Arffmann, E., *J. Nat. Cancer Inst.*, 25, 893—926, 1960.

286. Lane, A., Blickenstaff, D., and Ivy, A. C., *Cancer (Brussels)*, 3, 1044—1051, 1950.

287. Sugai, M., Witting, L. A., Tsuchiyama, H., and Kummerow, F. A., *Cancer Res.*, 22, 510—519, 1962.

288. Miller, J. A., Cramer, J. W., and Miller, E. C., *Cancer Res.*, 20, 950—962, 1960.

289. Miller, E. C., Miller, J. A., and Hartman, H., *Cancer Res.*, 21, 815—824, 1964.

290. McLean, A. E. M. and Marshall, W. J., *Biochem. J.*, 123, 28P, 1971.

291. Marshall, W. J. and McLean, A. E. M., *Proc. Nutr. Soc.*, 30, 66A, 1971.

292. Marshall, W. J. and McLean, A. E. M., *Biochem. J.*, 122, 569—573, 1971.

293. Arrhenius, E., *Xenobiotica*, 1, 487—495, 1971.

294. Mitchell, J. R., Jollow, D. J., Gillete, J. R., and Brodie, B. B., *Drug Metab. Dispos.*, 1, 418—423, 1973.

295. National Diet-Heart Study, *Circulation Suppl.*, (1), 37, 1968.

296. American Medical Association, *J.A.M.A.*, 222, 1647, 1972.

297. Marx, J. L., *Science*, 187, 526, 1975.

298. Van Den Bosch, H., Slotboom, A. J., and Van Deenen, L. L. M., *Biochim. Biophys. Acta*, 176, 632—637, 1969.

299. Van Den Bosch, H., Van Golde, L. M. C., Slotboom, A. J., and Van Deenen, L. L. M., *Biochim. Biophys. Acta*, 152, 694—703, 1968.

300. Jones, P. D., Holloway, P. W., Peluffo, R. O., and Wakil, S. J., *J. Biol. Chem.*, 244, 744—754, 1969.

301. Pande, S. V. and Mead, J. F., *J. Biol. Chem.*, 243, 352—361, 1968.

302. Demel, R. A., Bruckdorfer, K. R., and Van Deenen, L. L. M., *Biochim. Biophys. Acta*, 255, 311—320, 1972.

303. De Kruyff, B., Demel, R. A., Slotboom, A. J., Van Deenen, L. L. M., *Biochim. Biophys. Acta*, 307, 1—19, 1973.

# EFFECT OF PROCESSING ON NUTRITIVE VALUE OF FOOD: PROTEIN

## J. Mauron

## INTRODUCTION

The general objective of food processing is to protect and preserve food, to destroy microorganisms, to inactivate enzymes, to destroy inhibitors and toxic substances, to augment digestibility, to maintain or improve organoleptic properties, and to produce more desirable physical functions and aesthetic characteristics. However, the pursuit of the primary effect in processing often results in unwanted secondary effects, the so-called processing damage.[1,224] Because protein plays an essential role in nutrition as purveyor of the essential amino acids, particular attention must be given to protein deterioration in food processing. The detection of this type of damage is of increasing importance if we are to maintain a satisfactory nutrition of the population, since most of our food at the present time is processed in one way or another.

The chapter will be divided into three parts that correspond to three approaches. The first, phenomenological approach will give a very brief survey of some main, food-processing operations and their impact on food proteins. The second, causal approach will give some insight into the chemical mechanisms involved, and the third approach will be a methodological expounding of the means available to detect protein damage.

## IMPACT OF SOME FOOD PROCESSING OPERATIONS ON PROTEIN QUALITY (PHENOMENOLOGICAL APPROACH)[225]

The key variables that influence protein quality during processing and that can be controlled in the manufacture of a good product are temperature, moisture content, pH, composition of food product, and composition of gaseous phase. Because of the overwhelming importance of water content during processing, we shall consider moist and dry heat applications separately.

### Heat Treatments in the Presence of Water
#### Boiling and Cooking
These are essentially household operations that are sometimes also used in the food industry but generally under better-controlled conditions. During the ordinary household cooking of fish and meat, there is no loss of protein quality and no diminution of the essential amino acid content, in spite of some losses in the extractable substances that contain practically no essential amino acids.[2,10] Boiling of milk does not affect either amino acid content or availability.[11]

Egg causes a special problem because of the different heat sensitivity of egg white and yolk. Raw egg white is not well-digested when consumed alone — the digestibility coefficient is of the order of 50% only, whereas egg yolk is fully digestible even in the raw state.[12] Soft-boiled egg has a digestibility coefficient and biological value of nearly 100[13] due to the beneficial effect of heat denaturation of the proteins.

The beneficial effect of moist heat is the general rule when considering most vegetable proteins, especially the different kinds of beans, since it is common knowledge that very prolonged cooking is necessary to take full dietary benefits of a bean dish.[14,15] The increased nutritive value of heated legumes is mainly due to three factors: the denaturation of the proteins, the destruction of antidigestive and toxic factors, and the disruption of the vegetable tissues and starch granules.

*Pasteurization of Milk*

It is generally agreed that the heat required for normal pasteurization, whether by the "holder" method (143°F for 10 min) or the high-temperature short-time (HTST) procedures (161°F for 15 sec) has but little effect on milk proteins, except for partial denaturation of the whey proteins.[16,17,18] The nutritive value of milk proteins is not affected, as shown by numerous studies in infants,[19] school children, adults, and laboratory animals.[20,21] The term "pasteurization" is often used in a broader sense for any heat treatment intended to destroy all pathogenic germs. Pasteurization of milk at 110°C for 2 min does not effect amino acid availability.[11] The same is true of uperization (150°C for 2.4 sec).[1]

*Sterilization*

For sterilization to be successful, it depends upon the application of sufficient heat to a sealed container to render the content sterile. The intensity of the heat treatment depends very much on the physical state of the food. In fact, the heat transfer from the walls of the container to the center of the product in conventional heat sterilization is much less in the case of semisolid goods than it is with fluid material, which acts as the heat-transfer medium. New techniques, such as dithermal and electronic heating as well as aseptic canning, tend to circumvent these difficulties, but their use is still rather limited.

**Milk** — Conventional sterilization of fluid milk does reduce its biological value by 6%,[25] and there is a 10% drop in lysine and 13% in cystin content.[23,24] The drop in biological value is probably due to the drop in cystin content.

**Evaporated milk** — When conventional sterilization is applied to precondensed milk, as in evaporated milk manufacture, the heat effect on the milk protein is more pronounced. A loss of available lysine of 15 to 25% was found in conventional evaporated milk, whereas in a sweetened, condensed milk submitted to the same treatments (excluding, of course, the final sterilization) no change in amino acid availability was observed.[11] In spite of this average 20% loss in available lysine, evaporated milk shows the same protein efficiency ratio as sweetened, condensed milk when tested in a diet containing a methionine addition to compensate for the slight cystine loss in evaporated milk. When evaporated milk was compared to sweetened, condensed milk as a supplement to wheat flour, however, it was found to be inferior.[26] The explanation is that the 20% loss of available lysine in evaporated milk does not affect the protein value when milk is the only protein source because of the excess of lysine in milk, whereas in a diet in which lysine is limiting, this loss is great enough to lower the protein efficiency ratio. This explains why, in most studies on the nutritive value of evaporated milk, no or only very slight differences are found between evaporated milk and raw or pasteurized milk.[27-32]

Hodson[33] concluded from a very extensive rat growth study that there was about 10% loss in protein efficiency ratio due to sterilization in evaporated milk and that this effect is due to the loss in cystine. Indeed, when sulfur amino acids such as methionine are added to the diet, the reduction in the protein efficiency ratio observed in evaporated milk disappears.

**Meat** — In canning meat for human consumption the conventional conditions are generally more severe than in the case of milk preserves because the heat transfer through the solid or semisolid mass is more difficult. Commercial heat-processing methods applied in canning meat do not destroy significant amounts of amino acids other than cystine.[34-36]

Nevertheless, it has been observed that canning can lead to a small decrease in digestibility of beef protein from 98 to 94% and to a slight lowering of biological value (6 to 9%).[37] In other studies a small reduction in the availability of lysine and methionine

### Table 1
### MAIN THERMAL PROCESSING OPERATIONS IN THE PRESENCE OF WATER

| Treatment | Temperature | Time | Water | Effect on proteins | | | Ref. |
|---|---|---|---|---|---|---|---|
| | | | | Structure | Composition | Nutritive value | |
| Cooking and boiling | 100°C | Variable | Excess | Denaturation | Not affected | Increased digestibility (often) no or insignificant reduction of biological value | 1—15 |
| **Milk** | | | | | | | |
| Pasteurization | 61—65°C 71—73°C | 30 min 15 sec | 87% 87% | Denaturation of whey proteins (partial, ~10%) | Not affected | Not affected | 16—18 19—21 |
| Superpasteurization | 80—110°C | 2 min | 87% | Denaturation of whey proteins | Not affected | | 11 |
| Uperization | 150°C | 2.4 sec | 87% | Denaturation of whey proteins | Amino acid availability not changed | Not affected | 1 |
| Ultra-high temperature Stream injection | 150°C | 5,10,20 sec | 87% | (Denat. of whey proteins) | No destruction of cystine + methionine No lysine blocked | Not affected | 218 |
| Ultra-high temperature and sterilization | 130—150°C 110—112°C | 1 sec 15—20 min | 87% 87% | Denaturation of whey proteins, 70% Denaturation of whey proteins, 75% | Small reduction in availability of lysine and methionine | Small loss in digestibility and biological value | 18, 22 |
| Sterilization (bottles) | 118—122°C | 14—20 min | 87% | Denaturation of whey proteins, 75% | 10% Loss in lysine, 13% Destruction cystine | 6% Drop in biological value | 18, 23—25 |
| Sterilization of evaporated milk (cans) | 113°C | 15 min | 74% | Denaturation of whey proteins | 15—25% Drop in lysine availability | Slight or no drop in biological value. Inferior as supplement to wheat | 11, 26—33 |

Table 1 (continued)

## MAIN THERMAL PROCESSING OPERATIONS IN THE PRESENCE OF WATER

| Treatment | Temperature | Time | Water | Effect on proteins | | | Ref. |
|---|---|---|---|---|---|---|---|
| | | | | Structure | Composition | Nutritive value | |
| | | | | **Meat** | | | |
| Canning (sterilization) | Conventional conditions<br>235—250°F | 30—180 min according to can size | >60% | Denaturation | Almost no destruction of amino acids; small drop in cystine and in availability of lysine + methionine | Small drop in digestibility; 4%<br>Small drop in biological value (6—9%) | 34—40 |
| | | | | **Fish** | | | |
| Canning | Conventional conditions<br>235—250°F | 30—180 min according to can size | >60% | Denaturation | No destruction of amino acids | Slight drop in nutritive value (<10%) | 35—36 |

was observed for canned meat as compared to fresh meat,[38-40] and this small loss in amino acid availability may explain the lowering of biological value observed by other authors.[37] Similar observations were made with canned fish.[7,35-36] A summary of the preceding material is found in Table 1.

*Moist Heat Treatments of Vegetable Protein Sources*

In contrast to what is found with most animal protein foods — in which sterilization has a tendency to lower the biological value of the protein — autoclaving under certain conditions is beneficial to most vegetable protein sources, not only because of increased digestibility but also because of the destruction of naturally present antinutritional factors.[41,226]

**Soybeans** — Soybeans have been extensively studied, and it has been well-established that heat treatment is necessary in order to derive their full nutritional benefit. Soybean processing has reached a high degree of sophistication, but the essential fact that some moisture is indispensable for heat treatment to be effective was settled long ago.[42] It should be noticed that the relatively small amount of moisture present in the raw beans is sufficient to improve the nutritive value upon heating. Development of new equipment for soybean processing such as extrusion cooking allows more accurate control of moisture content and exact timing of the heat application so as to obtain optimal nutritive quality. In fact, in transgressing the optimal conditions and in applying excessive heat, the nutritive value of soy may be diminished, as is the case with animal protein foods. Thus it has been shown that overheating soy resulted in a reduction of nutritive value accompanied by a reduced availability of several amino acids but more particularly lysine and arginine.[43]

Studies with soy product heating must consider the inactivation of naturally occurring toxicants, such as the trypsin inhibitor, as well as nutritional heat damage. It would be useful to design a process that accomplishes this destruction with minimal damage. The data for heat damage[44] (lysine loss) indicate that the reaction rate constant assuming a first order reaction is 0.166 per hour with an activation energy of 30 kcal/g-mol in the wet state. The destruction of trypsin inhibitor occurs at a rate approximately 100 times faster with an activation energy of 18.5 kcal/g-mol.[45] Because lysine is more sensitive to the ultimate temperature reached (higher activation energy), trypsin inhibitor destruction should be performed at the lowest temperature possible. Data of Hackler et al.[45] substantiate this (Table 2). The PER (protein efficiency ratio) actually reflects the destruction of the sulfur-containing amino acids (cystine) which are limiting, but it can be used as an index of lysine loss in dried soy milk. During spray-drying experiments, trypsin inhibitor destruction increases as the air inlet temperature increases. The PER shows only small changes until the temperature of 277°C is reached but drops dramatically upon further temperature increase. When considering the balance between trypsin inhibitor destruction and PER decrease, an air inlet temperature of 227°C is optimum. The data also show that drum drying in air results in a significant reduction in trypsin inhibitor without affecting PER.

**Sunflower protein** — In this case, the nutritive value is again increased by moderate heating, whereas prolonged heating decreases the availability of lysine, arginine, and tryptophan.[46]

**Oilseed processing** — In this technology, heat is applied in the cooking stage and in the mechanical or hydraulic oil-extraction step. Moisture is relatively low in these operations, starting with the natural moisture content of the initial goods of 6 to 15% and ending with a moisture level of 4 to 3% in the final meal.

**Peanut oil meal** — Lysine availability was found to diminish with increasing heat treatment as did net protein utilization (NPU). The correlation is represented in Figure

## Table 2
## EFFECT OF PROCESSING SOY MILK[45]

| Process | Temperature | Duration (minutes) | Trypsin inhibitor retained (%) | Available lysine (g/16 g N) | PER |
|---|---|---|---|---|---|
| Cooking | | | | | |
| | 121°C | 0 | 100 | 6.0 | 0.65 |
| | 121°C | 4 | 20 | 5.8 | 2.21 |
| | 121°C | 8 | 16 | 5.7 | 2.20 |
| | 121°C | 16 | 12 | 5.8 | 2.11 |
| | 121°C | 32 | 5 | 5.6 | 1.97 |
| Spray-drying[a] (air inlet) | | | | | |
| | 166°C | | 10 | 5.4 | 2.22 |
| | 182°C | | 8 | 5.3 | 2.10 |
| | 227°C | | 4 | 4.9 | 1.99 |
| | 277°C | | 5 | 4.0 | 1.63 |
| | 316°C | | 3 | 1.9 | 0.16 |
| Drum drying[a] (drum temperature) | | | | | |
| Air | 150°C | | 5 | 5.5 | 2.19 |
| Vacuum drum | 108°C | | 10 | 5.3 | 2.22 |
| Freeze drying | — | | 10 | 5.6 | 2.14 |

[a]   Milk previously cooked at 121°C for 10 min. 15% inhibitor retention.

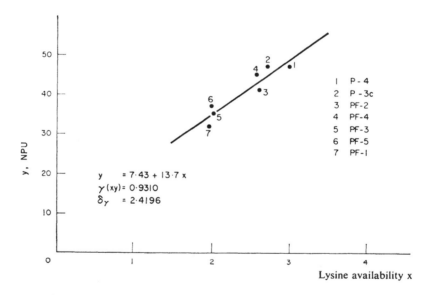

FIGURE 1.   Correlation between lysine availability (x) and NPU (y). x, available lysine g/16 g nitrogen; y, NPU; P, raw peanuts; PF, peanut meals. (From Mauron, J. and Mottu, F., *Ann. Nutr. Aliment.*, 14, 314, 1960. With permission.)

1. Although the sulfur amino acids are limiting in the raw peanuts, lysine becomes limiting in severely heated peanut meal.[49]

**Cottonseed oil meal**[47,48] — An enormous, potential protein source for developing countries is represented by cottonseed oil meal, a rather well-balanced protein. However, raw or unsufficiently cooked cottonseed meal is toxic to monogastric animals, although it can be made harmless by cooking. Prolonged, intense heating, on the other hand, impairs the nutritive value. A simplified explanation is that cottonseed meal contains a toxic factor, the aldehyde gossypol. This component is inactivated or detox-

Table 3
## AVAILABLE LYSINE LEVELS IN COTTONSEED MEALS PRODUCED BY DIFFERENT PROCESSING METHODS[48,51]

(g/16 g N)

| Screw press (commercial) | Prepress solvent extraction (commercial) | Hexane extraction (commercial) | Azeotrope extraction (acetone-hexane-water) (pilot plant) |
|---|---|---|---|
| 2.59 | 3.14 | 3.30 | 4.23 |
| 3.07 | 3.21 | 3.31 | 4.18 |
| 2.70 | 3.38 | 3.20 | 4.15 |
| 2.22 | 3.52 | 3.75 | 4.25 |
| 3.11 | 3.36 | 3.12 | 4.28 |

Table 4
## COMPARISON OF ACETONE-HEXANE-WATER AZEOTROPE AND COMMERCIAL HEXANE IN THE EXTRACTION OF COTTONSEED[48,53]

|  | Hexane extraction | Azeotrope extraction |
|---|---|---|
| Yield of neutral oil per ton of kernels (1b) | 494 | 512 |
| Residual oil in meal (%) | 1 | 0.1 |
| Total gossypol in meal (%) | 1.3 | 0.1—0.4 |
| Mortalities in swine receiving cottonseed meal (to market weight at 200 lb) (%) | 100 | 0.0 |

ified by heat in being bound to the protein, but the latter is damaged by this process, resulting in an inactivation of the free $\varepsilon$-amino groups of lysine.[50] Processing cottonseed meal in order to obtain an optimal nutritive value of the protein is therefore very tricky and must be elaborated for each type of cottonseed. Solvent extraction is now widely used for oil production, but in commercial operations the cooking stage remains necessary. Thus, lysine availability is still reduced and total gossypol high. Azeotrope extraction of the raw cottonseed flakes allows substantial reduction of the gossypol content without damaging lysine[51] (Table 3). The superiority of these azeotrope-extracted meals has been established[52] (Table 4).

## Dry Heat Application and Dehydration
It is difficult to draw a clear-cut dividing line between moist and dry heat treatments since, strictly speaking, we are always dealing with moist heat of some kind. This is even more obvious for dehydration, in which the initial heat is applied in the liquid state. What characterizes these heat treatments, however, is that the foodstuff reaches moisture values below 5% at the end of the procedure.

### Dehydration of Milk
Milk and milk products lend themselves to dehydration, which always involves some heat treatments. The two classical conventional dehydration procedures are roller-drying and spray-drying. The effect of these treatments on the nutritive value of the proteins in milk powder has been the object of considerable investigation and much controversy[1,62] (Tables 5 and 6). There are two main reasons for this. First, roller-

Table 5
## IN VITRO LYSINE AVAILABILITY IN MILK POWDERS

| | Destruction[a] (%) | Inactivation[b] (%) | Deterioration[c] (%) | Availability[d] (%) |
|---|---|---|---|---|
| Fresh milk reference value | 0 | 0 | 0 | 100 |
| Spray-dried milk reference value | 3.6 | −3.6 | 0 | 100 |
| Spray-dried milk | — | — | 0 | 100 |
| Roller-dried milk I[e] | 9.3 | 9.0 | 18.3 | 81.7 |
| Roller-dried milk II | 13.2 | 20.0 | 33.2 | 66.8 |
| Roller-dried milk III | 14.6 | 20.0 | 34.6 | 65.4 |
| Roller-dried milk IV | 17.0 | 29.3 | 46.3 | 53.7 |
| Roller-dried milk V | — | — | 62.9 | 37.1 |
| Roller-dried milk VI | 26.6 | 45.8 | 72.4 | 27.6 |

[a]  Difference between lysine content of fresh milk and that of the sample, determined after acid hydrolysis, expressed in percent of lysine content of fresh milk.
[b]  Difference between lysine deterioration and destruction (exclusively analytical concept).
[c]  Difference between amount of lysine liberated enzymically from fresh milk and that freed from the sample, expressed in percent of lysine liberated from fresh milk (= lysine made unavailable).
[d]  Lysine freed enzymically from sample, expressed as percent of lysine liberated from fresh milk.
[e]  Roman numerals indicate increasing heat treatment.

From Mauron, J., Mottu, F., Bujard, E., and Egli, R. H., *Arch. Biochem.*, 59(2), 444, 1955. With permission.

drying can be performed under a great variety of conditions using fluid milk on the drums or a precondensate, resulting in various degrees of heat damage. Second, milk dehydration essentially damages the amino acid lysine, which is not the limiting amino acid in milk protein. Since the usual methods of protein evaluation in fact measure the influence of the limiting amino acid, there is no wonder that, up to a certain point, lysine deterioration in milk powder does not influence classic nutritive value. According to Mauron and Mottu, who were using scorched, roller-dried milk powders, this happens when lysine availability has dropped to a level of about 30%[58] (Figure 2). Finally, it should be mentioned that storage of milk powder may provoke a continued drop in lysine availability. Under proper conditions this drop is small, but it is more pronounced for roller-dried powder than for spray-dried milk.[59]

### Dehydration of Eggs

It can be stated that in dehydrated egg, the rapid loss of functional properties upon improper processing precludes important nutritional damage in commercially attractive samples.[1,21]

### Dehydration of Meat and Fish

Commercial heat dehydration of meat is not extensively practiced at the present time because the products cannot rival other processed foods in quality and consumer acceptability at competitive prices. It may be said that only under the best possible conditions does conventional thermal meat dehydration cause no loss in protein value, but in general, freeze-dried meat is superior in nutrient content (including amino acids) to thermally processed or irradiated products.[63] Unfortunately, the superior quality of the freeze-dried products is not permanent but is subject to change during storage, which is quite critical for meat products.[64]

## Table 6
## THE EFFECT OF MILK DEHYDRATION

| Sample | Loss in available lysine (or content) (%) | Loss in methionine content (or availability) (%) | Nutritive value | Ref. |
|---|---|---|---|---|
| Spray-dried whole milk | 0—3.6 | 0 (Availability) | No reduction | 11, 58 |
| | 0—4.1 | — | — | 54 |
| | 3—10 | 0 | — | 18 |
| | — | — | No modification in biological value (N-balance) | 56 |
| Spray-dried whole milk without preheating | — | — | No modification in biological value (N-balance) | 55 |
| Skim milk powder (spray-dried) | 0 (Content) | — | No modification in PER[a] | 60 |
| Instantized skim milk powder | 0—3.1 (Content) | 0—4.9 | — | 61 |
| Spray-dried whey powder | — | — | Digestibility: 93.1—99.3 (egg = 100) | 57 |
| | — | — | Biological value: 91.0—93.9 (egg = 100) | 57 |
| Drum-dried whole milk[b] | 18.3—33.2 | 0—11 (Availability) | Decrease in PER 0—8% | 11, 58 |
| | 3—16 | — | — | 54 |
| | 5—40 | 0—10 (Availability) | — | 18 |
| | — | — | 8—30% Loss in biological value | 55 |
| | 2—23 | — | Reduced growth (3—25%) | 59 |
| | — | — | No modification in biological value (N-balance) | 56 |
| Drum-dried skim milk | | | | |
| Fresh milk sprayed on the roller | 0 (Content) | — | No reduction in growth test | 60 |
| Conventional (milk picked up from trough) | 20 (Content) | — | Reduced growth only when fed as supplement in lysine-deficient diets | 60 |
| Drum-dried whey powder | — | — | Digestibility: 74.9—81.3 (egg = 100) | 57 |
| | — | — | Biological value: 81.8—82.7 | 57 |

[a]  PER = protein efficiency ratio.
[b]  Drum = roller.

**Fish** — Dehydration of fish is performed on a huge scale to produce fish meal as animal feed, but only insignificant amounts are so far used in human foods. A great variety of methods exists to dehydrate fish (flame-drying, steam-tube drying, solvent

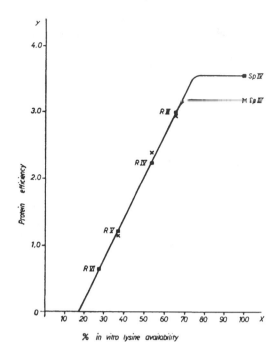

FIGURE 2. Relationship between PER and lysine availability. Sp, spray-dried milk; R, roller-dried milk; ■, DL-methionine supplement 0.2%; x, no methionine added. Each point represents the mean PER obtained with four rats. A difference of 0.338 PER unit between two means is significant at the 5% level. (From Mauron, J. and Mottu, F., *Arch. Biochem. Biophys.*, 77(2), 322, 1958. With permission.)

drying, etc.), so that a general statement about the protein quality of conventional dehydrated fish cannot be made. Evidence for damage to the proteins is reported in the older literature,[65,66] and the mechanism of damage has been extensively studied in laboratory samples produced by prolonged heating.[67-70] The laboratory studies on fish meal reveal the existence of two mechanisms of heat damage: one involving the fat part of the meal, the other independent of the presence of fat.[71] The former occurs at temperatures below 100°C, and lysine is lost by reaction with autoxidizing fat. The latter reaction occurs at high temperatures between 115 and 130°C, and the lysine loss, although greatly increased, is not influenced by fat content.

Myklestad et al.[72] heated fish meal prepared from herring at different temperatures, times, and moisture contents. The results (Table 7) show that a substantial decrease in available lysine only occurred when moisture content of the meal during heating was higher than 10%. In vivo studies, however, have shown only an insignificant loss in nutritive value because lysine is not limiting in fish meal.

However, these specially prepared samples are not representative of the meals processed by sound manufacturing practices. The latter results in uniform products, even when quite different processing methods are used, as shown in the study of Njaa et al.[73] on the protein quality of Norwegian herring meal (Table 8).

*Freeze Dehydration*

Although most foodstuffs are still dried by conventional means, freeze dehydration tends to gain importance in the preparation of heat-labile foodstuffs, delicacies, and

Table 7
EFFECT OF HEAT AND MOISTURE ON FISH MEAL[72,90]

| Conditions of treatment | | | Available lysine | NPU[a] | |
|---|---|---|---|---|---|
| Temperature (°C) | Moisture (%) | Time (min) | (%) | Rats | Chicks |
| 96 | 7.7 | 30 | 94 | — | 98.6 |
| | 8.8 | 60 | 96 | — | 102.0 |
| | 10.8 | 120 | 87 | — | 98.1 |
| | 36.8 | 60 | 87 | 97.7 | 98.6 |
| 116 | 6.4 | 120 | 94 | 95.3 | 96.8 |
| | 7.5 | 60 | 100 | 97.0 | 98.8 |
| | 8.4 | 30 | 96 | 97.4 | 99.7 |
| 132 | 2.5 | 120 | 97 | 91.8 | 97.1 |

[a]  NPU = net protein utilization.

complete dishes. Numerous investigations[74,75] show that proper application of lyophilization techniques will not damage the protein quality of foodstuffs (Table 9). However, it should be borne in mind that the superior qualities of the freeze-dried products are not permanent but are subject to change during storage.[76]

*Baking, Toasting, and Puffing of Cereals*

In baking and toasting, dry heat is applied, so that the moisture content of the baked goods rapidly decreases and might eventually reach levels at which heat damage to proteins becomes important. Loss of protein value in baking is especially severe in the crust, so the global loss in cookies and biscuits is very much dependent upon the thickness of the baked goods, as shown by the loss of available amino acids in biscuits as a function of thickness, heat intensity, and duration[77] (Table 10). The presence of sugar is still another factor influencing heat damage in biscuits, since it increases the loss in available lysine.[78] In ordinary bread 10 to 15% of lysine is lost in baking with a further loss of 5% as the bread turns stale. The greatest loss takes place in the crust.[79,80]

The ready-to-eat breakfast cereals are extremely popular in many countries. Some of these cereal products are submitted to intensive heat during processing (toasting, puffing) resulting in losses in the protein value (Table 11).[81,82] This is due to a sharp drop in lysine availability, whereas lysine content is much less affected. "Explosion puffing" of cereals also causes heavy losses in nutritive value of the proteins.[83] However, since the overall contribution of these puffed breakfast cereals to the protein intake of the Western populations is so small, the loss of biological value in the toasting operation is really not very significant in any practical sense.

**Newer Technological Processes Involving Alkaline Treatments**

There is an increased use in recent years of protein isolates in food technology. The isolates are produced by alkaline solubilization of oilseed protein, fish protein, etc., and by precipitation by acid or heat. These protein isolates may be used directly in food or be further transformed by sophisticated technologies such as spinning.[84] The latter procedure necessitates the solubilization of the protein at pH's slightly above 12.

It is therefore important to know that experiments by de Groot and Slump[85] have shown that strong alkali treatment of several types of food proteins such as casein, groundnut meal, and soy protein resulted in decreased protein quality, loss of amino acids, and formation of a new, unusual amino acid called lysinoalanine (LAL). These effects became more severe with increasing severity of alkali treatments such as higher

Table 8
NUTRITIVE VALUE OF HERRING MEALS PRODUCED BY DIFFERENT METHODS[73]

| Experiment number | Type of meal | Concentration of stickwater | Number of driers | Type of driers | NaNO$_2$[a] | HCHO[a] | BHT[a] | Light petrol extracted[a] | Nutritive value | |
|---|---|---|---|---|---|---|---|---|---|---|
| | | | | | | | | | Digestibility (apparent) | NPU |
| 1 | W[b] | — | 1 | Vacuum | | | | | 81.7 | 56.9 |
| | P[c] | — | 1 | Flame | | | | | 79.1 | 56.8 |
| | W | Pressure | 1 | Flame | | | | | 77.8 | 53.6 |
| | | Not concentrated | 2 | Flame | | | | | 78.1 | 52.1 |
| | | Pressure | 1 | Steam | | | | | 82.7 | 55.7 |
| | Control Ea[d] | | | | | | | | 82.6 | 68.0 |
| 2 | W | Vacuum | 1 | Flame | | | | | 84.3 | 57.1 |
| | P | | | Steam | | | | | 82.6 | 59.4 |
| | | — | 1 | Steam | | | | | 83.6 | 63.9 |
| | Control Ea | | | | | | | | 81.6 | 84.8 |
| 3 | W | Vacuum | 2 | Flame | — | — | | | 81.6 | 61.4 |
| | | Not concentrated | 2 | Flame | + | + | | | 78.8 | 55.9 |
| | | Vacuum | 1 | Flame | + | — | | | 82.1 | 59.6 |
| | | Pressure | 1 | Flame | — | + | | | 78.6 | 58.5 |
| | | Vacuum | 1 | Flame | — | — | | | 75.9 | 66.6 |
| 4 | W | Vacuum | 1 | Flame | + | — | | | 76.5 | 64.0 |
| 6 | W | Vacuum | 1 | Flame | | | — | — | 79.5 | 62.9 |
| | | | | | | | + | — | 80.0 | 64.9 |
| | | | | | | | + | + | 80.0 | 66.9 |
| | Control Ea | — | | | | | | | 83.8 | 91.3 |

a  +, with treatment; —, without treatment.
b  W = whole meal.
c  P = press cake meal.
d  Ea = spray-dried egg albumin.

From Njaa, L. R., Utne, F., and Braekkan, O. R., in *Proc. 7th Int. Congr. Nutrition*, Vol. 5, Kühnau, J., Ed., Vieweg und Sohn Gmbh, Brunswick, West Germany, 1967, 219. With permission.

### Table 9
### THE PROTEIN QUALITY OF SOME FREEZE-DRIED FOODS

| Food | Protein efficiency ratio (PER) |
|------|--------------------------------|
| Casein standard | 3.28 |
| Frozen shrimp | 3.02 |
| Freeze-dried shrimp | 3.24 |
| Frozen crab meat | 3.11 |
| Freeze-dried crab meat | 3.51 |
| Frozen chicken meat | 3.36 |
| Freeze-dried chicken meat | 3.29 |

Adapted from Goldblith, S. A., in *Aspects Théoriques et Industriels de la Lyophilisation,* Rey, L., Ed., Hermann, Paris, 1964, 569. With permission.

### Table 10
### LOSS OF AMINO ACID AVAILABILITY IN BISCUITS[77]

| Sample | Baking conditions | | | Percent loss in availability | | |
|--------|-------------------|---|---|------------------------------|---|---|
| | Thickness (mm) | Temperature (°C) | Duration (min) | Tryptophan | Methionine | Lysine |
| P[a] | — | — | — | 0 | 4 | 3 |
| F₁[b] | 4.9 | ~140 | 8 | 8 | 15 | 27 |
| F₂ | 3.7 | ~140 | 8 | 28 | 34 | 48 |
| F₃ | 4.0 | ~170 | 5 | 10 | 18 | 23 |
| F₄ | 3.8 | ~170 | 8 | 44 | 48 | 61 |
| F₅ | 7.6 | ~170 | 16 | 13 | 17 | 22 |

[a]   P = cooked and kneaded mass.
[b]   F = oven baked biscuits.

### Table 11
### THE NUTRITIVE VALUE OF CEREALS[82]

| Sample | PER |
|--------|-----|
| Boiled wheat | 1.78 |
| Cracked wheat, raw | 1.68 |
| Cracked wheat, toasted (200°C) | 1.12 |
| Puffed wheat | 0.69 |
| Rice, uncooked | 1.41 |
| Puffed rice | 0.55 |
| Corn, uncooked | 1.20 |
| Corn, toasted (150°C) | 0.82 |
| Gluten, uncooked | 1.39 |
| Gluten, toasted (150°C) | 0.96 |

pH and temperature and longer time of exposure. Later, the presence of LAL was confirmed in commercial samples of soy protein, first in $\alpha$-protein,[86] an unedible industrial soy preparation and later in edible, commercial, soy protein isolates[87] (Table 12).

It has been reported that, in addition to the loss in nutritive value, the presence of

Table 12
RESULTS OF LAL ASSAYS IN HOME-COOKED FOODS, FOOD
INGREDIENTS, AND COMMERCIAL FOOD PREPARATIONS[87]

| Name | Origin | LAL (μg/g proteins) |
|---|---|---|
| | **Home-cooked Food** | |
| Frankfurter | As purchased, before heating | None |
| | Boiled | 50 |
| | Fried | 50 |
| | Oven baked | 170 |
| | Charcoal broiled | 150 |
| Chicken thigh | Raw | None |
| | Charcoal broiled | 150 |
| | Retorted | 100 |
| | Cooked in microwave oven | 200 |
| | Oven baked | 110 |
| | Retorted in gravy | 170 |
| Pan scrapings | Pan frying of sirloin steak | 130 |
| Egg white | Fresh | None |
| | Boiled 3 min | 140 |
| | Boiled 10 min | 270 |
| | Boiled 30 min | 370 |
| | Pan fried 10 min at 150°C | 350 |
| | Pan fried 30 min at 150°C | 1,100 |
| | **Commercial Food Preparations** | |
| Corn chips | Commercial sample | 390 |
| Pretzels | Commercial sample | 500 |
| Hominy | Commercial sample | 560 |
| Tortillas | Commercial sample | 200 |
| Taco shells | Commercial sample | 170 |
| Milk, infant formula | Commercial sample, manufacturer A, batch 1 | 330 |
| | Commercial sample, manufacturer B, batch 1 | 550 |
| | Commercial sample, manufacturer A, batch 2 | 150 |
| | Commercial sample, manufacturer A, batch 3 | 640 |
| | Commercial sample, manufacturer B, batch 2 | 510 |
| | Commercial sample, manufacturer C | 490 |
| Milk, evaporated | Commercial sample, manufacturer D | 860 |
| | Commercial sample, manufacturer E | 590 |
| Milk, skim, evaporated | Commercial sample, manufacturer D | 520 |
| Milk, condensed | Commercial sample, manufacturer F | 540 |
| | Commercial sample, manufacturer G | 360 |
| Simulated cheese | Commercial sample, manufacturer H | 1,070 |
| | **Food Ingredients** | |
| Egg white solids, dried | Commercial sample, manufacturer I | 1,820 |
| | Commercial sample, manufacturer J | 1,530 |
| | Commercial sample, manufacturer K | 490 |
| | Commercial sample, manufacturer L | 160 |
| Calcium caseinate[a] | Commercial sample, supplier M | 1,000 |
| | Commercial sample, supplier N | 370 |
| Sodium caseinate | Commercial sample, supplier O | 600 |
| | Commercial sample, supplier P | 6,900 |
| | Commercial sample, supplier Q | 1,190 |
| | Commercial sample, supplier R | 430 |
| | Commercial sample, supplier S | 800 |

## Table 12 (continued)
### RESULTS OF LAL ASSAYS IN HOME-COOKED FOODS, FOOD INGREDIENTS, AND COMMERCIAL FOOD PREPARATIONS[87]

| Name | Origin | LAL (µg/g proteins) |
|---|---|---|
| Acid Casein | Commercial sample, supplier T | 140 |
| | Commercial sample, supplier U | 190 |
| | Commercial sample, supplier V | 70 |
| Masa harina | Commercial sample, | 480 |
| Hydrolyzed vegetable protein | A total of 18 commercial samples of different batches from 5 manufacturers | 40—500 |
| Whipping agent | Commercial sample, manufacturer's type 1 | 6,500 |
| | Commercial sample, manufacturer's type 2 | 50,000 |
| Soy protein isolate | A total of 45 commercial samples of different batches from 2 manufacturers | 0—370 |
| Yeast extract | Commercial sample | 120 |

[a] The identity of the manufacturer was not determined; therefore, the term supplier was used instead.

From Sternberg, M., Kim, C. Y., and Schwende, F., *Science*, 190, 993, 1975. With permission. Copyright 1975 by the American Association for the Advencement of Science.

LAL in a protein has a toxicological significance.[86] In fact, there have been reports of renal lesions characterized by cytoplasmic and nuclear enlargement of the tubular epithelium in the pars recta (so-called nephrocytomegalia) in rats fed $a$-protein as well as soy protein that was subjected in the laboratory to severe alkali treatment. However, other workers[88] have been unable to confirm nephrocytomegalia in rats fed either an edible, spun soy isolate or a severely alkali-treated sample. Subsequently, it has been shown[89] that free, synthetic LAL induces the pathological changes in the rat, but protein-bound LAL does not. In addition, these changes seem to be specific to the rat, since mice, hamsters, Japanese quails, dogs, and monkeys failed to exhibit renal cytomegalic effects even when fed synthetic LAL.

Finally, it should be noted that LAL has now been identified in food proteins that had not been subjected to alkali[87] (Table 12). LAL is generated in a variety of proteins when heated under nonalkaline conditions (Table 13). The quantities, however, are so small that they cannot reduce the nutritive value, and it is also very unlikely that they are of toxicological significance.

### Conclusions

Additional data on processing damage to protein can be found in the book of Harris and Karmas[90] and in an interpretative review in a paper by Bender.[91] From the wealth of the somewhat disordinate data, a few simple "rules" can be drawn:

1. Except for cystine, actual destruction of amino acids remains negligible in food processing.
2. The nutritive value of the proteins is often somewhat improved by moderate heating, especially in the case of vegetable proteins, whereas it is always impaired by intensive heat treatment.
3. Enzymic release of amino acids is reduced in severely heat-processed foods. The reduction is rather uniform for all the essential amino acids in foods low in carbohydrate, such as meat. It is very selective in foods rich in reducing carbohy-

Table 13
## FORMATION OF LAL IN PROTEINS BY HEATING UNDER NONALKALINE CONDITIONS

| Protein | Concentration (percent by volume) | Temperature (°C) | Time (hr) | pH | LAL (µg/g protein) |
|---|---|---|---|---|---|
| Bovine serum albumin | 1 | 120 | 1 | 6.0 | 3500 |
| Casein | 1 | 120 | 1 | 6.0 | 1700 |
| Lysozyme | 1 | 120 | 1 | 2.0 | None |
| | | | | 4.0 | 275 |
| | | | | 6.0 | 1000 |
| Ovalbumin | 1 | 120 | 1 | 2.0 | 150 |
| | | | | 3.0 | 250 |
| | | | | 4.6 | 310 |
| | | | | 6.0 | 570 |
| Soya globulin | 6 | 120 | 16 | 2 | <40 |
| | | | | 3 | <40 |
| | | | | 4 | 80 |
| | | | | 5 | 120 |
| | | | | 6 | 130 |
| | | | | 7 | 180 |
| | | 100 | 1 | 6.5 | <40 |
| | | | 2 | 6.5 | 80 |
| | | | 3 | 6.5 | 130 |

From Sternberg, M., Kim, C. Y., and Schwende, F. J., *Science,* 190, 994, 1975. With permission. Copyright 1975 by The American Association for the Advancement of Science.

drates, such as milk (in which lysine is most affected, followed by the sulfur amino acids).

4.    Heat damage to the protein will not become apparent in a biological test when the most damaged amino acid is not the limiting amino acid of the protein.
5.    In spite of this fact, a good correlation is generally found between the loss of free ε-amino lysine during heating and the fall in nutritive value, showing that it is a more general indicator of heat damage.
6.    Presence of reducing sugars in the food greatly increases heat damage, but does not appear to be a condition *sine qua non.*
7.    The presence of autoxidizing fats also increases heat damage. The presence of active aldehydes, such as gossypol and formaldehyde, greatly contributes to heat deterioration.
8.    High water content, such as in fluid foods, reduces heat damage, whereas intermediate moisture content augments the latter.
9.    At a given temperature the damage is proportional to the time of heating.
10.    Acid pH reduces typical Maillard-type damage, but increases hydrolysis phenomena.[221]

## THE MECHANISMS OF PROCESSING DAMAGE (CAUSAL APPROACH)

### Effect of Heat on Protein Structure

It is well known that heat affects native protein in changing the spacial arrangement of the protein molecule. Heat increases the thermal molecular oscillations that disrupt the binding forces and causes an unfolding of the molecule, which is then followed by a disruption of the disulfide bridges.[92] The whole sequence of events is referred to as "heat denaturation." It can be defined simply as a major change from the original

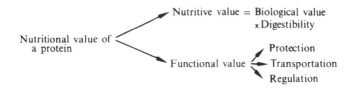

FIGURE 3. Nutritional value of a protein. (From Mauron, J., *International Encyclopaedia of Food and Nutrition*, Vol. 2, Bigwood, E. J., Ed., Pergamon Press, Oxford, 1972, 443. With permission.)

native structure (quaternary, tertiary, and secondary) without alteration of the amino acid sequence (primary structure). In principle, denaturation is a reversible process, but when it is performed by heat, the irreversible stage is quickly reached and heat denaturation of proteins often appears irreversible. In food chemistry the term "denaturation" should be used only in connection with changes involving the spacial arrangement of the protein molecule, including disulfide bonds, but never to describe irreversible chemical modifications of the amino acid side chains (primary structure), for which the term "deterioration" should be employed.

Although protein denaturation plays an important role in food technology (solubility and functional properties), it is of relatively little concern to the nutritionist. It is generally agreed that the disruption of the native protein structure by heat tends to increase the nutritive value of the protein because its susceptibility to enzymic attacks is augmented. Actually, the first step in protein digestion is a denaturation by the proteolytic enzymes. Normally, this takes place in the stomach with pepsin and hydrochloric acid. Heat denaturation of food proteins facilitates this first step of digestion and must therefore be considered a positive factor in nutrition. There might be exceptions to this rule, however, in all cases where the food protein has a specific function to perform in the digestive tract that is linked to its native structure. Thus, in the feeding of the calf, it has indeed been shown that the denaturation of the whey proteins has a detrimental effect on the thriving of the animal.[93] The same is true for the baby pig.[94]

The occurrence of similar phenomena cannot be completely discarded when the feeding of the newborn baby is considered. Thus it has been shown by Mellander[95] that the proteins of breast milk are less rapidly digested in the stomach of the baby than cow's milk proteins. They are also less prone to attack by trypsin. It may therefore be argued that some proteins in breast milk have a function to perform in the digestive tract.[96] These functions may comprise the transport of iron (lactotransferrine), the transfer of passive immunity (immunoglobulins), the destruction of certain microorganisms (lysozyme), and the activation of others (strepogenin for lactobacilli).

It is not known to what extent the heterologous proteins of cow's milk could perform similar tasks, but more thought should certainly be given to the possible functional role of proteins in the artificial feeding of infants. It should also be remembered that phosphopeptones derived from cow's milk casein were shown by Mellander[97] to form hydrosoluble chelates with iron and calcium. The latter are easily absorbed from the gut in this form. It has also been observed by Kirsch[98] that immunoglobulins from cow's milk pass in part intact through the digestive tract of the infant and can therefore display a protective effect in the intestine.

We propose, therefore, to extend the nomenclature as regards the nutritional value of proteins and to distinguish between the nutritive value proper and the functional value of a protein[1] (Figure 3).

First type : mild heat treatment + reducing sugar (carbonyl—groups)

Second type : severe heat treatment — without sugar

— with sugar ⟨ reducing / non reducing

— with oxidized lipids (carbonyl—groups)

Third type : alkali treatment    — carbonates
— ammonia
— strong bases

Fourth type : oxidations    — molecular $O_2$
— hydroperoxides ⎤
— free radicals ⎦ ←lipid oxidation
— $H_2O_2$
— photoxidation

FIGURE 4.    The main types of processing damage to protein.

## The Effect of Processing on Protein Composition

Under this heading we include all modifications of the amino acid side chains of the protein leading to changes in amino acid content or availability. For the chemical modifications of the primary structure (amino acid side chains), we use the word "deterioration." This term should be clearly distinguished from "denaturation" as defined above. Figure 4 summarizes the main types of processing damage to protein.

### Protein-Protein Interactions
### Formation of New Cross-Links Through Isopeptides (Figure 5)

Nutritional studies with pure proteins are necessarily limited, but it does appear that heat damage in animal tissues is largely of a protein-protein nature without other groups being involved, and that much of the fall in nutritional value is explained by a lower rate of proteolysis, the availability of all amino acids being affected.[99] Miller et al.,[100] for instance, showed that in severely heated cod muscle, cystine is heavily destroyed and lysine is barely destroyed, while the content of all the other amino acids is unchanged. Considerable impairment of the nutritive value has shown, however, that several or most essential amino acids must have been inactivated.

There has been considerable speculation as to what might be the chemical reactions leading to such changes in the nutritional value of heated protein. Conventional amino acid analysis has usually shown severe losses of cystine only,[101] whereas the availability of several amino acids was found to be impaired. This simultaneous inactivation of several amino acids suggests that new enzyme-resistant cross-links are formed between the side chains of the same protein molecule; thus, part of the latter becomes biologically unavailable due to masking of the sites of enzyme attachment.

Condensation between the carboxylic groups of glutamic and aspartic acid and the ε-NH₂ groups of lysine has been postulated for a long time as a new peptide link. Bjarnason and Carpenter[102] gave evidence, however, that the same linkages are more probably formed as a result of reaction of lysine groups with the amide groups of asparagine and glutamine resulting in the elimination of ammonia (Figure 5-1). The reaction of lysine with amides rather than with free carboxylic acid groups has also a thermodynamic advantage.

The isopeptide ε-(γ-glutamyl)-lysine, containing the cross-link hypothesized as the main cause of nutritional deterioration in heated proteins, has proved to be fully available as a source of lysine for both rats[103] and chicks.[104] It was shown, however, that it is not hydrolyzed in the gut but absorbed as such and hydrolyzed in the kidneys.[105]

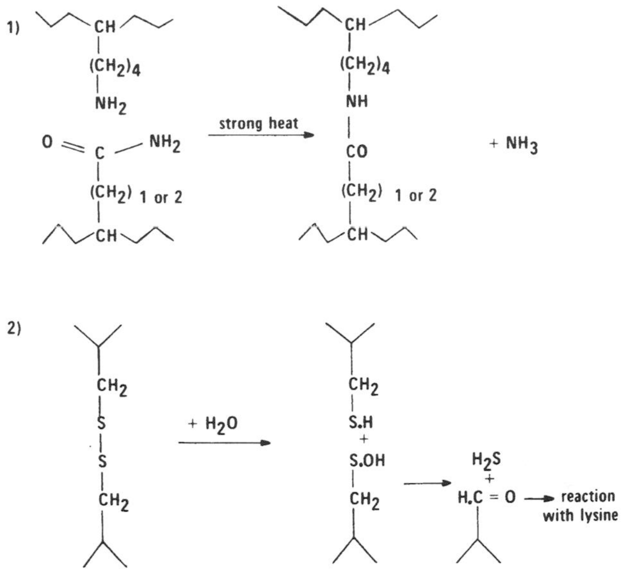

FIGURE 5. Reaction of pure proteins that have been severely heated. (From Carpenter, K. J., in *Nutrients in Processed Foods: Proteins*, White, P. L. and Fletcher, D. C., Eds., Publishing Sciences Group, Acton, Mass., 1974, 106. With permission.)

The presence of numerous such cross-linkages that are not split in the gut may still be expected to hinder the digestion of overheated protein and thus explain the reduced availability of most amino acids.

### Desulfhydration (Figure 5-2)

Cystine is the only amino acid that is always partially destroyed and not merely inactivated when a protein is intensively heated in the presence of moisture. Cystine in a peptide chain may break down with evolution of hydrogen sulfide in several ways, some of them leading to the free carbonyl groups that would combine readily with ε-NH$_2$ lysine groups.[102,106] This could explain why cystine destruction is generally accompanied by lysine inactivation.

### Alkaline Treatments (Figures 6 and 7)

These treatments induce chemical reactions in protein with several amino acids such as cystine,[107,108] serine, lysine, and arginine, leading to the formation of new cross-links and new amino acids such as lanthionine,[109] β-aminoalanine,[110] ornithinoalanine,[111] ornithine,[177] alloisoleucine,[178] and, especially important, lysinoalanine (LAL) (Table 12).[85,86]

### Protein-Carbohydrate Interactions
### The Mild Reaction with Reducing Sugars (Early Maillard Reaction[227])

The Maillard reaction (or nonenzymic browning reaction) occurs between reducing sugars and the free amino group of amino acids, peptides, and proteins. Other carbonyl groups (aldehydes and ketones) react in the same way. This reaction is encountered very frequently in food storage and processing, especially in milk-containing products. The velocity of the reaction is dependent on temperature and moisture content[112] (Figure 8).

It was first shown by Maillard[113] that glycine and glucose react, when heated in a

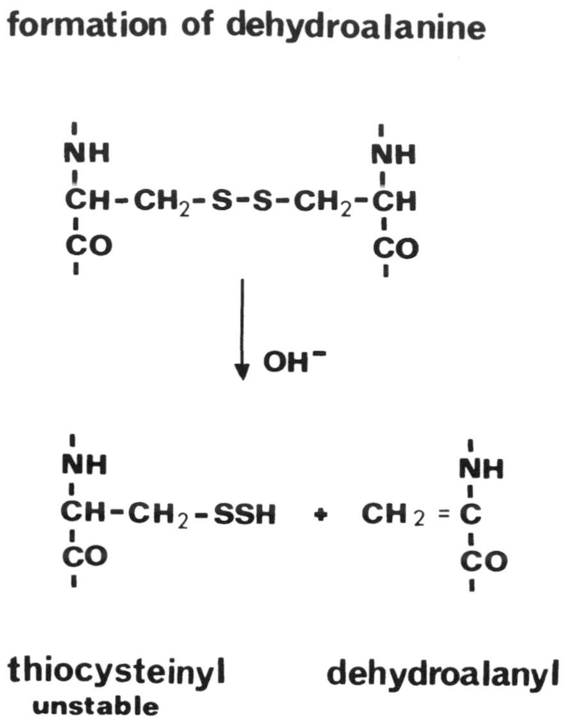

## formation of dehydroalanine

$$
\begin{array}{ccc}
| & & | \\
NH & & NH \\
| & & | \\
CH-CH_2-S-S-CH_2-CH \\
| & & | \\
CO & & CO \\
| & & |
\end{array}
$$

$\downarrow OH^-$

$$
\begin{array}{ccc}
| & & | \\
NH & & NH \\
| & & | \\
CH-CH_2-SSH & + & CH_2 = C \\
| & & | \\
CO & & CO \\
| & & |
\end{array}
$$

**thiocysteinyl**            **dehydroalanyl**
**unstable**

FIGURE 6.   Alkaline treatment of proteins: initial reaction. (From Mauron, J., in *Proc. 4th Int. Congr. Food Science and Technology*, Vol. 1, Instituto de Agronomica y Technologia de Alimentos, Valencia, Spain, 1974, 567. With permission.)

$$
\begin{array}{ccc}
| & | & | \\
NH & NH & NH \\
| & | & | \\
C=CH_2 & NH_2-(CH_2)_4-CH & NH_2-CO-CH_2-CH \\
| & | & | \\
CO & CO & CO \\
| & | & |
\end{array}
$$

**dehydroalanyl**    |    **lysyl -**    |    **aspartyl -amide**

$$
\begin{array}{cc}
| & | \\
NH & NH \\
| & | \\
CH-CH_2-NH-(CH_2)_4-CH & CH-CH_2-NH-CO-CH_2-CH \\
| & | \\
CO & CO \\
| & |
\end{array}
$$

$\downarrow HCl$            $\downarrow HCl$

$$
\begin{array}{cc}
NH_2 & NH_2 \\
| & | \\
CH-CH_2-NH-(CH_2)_4-CH & CH-CH_2-NH_2 \quad HOOC-CH_2-CH \\
| & | \\
COOH & COOH
\end{array}
$$

**lysinoalanine**            **ß·aminoalanine  aspartic ac.**

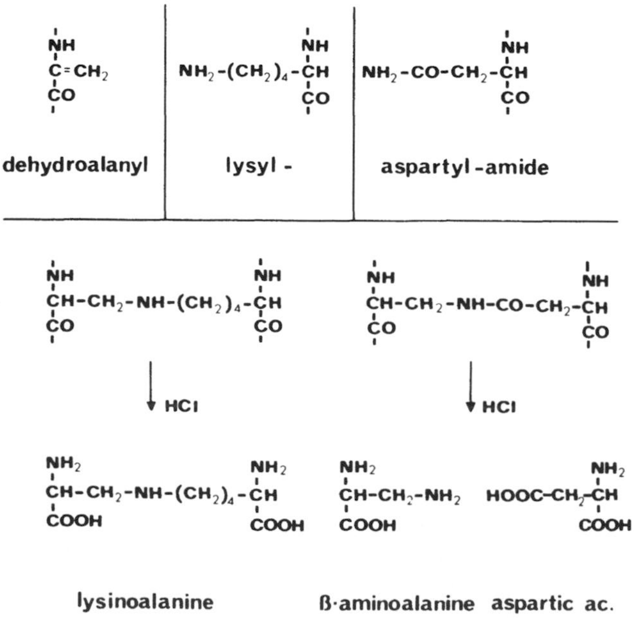

FIGURE 7.   Alkaline treatment of proteins: cross-linkage reaction. (From Mauron, J., in *Proc. 4th Int. Congr. Food Science and Technology*, Vol. 1, Instituto de Agronomica y Technologia de Alimentos, Valencia, Spain, 1974, 567. With permission.)

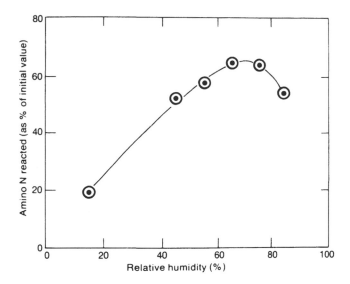

FIGURE 8. Influence of humidity on the rate of reaction of insulin with glucose. Insulin reacted with 1.5 equivalents of glucose per amino group for 16 days at 37°. (From Tannenbaum, S. E., *Nutrients in Processed Foods: Protein,* White, P. L. and Fletcher, D. C., Eds., Publishing Sciences Group, Acton, Mass., 1974, 137. With permission.)

concentrated aqueous solution, with the formation of brown pigments referred to as humins or melanoidins. The first coherent reaction scheme was put forward by Hodge.[114] This scheme is still essentially valid but needs some modifications, taking into account some of the research since performed[1] (Figure 9). A simplified scheme based on the work of Burton[115] is also given[116] in Figure 10.

It is generally agreed[114] that the first step in the carbonyl-amino reaction consists of a single condensation process between the carbonyl group and the free amino group. The condensation product is converted into the Schiff-base, which in turn is isomerized into the nitrogen-substituted glycosyl amine. Whereas glycosyl amines derived from amines show a certain stability, those from amino acids are immediately converted into the 1-amino-1-deoxy-2-ketose by the Amadori rearrangement (Figure 11). This first part of the Maillard reaction leading to the 1-amino-1-deoxy-2-ketose, a relatively stable compound, is thus straightforward and actually represents the main pathway of the Maillard reaction in heated milk when the conditions are relatively mild.

In food proteins most primary amino groups are represented by the ε-amino group of lysine. In heated milk, therefore, the main compound formed is the 1-amino-1-deoxy derivative of ε-lysine (ε-*N*-deoxy-lactylosyl-L-lysine).[117] The model compound ε-*N*-deoxyfructosyl-L-lysine was prepared by reacting protected L-lysine with glucose, and its biological and chemical properties were studied. Upon acid hydrolysis with 6 N·HCl the latter compound yields roughly 50% lysine, 20% furosine,[118] and 10% pyridosine,[119] the rest being destroyed.[120] It was also shown that deoxyfructosyl-lysine is totally inefficient as a source of lysine in nutrition; it represents, therefore, a blocked form of lysine that is biologically unavailable.[103,121] Furthermore, it was found that the greater part of the compound is excreted in an unmodified form in the urine and a very small part in the feces, the rest being degraded by the intestinal flora.[122]

The second part of the Maillard reaction is extremely complex and leads to the formation of reductones, furfurals, and unsaturated carbonyl compounds.[114] These different compounds can, in turn, react together to first form soluble, N-containing po-

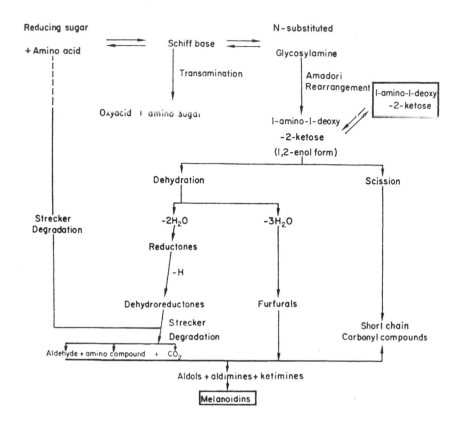

FIGURE 9.   Scheme of the Maillard reaction. (From Mauron, J., *J. Int. Vitaminol.*, 40(2), 217, 1970. With permission.)

lymers and then condense to form insoluble, brown polymers (melanoidins). This second part of the Maillard reaction leads to the destruction of lysine and of all $\alpha$-N terminal amino acids in the proteins.

The question has been raised whether, in addition to the loss in protein value, some of the compounds formed during the Maillard reaction could have deleterious effects on the organism. There is evidence that the brown, soluble compounds, the so-called premelanoidins, formed when free amino acids are heated with glucose, have some peculiar biological[123] and antinutritional[124] properties. The bound premelanoidins formed when proteins are heated, are biologically inert, however, since severely heated protein-glucose mixtures provoke no growth depression when added to well-balanced diets.[125,126]

In essence then, the Maillard reaction, as it occurs under relatively mild conditions in usual foodstuffs, decreases lysine availability and content of the protein of the food. Thus it reduces its nutritive value.

### The Reaction with Carbonyl Groups Under Severe Conditions (Late Maillard Reaction[227])

Many workers have shown just how little nutritional value is left in a protein autoclaved with glucose even for a short period.[125,127] It seems that under these conditions, the carbonyl compounds promote profuse cross-linking in the protein (through Strecker degradations and aldol condensation), which then shows very little value as a

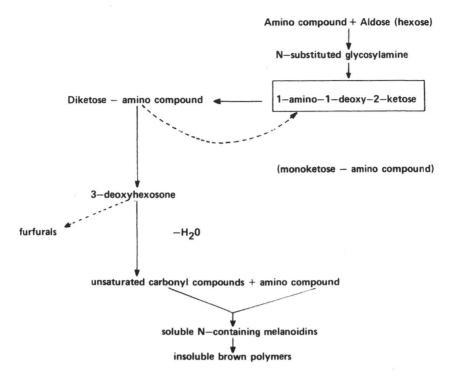

FIGURE 10. Simplified scheme of nonenzymatic browning. (From Mauron, J., in *Physical, Chemical, and Biological Changes in Food Caused by Thermal Processing*, Høyem, T. and Kvåle, M., Eds., Applied Science Publishers, London, 1977, 338. With permission.)

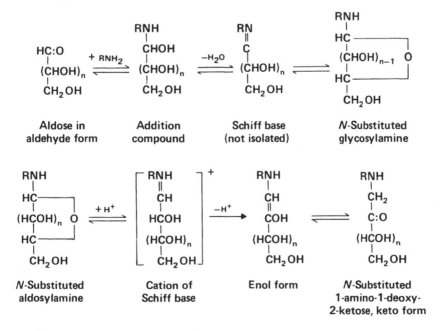

FIGURE 11. The initial steps of the Maillard reaction. (From Hodge, G. E., *Agric. Food Chem.*, 1(15), 931, 1953. With permission.)

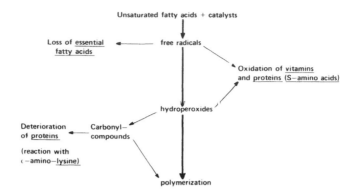

FIGURE 12.   Loss of nutrients by lipid oxidation. (From Mauron, J., in *Physical, Chemical, and Biological Changes in Food Caused by Thermal Processing*, Høyem, T. and Kvåle, M., Eds., Applied Science Publishers, London, 1977, 336. With permission.)

source of any amino acid.[127] The reactive lysine groups fall, but not in full proportion to the nutrition damage, which is of a more general nature.[128,223]

### Reaction with Sucrose

Although reducing sugars are the most active in deteriorating amino acids upon heating of proteins, it has been shown that sucrose could also participate in such a deterioration.[129] Aminolysis of the 1,2-glucosidic linkage by the ε-amino group of lysine has been described as a possible mechanism.[130] The splitting of the glucosidic linkage leads to the formation of a reducing group that can undergo a typical Maillard reaction with another molecule of lysine. It is easy to see how aminolysis could act as a trigger mechanism for the Maillard reaction.[1] However, Hurrell and Carpenter[215] could not confirm this mechanism and found that sucrose acts after being hydrolytically split.

### Protein-Lipid Interactions (Figure 12)

There is considerable literature on the reaction between oxidized fat and protein, but it is difficult to present simple conclusions as the patterns of oxidation of fat are complex.[99] Fat oxidation first involves the reaction between unsaturated fatty acids and catalysts to give free radicals. In the presence of oxygen these combine to form hydroperoxides and the hydroperoxides in turn can react in a number of different ways. They can either give carbonyl compounds of a type very similar to the types participating in the Maillard reaction, they can decompose, or the carbonyl compounds can further react to give polymers.[116]

In fact, the first reaction that occurs between the free radicals and the protein molecule is a formation of cross-links leading to a decrease in protein solubility and a resistance to the digestive enzymes and finally to the actual destruction of most amino acids.[131,136] The second type of reaction is the oxidation of sulfur amino acids by the hydroperoxides. Methionine is oxidized to methionine sulfoxide.[1,132,133] Free methionine sulfoxide is almost as good a methionine source as methionine itself,[134,135] depending on adaptation,[136] whereas peptide-bound sulfoxide is less effective than methionine[135] because of reduced availability due to resistance to enzymic hydrolysis.[137] Cystine is rapidly decomposed and is possibly also oxidized to cysteic acid,[116] an inefficient source of cystine.[138]

The third reaction occurs between the newly formed reactive carbonyl compounds and ε-aminolysine and is very similar to the browning reaction. This generally results in lysine becoming biologically unavailable.[139,140] Actual destruction of lysine has also been described, but it is accompanied by the destruction of other amino acids[141] ( = first reaction).

Finally, it should be noted that there is evidence for the formation of simple complexes between the oxidized lipid and the protein held by electrostatic forces with no involvement of the ε-amino groups.[142] The nutritive value of the protein in such complexes is only very slightly impaired[143] if at all.

*Protein-Aldehyde Interactions*

In addition to the carbonyl amino reactions already described, two reactions with specific aldehydes play a certain role in food technology: the reaction with gossypol in the processing of cottonseed meal[48,50] and the reaction with formaldehyde in the smoking of meat.[144] Both reactions result in the loss of lysine availability.

In spite of some recent progress the elucidation of the chemical mechanisms of heat damage to food proteins remains very incomplete.

## THE DETECTION OF HEAT EFFECTS (METHODOLOGICAL APPROACH)[228,229]

### The Determination of Protein Structure

The detailed investigation of any protein proceeds generally in three phases: isolation and purification, application of tests of homogeneity, and detailed characterization. Modern biophysics provides a whole set of sophisticated methods to do this, but their application is meaningful only in the case of native foodstuffs. In heated foods, proteins have partly lost their identity, and a homogeneity test must therefore fail. What can be detected, however, is the loss of the native protein structure. This is a specialized field of protein chemistry beyond the scope of this review. Two reference books on the subject may be cited.[145,146]

Protein denaturation[147] is much more important in food technology than in nutrition since the loss of the native structure destroys many functional properties of proteins (water binding, gel formation, whippability, solubility, spinnability, etc.) so important in the preparation of certain foods. A great many empirical methods, mostly in the field of viscosimetry and rheology, have therefore been developed to measure the functional properties of proteins in view of a precise application in food preparations. Here again we must refer to the specialized literature.[148]

A few indirect tests for protein denaturation that have a certain relationship with nutritional aspects (even if remote) are mentioned in Table 14. They comprise loss of solubility and of enzyme activity (Figure 13). These tests are only useful in following the initial phases of a heat treatment. Once the native protein structure has been lost, additional heat effects can obviously not be detected by these methods. Thus, to take an example, the presence of urease activity in soybean meal is a fair indication that the heat treatment has not been sufficient to destroy the toxic factors, but the absence of urease activity does not necessarily mean proper heating since overheating cannot be detected in this way. Detection of protein denaturation can be of direct nutritional significance when the native protein has antinutritional properties. The classic examples are the trypsin inhibitors.[166,212]

The more elaborate methods of analysis of protein mixtures such as chromatography, ultra-centrifugation, and the various forms of electrophoresis require that the preparations be free from turbidity and solubilized. Consequently, the protein food must be subjected to such procedures of fractionation as salting out, isoelectric precipitation, solubilization by additives, and so on. The tacit but unproven assumption inherent in such procedures is that these manipulations have no effect on the proteins.

## Table 14
## EXAMPLES OF INDIRECT TESTS
## FOR PROTEIN "DENATURATION"
## IN FOODSTUFFS

| Principle of method | Foodstuff | Ref. |
|---|---|---|
| **Solubility** | | |
| Solubility of N fractions | Milk | 149 |
| Soluble nitrogen | Soy | 150 |
| Solubility in water (8 hr; 40°C; pH 7.6) | Oil seeds | 151 |
| **Enzyme activity** | | |
| Alkaline phosphatase | Milk | 152 |
| | | 153 |
| Lipase | Milk | 154 |
| Peroxidase | Milk | 155 |
| Urease | Soy | 156 |
| | | 157 |
| **Protein inhibitor activity** | | |
| Trypsin inhibitor | Soy | 158 |

The use of gel electrophoresis for separating proteins in a mixture circumvents the reliance on such an assumption and renders the analysis of heated foodstuffs possible. Furthermore, the resolution and sensitivity of this method of separating protein has been extended by combining it with immunodiffusion into the analytical procedure known as immunoelectrophoresis.[167-169] Since proteins are antigenic, the fractions separated electrophoretically can be detected by antigen-antibody precipitin reactions, [170,171] which are both more specific and more sensitive than either chemical or optical detection methods.

Immunoelectrophoresis[172] has been shown to be useful in following progressive heat denaturation of whey proteins in milk powders (Figure 14).[1] Whereas about 12 well-formed precipitation arcs corresponding to the different whey proteins are found in a standard of reference, the number decreases steadily with increasing heat treatment due to the progressive loss of native protein structure.[17] In the case of small structural modifications, the protein has retained enough antigenic sites to react with the antiserum, but the electrophoretic mobility is decreased. Complete denaturation leads to the disappearance of the precipitation arc. For a given commodity such as milk, the method thus allows classification of the heat treatments according to the denaturating effect on protein.

The method can also be used to determine heat resistance of individual food proteins, provided that the latter has been previously isolated in the pure form to produce a specific antiserum. Figure 15 shows the resistance of $\beta$-lactoglobulin in industrial milks.[17] The major disadvantage of the procedure is its dependence on a specific antibody and the fact that proteins differ very much in their ability to stimulate antibody production. It is also true that the antigen-antibody precipitate may redissolve in an excess of antiserum so that the method has to be used with great discrimination. Thus in spite of its usefulness, the application of immunoelectrophoresis will remain limited to very specific problems.

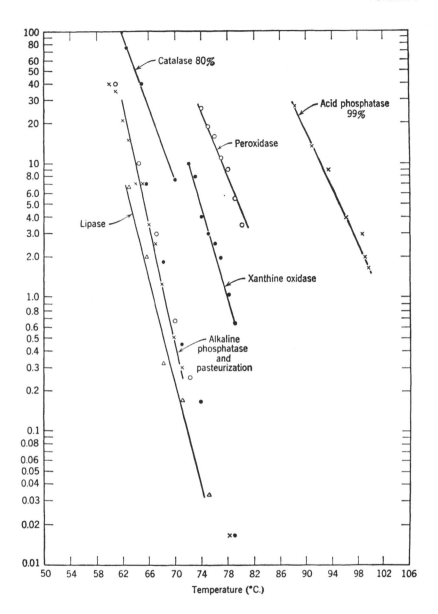

FIGURE 13. Time-temperature relationships for inactivation of milk enzymes. (From Jenness, R. and Palton, S., *Principles of Dairy Chemistry,* John Wiley & Sons, New York, 1959, 201. With permission.)

## The Determination of Protein Composition
### Amino Acid Analysis[174]

Ion exchange chromatography[173,175] of the acid hydrolysate of a food is the basic tool to detect nutritionally relevant modifications of the protein, i.e., changes in the essential amino acid content. In addition, this classic method is able to discriminate between different types of damage to protein.[176]

**Protein-protein interaction** — The internal peptide links formed between glutamic acid and ε-amino-lysine during severe heating of pure proteins[102] do not leave any trace on the chromatogram because the isopeptide linkage is split by acid hydrolysis.[176] Only the destruction of cystine[101] remains as a sign of the extensive heat damage. Isopeptides may be estimated, however, in enzymic digests of the protein.[219]

On the contrary, processing damage by alkali treatment is easily detected by conven-

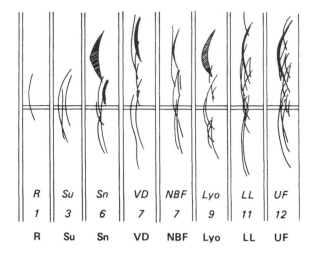

| R | Su | Sn | VD | NBF | Lyo | LL | UF |
|---|----|----|----|----|----|----|----|
| 1 | 3  | 6  | 7  | 7  | 9  | 11 | 12 |

R    Su    Sn    VD    NBF    Lyo    LL    UF

FIGURE 14.    Immunoelectrophoreses of milk powders. The lactoserum, prepared by ultracentrifugation and concentrated by ultrafiltration to a protein content of ∼ 5%, was used throughout. Antiserum: prepared from bovine lactoserum. R, scorched roller-dried milk; Su, standard spray-dried milk; Sn, low-temperature spray-dried milk; VD, vacuum-dried milk (60°C); NBF, low-temperature spray-dried, "humanized" milk; Lyo, milk, lyophilized on an industrial scale; LL, milk, lyophilized in the laboratory; UF, fresh fluid milk. (From Mauron, J. and Blanc, B., *Bibl. Nutr. Dieta,* 7, 72, 1965. With permission.)

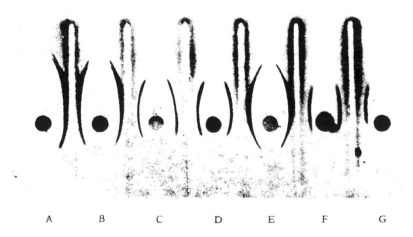

A          B          C          D          E          F          G

FIGURE 15.    Immunoelectrophoreses of industrial milks. The behavior of β-lactoglobuline. Antiserum: pure bovine β-lactoglobuline. A, B, "humanized" milk powders (low temperature spray); C, acidified whole milk powder (spray); D, acidified half skim milk powder (spray); E, acidified "humanized" milk powder (low temperature spray); F, sweetened condensed milk; G, sterilized, fluid "humanized" milk. (From Mauron, J. and Blanc, B., *Bibl. Nutr. Dieta,* 7, 75, 1965. With permission.)

tional amino acid analysis.[178] Lysinoalanine (LAL),[85,86] the main compound formed during these treatments and also found in small amounts in ordinary heated foods, emerges in the chromatogram just before lysine. It can also be determined by thin-layer chromatography.[179] Ornithinoalanine that is formed under even milder conditions such as boiling with carbonate, emerges before LAL.[111]

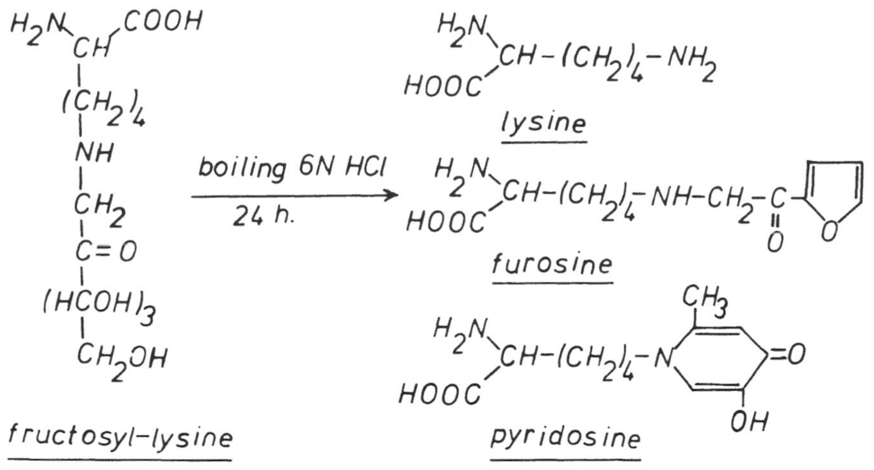

H₂N–CH(COOH)–(CH₂)₄–NH–CH₂–C=O–(HCOH)₃–CH₂OH

boiling 6N HCl, 24 h.

*fructosyl-lysine*

H₂N–(HOOC)CH–(CH₂)₄–NH₂  *lysine*

H₂N–(HOOC)CH–(CH₂)₄–NH–CH₂–C(=O)–(furan)  *furosine*

H₂N–(HOOC)CH–(CH₂)₄–N(ring: CH₃, =O, OH)  *pyridosine*

FIGURE 16. Compounds obtained by acid hydrolysis of ε-deoxy-fructosyl-lysine (ε-DF-lys). (From Mauron, J., in *Proc. 4th Int. Congr. Food Science and Technology*, Vol. 1, Instituto de Agronomica y Technologia de Alimentos, Valencia, Spain, 1974, 566. With permission.)

**Maillard reaction** — Heat damage of this kind due to an interaction of the protein with reducing sugars is easily detectable in the chromatogram of the basic amino acids by the presence of furosine[118] [ε-*N*-(2-furoyl-methyl)-L-lysine] and pyridosine[119] [ε-(1,4-dihydro-3-hydroxy-4-oxo-6-methyl-1-pyridyl)-L-norleucine]. Furosine appears after arginine in the ordinary run, whereas pyridosine is separated ahead of lysine.[176] The quantities and proportions of furosine and pyridosine found in an acid hydrolysate for given food are constant and proportional to the amount of lysine bound in the food as 1-deoxy-2-ketose[120] (Figure 16). Whenever furosine is found in a chromatogram, it indicates that part of the lysine appearing in the same chromatogram is unavailable in the food and that processing damage has therefore occurred that needs further investigation. In processed milk, furosine content can also be used for a quantitative determination[180,220] of the amount of lysine made unavailable during processing using the formula

$$\text{Percent lysine deteriorated} = \frac{3.1 \text{ fur} \times 100}{\text{lys} + 1.9 \times \text{fur}}$$

Another possibility to detect lysine deterioration in the Maillard reaction is to stabilize the carbonyl amino derivatives of lysine by hydrogenation and determine lysine afterwards in an acid hydrolysate. In this case lysine content will correspond to available lysine value.[181]

**Carbonyl amino reaction under severe conditions (late Maillard)** — This results in the formation of profuse cross-linkages,[127] resulting in undigestible peptides that are split to considerable extent by acid hydrolysis. This leaves only traces of furosine and pyridosine in the chromatogram that have, however, no relationship to the great loss in nutritive value.[128] A similar situation occurs when protein food is severely heated in the presence of nonreducing sugars. Amino acid destruction remains relatively small, and the furosine-like peaks appearing on the chromatogram have not yet been sufficiently investigated to be useful as a measure of this type of heat damage.[182]

**Protein-oxidized fat interaction** — This results generally in an inactivation of lysine that does not leave any trace in the chromatogram, but under extreme model conditions, actual amino acid destruction can take place.[141] The reaction with oxidized lipids

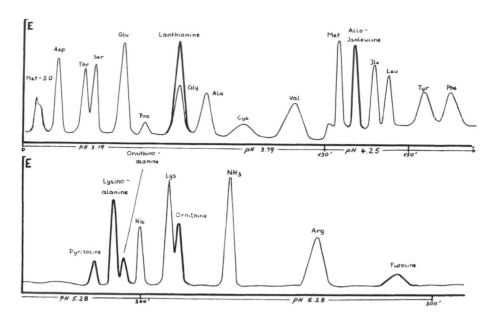

FIGURE 17.    Chromatogram showing markers for different types of protein damage. (From Mauron, J., in *Proc. 4th Int. Congr. Food Science and Technology,* Vol. 1, Instituto de Agronomica y Technologia de Alimentos, Valencia, Spain, 1974, 569. With permission.)

or other oxidative agents leads to the oxidation of methionine to methionine sulfoxide. Since the latter is partially unstable upon acid hydrolysis, it cannot be determined accurately in the usual chromatogram, but can be detected in an alkaline hydrolysate.[137,183] Under proper conditions it appears just ahead of aspartic acid. The markers for the different types of protein damage are shown in Figure 17 as they appear on the chromatogram.[176]

*Amino Acid Availability*

It has become increasingly apparent that the amount of amino acids available to the body after ingestion of food proteins may be less than indicated by the amino acid composition of the dietary protein.[184] In Table 15, a variety of chemical and biological procedures that have been developed to evaluate amino acid availability are tabulated. Despite considerable efforts the determination of the availability of all essential amino acids remains a formidable task.

The most useful chemical method is certainly that of Carpenter,[185] designed to determine available lysine. Unfortunately, it is not very accurate for foods that have undergone a typical Maillard reaction, such as milk.[122] Guanidination[192] is better in this respect, giving true (although uniformly somewhat low) values for all types of heat damage (Figure 18).[216]

In vitro enzymic digestion has been used to determine the availability of all amino acids.[194,213,222] It can give relative availability values as compared to a standard of reference or a direct estimate of nutritive value in the form of an index such as the PDR index[202] (pepsin digest residue amino acid), the PPD[203] index (pepsin pancreatin digest), or the PPDD index[194] (pepsin pancreatin digest dialysate). In order to evaluate heat damage to food proteins, the former procedure is preferred as it would indicate any relative loss in availability for each amino acid in the test sample as compared to the unheated or properly processed material. This information is of greater practical value than the estimate of the global nutritive value given by the indexes, although the

**Table 15**

**SOME METHODS TO MEASURE AMINO ACID AVAILABILITY**

| Method | Principle | Remarks | Ref. |
|---|---|---|---|
| | Chemical | | |
| Reaction with F-DNB (1-fluoro-2,4-dinitrobenzene) | Available lysine = FDNB - reactive lysine | Most generally useful method; some difficulties with starch and early Maillard reaction products (milk!) | 185 |
| | Available lysine = FDNB - reactive lysine with chromatographic separation of ε-DNP-lysine | Not very suitable for routine laboratory; improved separation | 186-189 |
| Reaction with F-DNB (1-fluoro-2,4-dinitrobenzene) "difference method" | Available lysine = total lysine minus inaccessible lysine (lysine in the hydrolysate of the F-DNB-treated protein) | Of limited value; not suitable for Maillard reaction products | 190 |
| Reaction with TNBS (trinitrobenzene sulfonic acid) | Available lysine = TNBS - reactive lysine | Not very specific; not suitable for Maillard reaction products | 191 |
| Guanidation (reaction with O-methyl-isourea) | Available lysine = homoarginine (Figure 18) | Most specific method, suitable for all kinds of heat damage; time consuming, not for routine screening | 192, 216 |
| Total lysine after borohydride treatment | Inaccessible lysine stabilized by hydrogenation, so that no lysine is liberated upon acid hydrolysis; available lysine = total lysine | Specific method for Maillard reaction products; slight under-estimation due to stabilization of available Schiff bases; not suitable for protein-protein interactions | 181, 193 |

**Table 15 (continued)**
## SOME METHODS TO MEASURE AMINO ACID AVAILABILITY

| Method | Principle | Remarks | Ref. |
|---|---|---|---|
| | Enzymatic | | |
| In vitro enzymic digestion with dialysis | Digestion of the sample with pepsin followed by pancreatin and determination of free amino acids in the dialyzate; difference between heated and unheated sample measures loss in availability | Extensively used to measure loss in lysine availability in milk products; results agree well with in vivo availability; theoretically sound for all types of damage; not suitable for routine use | 11, 194 |
| | Microbiological | | |
| Assay with Streptococcus zymogenes NCDO 592 | Classic bioassay with this proteolytic strain using a basal medium containing all the amino acids essential for growth except the one under test; sample predigested with papain | Generally useful method but validity definitely established for methionine only; conditions of predigestion must be well standardized; excellent for routine assays | 195, 196 |
| | In vivo tests | | |
| Rat growth (lysine) | Growth rate of rats is a measure of available lysine in a lysine deficient basal diet; body weight gain per day or per g food eaten is plotted against lysine consumed or percentage of lysine in diet | Standard of reference to check validity of other procedures; results may be influenced by the balance of the other amino acids and the gross composition of the food to be tested; not for routine use | 197, 198 |

| | | |
|---|---|---|
| Chick growth (lysine) | Growth rate of chicks is a measure of available lysine in a lysine deficient basal diet; body weight gain per day or per g food eaten is plotted against lysine consumed or percentage of lysine in diet | Standard of reference to check validity of other procedures; results may be influenced by the balance of the other amino acids and the gross composition of the food to be tested; not for routine use | 199 |
| Chick growth (methionine) | Live weight gain of young chicks is a measure of available methionine in a basal diet deficient in S-amino acids; weight gain or food conversion efficiency (FCE) is compared to percentage of methionine in diet | Reference method to calibrate in vitro procedures; values based on FCE slightly higher and probably more reliable because less dependent on appetite; validity confirmed by collaborative studies | 200, 201 |

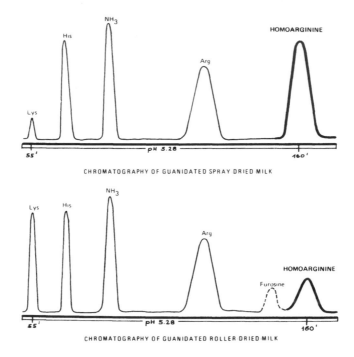

FIGURE 18. Chromatography of guanidated, spray-dried milk (top). Chromatography of guanidated, roller-dried milk (bottom). (From Mauron, J., in *Proc. 4th Int. Congr. Food Science and Technology,* Vol. 1, Instituto de Agronomica y Technologia de Alimentos, Valencia, Spain, 1974, 571. With permission.)

results show generally good agreement with feeding tests.[204] However, the latter are probably cheaper and easier for establishing global nutritive value. The sophisticated in vitro tests have therefore served to demonstrate the physiological basis of differences in protein quality but do not provide an economical means of routine quality control in practice, although they remain useful in solving methodological problems of amino acid availability.

An interesting alternative has been to carry out microbiological assays using a microorganism such as *Streptococcus zymogenes,* which is itself proteolytic.[195] Most work has been done on the assay of methionine in this way; a large number of samples can be assayed at the time, and the results have shown quite good correlations with corresponding animal assays on processed materials.[133,205] The only problem, however, is to maintain culture conditions so that absolute values remain constant from one assay to another. The availability of many other essential amino acids can be determined by this method,[206] but the laboratory experience is less extensive.

Nutritional bioassays,[99,184,207] in which weight gain is the response determined, provide a measure of available nutrients without any reliance having to be placed on the results of chemical analyses. Theoretically, this type of assay represents the standard of reference, but it is relatively unprecise, slow, and expensive. Nevertheless, animal growth assays have served to establish the validity of the simpler analytical methods (Table 16).

## The Biological Determination of the Nutritive Value

The methods used to determine the nutritive value of processed food proteins are obviously none other than the classic biological procedures of protein evaluation (pro-

Table 16

COMPARISON OF CHEMICAL, ENZYMIC AND BIOLOGICAL
METHODS TO MEASURE LYSINE AVAILABILITY[198]

| Method of preparation | Total after acid hydrolysis | FDNB-reactive[a] | Digestion in vitro and dialysis | Rat growth assay |
|---|---|---|---|---|
| Freeze-dried | 8.3 | 8.4 | (8.3)[b] | 8.4 |
| Spray-dried | 8.0 | 8.2 | 8.3 | 8.1 |
| Evaporated | 7.6 | 6.4 | 6.2 | 6.1 |
| Roller-dried 2[c] | 7.1 | 4.6 | 5.4 | 5.9 |
| Roller-dried 4 | 6.8 | 3.8 | 4.5 | 4.0 |
| Roller-dried 6 | 6.3 | 2.5 | 3.1 | 2.9 |
| Roller-dried 8 | 6.1 | 1.9 | 2.3 | 2.0 |

[a] Determined by the Carpenter[185] procedure.

[b] The actual values were all lower than given here because of the limitations of the procedure. The values listed were calculated "relative" to the freeze-dried sample, for which the true digestibility was assumed to be 100%.[11]

[c] The code numbers refer to samples prepared under increasingly severe conditions.

Modified from Mottu, F. and Mauron, J., *J. Sci. Food Agric.*, 18(2), 62, 1967. With permission.

tein efficiency ratio, digestibility, biological value, nutritive value, net protein utilization, and nitrogen balance sheet). Historically, they have been the first used to evaluate heat damage to proteins and are still employed to a considerable extent for that purpose.[208-210]

They are definitely useful in the sense that they constitute a test on the intact animal and will always detect gross nutritional damage. In addition, protein efficiency as well as slope ratio assays have the advantage of disclosing possible toxic effects of processing, since growth is extremely sensitive to toxic factors. On the other hand, it is obvious that these biological measures will not detect the heat damage involving amino acids that are not limiting in the particular protein. In other words, essential amino acids in excess of the requirements can be damaged to the point where they become limiting, without modification of the protein value. Multiple assays with various combinations of supplementary amino acids[211] can, however, overcome this difficulty and give information on all essential amino acids. In this form the biological measures are almost, although not quite, as efficient in detecting the cause of heat damage as is the determination of amino acid availability.

It is very difficult to generalize in giving advice as to what methods should or should not be used for the evaluation of a particular protein food. For the evaluation of a totally new type of food or new type of processing, the determination of amino acid availability as well as some tests on the intact animal are advisable. On the other hand, for the day-by-day quality control of a product produced by the same process from a single factory, a simple solubility or dye-binding test[217] might be adequate if there is no reason to suspect any variability in the raw materials subjected to processing. Between these two extremes we find the majority of cases for which the choice of tests will depend on previous knowledge and available laboratory facilities. In this respect, the chemical determination of available lysine is certainly the most useful laboratory method to rapidly evaluate the effect of heat processing on food proteins.

Finally, it should be noted that there is a great need for rapid methods of protein quality determination for the food processor. In one conference (February 1977) held at the University of Nebraska, the problem was clearly stated, and different approaches to possible solutions were discussed; however, no rapid shortcut can yet be envisaged.[214]

# REFERENCES

1. **Mauron, J.,** Influence of industrial and household handling on food protein quality, in *International Encyclopaedia of Food and Nutrition,* Vol. 2, Bigwood, E. J., Ed., Pergamon Press, Oxford, 1972, 417—473.

2. **Lobanov, D. I. and Bykova, S. W.,** Ablauf der Extraktion löslicher Stoffe beim Kochen des Fleisches, *Z. Unters. Lebensm.,* 69(4), 313—318, 1935.

3. **Jean-Blain, M.,** *Les Aliments d'Origine Animale Destinés à l'Homme,* Vigot, Paris, 1940.

4. **McCance, R. A. and Shipp, H. L.,** The chemistry of flesh foods and their losses on cooking, *Med. Res. Counc., G. B., Spec. Rep. Ser.* No. 187, 7, 1933.

5. **Baker, L. C.,** The Nation's food. VI. Fish as food. The cooking of fish, *Chem. Ind.,* 62, 356—359, 1943.

6. **Trémolières, J., Serville, Y., and Jacquot, R.,** *Manuel Élémentaire d'Alimentation Humaine,* Editions Sociales Françaises, Paris, 1964.

7. **Marks, A. L. and Nilson, H. W.,** Effect of cooking on the nutritive value of the protein of cod, *Commer. Fish. Rev.,* 8(12), 1—6, 1946.

8. **Martinek, W. A. and Goldberg, C. G.,** Nutritive value of baked croaker, *Commer. Fish. Rev.,* 9(4), 9—13, 1947.

9. **Kraybill, H. R.,** The nutritive aspect of meat and meat products, in *Protein and Amino Acids in Nutrition,* Sahyun, M., Ed., Reinhold, New York, 1948, 199—220.

10. **Schweigert, B. S., Tatman, I. E., and Elvehjem, C. A.,** Leucine, valine, and isoleucine contents of meats, *Arch. Biochem.,* 6, 177—184, 1945.

11. **Mauron, J., Mottu, F., Bujard, E., and Egli, R. H.,** The availability of lysine, methionine and tryptophan in condensed milk and milk powder. *In vitro* digestion studies, *Arch. Biochem.,* 59(2), 433—451, 1955.

12. **Terroine, E. F.,** *Métabolisme de l'Azote,* Vol. 1, Presses Universitaires de France, Paris, 1933.

13. **Henry, K. M., Kon, S. K., and Thompson, S. Y.,** The effect of the level of calcium intake on the biological value of a protein, *Biochem. J.,* 34, 998—1001, 1940.

14. **Terroine, E. F. and Valla, S.,** Comparative values of various protein foods for promoting growth, *Bull. Soc. Sci. Hyg. Aliment.,* 21, 105—174, 1933.

15. **Jacquot, R. and Rousier, M.,** Sur un nouveau mode de présentation des légumineuses. Valeur alimentaire du haricot "éclaté", *Bull. Acad. Med.,* 127, 439—441, 1943.

16. **Aurand, L. W., Brown, J. W., and Lecce, J. G.,** Effect of heat on the proteins of milk as revealed by gel and immunoelectrophoresis, *J. Dairy Sci.,* 46, 1177—1182, 1963.

17. **Mauron, J. and Blanc, B.,** Effet des traitements industriels sur la structure des protéines du lactosérum et rôle fonctionnel possible des protéines alimentaires, *Nutr. Dieta,* 7, 69—81, 1965.

18. **Rolls, B. A. and Porter, J. W. G.,** Some effects of processing and storage on the nutritive value of milk and milk products, *Proc. Nutr. Soc.,* 32, 9—15, 1973.

19. **Natvig, H. and Gram, L.,** The effect of raw certified milk and ordinary pasteurized milk on the growth and health of two uniform groups of infants, *Acta Paediatr. Scand.,* 44 (Suppl. 103), 104—105, 1955.

20. **Shahani, K. M. and Sommer, H. H.,** The protein and non-protein nitrogen fractions in milk. III. The effect of heat treatments and homogenization, *J. Dairy Sci.,* 34(11), 1035—1041, 1951.

21. **Harris, R. S. and V. Loesecke, S. B.,** *Nutritional Evaluation of Food Processing,* J. Wiley & Sons, New York, 1960, 174—176.

22. **Ford, J. E. and Porter, J. W. G.,** The availability of some essential amino acids in commercial sterilized milk, in *Proc. 17th Int. Dairy Congr.,* Vol. B, XVII Internationaler Milchwirtschaftskongress, Munich, 1966, 357—360.

23. **Dulcino, J. and Lontie, R.,** Modification of lysine in the course of thermal treatment of milk, in *Protides of the Biological Fluids,* Peeters, H., Ed., Elsevier, 1960, 100—104.

24. **Payne-Botha, S. and Bigwood, E. J.,** Amino-acid content of raw and heat-sterilized cow's milk, *Br. J. Nutr.,* 13(4), 385—389, 1959.

25. **Kon, S. K. and Henry, K. M.,** The effect of commercial sterilization on the nutritive value of milk, *J. Dairy Res.,* 9(1), 1—5, 1938.

26. **Mauron, J. and Mottu, F.,** Sweetened condensed vs. evaporated milk in improving the protein efficiency of wheat flour, *Agric. Food Chem.,* 10(6), 512—515, 1962.

27. **Henry, K. M., Houston, J., Kon, S. K., and Thompson, S. Y.,** The effects of commercial processing and of storage on some nutritive properties of milk. Comparison of full-cream sweetened condensed milk and of evaporated milk with the original raw milk, *J. Dairy Res.,* 13, 329—339, 1944.

28. **Cook, B. B., Morgan, A. F., Weast, E. O., and Parker, J.,** The effect of heat treatment on the nutritive value of milk proteins. I. Evaporated and powdered milks, *J. Nutr.,* 44, 51—61, 1951.

29. **Abbott, O. D., French, R. B., and Townsend, R. O.,** Effect of processing upon the nutritive value of milk as evaluated with rats, *Fl. Agric. Exp. Stn. Bull.,* 485, 4—12, 1951.

30. **Hodson, A. Z.,** Nutritive value of milk proteins. I. Stability during sterilization and storage of evaporated milk as determined by the rat repletion method, *Food Res.,* 17, 168—171, 1952.

31. **Schroeder, L. J., Iacobellis, M., and Smith, A. H.,** Heat processing and the nutritive value of milk and milk products, *J. Nutr.,* 49, 549—561, 1953.

32. **Sinios, A.,** Comparative studies on the nutrition of young infants with evaporated milk and collective human milk. A simultaneous contribution to the critical evaluation of nutritional statistics, *Z. Kinderheilk.,* 75, 634—642, 1954.

33. **Hodson, A. Z.,** Nutritive value of milk proteins. II. Stability during sterilization of evaporated milk as determined by the rat growth method, *Food Res.,* 19, 224—230, 1954.

34. **Beuk, J. F., Chornock, F. W., and Rice, E. E.,** The effect of severe heat treatment upon the amino acids of fresh and cured pork, *J. Biol. Chem.,* 175, 291—298, 1948.

35. **Neilands, J. B., Sirny, R. J., Sohljell, I., Strong, F. M., and Elvehjem, C. A.,** The nutritive value of canned foods. II. Amino acid content of fish and meat products, *J. Nutr.,* 39, 187—202, 1949.

36. **Dunn, M. S., Camien, M. N., Eiduson, S., and Malin, R. B.,** The nutritive value of canned foods. I. Amino acid content of fish and meat products, *J. Nutr.,* 39, 177—185, 1949.

37. **Mayfield, H. L. and Hedrick, M. T.,** The effect of canning, roasting and corning on the biological value of the proteins of western beef, finished on either grass or grain, *J. Nutr.,* 37, 487—494, 1949.

38. **Wilder, O. H. M. and Kraybill, H. R.,** Effect of cooking and curing on lysine content of pork luncheon meat, *J. Nutr.,* 33, 235—242, 1947.

39. **Guthneck, B. T., Bennett, B. A., and Schweigert, B. S.,** Utilization of amino acids from foods by the rat. II. Lysine, *J. Nutr.,* 49, 289—294, 1953.

40. **Schweigert, B. S. and Guthneck, B. T.,** Utilization of amino acids from foods by the rat. III. Methionine, *J. Nutr.,* 54, 333—343, 1954.

41. **Woodham, A. A.,** The effects of processing on the nutritive value of vegetable protein concentrates, *Proc. Nutr. Soc.,* 32, 23—29, 1973.

42. **Hayward, J. W., Steenbock, H., and Bohstedt, G.,** The effect of heat as used in the extraction of soy bean oil upon the nutritive value of the protein of soy bean oil meal, *J. Nutr.,* 11, 219—234, 1936.

43. **Riesen, W. H., Clandinin, D. R., Elvehjem, C. A., and Cravens, W. W.,** Liberation of essential amino acids from raw, properly heated, and overheated soy bean oil meal, *J. Biol. Chem.,* 167, 143—150, 1947.

44. **Taira, H., Taira, H., and Sakurai, Y.,** Amino acid contents of processed soybean. VIII. Effect of heating on total lysine and available lysine in defatted soybean flour, *Jpn. J. Nutr. Food,* 18(5), 359—361, 1966.

45. **Hackler, L. R., Van Buren, J. P., Steinkraus, K. H., El Rawi, I., and Hand, D. B.,** Effect of heat treatment on nutritive value of soymilk protein fed to weanling rats, *J. Food Sci.,* 30, 723—728, 1965.

46. **Renner, R., Clandinin, D. R., Morrison, A. B., and Robblee, A. R.,** The effects of processing temperatures on the amino acid content of sunflower seed oil meal, *J. Nutr.,* 50, 487—490, 1953.

47. **Altschul, A. M.,** *Processed Plant Protein Foodstuffs,* Academic Press, New York, 1958, 419—527.

48. **Frampton, V. L.,** Effects of processing on the nutritive quality of oilseed meals, in *Nutritional Evaluation of Food Processing,* 2nd ed., Harris, R. S. and Karmas, E., Eds., AVI Publishing, Westport, Conn., 1975, 187—204.

49. **Mauron, J. and Mottu, F.,** Problèmes nutritionnels que pose la lutte contre la malnutrition protéique dans les pays en voie de développement. III. Corrélation entre la teneur en lysine disponible et la valeur nutritive dans les tourteaux d'arachide, *Ann. Nutr. Aliment.,* 14, 309—315, 1960.

50. **Conkerton, E. J. and Frampton, V. L.,** Reaction of gossypol with free ε-amino groups of lysine in proteins, *Arch. Biochem. Biophys.,* 81, 130—134, 1959.

51. **Frampton, V. L.,** Cottonseed proteins; their status in nonruminant feeding, *Cereal Sci. Today,* 10, 557, 1965.

52. **Vix, H. L. E., Dupuy, H. R., and Lambu, M. G.,** Critical evaluation of the use of acetone in solvent extraction process, in *Conf. Protein Rich Food Prod. Oil Seeds,* U.S. Department of Agriculture, Agricultural Research Service, Washington, D.C., 1969, 71—72.

53. **King, W. H. and Frampton, V. L.,** Properties of oil extracted from cottonseed with acetone-hexane-water solvent mixture, *J. Am. Oil Chem. Soc.,* 38, 497—499, 1961.

54. **MacDonald, F. J.,** Available lysine content of dried milk, *Nature (London),* 209, 1134, 1966.

55. **Fairbanks, W. and Mitchell, H. H.,** The nutritive value of skim-milk powders with special reference to the sensitivity of milk proteins to heat, *J. Agric. Res.,* 51, 1107—1121, 1935.

56. **Henry, K. M., Houston, J., Kon, S. K., and Osborne, L. W.,** The effect of commercial drying and evaporation on the nutritive properties of milk, *J. Dairy Res.,* 10, 272—293, 1939.

57. **Riggs, L. K., Beaty, A., and Mallon, B.**, Nutritive value of whey powder protein, *J. Agric. Food Chem.*, 3(4), 333—337, 1955.
58. **Mauron, J. and Mottu, F.**, Relationship between *in vitro* lysine availability and *in vivo* protein evaluation in milk powders, *Arch. Biochem. Biophys.*, 77(2), 312—327, 1958.
59. **Erbersdobler, H. and Zucker, H.**, Untersuchungen zum Gehalt an Lysin und verfügbarem Lysin in Trockenmagermilch, *Milchwissenschaft*, 21, 564—568, 1966.
60. **Pion, R. and Rerat, A.**, Influence des Procédés de Fabrication sur la Valeur Nutritive des Poudres de Lait, in *Proc. 16th Int. Dairy Congr.*, Copenhagen, Vol. B, 1962, 993—1001.
61. **Posati, L. P., Holsinger, V. H., DeVilbiss, E. D., and Pallansch, M. J.**, Effect of instantizing on amino acid content of nonfat dry milk, *J. Dairy Sci.*, 57, 258—260, 1974.
62. **Porter, J. W. G. and Garton, G. A.**, Reviews of the progress of dairy science. Section D. Nutritive value of milk and milk products. I. Nutritive value of milk proteins. II. Nutritive value of milk fat, *J. Dairy Res.*, 31, 201—212, 1964.
63. **Thomas, M. and Calloway, D.**, Nutritional value of dehydrated food, *J. Am. Diet. Assoc.*, 39, 105—116, 1961.
64. **Gooding, E. G. B.**, The storage behaviour of dehydrated foods, in *Recent Advances in Food Science*, Vol. 2, Hawthorn, J. and Leitch, J. M., Eds., Butterworths, London, 1962, 22—38.
65. **Lopez-Matas, A. and Fellers, C. R.**, Composition and nutritive value of fresh, cooked, and processed swordfish, *Food Res.*, 13, 387—396, 1948.
66. **Deas, P. and Tarr, H. L. A.**, Amino acid composition of fishery products, *J. Fish. Res. Board Can.*, 7, 513—521, 1949.
67. **Bender, A. E., Miller, D. S., and Tunnah, E. J.**, The biological value of fish meals, *Proc. Nutr. Soc.*, 12, ii, 1953.
68. **Miller, D. S.**, The nutritive value of fish proteins, *J. Sci. Food Agric.*, 7, 337—343, 1956.
69. **Carpenter, K. J., Ellinger, G. M., Munro, M. I., and Rolfe, E. J.**, Fish products as protein supplements to cereals, *Br. J. Nutr.*, 11, 162—173, 1957.
70. **Yanez, E., Ballester, D., and Donoso, G.**, Effect of drying temperature on quality of fish protein, *J. Sci. Food Agric.*, 21(8), 426—428, 1970.
71. **Lea, C. H., Parr, L. J., and Carpenter, K. J.**, Chemical and nutritional changes in stored herring meal, Part 2, *Br. J. Nutr.*, 14, 91—113, 1960.
72. **Myklestad, O., Bjørnstad, J., and Njaa, L.**, Effects of heat treatment on composition and nutritive value of herring meal, *Fiskerdir. Norw. Skr. Ser. Teknol. Unders.*, 5(10), 1—15, 1972.
73. **Njaa, L. R., Utne, F., and Braekkan, O. R.**, Protein quality of herring meal, in *Proc. 7th Int. Congr. Nutr.*, Vol. 5, Kühnau, J., Ed., Vieweg und Sohn GmbH, Brunswick, West Germany, 1967, 218—222.
74. **Goldblith, S. A.**, Freeze-dehydration of foods, in *Aspects Théoriques et Industriels de la Lyophilisation*, Rey, L., Ed., Hermann, Paris, 1964, 555—572.
75. **De Groot, A. P.**, The influence of dehydration of foods on the digestibility and the biological value of the protein, *Food Technol. (Chicago)*, 17(3), 339—343, 1963.
76. **Calloway, D. H.**, Dehydrated foods, *Nutr. Rev.*, 20(9), 257—260, 1962.
77. **Mauron, J., Mottu, F., and Egli, R. H.**, Problèmes nutritionnels que pose la malnutrition protéique dans les pays en voie de développement. I. La détérioration des acides aminés lors de la préparation des biscuits riches en protéines, *Ann. Nutr. Aliment.*, 14(1), 135—150, 1960.
78. **Clark, H. E., Howe, J. M., Mertz, E. T., and Reitz, L.**, Lysine in baking powder biscuits, *J. Am. Diet. Assoc.*, 35, 469—471, 1959.
79. **Rosenberg, H. R. and Rohdenburg, E. L.**, The fortification of bread with lysine. I. The loss of lysine during baking, *J. Nutr.*, 45, 593—598, 1951.
80. **Jansen, G. R., Ehle, S. R., and Hause, N. L.**, Studies on the nutritive loss of supplemental lysine in baking. II. Loss in water bread and in breads supplemented with moderate amounts of nonfat dry milk, *Food Technol. (Chicago)*, 18(3), 372—375, 1964.
81. **Morgan, A. F. and King, F. B.**, Changes in biological value of cereal proteins due to heat treatment, *Proc. Soc. Exp. Biol. Med.*, 23, 353, 1926.
82. **Morgan, A. F., King, F. B., Boyden, R. E., and Petro, A.**, The effect of heat upon the biological value of cereal proteins and casein, *J. Biol. Chem.*, 90, 771—792, 1931.
83. **Sure, B.**, Nutritional values of proteins in various cereal breakfast foods, *Food Res.*, 16, 161—165, 1951.
84. **Anon.**, Soy fibers — A new approach to vegetable protein acceptability, *Nutr. Rev.*, 25(10), 305—307, 1967.
85. **De Groot, A. P. and Slump, P.**, Effects of severe alkali treatment of proteins on amino acid composition and nutritive value, *J. Nutr.*, 98, 45—56, 1969.
86. **Woodard, J. C. and Short, D. D.**, Toxicity of alkali-treated soy protein in rats, *J. Nutr.*, 103, 569—574, 1973.

87. Sternberg, M., Kim, C. Y., and Schwende, F. J., Lysinoalanine: Presence in foods and food ingredients, *Science*, 190, 992—994, 1975.
88. Van Beek, L., Feron, V. J., and De Groot, A. P., Nutritional effects of alkali-treated soy protein in rats, *J. Nutr.*, 104, 1630—1636, 1974.
89. De Groot, A. P., Slump, P., Feron, V. J., and Van Beek, L., Effects of alkali-treated proteins: Feeding studies with free and protein-bound lysinoalanine in rats and other animals, *J. Nutr.*, 106, 1527—1538, 1976.
90. Harris, R. S. and Karmas, E., *Nutritional Evaluation of Food Processing*, 2nd ed., AVI Publishing, Westport, Conn., 1975.
91. Bender, A. E., Processing damage to protein food, a review, *J. Food Technol.*, 7, 239—250, 1972.
92. Tanford, C., Protein denaturation, in *Advances in Protein Chemistry*, Vol. 23, Anfinsen, C. B., Anson, M. L., Edsall, J. T., and Richards, F. M., Eds., Academic Press, New York, 1968, 121—282.
93. Roy, J. H., The nutrition of intensively-reared calves, *Vet. Rec.*, 76, 511—526, 1964.
94. Braude, R., Newport, M. J., and Porter, J. W. G., Artificial rearing of pigs. III. The effect of heat treatment on the nutritive value of spray-dried whole-milk powder for the baby pig, *Br. J. Nutr.*, 25, 113—125, 1971.
95. Mellander, O., The nutritional significance of some peptides, *Voeding*, 16, 219—222, 1955.
96. Ballabriga, A., Hilpert, H., and Isliker, H., Immunity of the infantile gastrointestinal tract and implications on modern infant feeding, in *Nestlé Research News 1974/1975*, Nestlé Products Technical Assistance Co., Lausanne, Switzerland, 24—45.
97. Mellander, O., Protein quality, *Nutr. Rev.*, 13(6), 161—163, 1955.
98. Kirsch, W., Der Einfluss von Magen-Darm-Sekreten auf Immunglobuline aus Milch und Serum, *Helv. Paediatr. Acta*, 25, 119—126, 1970.
99. Carpenter, K. J. and Booth, V. H., Damage to lysine in food processing: its measurement and its significance, *Nutr. Abstr. Rev.*, 43(6), 424—451, 1973.
100. Miller, E. L., Carpenter, K. J., and Milner, C. K., Availability of sulphur amino acids in protein foods. III. Chemical and nutritional changes in heated cod muscle, *Brit. J. Nutr.*, 19, 547—564, 1965.
101. Miller, E. L., Hartley, A. W., and Thomas, D. C., Availability of sulphur amino acids in protein foods. IV. Effect of heat treatment upon the total amino acid content of cod muscle, *Br. J. Nutr.*, 19, 565—573, 1965.
102. Bjarnason, J. and Carpenter, K. J., Mechanisms of heat damage in proteins. II. Chemical changes in pure proteins, *Br. J. Nutr.*, 24, 313—329, 1970.
103. Mauron, J., Le comportement chimique des protéines lors de la préparation des aliments et ses incidences biologiques, *J. Int. Vitaminol.*, 40(2), 209—227, 1970.
104. Waibel, P. E. and Carpenter, K. J., Mechanisms of heat damage in proteins. III. Studies with ε-(γ-L-glutamyl)-L-Lysine, *Br. J. Nutr.*, 27(3), 509—515, 1972.
105. Finot, P. A., Mottu, F., Bujard, E., and Mauron, J., N-substituted lysines as sources of lysine in nutrition, in *Nutritional Improvement of Food and Feed Proteins*, Friedman, M., Ed., Plenum Press, New York, 1978, 549—570.
106. Carpenter, K. J., personnal communication, 1968.
107. Swan, J. M., Mechanism of alkaline degradation of cystine residues in proteins, *Nature (London)*, 179(4567), 965, 1957.
108. Catsimpoolas, N. and Wood, J. L., The reaction of cyanide with bovine serum albumin, *J. Biol. Chem.*, 239(12), 4132—4137, 1964.
109. Horn, M. J., Breese-Jones, D., and Ringel, S. J., Isolation of a new sulfur-containing amino acid (lanthionine) from sodium carbonate treated wool, *J. Biol. Chem.*, 138, 141—149, 1941.
110. Asquith, R. S., Booth, A. K., and Skinner, J. D., The formation of basic amino acids on treatment of proteins with alkali, *Biochim. Biophys. Acta*, 181, 164—170, 1969.
111. Ziegler, K., Melchert, I., and Lürken, C., Nδ-(2-amino-2-carboxyethyl)-ornithine, a new amino-acid from alkali-treated proteins, *Nature (London)*, 214, 404—405, 1967.
112. Lea, C. H., Chemical changes in the preparation and storage of dehydrated foods, in *Fundamental Aspects of Dehydration of Foodstuffs*, Society of Chemical Industry, London, 1958, 178—196.
113. Maillard, L. C., Réaction générale des acides aminés sur les sucres. Ses conséquences biologiques, *C. R. Soc. Biol. Paris*, 72, 599—601, 1912.
114. Hodge, J. E., Dehydrated foods. Chemistry of browning reactions in model systems, *Agric. Food Chem.*, 1, 928—943, 1953.
115. Burton, H. S. and McWeeny, D. J., Non-enzymatic browning: routes to the production of melanoidins from aldoses and amino-compounds, *Chem. Ind.*, 11, 462—463, 1964.
116. Tannenbaum, S., Industrial processing, in *Nutrients in Processed Foods: Proteins*, White, P. L. and Fletcher, D. C., Eds., Publishing Sciences Group, Acton, Mass., 1974, 131—138.

117. **Finot, P. A. and Mauron, J.,** Le blocage de la lysine par la réaction de Maillard. I. Synthèse de *N*-(désoxy-1-D-fructosyl-l)- et *N*-(désoxyl-1-D-lactulosyl-l)-L-lysines, *Helv. Chim. Acta,* 52(6), 1488—1495, 1969.

118. **Finot, P. A., Bricout, J., Viani, R., and Mauron, J.,** Identification of a new lysine derivative obtained upon acid hydrolysis of heated milk, *Experientia,* 24(11), 1097—1099, 1968.

119. **Finot, P. A., Viani, R., Bricout, J., and Mauron, J.,** Detection and identification of pyridosine, a second lysine derivative obtained upon acid hydrolysis of heated milk, *Experientia,* 25(2), 134—135, 1969.

120. **Finot, P. A. and Mauron, J.,** Le blocage de la lysine par la réaction de Maillard. II. Propriétés chimiques des dérivés *N*-(désoxy-1-D-fructosyl-l) et *N*-(désoxy-1-D-lactulosyl-l) de la lysine, *Helv. Chim. Acta,* 55(4), 1153—1164, 1972.

121. **Mauron, J.,** The analytical, nutritional and toxicological implications of protein food processing, *Proc. IV. Int. Congr. Food Sci. Technol.,* Vol. I, 1974, 564—577.

122. **Finot, P. A.,** Non-enzymic browning, in *Proteins in Human Nutrition,* Porter, J. W. G. and Rolls, B. A., Eds., Academic Press, London, 1973, 501—514.

123. **Chichester, C. O.,** Protein and amino acid interactions with other macronutrients, in *Nutrients in Processed Foods: Proteins,* White, P. L. and Fletcher, D. C., Eds., Publishing Sciences Group, Acton, Mass., 1974, 127—129.

124. **Adrian, J.,** Nutritional and physiological consequences of the Maillard reaction, *World Rev. Nutr. Diet.,* 19, 71—122, 1974.

125. **Boctor, A. M. and Harper, A. E.,** Measurement of available lysine in heated and unheated foodstuffs by chemical and biological methods, *J. Nutr.,* 94, 289—296, 1968.

126. **Atkinson, J. and Carpenter, K. J.,** Nutritive value of meat meals. I. Possible growth depressant factors, *J. Sci. Food Agric.,* 21(7), 360—365, 1970.

127. **Valle-Riestra, J. and Barnes, R. H.,** Digestion of heat-damaged egg albumen by the rat, *J. Nutr.,* 100, 873—882, 1970.

128. **Erbersdobler, H.,** Rise of amino acids in portal plasma after feeding rats adapted to high protein intake on heat-damaged proteins, *Z. Tierphysiol. Tierernahr. Futtermittelkd.,* 25, 119—121, 1969.

129. **Evans, R. J. and Butts, H. A.,** Studies on the heat inactivation of lysine in soy bean oil meal, *J. Biol. Chem.,* 175, 15—20, 1948.

130. **El-Nockrashy, A. S. and Frampton, V. L.,** Destruction of lysine by nonreducing sugars, *Biochem. Biophys. Res. Commun.,* 28(5), 675—681, 1967.

131. **Desai, I. D. and Tappel, A. L.,** Damage to proteins by peroxidized lipids, *J. Lipid Res.,* 4(2), 204—207, 1963.

132. **Tannenbaum, S. R., Barth, H., and Le Roux, J. P.,** Loss of methionine in casein during storage with autoxidizing methyl linoleate, *J. Agric. Food Chem.,* 17(6), 1353—1354, 1969.

133. **Miller, E. L., Carpenter, K. J., and Milner, C. K.,** Availability of sulphur amino acids in protein foods. III. Chemical and nutritional changes in heated cod muscle, *Br. J. Nutr.,* 19, 547—564, 1965.

134. **Njaa, L. R.,** Utilization of methionine sulphoxide and methionine sulphone by the young rat, *Br. J. Nutr.,* 16, 571—577; 1962.

135. **Ellinger, G. M. and Palmer, R.,** The biological availability of methionine sulphoxide, *Proc. Nutr. Soc.,* 28, 42A, 1969.

136. **Miller, S. A., Tannenbaum, S. R., and Seitz, A. W.,** Utilization of L-methionine sulfoxide by the rat, *J. Nutr.,* 100, 909—916, 1970.

137. **Cuq, J. L., Provansal, M., Guilleux, F., and Cheftel, C.,** Oxidation of methionine residues of casein by hydrogen peroxide. Effects on *in vitro* digestibility, *J. Food Sci.,* 38, 11—13, 1973.

138. **Bennett, M. A.,** Metabolism of sulphur. VII. A quantitative study of the replaceability of L-cystine by various sulphur-containing amino acids in the diet of the albino rat, *Biochem. J.,* 33, 885, 1939.

139. **Andrews, F., Bjorksten, J., Trenk, F. B., Henick, A. S., and Koch, R. B.,** The reaction of an autoxidized lipid with proteins, *J. Am. Oil Chem. Soc.,* 42, 779—781, 1965.

140. **Lea, C. H., Parr, L. J., and Carpenter, K. J.,** Chemical and nutritional changes in stored herring meal (2), *Br. J. Nutr.,* 14, 91—113, 1960.

141. **Roubal, W. T. and Tappel, A. L.,** Damage to proteins, enzymes, and amino acids by peroxidizing lipids, *Arch. Biochem. Biophys.,* 113, 5—8, 1966; Polymerization of proteins induced by free-radical lipid peroxidation, *Arch. Biochem. Biophys.,* 113, 150—155, 1966.

142. **Narayan, K. A., Sugai, M., and Kummerow, F. A.,** Complex formation between oxidized lipids and egg albumin, *J. Am. Oil Chem. Soc.,* 41, 254—259, 1964.

143. **Mareckova, O., Vacrikova, J., Pokorny, J., and Vavrinkova, H.,** Die biologische Bedeutung von Komplexen oxydierter Lipide mit Eiweiss. IV. Die enzymatische Hydrolyse der Eiweisskomponente *in vivo, Nahrung,* 12(8), 769—773, 1968.

144. **Dvorak, Z. and Vognarova, I.,** Available lysine in meat and meat products, *J. Sci. Food Agric.,* 16(6), 305—312, 1965.

145. Haschemeyer, R. H. and Haschemeyer, A. E. V., *Proteins, A Guide to Study by Physical and Chemical Methods,* John Wiley & Sons, New York, 1973.

146. Bezkorovainy, A., *Basic Protein Chemistry,* Charles C Thomas, Springfield, Ill., 1970.

147. Joly, M., *A Physico-chemical Approach to the Denaturation of Proteins,* Academic Press, New York, 1965, 1—189.

148. Sone, T., *Consistency of Foodstuffs,* Reidel Publishing, Dordrecht, Holland, 1972.

149. Rowland, S. J., The determination of the nitrogen distribution in milk, *J. Dairy Res.,* 9, 42—46, 1938.

150. Smith, A. K., Belter, P. A., and Johnsen, V. L., Peptization of soybean meal protein. Effect of method of dispersion and age of beans, *J. Am. Oil Chem. Soc.,* 29, 309—312, 1952.

151. Delort-Laval, J., Cuisson et qualité du tourteau de soja, in *Proc. 7th Int. Congr. Nutr.,* Vol. 5, Vieweg and Sohn, Brunswick, West Germany, 1967, 261—267.

152. Sanders, G. P. and Sager, O. S., Heat inactivation of milk phosphatase in dairy products, *J. Dairy Sci.,* 31, 845—857, 1948.

153. Haab, W. and Smith, L. M., Variations in alkaline phosphatase activity of milk, *J. Dairy Sci.,* 39, 1644—1650, 1956.

154. Frankel, E. N. and Tarassuk, N. P., The specificity of milk lipase. I. Determination of the lipolytic activity in milk toward milk fat and simpler esters, *J. Dairy Sci.,* 39, 1506—1516, 1956.

155. Aurand, L. W., Roberts, W. M., and Cardwell, J. T., A method for the estimation of peroxidase activity in milk, *J. Dairy Sci.,* 39, 568—573, 1956.

156. Caskey, C. D., Jr. and Knapp, F. C., Method for detecting inadequately heated soybean oil meal, *Ind. Eng. Chem. Anal. Ed.,* 16(10), 640—641, 1944.

157. Croston, C. B., Smith, A. K., and Cowan, J. C., Measurement of urease activity in soybean oil meal, *J. Am. Oil Chem. Soc.,* 32, 279—282, 1955.

158. Van Buren, J. P., Steinkraus, K. H., Hackler, L. R., El Rawi, I., and Hand, D. B., Indices of protein quality in dried soymilks, *J. Agric. Food Chem.,* 12, 524—528, 1964.

159. Hetrick, J. H. and Tracy, P. H., Effect of high-temperature short-time heat treatments on some properties of milk. II. Inactivation of the lipase enzyme, *J. Dairy Sci.,* 31, 881—887, 1948.

160. Hetrick, J. H. and Tracy, P. H., Effect of high-temperature short-time treatments on some properties of milk. I. Inactivation of the phosphatase enzyme, *J. Dairy Sci.,* 31, 867—879, 1948.

161. Lear, S. A. and Foster, H. G., The rate of phosphatase inactivation in milk, *J. Dairy Sci.,* 32, 509—514, 1949.

162. Mullen, J. E. C., The acid phosphatase of cows' milk, *J. Dairy Res.,* 17, 288—295, 1950.

163. Burstein, A. I. and Frum, F. S., Kinetik der Milchkatalase beim Erhitzen, *Z. Unters. Lebensm.,* 62, 489—509, 1931.

164. Picn, J., Le contrôle de la pasteurisation du lait et de la crème, *Lait,* 25, 311—320, 1945.

165. Jenness, R. and Patton, S., *Principles of Dairy Chemistry,* John Wiley & Sons, New York, 1959, 201.

166. Laskowski, M. and Laskowski, M., Jr., Naturally occurring trypsin inhibitors, in *Advances in Protein Chemistry,* Vol. 9, Anson, M. L., Bailey, K., and Edsall, J. T., Eds., Academic Press, New York, 1954, 203—242.

167. Grabar, P. and Williams, C. A., Jr., Méthode immuno-électrophorétique d'analyse de mélanges de substances antigéniques, *Biochim. Biophys. Acta,* 17, 67—74, 1955.

168. Grabar, P., The use of immunochemical methods in studies on proteins, in *Advances in Protein Chemistry,* Vol. 13, Anfinsen, C. B., Anson, M. L., Bailey, K., and Edsall, J. T., Eds., Academic Press, New York, 1958, 1—33.

169. Grabar, P., Immunoelectrophoretic analysis, *Methods Biochem. Anal.,* 7, 1—38, 1959.

170. Ouchterlony, O., Antigen-antibody reactions in gels, *Acta Pathol. Microbiol. Scand.,* 26, 507—515, 1949.

171. Ouchterlony, O., Diffusion-in-gel methods for immunological analysis, *Prog. Allergy,* 5, 1—78, 1958.

172. Ouchterlony, O., *Handbook of Immunodiffusion and Immunoelectrophoresis,* Ann Arbor Science Publishing, Ann Arbor, Michigan, 1967.

173. Spackmann, D. H., Stein, W. H., and Moore, S., Automatic recording apparatus for use in the chromatography of amino acids, *Anal. Chem.,* 30, 1190—1206, 1958.

174. Light, A. and Smith, E. L., Amino acid analysis of peptides and proteins, in *The Proteins, Composition, Structure, and Function,* Vol. 1, 2nd ed., Neurath, H., Ed., Academic Press, New York, 1963, 1—44.

175. Jacobs, S., An improved system for automatic amino-acid analysis, *Analyst,* 95(4), 370—378, 1970.

176. Mauron, J., Ernährungsphysiologische Beurteilung verarbeiteter Eiweissstoffe, *Dtsch. Lebensm. Rundsch.,* 71(1), 27—35, 1975.

177. Parisot, A. and Derminot, J., Formation of amino acids in wool treated with 0,1 N sodium hydroxide at various temperatures, *Bull. Inst. Textiles Fr.,* 24(149), 603—615, 1970.

178. **Provansal, M.**, Contribution à l'Étude des Modifications Chimiques des Proteines sous l'Influence de Traitement Technologiques Alimentaires. Effets des Traitements Alcalins sur la Valeur Nutritionnelle d'Aliments Protéiques, Ph.D. thesis, Academie de Montpellier, Université des Sciences et Techniques du Languedoc, 1974.

179. **Sternberg, M., Kim, C. Y., and Plunkett, R. A.**, Lysinoalanine determination in proteins, *J. Food Sci.*, 40, 1168—1170, 1975.

180. **Finot, P. A. and Bujard, E.**, unpublished data, Nestlé Products Technical Assistance Co., La Tour de Peilz, Switzerland, 1977.

181. **Hurrell, R. F. and Carpenter, K. J.**, Mechanisms of heat damage in proteins. IV. The reactive lysine content of heat-damaged material as measured in different ways, *Br. J. Nutr.*, 32, 589—604, 1974.

182. **Finot, P. A.**, unpublished data, Nestlé Products Technical Assistance Co., La Tour de Peilz, Switzerland, 1973.

183. **Neumann, N. P.**, Analysis for methionine sulfoxides, in *Methods in Enzymology*, Vol. 2, Hirs, C. H. W., Ed., Academic Press, New York, 1967, 487—490.

184. **Morrison, A. B. and McLaughlan, J. M.**, Availability of amino acids in foods, *International Encyclopaedia of Food and Nutrition*, Vol. 2, Bigwood, E. J., Ed., Pergamon Press, Oxford, 1972, 389—415.

185. **Carpenter, K. J.**, The estimation of the available lysine in animal-protein foods, *Biochem. J.*, 77, 604—610, 1960.

186. **Baliga, B. P., Bayliss, M. E., and Lyman, C. M.**, Determination of free lysine ε-amino groups in cottonseed meals and preliminary studies on relation to protein quality, *Arch. Biochem. Biophys.*, 84, 1—6, 1959.

187. **Raghavendar Rao, S., Carter, F. L., and Frampton, V. L.**, Determination of available lysine in oilseed meal proteins, *Anal. Chem.*, 35(12), 1927—1930, 1963.

188. **Slump, P.**, Characterization of the Nutritive Value of Food Proteins by Amino Acid Composition and the Effect of Heat and Alkali Treatment on the Availability of Amino Acids, Ph.D. thesis, University of Amsterdam, 1969.

189. **Ruderus, H. and Kilberg, R.**, Rep. No. 33, Department of Applied Microbiology, Karolinska Institute, Stockholm, 1970.

190. **Roach, A. G., Sanderson, P., and Williams, D. R.**, Comparison of methods for the determination of available lysine value in animal and vegetable protein sources, *J. Sci. Food Agric.*, 18(7), 274—278, 1967.

191. **Kakade, M. L. and Liener, I. E.**, Determination of available lysine in proteins, *Anal. Biochem.*, 27, 273—280, 1969.

192. **Mauron, J. and Bujard, E.**, Guanidination, an alternative approach to the determination of available lysine in foods, in *Proc. 6th Int. Congr. Nutr.*, Mills, C. F. and Passmore, R., Eds., Livingstone, Edinburgh, 1964, 489.

193. **Finot, P. A., Bujard, E., Mottu, F., and Mauron, J.**, Availability of the true Schiff's bases of lysine. Chemical evaluation of the Schiff's base between lysine and lactose in milk, in *Protein Crosslinking*, Freidman, M., Ed., Plenum Press, New York, 1977, 343—365.

194. **Mauron, J.**, Nutritional evaluation of proteins by enzymatic methods, in *Evaluation of Novel Protein Products*, Bender, A. E., Kihlberg, R., Löfqvist, B., and Munck, L., Eds., Pergamon Press, Oxford, 1970, 211—234.

195. **Ford, J. E.**, A microbiological method for assessing the nutritional value of proteins. II. The measurement of "available" methionine, leucine, isoleucine, arginine, histidine, tryptophan and valine, *Br. J. Nutr.*, 16, 409—425, 1962.

196. **Ford, J. E.**, A microbiological method for assessing the nutritional value of proteins. III. Further studies on the measurement of available amino acids, *Br. J. Nutr.*, 18, 449—460, 1964.

197. **Gupta, J. D., Dakroury, A. M., Harper, A. E., and Elvehjem, C. A.**, Biological availability of lysine, *J. Nutr.*, 64, 259—270, 1958.

198. **Mottu, F. and Mauron, J.**, The differential determination of lysine in heated milk. II. Comparison of the *in vitro* methods with the biological evaluation, *J. Sci. Food Agric.*, 18(2), 57—62, 1967.

199. **Carpenter, K. J., March, B. E., Milner, C. K., and Campbell, R. C.**, A growth assay with chicks for the lysine content of protein concentrates, *Br. J. Nutr.*, 17, 309—323, 1963.

200. **Miller, E. L., Carpenter, K. J., and Morgan, C. B.**, Availability of sulphur amino acids in protein foods. II. Assessment of available methionine by chick and microbiological assays, *Br. J. Nutr.*, 19, 249—267, 1965.

201. **Carpenter, K. J., McDonald, I., and Miller, W. S.**, Protein quality of feedingstuffs. V. Collaborative studies on the biological assay of available methionine using chicks, *Br. J. Nutr.*, 27(1), 7—17, 1972.

202. **Sheffner, A. L., Eckfeldt, G. A., and Spector, H.**, The pepsin-digest-residue (PDR) amino acid index of net protein utilization, *J. Nutr.*, 60, 105—120, 1956.

203. **Akeson, W. R. and Stahmann, M. A.**, A pepsin pancreatin digest index of protein quality evaluation, *J. Nutr.*, 83, 257—261, 1964.

204. **Mauron, J.**, The analysis of food proteins, amino acid composition and nutritive value, in *Proteins in Human Nutrition*, Porter, J. W. G. and Rolls, B. A., Eds., Academic Press, London, 1973, 131—154.

205. **Waterworth, D. G.**, The nutritive quality and available amino acid composition of some animal protein concentrates, *Br. J. Nutr.*, 18, 503—517, 1964.

206. **Ford, J. E. and Salter, D. N.**, Analysis of enzymically digested food proteins by Sephadex-gel filtration, *Br. J. Nutr.*, 20, 843—860, 1966.

207. **Erbersdobler, H.**, Amino acid availability, in *Protein Metabolism and Nutrition*, Cole, D. J. A., Boorman, K. N., Buttery, P. J., Lewis, D., Neale, R. J., and Swan, H., Eds., Butterworths, London, 1976, 139—158.

208. **Den Hartog, C. and Pol, G.**, Biological evaluation of protein quality, in *International Encyclopaedia of Food and Nutrition*, Vol. 11, Bigwood, E. J., Ed., Pergamon Press, Oxford, 1972, 307—388.

209. **Pellet, P. L.**, *Evaluation of Protein Quality*, Publ. No. 1000, National Academy of Sciences — National Research Council, Washington, D.C., 1963.

210. **Hegsted, D. M. and Chang, Y. O.**, Protein utilization in growing rats. I. Relative growth index as a bioassay procedure, *J. Nutr.*, 85, 159—168, 1965.

211. **Bender, A. E.**, Recent work on proteins, with special reference to peptide biosynthesis and nutritive value, *J. Sci. Food Agric.*, 5, 305—318, 1954.

212. **Wolf, W. J.**, Physical and chemical properties of soybean proteins, *J. Am. Oil Chem. Soc.*, 54, 112A—117A, 1977.

213. **Stahmann, M. A. and Woldegiorgis, J. G.**, Enzymatic methods for protein quality determination, in *Protein Nutritional Quality of Foods and Feeds*, Part I, Friedman, M., Ed., Marcel Dekker, New York, 1975, 211.

214. **Satterlee, L. D.**, Rapid determination of protein quality. Overview, *Food Technol. (Chicago)*, 31, 69—96, 1977.

215. **Hurrell, R. F. and Carpenter, K. J.**, Mechanisms of heat damage to proteins. VIII. The role of sucrose in the susceptibility of protein foods to heat damage, *Br. J. Nutr.*, 38, 285—297, 1977.

216. **Maga, J. A.**, Measurement of available lysine using the guanidination reaction, *J. Food Sci.*, 46, 132—134, 1981.

217. **Hurrell, R. F., Lerman, P., and Carpenter, K. J.**, Reaction lysine in foodstuffs as measured by a rapid dye-binding procedure, *J. Food Sci.*, 44, 1221—1227, 1979.

218. **Hurrell, R. F., Deutsch, R., and Finot, P. A.**, Effect of ultra-high-temperature steam injection on sulfur-containing amino acids of skim milk, *J. Dairy Sci.*, 63, 298—300, 1980.

219. **Weder, J. K. P. and Scharf, U.**, Analysis of food proteins — a new method for the rapid estimation of the isopeptides N'-($\beta$-L-aspartyl)-L-lysine and N'-($\gamma$-glutamyl)-L-lysine, *Z. Lebensm. Unters. Forsch.*, 172, 9—11, 1981.

220. **Bujard, E. and Finot, P. A.**, Mesure de la disponibilité et du blocage de la lysine dans les laits industriels, *Ann. Nutr. Alim.*, 32, 291—305, 1978.

221. **Underwood, J. C., Lento, H. G., Jr., and Willits, C. O.**, Browning of sugar solutions, *Food. Res.*, 24, 181—184, 1959.

222. **Pieniazek, D., Rakowska, M., Szkilladziowa, W., and Grabarek, Z.**, Estimation of available methionine and cystine in proteins of food products by in vivo and in vitro methods, *Br. J. Nutr.*, 34, 175—190, 1975.

223. **Pieniazek, D., Rakowska, M., and Kunachowicz, H.**, The participation of methionine and cysteine in the formation of bonds resistant to the action of proteolytic enzymes in heated casein, *Br. J. Nutr.*, 34, 163—173, 1975.

224. **Tannenbaum, S. R.**, *Nutritional and Safety Aspects of Food Processing*, Marcel Dekker, New York, 1979.

225. **Bender, A. E.**, *Food Processing and Nutrition*, Academic Press, London, 1978.

226. **Hellendorn, E. W., de Groot, A. P., Slump, P., et al.**, Effect if sterilisation and three years storage on the nutritive value of canned prepared meals, *Voeding*, 30, 44—63, 1969.

227. **Mauron, J.**, The Maillard Reaction in food; a critical review from the nutritional standpoint, in *Maillard Reactions in Food; Chemical, Physiological and Technological Aspects*, Vol. 4, Eriksson, C., Ed., Pergamon Press, Oxford, 1981.

228. **Mauron, J.**, General principles involved in measuring specific damage of food components during thermal processes, in *Physical, Chemical and Biological Changes in Food Caused by Thermal Processing*, Høyem, T. and Kvåle, M., Eds., Applied Science Publishers, London, 1977, 328—359.

229. **Mauron, J.**, Methodology to detect nutritional damage during thermal food processing, in *Food and Health: Science and Technology*, Birch, G. G., et al., Eds., Applied Science Publishers, London, 1980, 389—413.

# EFFECT OF PROCESSING ON NUTRIENT CONTENT OF FOOD: VITAMINS

## Elmer De Ritter

Broadly defined, "processing" includes everything that is done to a food from the time it is removed from its source until it is consumed. The primary reason for processing foods is for preservation in order to free man from total dependence on geography and climate in providing for his nutritional needs and wants. Foods are also processed for other reasons such as to remove inedible or less-digestible portions, to destroy harmful bacteria, to make foods more palatable or nutritious, or to make them more convenient for the consumer.

Losses of vitamin content result from many processing operations; the amount of loss is dependent on the susceptibility of the particular vitamin to the stress involved. The main factors contributing to vitamin losses are (1) oxidation (air exposure), (2) heat (temperature and time), (3) catalytic effects of metals, (4) pH, (5) action of enzymes, (6) moisture, (7) irradiation (light or ionizing radiation), and (8) various combinations of these factors.

Variations in the vitamin content of raw food materials can affect the content of vitamins in the final food product to a considerable extent. Raw foods may vary widely in vitamin content because of climatic and soil conditions, genetic variations, and maturity at the time of harvest. This is especially true for some fresh fruits and vegetables. Meat products may vary in vitamin content due to differences in levels of the vitamins in animal diets. These differences in vitamin content of raw foods may have as much or more influence on vitamin levels in processed foods as the processing itself. In addition, home preparation of foods by heating or cooking can result in appreciable losses of vitamins besides those losses incurred through processing and storage.

The extensive literature dealing with the influence of processing on the vitamins in foods reveals a wide range of values for any given process. In addition to variations noted above in the foodstuffs before processing, the conditions of processing may vary from one study to another, and differences in analytical methodology can also introduce variations in the results. For some of the vitamins the analytical methods used are not always as accurate as one would desire. For example:

1. The Carr-Price colorimetric method for vitamin A tends to overestimate the true vitamin A value if significant amounts of *cis*-isomers or anhydro-vitamin A or retrovitamin A are present.
2. Complete separation and measurement of the various isomers of $\beta$-carotene and of other carotenoids having some vitamin A activity is a difficult analytical problem.
3. Complete release of pantothenic acid from bound forms in foodstuffs prior to microbiological assay requires a double-enzyme digestion; the two enzymes have not been available commercially.
4. Vitamin $B_6$ occurs in foods as pyridoxol, pyridoxamine, and pyridoxal, which may be in the free or chemically bound state; differences in biological activity of the three forms have been shown for animals and test microorganisms; also, vitamin $B_6$ in dilute solutions is sensitive to light.
5. Vitamin $B_{12}$ is found at very low levels and in various forms in foods, and microbiological assays with different organisms have frequently shown significant differences.
6. Folic acid occurs in a number of forms with varying potencies for different test

organisms, and different extraction methods may liberate varying amounts of bound forms of the vitamin.

Since variations in the natural content of the raw food, in processing conditions, and in analytical methodology influence the vitamin content of the processed food, it is evident that a tabulated value for the content of any vitamin in a particular food product can only represent an average situation for that product and process.

## STABILITY CHARACTERISTICS OF VITAMINS

### Fat-Soluble Vitamins

**Vitamin A and beta-carotene (provitamin A)** — These vitamins are sensitive to air, oxidizing agents, and ultraviolet light, and decomposition is accelerated by increased temperature and catalyzed by mineral ions. At pH 4.5 and lower, partial isomerization occurs with an attendant partial loss of vitamin A activity due to the lower potency of *cis*-isomers as compared to the all-*trans* forms. The addition of food-approved antioxidants tends to stabilize vitamin A and carotene. Dry concentrates of vitamin A and carotene for food fortification are stabilized both by antioxidants and by protective coatings that provide an oxygen barrier. In situations where added vitamin A is subjected to a high moisture stress, vitamin A palmitate tends to be more stable than vitamin A acetate.

**Vitamin D** — This vitamin is sensitive to the same factors that affect vitamin A. Under comparable conditions, vitamin D usually shows stability equal to or better than that of vitamin A. Thus, an oil solution of vitamins A and D per se or incorporated into an emulsion or dry preparation will normally exhibit stability of vitamin D as good as or better than that of vitamin A.

**Vitamin E** — The vitamin E that occurs naturally in foods is in the form of free tocopherols, of which $\alpha$-tocopherol has the highest vitamin E activity. The tocopherols are unstable in air and sensitive to heavy metal salts and bleaching agents. Heat stability in the absence of air is good. Esterified forms, e.g., tocopheryl acetate, are much more resistant to air oxidation and more stable at very high temperatures such as those encountered in cooking oils.

**Vitamin K** — Vitamin K is fairly stable to heat and air but highly sensitive to light and alkali.

### Water-Soluble Vitamins

**Thiamin** — Thiamin is stable at strongly acid pH and becomes progressively less stable as pH increases; losses are increased as temperature and time increase. Oxygen, oxidizing agents, ultraviolet and gamma radiation, and thiaminases in vegetable and animal products, especially certain sea foods, can cause destruction of thiamin. Metal ions such as copper catalyze breakdown reactions. Sulfite can cleave and inactivate the thiamin molecule, a reaction that is very slow at pH 3, very rapid at pH 5, and immediate at pH 6. Proteins tend to have a sparing action. The chemistry of thiamin degradation in food products and model systems has been discussed by Dwivedi and Arnold[1] in a review covering reaction mechanisms and the nature of the degradation products at various pH levels.

**Riboflavin** — Riboflavin is stable at acid pH but unstable in alkaline solution; it is decomposed by light.

**Pyridoxine** — Pyridoxine is stable to heat in solution but can be decomposed in the presence of mineral salts or oxides; it is sensitive to light in dilute solution, particularly at neutral or alkaline pH.

**Niacin and Niacinamide** — These vitamin forms are stable in air and light and over the normal pH range of food products.

**Pantothenic acid** — Pantothenic acid shows good stability at pH 6 but becomes progressively less stable as pH decreases below 6 or increases above 7. Increasing temperature and time of heating increases the rate of decomposition.

**Biotin** — Biotin is stable in acid solution, in air, and to heat but is less stable in alkaline solution.

**Folic acid** — Folic acid is unstable in acid medium and is decomposed by sunlight and heat.

**Cyanocobalamin** — This vitamin is most stable in aqueous solution at pH 4.5 to 5.0; decomposition is accelerated by oxidizing and reducing agents.

**Ascorbic acid** — Ascorbic acid oxidizes readily in solution with a peak rate of decomposition in acid solution at pH of about 4; metal ions, e.g., copper and iron, catalyze the decomposition. It is stable in the absence of moisture. Ascorbic acid is sensitive to UV-, X-, and gamma-radiation; these reactions are catalyzed by metal ions and oxygen.

## EFFECT OF PROCESSING ON THE VITAMIN CONTENT OF FOODS

### Refining and Processing of Cereal Grains

Following is a brief description of cereal-refining processes.[2]

**Wheat** — The composition and quality of individual lots of wheat vary according to variety and environmental conditions under which they are grown. Blends of various lots may be made to achieve the desired quality characteristics in the milled products. The milling operations include cleaning, tempering, breaking, bolting (sieving), purification, and reduction. The products from hard wheat are farina, patent flour, first-clear flour, second-clear flour, germ, shorts, and bran. Similar milling processes for soft and durum wheat provide products with properties differing from those of hard-wheat products. Additives such as maturing agents, bleaching agents, and self-rising ingredients are frequently blended into wheat flours at the mill. Flour for home use is enriched at the mill with vitamins and iron. Flour for bakers is normally enriched at the bakery.

**Corn** — In the dry-milling process shelled corn is cleaned, tempered (steeped), degerminated, graded, aspirated to remove bran, ground, and bolted. The products consist of coarse, medium, and fine grits that may be removed as such or may be subjected to further grinding, sifting, and aspirating to produce meal and flour. The flattened germs generally are utilized for the production of corn oil. In the wet-milling process the object is to separate the various components of the corn to be utilized for industrial purposes, i.e., for processing into cornstarch, corn sugar or syrup, dextrin, corn oils, and animal-feed products.

**Rice[3]** — The objective of rice milling is to remove hull, bran, and germ with a minimum breakage of the endosperm kernels. Rough rice from the field is cleaned and passed through shelling stones to loosen the hulls and then through a "stone reel" to remove fines. After removal of the large pieces of hulls by suction in a monitor (aspirator), hulled and unhulled rice are separated in a paddy machine. The grain with hulls removed (but with most of the bran and germ intact) is called brown rice. The unhulled rice passes through a second set of shelling stones with smaller tolerances before reentering the main stream. Bran and germ are removed from the brown rice in hullers and/or pearling cones. After cooling, polishing, and removal of the smallest endosperm particles as brewers rice, the white rice is graded by size into head rice (mainly whole kernels), second-head rice (the larger broken pieces plus some whole kernels), and screenings rice (more finely broken fragments). Parboiling[4] and drying of rice before milling causes vitamins and minerals in the bran and hull to permeate the endosperm, thereby enhancing the content of nutrients in the milled rice. The yellow to amber color and less satisfactory keeping qualities of the milled rice after parboiling have limited the acceptance of this product in some areas of the world. Quick-cooking rice[5] usually is made by subjecting the milled rice to moist heat to gelatinize the starch, followed by dry heating to provide a porous structure that permits rapid rehydration. Canned cooked rice is prepared by soaking, cooking 4 to 5 min in excess water, draining, filling into cans, vacuum sealing, and retorting. A flash process[6] involving steam-injection heating and filling under pressure at 250 to 255°F is also used for canning rice.

**Oats** — Milling involves the following principal steps: cleaning; grading or sizing; drying; hulling; separating the hulls and unhulled oats from the groats; steaming the groats; rolling the groats into flakes; and packaging. The bulk of the bran, aleurone layer, and germ remain with the portion used as human food. Hence, rolled oats and oatmeal are whole-grain cereal products from the nutritional standpoint.

**Barley** — Barley is cleaned and then processed by gradual removal of the hull and outer portion of the kernel by abrasive action in a series of pearling machines, followed by removal of the hulls, and aspiration of fine particles after each machine. After the third pearling the product may be classified and sold as pot or Scotch barley. After two or three additional pearling operations, the small, round, white pearl barley is obtained. Some flour is produced in manufacturing pearl barley. The latter may also be ground to yield granular barley grits and/or barley flour. These two products can also be made by roller milling, bolting, and purification similar to the wheat-milling process.

**Rye** — Rye is milled into flour by a process similar to that used for wheat, using a succession of five to seven breaking rolls. After each break the chopped material is separated in a bolter into flour, middlings, and tailings. The tailings go to the next break rolls, and the middlings are ground to flour. The highest grade flour is produced by the first-break rolls. Three main grades of rye flour are produced, namely, white (light or patent), medium, and dark.

**Triticale** — This hybrid cereal produced by cross-breeding of wheat and rye is milled by a process similar to that used for wheat and rye.

**Buckwheat** — Buckwheat is milled into flour by a roller-milling process similar to but much shorter than that used for production of wheat flour.

**Ready-to-serve cereal breakfast foods** — These may be made from whole grain or milled products or from fabricated mixtures by flaking, shredding, puffing, and toasting processes. In the manufacture of flaked cereals, the grain product is usually tempered, or cooked and tempered, flavored, flaked, dried, and toasted. Cooking temperatures, tempering times, and moisture content of the material going to the rolls differ for each cereal product. For puffed products the cooked grain or dough to be puffed is enclosed in a pressure chamber or puffing gun and heated to increase the vapor pressure. Sudden opening of the gun releases the pressure, and the expansion of water vapor and other gases results in the explosion of the product particles to several times their original volume. The shredding process for wheat involves cooking of the grains under pressure with stirring, draining, curing, passing through shredding rollers, cutting the layered product into biscuits, baking, and drying. Many ready-to-serve breakfast foods contain added vitamins and minerals. The vitamin and mineral mixture may be mixed with the moist cereal with or without the use of an adhesive binder such as sugar syrup, salt solution, dextrins, oils, or fats. Another method of addition is to spray a suspension, emulsion, or solution of the vitamins onto the cereal. The vitamin contents of raw and processed cereal grain products are summarized in Table 1.

## Table 1
## EFFECT OF MILLING ON VITAMIN CONTENT OF CEREAL GRAINS[3,7-11,19]

| Product | Vitamin A* (IU) | α-Tocopherol[b] (mg) | Thiamin (mg) | Riboflavin (mg) | Niacin (mg) | Ascorbic acid (mg) | Pantothenic acid (mg) | Vitamin B6 (mg) | Folic[c] acid (µg) | Biotin (µg) |
|---|---|---|---|---|---|---|---|---|---|---|
| **Barley** | | | | | | | | | | |
| Pearled light | 0 | 0.04 | 0.12 | 0.05 | 3.1 | 0 | 0.50 | 0.22 | 40.4 | 14.4 |
| Pearled pot or Scotch | 0 | 0.08 | 0.21 | 0.07 | 3.7 | 0 | — | 0.29 | 31 | — |
| **Buckwheat** | | | | | | | | | | |
| Whole grain | 0 | — | 0.60 | — | 4.4 | 0 | — | — | — | — |
| Flour, dark | 0 | — | 0.58 | 0.15 | 2.9 | 0 | 1.45 | 0.58 | — | — |
| Flour, light | 0 | 0.32 | 0.08 | (0.04) | (0.4) | 0 | — | — | — | — |
| **Corn** | | | | | | | | | | |
| Raw, white and yellow | 400 | •1.43 | 0.15 | 0.12 | 1.7 | 12 | 0.54 | 0.16 | 26.8 | 11.0 |
| Flour | 340 | — | 0.20 | 0.06 | 1.4 | 0 | — | — | — | — |
| Grits, degermed | | | | | | | | | | |
| Unenriched | | | | | | | | | | |
|   Dry | 440 | 0.31 | 0.13 | 0.04 | 1.2 | 0 | 0.34 | 0.15 | 3.8 | 0.7 |
|   Cooked | 60 | — | 0.02 | 0.01 | 0.2 | 0 | — | — | — | — |
| Enriched | | | | | | | | | | |
|   Dry | 440 | 0.31 | 0.44[d] | 0.26[d] | 3.5[d] | 0 | 0.34 | 0.15 | 3.8 | 0.7 |
|   Cooked | 60 | — | 0.04[d] | 0.03[d] | 0.4[d] | — | — | — | — | — |
| Meal, yellow | | | | | | | | | | |
| Whole-ground, unbolted | 510 | 0.57 | 0.38 | 0.11 | 2.0 | 0 | 0.58 | 0.25 | 6.4 | 6.6 |
| Bolted | 480 | — | 0.30 | 0.08 | 1.9 | 0 | — | — | — | — |
| Degermed | | | | | | | | | | |
| Unenriched | | | | | | | | | | |
|   Dry | 440 | — | 0.14 | 0.05 | 1.0 | 0 | — | — | — | — |
|   Cooked | 60 | — | 0.02 | 0.01 | 0.1 | 0 | — | — | — | — |
| Enriched | | | | | | | | | | |
|   Dry | 440 | — | 0.44[d] | 0.26[d] | 3.5[d] | 0 | — | — | — | — |
|   Cooked | 60 | — | 0.06 | 0.04[d] | 0.5[d] | 0 | — | — | — | — |

Table 1 (continued)

## EFFECT OF MILLING ON VITAMIN CONTENT OF CEREAL GRAINS[3,7-11,19]

| Product | Vitamin A (IU) | α-Tocopherol[b] (mg) | Thiamin (mg) | Riboflavin (mg) | Niacin (mg) | Ascorbic acid (mg) | Pantothenic acid (mg) | Vitamin B6 (mg) | Folic acid (μg) | Biotin (μg) |
|---|---|---|---|---|---|---|---|---|---|---|
| Self-rising | | | | | | | | | | |
| Whole-ground | 450 | — | 0.28 | 0.08 | 1.8 | 0 | — | — | — | — |
| Degermed | 420 | — | 0.13 | 0.05 | 0.9 | 0 | — | — | — | — |
| **Oats** | | | | | | | | | | |
| Oatmeal or rolled oats | | | | | | | | | | |
| Dry | 0 | 1.71 | 0.60 | 0.14 | 1.0 | 0 | 1.50 | 0.14 | 29.3 | 19.0 |
| Cooked | 0 | 0.19 | 0.08 | 0.02 | 0.1 | 0 | — | — | — | — |
| **Rice** | | | | | | | | | | |
| Brown | | | | | | | | | | |
| Raw | 0 | 0.68 | 0.34 | 0.05 | 4.7 | 0 | 1.10 | 0.55 | 20.2 | 12.0 |
| Cooked | 0 | — | 0.09 | 0.02 | 1.4 | 0 | — | — | — | — |
| White, unenriched | | | | | | | | | | |
| Raw | 0 | 0.10 | 0.07 | 0.03 | 1.6 | 0 | 0.55 | 0.17 | 14.1 | 5.0 |
| Cooked | 0 | 0.09 | 0.02 | 0.01 | 0.4 | 0 | — | — | — | — |
| White, enriched | | | | | | | | | | |
| Raw | 0 | 0.10 | 0.44[d] | 0.03 | 3.5 | 0 | 0.55 | 0.17 | 14.1 | 5.0 |
| Cooked | 0 | 0.09 | 0.11[d] | 0.01 | 1.0 | 0 | — | — | — | — |
| Parboiled, long grain | | | | | | | | | | |
| Dry | 0 | 0.15 | 0.44 | 0.04 | 3.5 | 0 | 0.90 | 0.43 | 19.0 | 10.0 |
| Cooked | 0 | — | 0.11 | 0.01 | 1.2 | 0 | — | — | — | — |
| Precooked (instant) | | | | | | | | | | |
| Enriched | | | | | | | | | | |
| Dry | 0 | — | 0.44[d] | — | 3.5[d] | 0 | 0.29 | 0.034 | — | — |
| Cooked | 0 | — | 0.13[d] | — | 1.0[d] | 0 | — | — | — | — |
| Rice bran | 0 | — | 2.26 | 0.25 | 29.8 | 0 | 2.8 | 2.5 | 150 | 60 |
| Rice polish | 0 | — | 1.84 | 0.18 | 28.2 | 0 | 3.3 | 2.0 | 190 | 57 |
| Rice flakes, enriched | 0 | — | 0.35[d] | 0.05 | 5.4[d] | 0 | 0.34 | 0.125 | — | — |
| Puffed rice, enriched | 0 | — | 0.44[d] | 0.04 | 4.4[d] | 0 | 0.38 | 0.075 | — | — |

| | | | | | | | | | | |
|---|---|---|---|---|---|---|---|---|---|---|
| **Rye** | | | | | | | | | | |
| Whole grain | 0 | 1.04 | 0.43 | 0.22 | 1.6 | 0 | — | — | 33.6 | — |
| Flour | | | | | | | | | | |
| Light | 0 | 0.35 | 0.15 | 0.07 | 0.6 | 0 | 0.72 | 0.09 | — | — |
| Medium | 0 | 0.79 | 0.30 | 0.12 | 2.5 | 0 | — | — | 16.3 | — |
| Dark | 0 | 1.41 | 0.61 | 0.22 | 2.7 | 0 | 1.34 | 0.30 | — | — |
| **Wheat** | | | | | | | | | | |
| Whole grain | | | | | | | | | | |
| Hard red spring | 0 | 1.35 | 0.57 | 0.12 | 4.3 | 0 | — | — | 14.4 | 12 |
| Hard red winter | 0 | — | 0.52 | 0.12 | 4.3 | 0 | — | — | 40.8 | 12 |
| Soft red winter | 0 | 1.24 | 0.43 | 0.11 | (3.6) | 0 | — | — | 30.6 | 14 |
| White | 0 | — | 0.53 | 0.12 | 5.3 | 0 | — | — | 37.9 | — |
| Durum | 0 | 0.99 | 0.66 | 0.12 | (4.4) | 0 | — | — | 27.0 | — |
| Flour | | | | | | | | | | |
| Whole (from hard wheat) | 0 | 0.82 | 0.55 | 0.12 | 4.3 | 0 | 1.10 | 0.34 | 36.0 | 9 |
| 80% Extraction (from hard wheat) | 0 | — | 0.26 | 0.07 | 2.0 | 0 | — | — | — | — |
| Straight (hard wheat) | 0 | — | 0.12 | 0.07 | 1.4 | 0 | — | — | — | — |
| Straight (soft wheat) | 0 | — | 0.08 | 0.05 | 1.2 | 0 | — | — | — | — |
| Patent | | | | | | | | | | |
| All-purpose (family) | 0 | 0.03 | 0.06 | 0.05 | 0.9 | 0 | 0.47 | 0.06 | 8.1 | 0.9 |
| Bread | 0 | 0.28 | 0.08 | 0.06 | 1.0 | 0 | 0.50 | 0.06 | 6.7 | — |
| Cake or pastry | 0 | — | 0.03 | 0.03 | 0.7 | 0 | 0.32 | 0.045 | 5.0 | — |
| Gluten (45% gluten, 55% patent) | 0 | — | — | — | — | 0 | — | — | 27.0 | 22 |
| Bran, crude | 0 | 1.71 | 0.72 | 0.35 | 21.0 | 0 | 2.9 | 0.82 | 155 | 49 |
| Germ, crude | 0 | 11.7 | 2.01 | 0.68 | 4.2 | 0 | 1.2 | 1.15 | 260 | — |
| Cereal (hot) | | | | | | | | | | |
| Rolled, dry | 0 | — | 0.36 | 0.12 | 4.1 | 0 | — | — | — | — |
| Rolled, cooked | 0 | — | 0.07 | 0.03 | 0.9 | 0 | — | — | — | — |
| Whole meal, dry | 0 | 1.17 | 0.51 | 0.13 | 4.7 | 0 | 0.87 | 0.39 | 40.0 | 16.0 |
| Whole meal, cooked | 0 | — | 0.06 | 0.02 | 0.6 | 0 | — | — | — | — |
| Cereal (ready to eat) | 0 | — | — | — | — | 0 | — | — | — | — |
| Bran (plus sugar and malt extract) | 0 | — | 0.10 | 0.29 | 17.8 | Trace | — | — | — | — |

## Table 1 (continued)
## EFFECT OF MILLING ON VITAMIN CONTENT OF CEREAL GRAINS[3,7-11,19]

| Product | Vitamin A[a] (IU) | α-Tocopherol[b] (mg) | Thiamin (mg) | Riboflavin (mg) | Niacin (mg) | Ascorbic acid (mg) | Pantothenic acid (mg) | Vitamin B₆ (mg) | Folic[c] acid (μg) | Biotin (μg) |
|---|---|---|---|---|---|---|---|---|---|---|
| Bran (plus sugar and defatted wheat germ) | 0 | — | 0.28 | 0.21 | 14.0 | 0 | — | — | — | — |
| Bran flakes | 0 | 1.13 | 0.40[d] | 0.17 | 6.2 | 0 | 0.47 | 0.29 | — | — |
| Shredded wheat | 0 | 0.24 | 0.22 | 0.11 | 4.4 | 0 | 0.71 | 0.24 | 55.0 | — |
| Parboiled (Bulgur) | | | | | | | | | | |
| Dry (club wheat) | 0 | — | 0.30 | 0.10 | 4.2 | 0 | — | — | — | — |
| Dry (hard red winter) | 0 | 0.06 | 0.28 | 0.14 | 4.5 | 0 | 0.66 | 0.23 | — | — |
| Canned (hard red winter) | 0 | — | 0.05 | 0.03 | 2.4 | 0 | — | — | — | — |

*Note:* Values per 100 g of edible portion. Values in parentheses are estimates.

[a] Includes vitamin A value of provitamin A carotenoids.
[b] See Reference 8 for content of other tocopherols and tocotrienols.
[c] Folic acid assay by *L. casei*; see Reference 10 for values obtained with *S. faecalis*.
[d] Nutrient added.

**Sprouted wheat flour** — Lemar and Swanson[12] determined the effect of sprouting of wheat flour on the thiamin and riboflavin contents. Sprouted flours had a mean thiamin content of 0.62 mg/100 g as compared to 0.56 mg/100 g for the control flour. Vacuum drying of both ¼-in. and 1-in. sprouts yielded higher thiamin content than convection drying. Riboflavin content was increased from 0.11 mg/100 g in the control flour to 0.16 mg/100 g in sprouted flours. Due to the better heat stability of riboflavin, the method of drying had no effect on the riboflavin content of the sprouted flour.

**Fortified flour in baking of bread** — In 1942, Schultz et al.[13] studied the stability of thiamin during baking of bread containing either synthetic thiamin, high-vitamin baker's yeast, or whole wheat as sources of the vitamin. The loss of thiamin was influenced markedly by the time of baking. Under normal baking conditions the loss of thiamin was about 20% for all three sources of the vitamin. Riboflavin and niacin, the two other vitamins currently used in enriched bread, are much more heat stable than thiamin. Hennessey et al.[14] reported excellent recoveries of pyridoxine hydrochloride added to flour and baked into bread. Keagy et al.[15] measured the stability of natural and added folic acid in bread making and found losses of about 33% of the natural vitamin but only 11% of added folic acid. In 1974, the Food and Nutrition Board of the National Academy of Sciences[16] proposed an expanded fortification guide for cereal-grain products that included the present vitamins, thiamin, riboflavin, and niacin and, in addition, vitamin A, vitamin B$_6$, and folic acid. Addition of the minerals, calcium, magnesium, iron, and zinc, was also recommended. Rubin et al.[17] reported stability data on vitamins in two bread tests in which the bread was mixed and baked in the laboratory of a commercial bakery. One sample contained all of the NRC vitamins and minerals, and the other omitted the addition of calcium and magnesium. The stability of the vitamins on baking and in the baked bread kept for 5 days at room temperature is shown in Table 2. Only vitamin A and folic acid showed small losses in the presence of all four minerals; without Ca and Mg the vitamin A loss was only 5% and folic acid was stable. The other vitamins showed no significant losses.

## Refining and Processing of Soybeans[18]

**Whole beans** — Only small amounts are consumed in the U.S. in the form of canned soybeans in tomato sauce, canned green soybeans, or soy-milk used by vegetarians or infants allergic to cow's milk.

**Full fat soy flour** — Beans are steamed, dried, cracked between corrugated rolls, dehulled by screening and aspiration, and ground.

**Defatted flakes, grits, and flour** — Soybeans are cleaned, cracked, dehulled, conditioned, and extracted with hexane to remove the oil, desolventized, and heat treated. The flakes are ground and classified as grits and flours.

**Soy protein concentrates** — The protein content of defatted soybean flakes or flour is raised by removal of soluble sugars and other low-molecular weight components by processes involving washing with alcohol or acid at pH 4.5 or with water after toasting of the flakes.

**Soy protein isolates (proteinates)** — These are the most refined forms of soy protein, having the water-insoluble polysaccharides removed in addition to the water-soluble components. This is accomplished by extraction of the protein with dilute alkali (pH 7 to 9), filtering to remove insoluble polysaccharides, precipitation of the proteins at pH 4.5, centrifuging, washing, concentrating, and drying. Alternatively, the washed curd may be resolubilized at about pH 7 and then spray dried.

**Oriental soybean foods** — Tofu is made from the oil-protein complex by precipitation with calcium. Miso is prepared by fermenting a paste of soybeans with or without rice or barley. Natto is made by fermenting soybeans with *Bacillus natto*. Soy sauce is made by fermenting soybeans, wheat, and salt or by acid hydrolysis of defatted soy-

Table 2
STABILITY OF VITAMINS IN BREAD (38% $H_2O$)
FORTIFIED WITH COMPLETE NRC PROPOSED
VITAMIN - MINERAL SUPPLEMENT (A) AND THE
SAME SUPPLEMENT WITHOUT CALCIUM AND
MAGNESIUM (B)

| | Level added per lb | Percent retention | | | |
|---|---|---|---|---|---|
| | | On baking | | 5 days at RT | |
| | | A | B | A | B |
| Vitamin A | 992 IU | 83 | 95 | 83 | 95 |
| Thiamin | 1.8 mg | 101 | 101 | 101 | 100 |
| Riboflavin | 1.1 mg | 105 | 101 | 108 | 100 |
| Vitamin $B_6$ | 1.2 mg | 100 | 105 | 100 | 105 |
| Niacin | 15.0 mg | 100 | 102 | 100 | 106 |
| Folic acid | 0.19 mg | 94 | 105 | 80 | 102 |

From Rubin, S. H., Emodi, A., and Scialpi, L., *Cereal Chem.*, 54, 896, 1977. With permission of American Association of Cereal Chemists, Inc.

bean meal or other plant protein materials. The vitamin contents of the various soybean products are listed in Table 3.

## Heat Processing

Heat processing of foods is carried out to increase storage life and to minimize the occurrence of diseases caused by food-carried bacteria. Examples of heat processing include blanching, pasteurization, and sterilization. Although such processing make foods available throughout the year instead of only during short harvesting periods, the thermal treatments entail some losses of vitamins.

*Blanching*

This is a heat process frequently applied to foodstuffs prior to freezing, drying, or canning. Blanching prior to freezing or drying is used primarily to inactivate enzymes that can lead to quality deterioration in storage. When applied prior to canning, blanching involves treatment with boiling water or steam. Microwave heating and hot-gas blanching are also used.

Vitamin losses during blanching can be caused by thermal effect, leaching and oxidation. In water blanching, the loss of water-soluble vitamins increases with time of contact, but fat-soluble vitamins are influenced to a much smaller extent. Steam blanching results in better retention of water-soluble vitamins. Microwave blanching should yield retention of vitamins at least equal to that achieved by steam blanching. Reviews of nutrient losses in blanching operations have been presented by Lee,[21] Feaster,[22] and Lund.[23] The retentions of vitamins in a number of foodstuffs blanched under various conditions are given in Table 4.

*Pasteurization*

In the pasteurization process, the foodstuff is subjected to a temperature high enough to destroy only pathogenic bacteria and to inactivate the most troublesome enzymes. This may be accomplished by a holding process, e.g., 30 min at 60 to 65°C for milk, or by a high-temperature, short-time (HTST) heating. Shapton et al.[35] have summarized the pasteurization treatments used for various food products. Tempera-

## Table 3
## VITAMIN CONTENT OF SOYBEAN PRODUCTS[7,18,20]

| Product | Vitamin A (IU) | α-Tocopherol (mg) | Thiamin (mg) | Riboflavin (mg) | Niacin (mg) | Ascorbic acid (mg) | Pantothenic acid (mg) | Vitamin B6 (mg) | Vitamin B12 (mg) | Folic acid (μg) | Biotin (μg) |
|---|---|---|---|---|---|---|---|---|---|---|---|
| Soybeans | | | | | | | | | | | |
| Immature seeds, raw | 690 | — | 0.44 | 0.16 | 1.4 | 29 | 1.2 | 0.35 | 0 | — | 50 |
| Mature seeds, dry | 80 | — | 1.10 | 0.31 | 2.2 | — | 1.2 | 0.64 | 0 | 450 | 60 |
| Fermented products | | | | | | | | | | | |
| Natto (soybeans) | 0 | — | 0.07 | 0.50 | 1.1 | 0 | — | — | — | — | — |
| Miso (plus cereal) | 40 | — | 0.06 | 0.10 | 0.3 | 0 | — | — | — | — | — |
| Sprouted seeds, raw | 80 | — | 0.23 | 0.20 | 0.8 | 13 | — | — | — | — | — |
| Soybean curd (tofu) | 0 | — | 0.39 | 0.37 | 0.55 | 0 | — | — | — | — | — |
| Soybean flours | | | | | | | | | | | |
| Full-fat | 110 | — | 0.85 | 0.31 | 2.1 | 0 | 1.75 | 0.57 | 0 | 407 | 70 |
| High-fat | — | — | 0.89 | 0.36 | 2.3 | 0 | 1.95 | 0.64 | 0 | — | — |
| Low-fat | 80 | — | 0.83 | 0.36 | 2.6 | 0 | 2.08 | 0.68 | 0 | — | — |
| Defatted | 40 | — | 1.09 | 0.34 | 2.6 | 0 | 2.22 | 0.72 | 0 | — | — |
| Soybean milk | | | | | | | | | | | |
| Fluid | 40 | — | 0.08 | 0.03 | 0.2 | 2.2 | — | — | — | — | — |
| Soybean oil | — | 10.4 | — | — | — | — | — | — | — | — | — |
| Soysauce | 0 | — | 0.88 | 0.37 | 6.0 | 0 | — | — | — | — | — |
| Soybean protein concentrate | 0 | — | — | 0.18 | 1.16 | 6 | 0.21 | 0.26 | 0 | 360 | 50 |
| Soybean protein isolate | 0 | — | — | 0.15 | 0.6 | 1 | 0.57 | 0.16 | 0 | 90 | 10 |

*Note:* Values per 100 g edible portion.

## Table 4
## EFFECT OF BLANCHING ON VITAMINS IN FOODS

| Food product | Blanching process* | Percent retention | Ref. |
|---|---|---|---|
| | **Carotene** | | |
| Carrots | W, 1—30 min/212°F | 103 | 25 |
| Peas | W, 3—9 min/200°F | 100 | 26 |
| Spinach | W, 0.5—2 min/212°F | 98 | 24 |
| | **Ascorbic acid** | | |
| Asparagus | W, 4 min/150°F | 89 | 31 |
| | W, 6 min/190°F | 89 | 31 |
| | W, 1.5 min/167°F | 94 | 31 |
| | Commercial | 96—100 | 27 |
| Beans (green) | Commercial | 74 | 27 |
| Beets | S | 85 | 32 |
| | W | 63 | 32 |
| Brussels sprouts | S, 11 min/190°F | 84 | 28 |
| | W, 9 min/190°F | 76 | 28 |
| | W, 6 min/212°F | 57 | 29 |
| | M, 1 min + W, 4 min/212°F | 71 | 29 |
| | M, 3 min + W, 2 min/212°F | 65 | 29 |
| Cabbage | S | 82 | 32 |
| | W | 48 | 32 |
| Carrots | S | 72 | 32 |
| | W | 55 | 32 |
| | M | 100 | 33 |
| Kale | S | 80 | 32 |
| | W | 56 | 32 |
| Peas | W, 3 min/200°F | 67 | 26 |
| | W, 9 min/200°F | 42 | 26 |
| | W, 4.5 min/190—200°F | 76—99 | 30 |
| | W, 18.5 min/190—200°F | 60—68 | 30 |
| | Commercial | 78 | 27 |
| Potatoes | S | 77 | 32 |
| | W | 62 | 32 |
| Spinach | S, 2.75 min/205°F | 97 | 27 |
| | W, 2.75 min/188°F | 72 | 27 |
| | W, 12 min/160°F | 67 | 27 |
| | W, 45 min/160°F | 6 | 27 |
| | **Thiamin** | | |
| Asparagus | W, 1.5 min/170°F | 100 | 34 |
| | Commercial | 91 | 27 |
| Beans (green, whole) | W, 6 min/170—180°F | 94 | 34 |
| | Commercial | 94 | 27 |
| Beans (green, cut) | W, 6 min/180°F | 83 | 34 |
| Lima beans | W, 12 min/208°F | 64 | 34 |
| Peas (Alaska) | W, 6—7 min/170—190°F | 64—100 | 34 |
| Peas | W, 4.5 min/190—200°F | 94—97 | 30 |
| | W, 18.5 min/190—200°F | 68—71 | 30 |
| | Commercial | 90 | 27 |
| Spinach | S, 2.75 min/205°F | 100 | 27 |
| | W (rotary) 2.5 min/206°F | 77 | 27 |
| | **Riboflavin** | | |
| Asparagus | Commercial | 92 | 27 |
| Beans (green) | Commercial | 97 | 27 |

Table 4 (continued)
## EFFECT OF BLANCHING ON VITAMINS IN FOODS

| Food product | Blanching process[a] | Percent retention | Ref. |
|---|---|---|---|
| Peas | W, 3 min/200°F | 70 | 26 |
| | W, 6 min/200°F | 70 | 26 |
| | W, 9 min/200°F | 50 | 26 |
| | Commercial | 92 | 27 |
| Spinach | S, 2.75 min/205°F | 102 | 27 |
| | W (rotary) 2.5 min/206°F | 82 | 27 |
| | Niacin | | |
| Asparagus | Commercial | 95—96 | 27 |
| Beans (green) | Commercial | 97 | 27 |
| Lima beans | W, 8 min/200°F | 60 | 26 |
| Peas | Commercial | 71 | 27 |

[a]  W = water; S = steam; M = microwave.

tures may range from as low as 60°C in a 30-min holding process to 95 to 100°C in a flash process. Most products that are pasteurized have a low natural pH or have been fermented to produce an acid environment.

Thermal losses of vitamins in the relatively mild heat treatments involved in pasteurization tend to be small, but oxidation losses can be high. To minimize oxidative effects, pasteurization of liquids such as fruit juices, beer, wine, etc., is usually done in indirect heat exchangers rather than in open-film pasteurizers, and fluids are often deaerated prior to pasteurization.

Pasteurization (low level)-radiation treatment of foods may also be used to prolong the shelf life of perishables, such as fruits, vegetables, meat, fish, poultry, and prepared foods, by destruction of microorganisms. Enzymes, however, are generally resistant to radiation, and other means such as heat treatment are desirable to inactivate them.

Ford et al.[36] reported losses of thiamin, ascorbic acid, and vitamin $B_{12}$ during pasteurization of milk to be 10, 10, and 0%, respectively, in the HTST process and 10, 20, and 10%, respectively, in the holding process. Vitamins A, D, $B_6$, pantothenic acid, riboflavin, biotin, niacin, and folic acid showed no loss in either process. In the case of vitamin C-fortified orange juice, hot-packed into cans at 190°F from a frozen base, the loss of vitamin C was only 5.3%.[37]

*Sterilization (Canning)*
The sterilization process will ideally produce a sterile food, i.e., one in which there are no viable microorganisms present. Since some microorganisms and their spores are extremely heat resistant, it is generally not feasible to achieve complete sterility by heat processing because of the unacceptable changes that would result in the organoleptic and nutrient values of the food. Consequently, the use of heat processing for sterilization of foods is supplemented by proper packaging and temperature of storage so that any remaining microorganisms or spores will not grow in the food during storage. Such heat-processed foods are considered to be "commercially sterile."

Brody[38] has reviewed the various methods for commercial sterilization of foods. The destruction of vitamins during the heating process depends on the time/temperature conditions and the rate of heat transfer into the product. Agitation of retorts to achieve increased rates of heat transfer has been investigated actively. The use of higher temperatures for shorter times has also increased, resulting in greater retention of vitamins in canned foods. Data on the content of raw and canned foods have been tabulated by Watt and Merrill[7] and by Orr.[8] Calculation of the percent retention of vitamins through the canning process has been made from these data and tabulated in Table 5 for a number of vegetables, fruits, meats, and fish. Differences in the moisture content of the edible portion before and after canning were taken into account where available in calculating the retention values. It must be noted that the losses of vitamins include losses from the blanching operation as well as for subsequent handling and sterilization in the cans. It is evident from the data in Table 5 that in most cases, there are very considerable losses of vitamins in the canning process.

### Kinetic Parameters for Thermal Degradation

The definition of the effect of time and temperature on the rate and extent of loss of vitamins in heat processing requires two parameters: (1) the rate constant ($R_r$) for loss at a reference temperature ($T_r$) and (2) the dependence of the rate of loss on temperature or the Arrhenius activation energy ($E_a$). In food processing it is customary to express these two parameters as (1) the time ($D_r$) required at $T_r$ for a 90% reduction in concentration of the vitamin, and (2) the number of degrees Fahrenheit temperature change (z value) necessary to cause a tenfold change in the D value.

The only vitamin that has been studied extensively in foods from a kinetic standpoint is thiamin; even for this nutrient the studies have been limited to relatively few foodstuffs. Kinetic parameters for thiamin in foods have been reported by Bendix et al.,[39] Felicotti and Esselen,[40] and Mulley et al.[41] Ramakrishnan and Francis[42] have investigated the thermal degradation of carotenoids in paprika. Garrett[43] has reported on the kinetics of breakdown of a number of vitamins in multivitamin supplements. These studies included vitamin A, thiamin, ascorbic acid, pantothenic acid, vitamin $B_{12}$, and folic acid. The kinetic parameters, $E_a$ and $D_{121°C}$, determined in these studies are listed in Table 6. A review of the thermal degradation of thiamin in food has been published by Farrer.[44]

### Preservation by Freezing

On the basis of retention of vitamins, the freezing process is the best method of food preservation. The technology of preservation by freezing has been described by Tressler et al.[45] Fennema[46] summarized literature data on retention of vitamins during the freezing process. In just the freezing operation itself, losses of vitamins are small or negligible. Losses for various vegetables average from 3 to 14% for ascorbic acid and from 3 to 8% for thiamin. Losses of carotene, riboflavin, and niacin from vegetables are at most a few percent. In freezing of orange juice concentrate, the loss of vitamin C is very small if aeration is avoided.[47] Loeffler[48] reported little loss of ascorbic acid in freezing of strawberry and raspberry purees. Losses of thiamin, riboflavin, niacin, pantothenic acid, and pyridoxine have been reported[46] to be negligible in freezing animal tissues, except in the case of pork chops where Lee et al.[49] and Lehrer et al.[50] found losses of these vitamins in the range of 20% on freezing and thawing.

Freezing preservation of foods involves preliminary processing such as blanching, washing, peeling, trimming, and grinding, all of which may contribute to losses of vitamins. Exposure to air can result in vitamin losses, particularly of vitamin C. Vitamin losses can continue during frozen storage and are dependent on the temperature of storage as well as the effectiveness of the packaging in preventing air penetration. These are discussed in greater detail later in this chapter.

### Dehydration

Dehydration is used as a method of preservation for many foods and involves many types of processes. The procedure is designed to reduce the availability of water by

## Table 5
## EFFECT OF CANNING ON VITAMINS IN FOODS[7,8]

| Product | Vitamin A | Thiamin | Riboflavin | Niacin | Ascorbic acid | Pantothenic acid | Vitamin B6 | Biotin |
|---|---|---|---|---|---|---|---|---|
| **Vegetables** | | | | | | | | |
| Asparagus, green | 90 | 33 | 50 | 53 | 46 | 31 | 36 | — |
| Beans, green | 78 | 38 | 46 | 61 | 21 | 39 | 50 | — |
| Beans, lima | 73 | 14 | 46 | 40 | 23 | 28 | — | — |
| Beets | 100 | 34 | 61 | 26 | 31 | 67 | 91 | 60 |
| Carrots | 138 | 34 | 62 | 69 | 26 | 46 | 20 | 37 |
| Corn | 86 | 21 | 44 | 55 | 35 | 41 | 70 | 22 |
| Peas | 106 | 25 | 42 | 27 | 29 | 20 | 31 | — |
| Potatoes | — | 44 | 56 | 44 | 72 | — | 41 | 33 |
| Spinach | 100 | 20 | 61 | 50 | 28 | 22 | 25 | 33 |
| Tomatoes | 100 | 83 | 75 | 100 | 74 | 70 | 90 | 45 |
| **Fruits (water pack)** | | | | | | | | |
| Apples | 104 | 69 | 52 | — | 26 | 85 | 100 | — |
| Apricots | 68 | 70 | 52 | 70 | 42 | 38[a] | 77[a] | — |
| Blackberries | 74 | 70 | 53 | 53 | 35 | 32 | 48 | — |
| Blueberries | 43 | 36 | 18 | 43 | 54 | 44 | 58 | — |
| Cherries | | | | | | | | |
| Sour, red | 71 | 63 | 35 | 52 | 52 | 73 | 68 | — |
| Sweet | 59 | 43 | 36 | 54 | 32 | — | 94 | — |
| Grapefruit | 100 | 78 | 100 | 100 | 84 | 42 | 59 | — |
| Peaches | 35 | 51 | 61 | 61 | 44 | 29 | 79 | — |
| Pears | — | 55 | 55 | 100 | 27 | 31 | 82 | — |
| Pineapple | 75 | 93 | 70 | 100 | 43 | 88 | — | — |
| **Meats and fish** | | | | | | | | |
| Bacon | — | 55 | 79 | 72 | — | — | — | — |
| Mackerel | 96 | 40 | 61 | 71 | — | — | 54 | — |
| Salmon | 91 | 27 | 100 | 100 | — | 42 | 43 | — |
| Swordfish | 103 | 21 | 103 | 146 | — | — | — | — |

*Note:* Values are in percent retention.

a Syrup pack.

Table 6
## KINETIC PARAMETERS FOR THERMAL DEGRADATION OF VITAMINS IN FOODS OR FOOD SUPPLEMENTS

| Vitamin | Medium | pH | Temperature | $E_a$ Kcal/mole | $D_{121°C}$ | | Ref. |
|---|---|---|---|---|---|---|---|
| Thiamin | Whole peas | Natural | 104—132 | 21.2 | 164 | min | 39 |
| Thiamin | Puree of: | | | | | | |
| | Carrots | 5.9 | 109—149 | 27 | 158 | min | 40 |
| | Green beans | 5.8 | 109—149 | 27 | 145 | min | 40 |
| | Peas | 6.6 | 109—149 | 27 | 163 | min | 40 |
| | Spinach | 6.5 | 109—149 | 27 | 134 | min | 40 |
| | Beef heart | 6.1 | 109—149 | 27 | 115 | min | 40 |
| | Beef liver | 6.1 | 109—149 | 27 | 124 | min | 40 |
| | Lamb | 6.2 | 109—149 | 27 | 120 | min | 40 |
| | Pork | 6.2 | 109—149 | 27 | 157 | min | 40 |
| Thiamin | Phosphate buffer | 6.0 | 121—138 | 29.4 | 156.8 | min | 41 |
| | Pea puree | Natural | 121—138 | 27.5 | 246.9 | min | 41 |
| | Beef puree | Natural | 121—138 | 27.4 | 254.2 | min | 41 |
| Thiamin | Liquid multivitamin | 3.2 | 4—65 | 26 | 1.35 | days | 43 |
| D-Pantothenic acid | Liquid multivitamin | 3.2 | 4—65 | 21 | 4.46 | days | 43 |
| Ascorbic acid | Liquid multivitamin | 3.2 | 4—65 | 23.1 | 1.12 | days | 43 |
| Vitamin $B_{12}$ | Liquid multivitamin | 3.2 | 4—65 | 23.1 | 1.94 | days | 43 |
| Folic acid | Vitamin preparation | 3.2 | 4—65 | 16.8 | 1.95 | days | 43 |
| Vitamin A | Vitamin preparation | 3.2 | 4—65 | 14.6 | 12.4 | days | 43 |

removing it in sufficient amounts so as to prevent microbiological deterioration during storage under proper conditions. Fruits, vegetables, juices, meats, fish, milk, and eggs are among the foodstuffs commonly subjected to dehydration processes. Sun drying is one of the oldest methods used by man, but many types of drying equipment have been developed, including drum, vacuum (shelf or continuous), belt, spray, rotary, cabinet, freeze, kiln, and tunnel driers. More recent processes include osmotic dehydration via a concentrated sugar solution,[51] extraction of water by solvents,[52,53] foam spray drying,[54] and foam mat drying.[55] More detailed descriptions of dehydration processes and their effects on nutrients have been given by von Loesecke,[56] Desrosier,[57] Brooker et al.,[58] Van Arsdel et al.,[59] Charm,[60] Williams-Gardner,[61] Masters,[62] Labuza,[63] and Bluestein and Labuza.[64]

The most labile vitamin in dehydration processes appears to be ascorbic acid. The decomposition reaction is very sensitive to the temperature of processing and to the water activity in the foodstuff. Lee and Labuza[65] have shown that the viscosity of the aqueous environment is also one of the most important factors in controlling the destruction of vitamin C. The higher the viscosity, the lower is the rate of loss. Addition of sulfite prior to drying protects ascorbic acid, but the sulfite cleaves the thiamin molecule and destroys its activity. Data on retention of ascorbic acid by drying are highly variable. Chace[66] reported better retention of ascorbic acid in rapid drying at high temperatures than in slower drying at lower temperatures. Bluestein and Labuza[64] summarized data on simulated two-stage drying of vegetables in which losses of ascorbic acid ranged from 16 to 37%, depending on time-temperature and dryer construction. Other studies have revealed losses of ascorbic acid in dehydrated vegetables ranging from very low to practically 100%, but other steps in the processing before dehydration may be the major sources of loss. Kaufman et al.[67] reported no significant loss of ascorbic acid on vacuum drying of tomato concentrates. Henshall[68] reported retentions of ascorbic acid of 92 to 97% after fruit juices were concentrated and frozen. Good retention of the vitamin requires deaeration of the pressed juice and evaporation at low temperature.

Of the B vitamins, thiamin is usually the most sensitive to temperature. Thomas and Calloway[69] found 95% retention of thiamin in freeze-dried beef, pork, and chicken. Karmas et al.,[70] on the other hand, reported only 70% retention of thiamin in freeze-dried pork; Calloway[71] recovered only 30 to 50% on air drying of pork. Harris and von Loesecke[72] reported retentions of thiamin in the drying step only of vegetables of 97% for peas, 96% for corn, 91% for cabbage, and 95% for beans. These authors found 73 to 86% retention of thiamin in evaporation of milk.

Stability data on other B vitamins are scanty. Hein and Hutchings[73] reported retentions of riboflavin, niacin, and pantothenic acid generally over 90% in the drying operation involving nine vegetables. Rowe et al.[74] found riboflavin retentions of 92 to 96% in freeze-dried chicken. Miller et al.[75] reported about 80% retention of thiamin, pyridoxine, niacin, and folic acid after drum drying of bean powders. When the beans were acid treated to pH 3.5, the niacin retention was almost complete and the $B_6$ remained at 80%, while thiamin retention decreased to 65% and folic acid to 40%. Klose et al.[76] observed that thiamin, riboflavin, pantothenic aicd, and nicotinic acid were stable in the spray drying of eggs.

In the case of fat-soluble vitamins, Hartman and Dryden[77] reported little or no loss of vitamins A and D during spray drying, drum drying, or evaporation of milk. Hauge and Zscheile[78] and Klose et al.[76] found little or no loss of vitamin A in spray drying of eggs. Denton et al.[79] confirmed these results and also found no loss of vitamin D or riboflavin in spray-dried eggs. Della Monica and McDowell[80] studied three methods of drying carrots, namely tray air drying, explosion puffing, and freeze drying; the retentions of total β-carotene were 74, 81, and 85%, respectively. Vitamin E losses during drying have not been reported.

### Fermentation Processing

The fermentation process involves the use of microorganisms or enzymes to oxidize carbohydrates in foods anaerobically or partially anaerobically. Foods are fermented for preservation, enhancement of flavor or nutritive value, or preparation of beverages. Although fermentation processes have been used in the home for many centuries, they are still of major importance in the food industry today. Some of the more important fermented foods are cheeses, yogurt, buttermilk, sour cream, pickled and salted vegetables, Oriental fermented foods made from soy beans, rice, wheat, beans, and other high-protein sources (including fish), and beverages such as wines and beers. The vitamin content of foods undergoing fermentation may be changed by chemical destruction, by gain or loss due to microbial growth, or by partition into solid and liquid phases such as in whey and curd in cheese manufacture.

The vitamin contents of a number of foodstuffs prior to fermentation and of the resultant products produced by fermentation processes are listed in Table 7. In the case of milk products the first step before a fermentation process is usually pasteurization. Pasteurization results in little or no loss of vitamin A or niacin, 3 to 20% loss of thiamin, 10 to 20% loss of ascorbic acid, and possibly small losses of riboflavin due to light exposure.[77,81-83] In the manufacture of cheese, the greatest loss of water-soluble vitamins occurs at the whey-separation stage. Kon[84] found the following percentages of vitamins in the whey, the balance (except for vitamin C) remaining in the curd: vitamin A, 6%; thiamin, 85%; riboflavin, 74%; and vitamin C, 84% (curd, 6%). Kon and Thompson[85] reported 90% of the niacin lost in the whey separation.

In fermented milk products such as sour cream, buttermilk, or yogurt, the nutritional value is closely comparable to that of the milk products from which they are prepared. The riblflavin content may actually be increased as a result of fermentation.[86]

In the lactic acid fermentation of chopped or shredded cabbage plus salt, the reten-

Table 7
VITAMIN CONTENT OF FOODS BEFORE AND AFTER FERMENTATION PROCESSING[7,8,10]

| Product | Vitamin A (IU) | Thiamin (mg) | Riboflavin (mg) | Niacin (mg) | Ascorbic acid (mg) | Pantothenic acid (mg) | Vitamin B6 (mg) | Vitamin B12 (µg) | Folic acid (µg) | Biotin (µg) |
|---|---|---|---|---|---|---|---|---|---|---|
| Milk, cow | | | | | | | | | | |
| Whole | 150 | 0.03 | 0.17 | 0.1 | 1 | 0.34 | 0.04 | 0.4 | 0.29 | 4.7 |
| Skim | Trace | 0.04 | 0.18 | 0.1 | 1 | 0.37 | 0.042 | 0.4 | 0.6 | — |
| Cream, heavy | 1540 | 0.02 | 0.11 | Trace | 1 | 0.26 | — | 0.18 | — | — |
| Dry, whole | 1130 | 0.29 | 1.46 | 0.7 | 6 | 2.4 | 0.27 | 2.3 | 2.1 | — |
| Dry, skim | 30 | 0.35 | 1.78 | 0.9 | 7 | 3.6 | 0.38 | 3.2 | 3.4 | 35 |
| Buttermilk | | | | | | | | | | |
| Fluid, cultured (made from skim milk) | Trace | 0.04 | 0.18 | 0.1 | 1 | 0.31 | 0.036 | 0.22 | 11.1 | — |
| Dried | 220 | 0.26 | 1.72 | 0.9 | — | 3.2 | 0.30 | 2.0 | — | — |
| Cheeses | | | | | | | | | | |
| Natural | | | | | | | | | | |
| Blue or Roquefort | (1240) | 0.03 | 0.61 | 1.2 | 0 | 1.80 | 0.17 | 1.4 | — | — |
| Brick | (1240) | — | 0.45 | 0.1 | 0 | 0.29 | 0.07 | 1.0 | — | — |
| Camembert (domestic) | (1010) | 0.04 | 0.75 | 0.8 | 0 | 1.25 | 0.22 | 1.3 | — | — |
| Cheddar (domestic) | (1310) | 0.03 | 0.46 | 0.1 | 0 | 0.50 | 0.08 | 1.0 | 16 | 3.6 |
| Cottage | | | | | | | | | | |
| Creamed | (170) | 0.03 | 0.25 | 0.1 | 0 | — | — | — | — | — |
| Uncreamed | (10) | 0.03 | 0.28 | (0.1) | 0 | 0.22 | 0.04 | 1.0 | — | — |
| Cream | (1540) | (0.02) | 0.24 | 0.1 | 0 | 0.27 | 0.055 | 0.22 | — | — |
| Limburger | (1140) | 0.08 | 0.50 | 0.2 | 0 | 1.18 | 0.086 | 1.04 | — | — |
| Parmesan | (1060) | 0.02 | 0.73 | 0.2 | 0 | 0.53 | 0.096 | — | — | — |
| Swiss (domestic) | (1140) | 0.01 | (0.40) | (0.1) | 0 | 0.37 | 0.075 | 1.8 | — | — |
| Pasteurized process | | | | | | | | | | |
| American | (1220) | 0.02 | 0.41 | Trace | 0 | 0.40 | 0.080 | 0.8 | — | 4.6 |
| Swiss | (1100) | (0.01) | 0.41 | 0.1 | 0 | 0.26 | 0.043 | 1.2 | — | — |
| Cheese food, American | (980) | (0.02) | 0.58 | 0.2 | 0 | — | — | 0.65 | — | — |
| Cheese spread, American | (870) | 0.01 | 0.54 | 0.1 | 0 | 0.313 | 0.059 | 0.40 | — | — |
| Yogurt | | | | | | | | | | |
| From partially skimmed milk | 70 | 0.04 | 0.18 | 0.1 | 1 | — | 0.046 | 0.11 | — | — |
| From whole milk | 140 | 0.03 | 0.16 | 0.1 | 1 | — | — | — | — | — |

| | | | | | | | | | |
|---|---|---|---|---|---|---|---|---|---|
| Grapes | 100 | 0.05 | 0.03 | 0.3 | 4 | 0.075 | 0.08 | 0 | — | 1.6 |
| Wines | | | | | | | | | | |
|   Dessert (18.8% alcohol by volume) | — | 0.01 | 0.02 | 0.2 | — | 0.03 | 0.04 | 0 | — | — |
|   Table (12.2% alcohol by volume) | — | Trace | 0.01 | 0.1 | — | — | — | — | — | — |
| Cabbage (fresh) | 165 | 0.05 | 0.07 | 0.3 | 51 | 0.21 | 0.16 | 0 | — | 2.4 |
| Sauerkraut, canned solids and liquid | 50 | 0.03 | 0.04 | 0.2 | 14 | 0.093 | 0.13 | 0 | — | — |
| Cucumbers, not pared | 250 | 0.03 | 0.04 | 0.2 | 11 | 0.25 | 0.042 | 0 | — | — |
| Pickles | — | — | — | — | — | — | 0.007 | 0 | — | — |
|   Dill | 100 | Trace | 0.02 | Trace | 6 | — | — | — | — | — |
|   Fresh (bread and butter) | 140 | Trace | 0.03 | Trace | 9 | — | — | — | — | — |
|   Sour | 100 | Trace | 0.02 | Trace | 7 | — | — | — | — | — |

*Note:* Values per 100 g edible portion. Values in parentheses are estimates.

tion of vitamin C is good, but a slow, progressive loss occurs during storage in the vat after fermentation is complete. Further destruction in the canning operation ranges from 25 to 33%.[87] Camillo et al.[88] reported nutrient changes during the manufacture of pickles. Losses of B vitamins ranged from 75 to 85% for salt-stock pickles and 33 to 87% for genuine dill pickles. Losses of vitamin C were about 100%, but $\beta$-carotene was higher in the salt-stock pickles than in the fresh cucumbers, although the level of $\beta$-carotene was not high enough to be of nutritional significance.

Hesseltine[89] and Pederson[90] have described the characteristics of various fermented foods made from soybeans and other high protein sources usually by a mold fermentation process. Tempeh, which is made using *R. oligosporus,* suffered a loss of thiamin of 50% or more, but riboflavin content was more than doubled, and niacin and vitamin $B_{12}$ contents were greatly increased during manufacture.[91-93] Natto is a product of fermentation of soybeans with *Bactillus subtilis.* Hayashi[94] found the thiamin content of natto to be equal to that of the soybeans before cooking, and the riboflavin content was found to be considerably higher than that originally present in the soybeans. Sano[95] reported about a threefold increase of thiamin and riboflavin and almost a fivefold increase of vitamin $B_{12}$ in natto as compared to the original soybeans. Sufu is a mold-fermented product of soybean curd or tofu. Chang and Murray[96] reported that when soybean curd was separated from the milk, 50% of the thiamin and 25% of the niacin were retained, whereas the riboflavin content of the curd was similar to that of the original soybeans. Miller et al.[97] found only about 20% retention of all three of these vitamins in the preparation of soybean curd.

### Salting, Curing, or Smoking
#### Salting
At high concentrations, salt exhibits an important bacteriostatic action and is used for preservation of meat, poultry, and especially fish.[98] Salt is added either in the dry form or as a brine solution. A low content of salt (0.5 to 1%) in fish flesh largely eliminates exudation of free liquid after the fish have been frozen and thawed. This very likely reduces the losses of water-soluble vitamins that would be expected to be higher at higher salt levels where exudation of liquid is greater. Although the vitamin contents of processed fish have been reported by Cutting,[99] Tarr,[100,101] and Sorasuchart,[102] comparative data on identical raw products are generally not available to permit evaluation of vitamin losses that have been assumed to be small in the salting processes.

#### Curing
Curing involves the treatment of meat with salt and other additives such as nitrite and/or nitrate, sugar, and other substances; the objectives are to develop stable, attractive color and characteristic flavor and to preserve the meat by inhibiting bacteriological spoilage. Curing agents are added in various ways, including dry rubbing, immersion into curing brine, arterial pumping, needle injection (stitch pumping), and combinations of these methods. Detailed descriptions of curing processes have been given by Lawrie,[103] Brissey and Goeser,[104] and Bard and Townsend.[105]

Losses of vitamins in curing of ham and bacon have been reported to range from 1 to 26% for thiamin, 1 to 11% for riboflavin, and 1 to 19% for niacin.[106-108] Vitamin C (sodium ascorbate) or sodium erythorbate are used extensively in curing processes to accelerate the curing process. Shortening of the curing time results in reduced shrinkage from water loss and rendering. The vitamin C or erythorbate also serves as an antioxidant to preserve color and flavor. Newmark et al.,[109] reported data on the stability of ascorbate added in curing of bacon at levels of 500, 1000, 1500 and 2000 ppm. Retention of ascorbate in the curing process averaged 58, 71, 86, and 83% at

Table 8
VITAMIN CONTENT OF CURED AND/OR SMOKED MEATS AND FISH[7,8,10]

| Product | Thiamin (mg) | Riboflavin (mg) | Niacin (mg) | Pantothenic acid (mg) | Vitamin B₆ (mg) | Vitamin B₁₂ (μg) | Folic acid (μg) | Biotin (μg) |
|---|---|---|---|---|---|---|---|---|
| | | | Meats | | | | | |
| Bacon, raw | 0.36 | 0.11 | 1.8 | 0.33 | 0.125 | 0.7 | — | 7.6 |
| Bacon, Canadian, unheated | 0.83 | 0.22 | 4.7 | — | — | — | — | — |
| Bologna | 0.16 | 0.22 | 2.6 | — | 0.10 | — | — | — |
| Frankfurters, raw | 0.16 | 0.20 | 2.7 | 0.43 | 0.14 | 1.3 | — | — |
| Ham, aired, raw, medium fat | 0.77 | 0.19 | 4.1 | 0.53 | 0.32 | 0.5 | 10.6 | 5.0 |
| Liverwurst, smoked | 0.17 | 1.44 | 8.2 | 2.78 | 0.19 | 13.9 | — | — |
| Pork sausage, raw | 0.43 | 0.17 | 2.3 | 0.68 | 0.165 | 0.54 | 11.6 | — |
| Salami | 0.37 | 0.25 | 5.3 | — | 0.123 | 1.4 | — | — |
| | | | Fish | | | | | |
| Halibut (Greenland) smoked | — | 0.17 | 1.5 | 0.72 | — | 0.6 | — | — |
| Herring (fat) cold smoked | — | 0.28 | 4.2 | 0.88 | 0.20 | 15.0 | — | — |
| Herring (fat) hot smoked | — | 0.26 | 4.7 | 0.99 | 0.32 | 14.0 | — | — |
| Mackerel (Autumn) smoked | — | 0.37 | 6.6 | 0.52 | 0.41 | 12.0 | — | — |
| Salmon, smoked | 0.11 | 0.19 | 5.0 | 0.71 | 0.70 | 7.0 | — | — |

*Note:* Values per 100 g edible portion.

these four levels of addition. Storage losses of ascorbate in the freezer for these bacons in vacuum packages or opened packages averaged about 1% per week. During refrigerator storage, ascorbate losses averaged about 8% per week in vacuum packages and 11% in packages opened to the air. Losses of ascorbate on frying averaged 26% of the amount present before frying. The vitamin contents of a number of cured meat products are listed in Table 8.

*Smoking*

The smoking process involves exposure of the food product to heat, flowing gases, and smoke components under controlled conditions of quantity and quality of smoke, heat transfer, humidity, and circulation of gases. Certain components of curing smoke such as phenolics have antioxidant activity that serves to protect against loss of nutritive value. The heating and drying effects and particularly the chemical components of the smoke exert a bactericidal activity that is also of significance in protecting against losses of nutrients via biological degradation. Reviews on the smoking process have been made by Draudt,[110] Cutting,[111] and Gorbatov.[112] The vitamin contents of smoked liverwurst and of a number of types of fish are listed in Table 8. Losses of thiamin in curing and smoking of ham have been found to be 15 to 20%, while losses of riboflavin and niacin were not more than 5%.[106,113] Jackson et al.[108] reported losses of thiamin, riboflavin, and niacin of 26, 11, and 19%, respectively, in brine-immersed and smoked bacon.

Chemical Additives

Chemical additives have been defined as nonnutritive substances added to foods, generally in small quantities, to improve appearance, flavor, texture, or storage properties. They may be categorized as preservatives, colors, flavoring agents, processing aids, or chemicals that affect the functional properties, moisture, or pH of the food. Desrosier[57] has listed a large number of chemical additives used in foods, but only a limited number of interactions of additives with vitamins has been studied. In some cases, an additive has a deleterious effect and in other cases, a protective effect on one or more vitamins. These effects have been reviewed by Cort.[114]

*Deleterious Substances*

**Sulfites** — Sodium bisulfite and sulfur dioxide are particularly destructive of thiamin, which is cleaved at the methylene bridge into its thiazole and pyrimidine moieties. Williams et al.[115] reported that this cleavage of thiamin by sulfite proceeds momentarily at pH 6 and is complete overnight at pH 5, but at pH 3 the vitamin may be kept in solution with sulfite for months without serious loss of potency.

**Alkalies** — Thiamin becomes increasingly unstable as pH increases and is very unstable in the alkaline range. For example, in baking a chocolate cake at pH 9, the retention of thiamin is only about 5% or less. On the basis of studies in model systems, one would expect losses of pantothenic acid to increase as the pH increases above 7. However, in contrast to thiamin, which is rather unstable in pH range of 5 to 7, pantothenic acid has excellent stability in that pH range. In a study of blanching and other treatments of summer squash, Sistrunk and Cash[116] found a higher loss of ascorbic acid at pH 7.5 than at pH 5.

**Acids** — In liquid or semiliquid foods acidified to pH 4 or lower, vitamin A tends to isomerize and becomes somewhat less stable. Pantothenic acid and folic acid also become less stable as the pH drops below 4.

**Copper and iron** — Ferric and cupric ions catalyze the destruction of ascorbic acid. They also react with tocopherol to form the inactive p-tocopherylquinone. Breakdown of tocopherols in vegetable oils decreases the oxidative stability of the oils. Oxidized oils have been shown by Aylward and Haisman[117] to oxidize vitamin A and carotene. Cupric ions are also deleterious to thiamin and folic acid.

*Beneficial Substances*

**Sulfites** — The activity of sodium metabisulfite or sulfite in scavenging oxygen in solutions tends to increase the stability of ascorbic acid. Bolin and Stafford[118] reported a protective effect of sulfur dioxide on both ascorbic acid and β-carotene in apricots.

**Ascorbic acid** — This vitamin, being easily oxidized, tends to stabilize vitamin A, vitamin E, thiamin, and folic acid.

**Antioxidants** — The commonly used antioxidants for foods such as BHA, BHT, and α-tocopherol are effective protecting agents for vitamin A, vitamin D, and β-carotene. Further protection to these fat-soluble vitamins is provided in various concentrate forms by coatings such as gelatin, which serves as an oxygen barrier to supplement the effect of added antioxidants.

**Radiation Treatment**

Three types of ionizing radiation used in processing of foods are electrons, X-rays produced by electrons in an X-ray target, and gamma rays from $^{60}$Co or $^{137}$Cs. In general, irradiated foods are as nutritious as food processed by conventional thermal treatments. Radappertization, a process analogous to thermal sterilization, refers to exposure to ionizing radiation of food in hermetically sealed packaging at doses necessary to kill all organisms of food spoilage or of public health significance. These doses are greater than 1 Mrad. Radicidation, analogous to pasteurization, involves exposure of food to ionizing radiation at doses necessary to kill all nonspore-forming pathogens. Doses are generally less than 1 Mrad. A dose of one rad is equal to 100 ergs of energy absorbed per gram of matter; 1000 rads is equal to 1 kilorad or krad; and 1 million rads is equal to 1 megarad or Mrad.

Detailed information on the processing of foods by ionizing radiation is given in the proceedings of symposia on this subject in 1966 and 1973, published by the International Atomic Energy Agency[118a,118b] and in Hearings on Food Irradiation conducted by the Joint Committee on Atomic Energy of the U.S. Congress.[118c]

The extent of destruction of a vitamin exposed to ionizing radiation depends on the sensitivity of the particular vitamin, the amount of energy to which it is exposed, and the nature of the medium in which the vitamin is contained. Data on the effect of ionizing radiation on vitamins in a number of mixed, animal diets is given in Table 9. Data on other food products are listed in Table 10. Of the water-soluble vitamins listed, thiamin and pyridoxine are most sensitive. Ascorbic acid is also radiosensitive, although like thiamin it is less sensitive in foods than as the pure compound. Retention of vitamin C in oranges, tangerines, tomatoes, and papaya exposed to low-dose irradiation (40 to 300 Krad) has been reported to range from 72 to 100%.[127,128] Green beans, carrots, and corn exposed to 4.8 Mrad retained 73, 78, and 71%, respectively, of their ascorbic acid content.[69,129]

Fat-soluble vitamins are also sensitive to ionizing radiation. Kung et al.[130] studied the irradiation of whole milk with 440 Krad and found losses of 40% of carotenoids, 70% of vitamin A, and 60% of tocopherols. Carotene losses can be reduced by the addition of ascorbic acid. The biological activity of vitamin D for the chick is decreased by gamma irradiation of the complete diet with 2.79 Mrad at ambient temperature.[131] Vitamin K in alfalfa-leaf meal and fresh spinach was stable when these products were irradiated with 2.79 Mrad at ambient temperature.[132]

On the basis of more than 10 years of research sponsored by the U.S. Army, the Army Surgeon General[132a] concluded that "foods irradiated up to absorbed doses of 5.6 Mrad with a cobalt[60] source of gamma radiation or with electrons with energies up to 10 million electron volts have been found to be wholesome; i.e., safe and nutritionally adequate." Reber et al.[133] have prepared an annotated bibliography of reports which support this statement.

## Packaging and Storage

Food packaging materials include glass, metals such as tin-coated steel or aluminum, paper, plastics, and various combinations, including (1) laminated plastics of various types, (2) plastic, silicone, or wax coatings over metals, woods, or paper, (3) rigid paper cans with metal tops and bottoms, (4) thin metal coating on plastic film, (5) thin plastic coating on metal foil, and (6) multicomponent barrier materials made up of as many as seven components including paper, textiles, metals, plastics, waxes, and resins. These packaging materials are designed to afford protection of foods from the various deleterious factors to which the packages are exposed during the customary storage before consumption. These environmental factors that can lead to losses of vitamins include temperature, light, oxygen, moisture, and biological agents. Karel and Heidelbaugh[134] have described in detail the various packaging materials and their interaction with the above environmental factors. More recently, Kramer[135] has reviewed the storage retention of nutrients.

## STORAGE STABILITY OF VARIOUS FOOD PRODUCTS

### Canned Foods

The stability of carotene, thiamin, riboflavin, niacin, and ascorbic acid in a number of canned food products stored for 12 or 24 months at 50, 65, or 80°F is listed in Table 11. It is evident that low-temperature storage yields better retention of vitamins in canned foods.

### Enriched Bakery Products

Thiamin and niacin have good stability in enriched bread under normal conditions

## Table 9
### EFFECTS OF TREATMENT WITH IONIZING RADIATION ON VITAMINS IN ANIMAL DIETS[119-122]

| Food product | Treatment | Percent retention | | | | | | | | | | |
|---|---|---|---|---|---|---|---|---|---|---|---|---|
| | | Vitamin A | Carotene | Vitamin E | Thiamin | Riboflavin | Niacin | Pantothenic acid | Vitamin B$_6$ | Vitamin B$_{12}$ | Folic acid | Biotin |
| Animal diets | | | | | | | | | | | | |
| Cat | ($^{60}$Co) 2.5 Mrad | 7 | 36 | 121 | 56 | 98 | 94 | 88 | 55 | 102 | 78 | 116 |
| Chick | ($^{60}$Co) 2 Mrad | 88 | 75 | 32 | 104 | 119 | 100 | 95 | 91 | 82 | — | 79 |
| Chick | ($^{60}$Co) 3 Mrad | 79 | 69 | 31 | 104 | 105 | 100 | 92 | 91 | 91 | — | 79 |
| Chick (air packed) | ($^{60}$Co) 5 Mrad | 72 | 50 | 49 | 72 | 100 | 103 | 110 | 73 | 100 | 118 | 100 |
| Chick (vacuum packed) | ($^{60}$Co) 5 Mrad | 65 | 61 | 90 | 66 | 108 | 97 | 100 | 78 | 100 | 102 | 100 |
| Guinea pig | ($^{60}$Co) 2.5 Mrad | 94 | 95 | 76 | 90 | 94 | 102 | 79 | 122 | 112 | 92 | 107 |
| Mouse | ($^{60}$Co) 6 ± 0.5 Mrad | 99 | 107 | 78 | 87 | 109 | 103 | — | 79 | — | — | — |

## Table 10
### EFFECTS OF TREATMENT WITH IONIZING RADIATION ON WATER-SOLUBLE VITAMINS IN FOODS[122-126]

| Food product | Treatment | Percent retention | | | | | |
|---|---|---|---|---|---|---|---|
| | | Thiamin | Riboflavin | Niacin | Pyridoxine | Pantothenic acid | Vitamin B$_{12}$ |
| Meat | | | | | | | |
| Beef (enzyme inactivated) | $^{60}$Co (4.7—7.1 Mrad) | 40 | 96 | 104 | 90 | — | — |
| | Electron (10 MeV) (4.7—7.1 Mrad) | 60 | 96 | 105 | 84 | — | — |
| Pork (canned) | 4.5 Mrad at −80 ± 5°C | 85 | 78 | 78 | 98 | — | — |
| Seafood | | | | | | | |
| Clams (air packed) | 450 krad | 80 | 99 | 84 | 63 | 115 | 92 |
| Clams (vacuum packed) | 350 krad | 67 | 111 | 97 | 93 | 115 | 91 |
| Haddock (air packed) | 250 krad | 37 | 105 | 106 | 125 | 164 | 110 |
| Haddock (vacuum packed) | 150 krad | 78 | 100 | 100 | 115 | 178 | 90 |

**Wheat products**

| Product | Dose | Carotene 12 months | Carotene 24 months | Thiamin 12 months | Thiamin 24 months | Riboflavin 12 months | Riboflavin 24 months | Niacin 12 months | Niacin 24 months | Ascorbic acid 12 months | Ascorbic acid 24 months |
|---|---|---|---|---|---|---|---|---|---|---|---|
| Wheat | 20 krad | — | — | — | 88 | 91 | 88 | — | — | — | — |
| | 200 krad | — | — | — | 88 | 87 | 91 | — | — | — | — |
| Flour | 30—50 krad | — | — | — | 100 | 100 | 89 | 100 | — | — | — |
| Bread (from irradiated flour) | 30—50 krad | — | — | — | 100 | 100 | 117 | 100 | — | — | — |

Table 11

## RETENTION OF VITAMINS DURING STORAGE OF CANNED FOODS[136]

| Product | Storage temperature (°F) | Percent retention | | | | | | | | | |
|---|---|---|---|---|---|---|---|---|---|---|---|
| | | Carotene | | Thiamin | | Riboflavin | | Niacin | | Ascorbic acid | |
| | | 12 months | 24 months | 12 months | 24 months | 12 months | 24 months | 12 months | 24 months | 12 months | 24 months |
| Apricots | 50 | 94 | 91 | — | — | — | — | — | — | 96 | 94 |
| | 65 | 85 | 84 | — | — | — | — | — | — | 93 | 90 |
| | 80 | 83 | 76 | — | — | — | — | — | — | 85 | 56 |
| Asparagus, green | 50 | 97 | 88 | 89 | 85 | 92 | 81 | 89 | 93 | 97 | 93 |
| | 65 | 88 | 84 | 79 | 72 | 87 | 77 | 85 | 91 | 94 | 91 |
| | 80 | 85 | 76 | 66 | 54 | 83 | 72 | 84 | 87 | 89 | 86 |
| Asparagus, white | 50 | — | — | 82 | 72 | — | — | 96 | 96 | 96 | 90 |
| | 65 | — | — | 74 | 65 | — | — | 94 | 98 | 94 | 87 |
| | 80 | — | — | 62 | 52 | — | — | 97 | 97 | 87 | 82 |
| Beans, green | 50 | — | — | 92 | 82 | 72 | 62 | 83 | 86 | 92 | 88 |
| | 65 | — | — | 86 | 80 | 69 | 57 | 81 | 86 | 90 | 81 |
| | 80 | — | — | 78 | 67 | 62 | 42 | 80 | 86 | 85 | 74 |
| Beans, lima | 50 | — | — | 88 | 87 | 95 | 75 | 101 | 99 | 100 | 86 |
| | 65 | — | — | 82 | 76 | 91 | 75 | 100 | 97 | 98 | 83 |
| | 80 | — | — | 74 | 66 | 88 | 70 | 99 | 100 | 95 | 78 |
| Carrots | 50 | 94 | 90 | — | — | — | — | — | — | — | — |
| | 65 | 97 | 95 | — | — | — | — | — | — | — | — |
| | 80 | 93 | 91 | — | — | — | — | — | — | — | — |
| Corn, white | 50 | — | — | 97 | 94 | — | — | 82 | 84 | 98 | 90 |
| | 65 | — | — | 85 | 89 | — | — | 85 | 86 | 92 | 88 |
| | 80 | — | — | 78 | 71 | — | — | 88 | 88 | 86 | 78 |

## Table 11 (continued)
## RETENTION OF VITAMINS DURING STORAGE OF CANNED FOODS[136]

| Product | Storage temperature (°F) | Percent retention | | | | | | | | | |
|---|---|---|---|---|---|---|---|---|---|---|---|
| | | Carotene | | Thiamin | | Riboflavin | | Niacin | | Ascorbic acid | |
| | | 12 months | 24 months | 12 months | 24 months | 12 months | 24 months | 12 months | 24 months | 12 months | 24 months |
| Corn, yellow | 50 | 85 | 69 | 90 | 89 | 84 | 71 | 89 | 91 | 98 | 92 |
| | 65 | 87 | 72 | 86 | 76 | 80 | 68 | 89 | 90 | 94 | 89 |
| | 80 | 84 | 87 | 74 | 60 | 78 | 61 | 91 | 96 | 89 | 81 |
| Grapefruit juice | 50 | — | — | 99 | 99 | — | — | — | — | 95 | 94 |
| | 65 | — | — | 100 | 94 | — | — | — | — | 91 | 82 |
| | 80 | — | — | 93 | 84 | — | — | — | — | 75 | 57 |
| Grapefruit, segments | 50 | — | — | — | — | — | — | — | — | 94 | 87 |
| | 65 | — | — | — | — | — | — | — | — | 91 | 77 |
| | 80 | — | — | — | — | — | — | — | — | 73 | 46 |
| Orange juice | 50 | — | — | 100 | 100 | — | — | — | — | 97 | 95 |
| | 65 | — | — | 98 | 94 | — | — | — | — | 92 | 80 |
| | 80 | — | — | 89 | 83 | — | — | — | — | 77 | 50 |
| Peaches | 50 | 95 | 75 | 92 | 88 | — | — | 101 | 98 | 98 | 98 |
| | 65 | 90 | 64 | 90 | 100 | — | — | 102 | 98 | 85 | 80 |
| | 80 | 86 | 63 | 81 | 86 | — | — | 101 | 99 | 72 | 53 |
| Peas, Alaska | 50 | 97 | 95 | 91 | 89 | 91 | 80 | 82 | 99 | 91 | 90 |
| | 65 | 95 | 93 | 86 | 85 | 84 | 73 | 77 | 87 | 89 | 88 |
| | 80 | 91 | 89 | 75 | 68 | 82 | 68 | 82 | 85 | 84 | 81 |
| Peas, sweet | 50 | 98 | 94 | 93 | 91 | 93 | 88 | 95 | 96 | 94 | 92 |
| | 65 | 92 | 90 | 88 | 85 | 89 | 84 | 87 | 95 | 92 | 89 |
| | 80 | 91 | 90 | 73 | 72 | 84 | 81 | 90 | 95 | 88 | 81 |
| Pineapple juice | 50 | — | — | 93 | 100 | — | — | — | — | 110 | 108 |
| | 65 | — | — | 93 | 100 | — | — | — | — | 108 | 100 |
| | 80 | — | — | 87 | 93 | — | — | — | — | 93 | 79 |
| Pineapple, sliced | 50 | — | — | 97 | 102 | — | — | — | — | 100 | 83 |
| | 65 | — | — | 96 | 103 | — | — | — | — | 95 | 78 |
| | 80 | — | — | 89 | 89 | — | — | — | — | 74 | 53 |
| Plums, purple | 50 | 102 | 90 | — | — | 84 | 84 | 95 | 86 | — | — |
| | 65 | 100 | 98 | — | — | 82 | 82 | 93 | 91 | — | — |
| | 80 | 97 | 86 | — | — | 78 | 76 | 103 | 95 | — | — |

| | | | | | | | | | | |
|---|---|---|---|---|---|---|---|---|---|---|
| Spinach | 50 | 91 | 80 | 96 | 90 | 92 | 82 | 100 | 96 | 93 | 90 |
| | 65 | 90 | 80 | 89 | 82 | 89 | 80 | 103 | 100 | 91 | 88 |
| | 80 | 84 | 81 | 76 | 71 | 85 | 69 | 99 | 101 | 86 | 81 |
| Tomatoes | 50 | 94 | 75 | 94 | 91 | 94 | 96 | 91 | 88 | 95 | 89 |
| | 65 | 98 | 75 | 93 | 87 | 95 | 98 | 93 | 88 | 94 | 87 |
| | 80 | 95 | 74 | 82 | 70 | 91 | 97 | 93 | 85 | 82 | 70 |
| Tomato juice | 50 | 98 | 94 | 95 | 103 | 88 | 92 | 99 | 92 | 100 | 102 |
| | 65 | 100 | 97 | 93 | 95 | 84 | 94 | 99 | 91 | 97 | 92 |
| | 80 | 99 | 98 | 85 | 77 | 83 | 94 | 99 | 90 | 86 | 74 |

in the trade. Some authors[137,138] have reported that riboflavin in enriched bread and rolls is sensitive to light and that waxed paper wrapping gives better protection than cellophane. Birdsall and Teply[139] found better retention of riboflavin in partially baked rolls exposed in a brightly lighted store when aluminum foil was used rather than waxed paper; cellophane wrapping provided even less protection to riboflavin. Morgareidge,[140] on the other hand, found no difference in the retention of riboflavin in bread wrapped in unprinted cellophane, printed cellophane, or waxed paper. Stephens and Chastain[141] found little loss of riboflavin in cellophane-packaged, partially baked rolls under simulated grocery conditions.

## Dairy Products

Ascorbic acid and riboflavin in fresh milk are destroyed by exposure to light. Sattar and De Man[142] exposed fresh milk at 4°C to 100 ft candles of light comparable to that of a typical supermarket display cabinet. Four containers were studied, namely, (1) black-pigmented polyethylene pouch, (2) standard paperboard carton, (3) plastic jug, and (4) clear polyethylene. After 12 hr of exposure the losses of ascorbic acid were (1) 13%, (2) 24%, (3) 86%, and (4) 22%.

Bauernfeind and Allen[143] studied the stability of vitamin A in enriched, nonfat dry milk (5000 IU/100g) that was stored in various packages. The moisture level of the milk powders was approximately 3.5%. In 12 months at 75°F the retention of vitamin A was best in vacuum-packed tin cans (96%), followed by laminated pouches (92%), tin cans with air pack (90%), polyethylene bags in cardboard cylinders (90%), cardboard cylinders with metal ends (89%), and polyethylene bags without protection from light (81%). A direct correlation was noted between moisture pick up and vitamin A loss during prolonged storage of nonfat dry milk. Cox et al.[144] also demonstrated better vitamin A stability in this product with gas packaging as compared to air packaging, and also found improved stability of vitamin A if an antioxidant was added. Bauernfeind and Pinkert[145] found 93% retention of vitamin C in dry whole milk stored for 12 months at 74°F in a gas pack as compared to 75% in an air pack.

The retention of vitamin A during storage of butter has been reported by Deuel and Greenberg[146] to range from 66 to 98% in 12 months at 5°C and from 64 to 68% in 5 months at 28°C. In fortified margarines the retention of vitamin A was found by Marusich et al.[147] to be 89 to 100% in 6 months at 5°C and 83 to 100% in 6 months at 23°C. In the same storage tests the retentions of β-carotene in margarine were reported to be 98 and 89%, respectively.

## Fresh Fruits and Vegetables

After harvesting, fresh fruits and vegetables are subject to nutritive losses on aging. Refrigeration is the most commonly used procedure for extending the shelf life of most fruits and vegetables. Bratley[148] has found, for example, that tangerines lost little ascorbic acid in 8 weeks at 0°C, but in 8 weeks at 7 to 9°C, they lost almost half of their initial ascorbic acid content. Oranges, on the other hand, suffered only a slight loss of vitamin C after storage for 3 to 6 days at 10°C plus 7 days at 21°C.[149] Scott and Kramer[150] measured losses of ascorbic acid in one lot of asparagus and found 50% loss in 1 week at 0°C and 90% loss after 1 week at 21°C. Allison and Driver[151] reported losses of ascorbic acid from 20 varieties of potatoes ranging from 10 to 16 mg/100 g. Other water-soluble vitamins are generally more stable than vitamin C.

Dark green, leafy vegetables are rich in carotene but require storage at low temperature and low humidity for good retention of carotene. Ezell and Wilcox[152] studied losses of carotene in kale and collards stored for 4 days at 32, 50, and 72°F with slow, moderate, and rapid rates of wilting. There was little or no loss of carotene in storage at 32°F and a slow rate of wilting. Increasing the rate of wilting increased carotene losses even at 32°F and at 72°F losses were about 76% for kale and 82% for collards subjected to rapid wilting.

Packaging of fresh fruits and vegetables is designed primarily to protect the characteristics of the products that are important for consumer acceptance. Optimal conditions of storage have been described by Smith[153] and by Wright et al.[154] Mapson[155] stated that wilting and mechanical damage are important factors affecting nutritional quality. The oxygen concentration during storage of tomatoes influences the β-carotene content.[156] Smith[153] found that oxygen and carbon dioxide concentrations influence the ascorbic acid content of lemons and that high $CO_2$ levels are very destructive of vitamin C.

## Dehydrated Foods

Packaging can influence the rate of nonenzymatic browning and oxidation that are, in general, the predominant mechanisms of loss of nutritional value in stored dehydrated foods. The browning reaction is not affected by oxygen, but is influenced by the moisture content of the product. The rate of browning increases above a water activity of 0.4 and reaches a maximum at about water activity = 0.65. The rate of oxidation can be slowed by protecting the product from air, light, and other prooxidants. This can be accomplished by various methods including: (1) use of packaging materials of low permeability to moisture and gases, (2) use of chemically inert packaging materials, (3) packing under vacuum or inert gas, (4) addition of an in-package desiccant, and (5) use of an in-package oxygen scavenger.

A series of studies on dehydrated fruits and vegetables conducted by the Research Staff of Continental Can Co.[157] included the following types of packaging: (1) cans sealed under air, (2) cans sealed under inert gases, and (3) cartons with laminated inner bags heat-sealed under air. In these tests, thiamin and riboflavin were not affected by packaging variation. In tomato flakes and cranberries, ascorbic acid stability was independent of the method of packaging, but in apple nuggets, cabbage, rutabagas, and potatoes, ascorbic acid was more stable in gas-packed cans. Moisture-proof packaging is especially important for good retention of ascorbic acid in dehydrated foods. The combination of in-package desiccation and packing under nitrogen was reported to yield excellent retention of ascorbic acid.[158,159] To achieve good stability of carotene, protection from moisture, oxygen, and light is necessary.

Storage temperature is an important factor governing the retention of vitamins in dehydrated foods. To achieve 90% retention of carotene and vitamin C in dehydrated vegetables in good, tight, film pouches for 1 year requires storage at 32°F or less. At 68°F there is often a loss of as much as 50% of these vitamins in 6 months.[160] To maintain 90% of the thiamin in dehydrated pork for just 1 month requires storage at 55°F or below.[161] Klose et al.[76] studied vitamin A losses in dehydrated eggs and found losses in 1 year of more than 25% at 0°F and about 50% at 10°F. Thiamin was found to be considerably more stable in the dehydrated eggs, with less than 10% loss in 1 year at 0°F. Riboflavin, niacin, pantothenic acid, and vitamin D in the eggs were stable for up to 9 months even at ambient temperatures.

## Frozen Foods

The general premise of the frozen food industry is that most frozen products will retain good quality for at least 1 year, if held at 0°F or below. This appears to be true in many cases for good vitamin retention as well. Ascorbic acid in frozen fruits and vegetables is normally the most labile vitamin and has been studied most extensively. Ascorbic acid in frozen peas has excellent stability during 1 year at 0°F but suffers high losses at 10°F in 1 year or at 20°F in 2 months.[162] Asparagus, green beans, lima beans, and peas retain at least 90% of their vitamin C content for 12 months if stored at −5°F, but broccoli, cauliflower, spinach, and peaches may lose 20 to 50% of their vitamin C under these storage conditions.[163,164] The vitamin C in orange juice concentrate is much more stable, and this product can be held at 40°F for as long as 2 years without losing more than 10% of its vitamin C.[165]

The type of packaging used is important in regards to the stabilization of vitamin C in frozen fruits and vegetables. Oxygen permeability is an important factor,[162] but water-vapor permeability has much less effect on ascorbic acid retention,[166,167] although it is of primary importance in protecting organoleptic quality. In the case of frozen meats, fish, and poultry, packaging is designed to prevent desiccation and oxidation that can destroy sensitive vitamins including tocopherol. Instability of tocopherol even during frozen storage has been reported by Bunnell et al.,[168] who found 68% loss of tocopherol on storage of French-fried potatoes for 1 month at −12°C.

There is normally little or no loss of thiamin during frozen storage due to thermal effects, but either destruction or synthesis by enzyme and microbiological activity can occur. Cook et al.[169] found no significant loss of thiamin from turkey tissues in 3 to 9 months at −9°F, and Morgan et al.[170] found similar results for chicken stored frozen for 8 months. Hartzler et al.[171] stored various pork cuts for 5 to 9 months at −6 to −9°F and found a very slight loss of thiamin from shoulder and loin but no loss from liver. Lehrer et al.,[50] on the other hand, reported losses of thiamin of 21 and 40% after frozen storage of pork chops for 3 and 4 months, respectively.

### Foods with Added Vitamin A

Bauernfeind and Cort[172] have reported stability data on a large number of food products containing added vitamin A and stored in various types of packages at room temperature (70 to 75°F). The vitamin A sources used for nutrification included pure vitamin A, oil concentrates, emulsions, beadlets, and spray-dried powders. In most products the stability of vitamin A after 6 or 12 months could be rated as good to excellent. A very small number of food products had losses in the range of 24 to 40% in 6 months.

## KINETICS OF VITAMIN DEGRADATION DURING STORAGE OF FOODS

The determination of the kinetic parameters describing the stability of vitamins during processing and storage is of importance in predicting the stability of the vitamins under a particular set of conditions or in selecting the type of container required to maintain the desired levels of the vitamins over the shelf-life storage period. Farrer[44] has studied extensively the kinetics of degradation of thiamin. Lund[23] has discussed the problem of predicting nutrient retention in heat-processed foods, and Labuza[63] commented on the need for kinetic data as related to dehydration and storage.

More recently, Singh et al.[173,174] conducted kinetic studies of light-induced losses of riboflavin in whole milk and of ascorbic acid during storage of infant formula. Lee et al.[175] developed a mathematical model describing the rate of destruction of ascorbic acid in tomato juice as functions of storage temperature, pH, and copper content. A computer simulation program was developed to use this mathematical model to predict the stability of ascorbic acid in tomato juice. Good agreement was obtained between predictions and results obtained from shelf-life tests. With the advent of nutritional labeling, it obviously becomes important to generate adequate kinetic data on the decomposition of vitamins to serve as a basis for the establishment of label claims.

## PREPARATION OF FOODS FOR SERVING

The final steps in the food-processing chain are the operations involved in preparing the foods for serving. Significant losses of vitamins can occur in each of the various stages of food preparation including (1) preliminary trimming, washing, soaking, slicing, or chopping, (2) the cooking process, (3) holding of the cooked food on a steam table, in a warming oven or insulated transport equipment, or under an infrared lamp, (4) storage of prepared food in refrigerator or freezer, and (5) reheating of stored food.

The methods of cooking of foods of animal origin include broiling, frying, braising, roasting, broasting, pressure cooking, infrared cooking, and electronic (microwave) cooking. Foods of plant origin are cooked by boiling, pressure cooking, steam cooking, baking, and frying. Losses of vitamins can be due to the cooking conditions (thermal, oxidative, light effects, etc.) and also to the discarding of drippings from foods of animal origin or of cooking water for foods of plant origin. Time-temperature relations are of obvious importance as factors influencing vitamin losses during food preparation. Where losses due to solution or oxidation are involved, an increase in the surface to weight ratio due to slicing, chopping, or grinding will tend to increase vitamin losses.

A comprehensive review of the effect of food-service practices in commercial establishments on the retention of nutrients has been made by Lachance.[176] A similar review of the effects of food-preparation practices in the home on the nutrient content of foods has been made by Lachance and Erdman.[177] Several recent publications have compared microwave vs. conventional oven cooking as to their effects on vitamin retention in meats. Bowers et al.[178] studied the vitamin $B_6$ content of pork muscle cooked to internal temperatures of 75 or 85°C in microwave and conventional electric ovens. On a moisture-free basis the vitamin contents of the pork, cooked to 75 and 85°C in the microwave oven, were 12.3 and 12.6 $\mu g/g$, respectively; the corresponding values for conventional cooking were 13.2 and 14.4 $\mu g/g$. Baldwin et al.[179] measured retention of thiamin, riboflavin, and niacin in beef, pork, and lamb roasts cooked in two 2450 MHz microwave ovens; one operated at 220 V (1050 W cooking power) and the other at 115V (492 W cooking power), and by a conventional gas oven (163 ± 3°C). Retention of all three vitamins in the cooked meat was lowest with the 115 V-microwave oven. Differences in vitamin retention between the 220 V-microwave-oven and the gas-oven cooking were small. Ziprin and Carlin[180] reported no significant difference in the thiamin content of beef and beef-soy loaves cooked in microwave or conventional oven.

De Ritter et al.[181] measured eight vitamins in various frozen convenience dinners and pot pies (14 products of 10 different types) before and after normal oven heating in accordance with package directions. Losses of vitamin A activity (preformed vitamin A + carotene) during the normal preparation of these products for eating averaged only 3% with a range of 0 to 55%. Vitamin E losses averaged 13% (range = 0 to 33%). Among the water-soluble vitamins, riboflavin and niacin showed no significant losses. Average losses and ranges for others were: thiamin, 30% (0 to 85%); vitamin $B_6$, 7% (0 to 25%); vitamin $B_{12}$, 4% (0 to 50%); and ascorbic acid in ten products having significant levels, 77% (49 to 91%).

# REFERENCES

1. Dwivedi, B. K. and Arnold, R. G., Chemistry of thiamine degradation in food products and model systems: a review, *J. Agric. Food Chem.,* 21, 54—60, 1973.
2. Geddes, W. F., Technology of cereal grains, in *The Chemistry and Technology of Food and Food Products,* Vol. II, Jacobs, M. B., Ed., Interscience, New York, 1944, 451—515.
3. Houston, D. F. and Kohler, G. O., *Nutritional Properties of Rice,* National Academy of Sciences, Washington, D.C., 1970.
4. Jones, J. W., Zeleny, L., and Taylor, J. W., Effect of Parboiling and Related Treatments on the Milling, Nutritional and Cooking Quality of Rice, Circular No. 752, U.S. Department of Agriculture, Washington, D.C., 1946.
5. Kester, E. B., Rice processing, in *Chemistry and Technology of Cereals as Food and Feed,* Matz, S. A., Ed., AVI Publishing, Westport, Conn., 1959, 427—461.
6. Cain, R. F., Water soluble vitamins: changes during processing and storage of fruits and vegetables, *Food Technol.* 21, 998—1007, 1967.
7. Watt, B. K. and Merrill, A. L., Composition of foods, raw processed, prepared, in *Agric. Handb. No. 8,* U.S. Department of Agriculture, Washington, D.C., 1975.
8. Orr, M. L., Pantothenic Acid, Vitamin $B_6$ and Vitamin $B_{12}$ in Foods, Home Econ. Res. Rep. No. 36, U.S. Department of Agriculture, Washington, D.C., 1969.
9. Bauernfeind, J. C., The tocopherol content of food and influencing factors, *Crit. Rev. Food Sci. Nutr.,* 8, 337—382, 1977.
10. Toepfer, E. W., Zook, E. G., Orr, M. L., and Richardson, L. R., Folic acid content of foods, *Agric. Handbook No. 29,* U.S. Department of Agriculture, Washington, D.C., 1951.
11. Scheiner, J. and DeRitter, E., Biotin content of feedstuffs, *J. Agric. Food Chem.,* 23, 1157—1162, 1975.
12. Lemar, L. E. and Swanson, B. G., Nutritive value of sprouted wheat flour, *J. Food Sci.,* 41, 719—720, 1976.
13. Schultz, A. S., Atkin, L., and Frey, C. N., The stability of vitamin $B_1$ in the manufacture of bread, *Cereal Chem.,* 19, 532—538, 1942.
14. Hennessy, D. J., Steinberg, A. M., Wilson, G. S., and Keaveney, W. P., Fluorometric determination of added pyridoxine in enriched white flour and bread baked from it, *J. Assoc. Off. Agric. Chem.,* 43, 765—768, 1960.
15. Keagy, P. M., Stokstad, E. L. R., and Fellers, D. A., Folacin stability during bread processing and family flour storage, *Cereal Chem.,* 52, 348, 1975.
16. National Academy of Sciences, *Proposed Fortification Policy for Cereal Grain Products,* National Academy of Sciences, Washington, D.C., 1974.
17. Rubin, S. H., Emodi, A., and Scialpi, L., Micronutrient additions to cereal grain products, *Cereal Chem.,* 54, 895—904, 1977.
18. Smith, A. K. and Circle, S. J., *Soybeans: Chemistry and Technology, Vol. I, Proteins,* AVI Publishing, Westport, Conn., 1972.
19. Frigg, M., Bio-availability of biotin in cereals, *Poult. Sci.,* 55, 2310—2318, 1976.
20. Wolf, W. J., Effects of refining operations on legumes, in *Nutritional Evaluation of Food Processing,* 2nd ed., Harris, R. S. and Karmas, E., Eds., AVI Publishing, Westport, Conn., 1975, 158—187.
21. Lee, F. A., The blanching process, *Adv. Food Res.,* 8, 63—109, 1958.
22. Feaster, J. F., Effects of commercial processing on the composition of fruits and vegetables. Washing, trimming, and blanching, in *Nutritional Evaluation of Food Processing,* Harris, R. S., and von Leosecke, H. W., Eds., John Wiley & Sons, New York, 1960, 109—172.
23. Lund, D. B., Effects of blanching, pasteurization, and sterilization on nutrients, in *Nutritional Evaluation of Food Processing,* 2nd ed., Harris, R. S., and Karmas, E., Eds., AVI Publishing, Westport, Conn., 1975, 205—240.
24. Zscheile, F. P., Beadle, B. W., and Kraybill, H. R., Carotene content of fresh and frozen green vegetables, *Food Res.,* 8, 299—313, 1943.
25. Lee, F. A., Vitamin retention in blanched carrots. Alcohol-insoluble solids as a reference base, *Ind. Eng. Chem. Anal. Ed.,* 17, 719—720, 1945.
26. Guerrant, N. B., Vavich, M. G., Fardig, O. B., Ellenberger, H. A., Stern, R. M., and Coonen, N. H., Nutritive values of canned foods. XXIII. Effect of duration and temperature of blanch on vitamin retention by certain vegetables, *Ind. Eng. Chem.,* 39, 1000—1007, 1947.
27. Lamb, F. C., Pressley, A., and Zuch, T., Nutritive values of foods. XXI. Retention of nutrients during commercial production of various canned fruits and vegetables, *Food Res.,* 12, 273—287, 1947.
28. Dietrich, W. C. and Neumann, H. J., Blanching brussels sprouts, *Food Technol.,* 19, 1174—1177, 1965.

29. **Dietrich, W. C., Huxsoll, C. C., and Guadagni, D. G.,** Comparison of microwave, conventional, and combination blanching of brussels sprouts for frozen storage, *Food Technol.,* 24, 613—617, 1970.

30. **Feaster, J. F., Mudra, A. E., Ives, M., and Tompkins, M. D.,** Effect of blanching times on vitamin retention in canned peas, *Canner,* 108, 27—30, 1949.

31. **Wagner, J. R., Strong, F. M., and Elvehjem, C. A.,** Nutritive value of canned foods. XIV. Effect of commercial canning operation on the ascorbic acid, thiamine, riboflavin, and niacin content of vegetables, *Ind. Eng. Chem.,* 39, 985—990, 1947.

32. **von Loesecke, H. W.,** Vegetable preparation and processing, *West. Canner Packer,* 34(7), 35—38, 1942.

33. **Proctor, B. E. and Goldblith, S. A.,** Radar energy for rapid food cooking and blanching, and its effect on vitamin content, *Food Technol.,* 2, 95—104, 1948.

34. **Clifcorn, L. E. and Heberlein, D. J.,** Thiamine content of vegetables. Effect of commercial canning, *Ind. Eng. Chem.,* 36, 168—171, 1944.

35. **Shapton, D. A., Lovelock, D. W., and Laurita-Longo, R.,** The evaluation of sterilization and pasteurization processes from measurements in degrees celcius (°C), *J. Appl. Bacteriol.,* 34, 491—500, 1971.

36. **Ford, J. E., Porter, J. W. G., Thompson, S.Y., Toothill, J., and Edwards-Webb, J.,** Effects of ultra-high temperature processing and of subsequent storage on the vitamin content of milk, *J. Dairy Res.,* 36, 447—454, 1969.

37. **Fenton-May, R.,** Fortification of beverages, in *Technology of Fortification of Foods,* National Academy of Sciences, Washington, D.C., 1975, 100—110.

38. **Brody, A. L.,** Food canning in rigid and flexible packages, *Crit. Rev. Food Technol.,* 2, 187—244, 1971.

39. **Bendix, G. H., Heberlein, D. G., Ptak, L. R., and Clifcorn, L. E.,** Thiamine destruction in peas, corn, lima beans, and tomato juice from 104.5° to 132°C (220°—270°F), *J. Food Sci.,* 16, 494—503, 1951.

40. **Feliciotti, E. and Esselen, W. B.,** Thermal destruction rates of thiamine in puréed meats and vegetables, *Food Technol.,* 11, 77—84, 1957.

41. **Mulley, E. A., Stumbo, C. R., and Hunting, W. M.,** Kinetics of thiamine degradation by heat: A new method for studying reaction rates in model systems and food products. Effect of pH and form of the vitamin on its rate of destruction, *J. Food Sci.,* 40, 985—992, 1975.

42. **Ramakrishnan, T. V. and Francis, F. J.,** Color degradation in paprika, *J. Food Sci.,* 38, 25—28, 1973.

43. **Garrett, E. R.,** Prediction of stability in pharmaceutical preparations. II. Vitamin stability in liquid multivitamin preparations, *J. Am. Pharm. Assoc.,* 45, 171—178, 1956.

44. **Farrer, K. T. H.,** The thermal destruction of vitamin $B_1$ in foods, *Adv. Food Res.,* 6, 257—311, 1955.

45. **Tressler, D. K., Van Arsdel, W. B., and Copley, M. J.,** *The Freezing Preservation of Foods,* Vol. 1, 2, 3, and 4, 4th ed., AVI Publishing, Westport, Conn., 1968.

46. **Fennema, O.,** Effects of freeze-preservation on nutrients, in *Nutritional Evaluation of Food Processing,* 2nd ed., Harris, R. S., and Karmas, E., Eds., AVI Publishing, Westport, Conn., 1975, 244—288.

47. **Tressler, D. K.,** Nutritive values of fruit and vegetable juices, in *Fruit and Vegetable Juice Processing Technology,* Tressler, D. K. and Joslyn, M. A., Eds., AVI Publishing, Westport, Conn., 1961, 447—485.

48. **Loeffler, H. J.,** Retention of ascorbic acid in strawberries and raspberries during the manufacture of Velva Fruit, *Food Res.,* 11, 69—83 and 507—515, 1946.

49. **Lee, F. A., Brooks, R. F., Pearson, A. M., Miller, J. I., and Wanderstock, J. J.,** Effect of rate of freezing on pork quality, appearance, palatability, and vitamin content, *J. Am. Diet. Assoc.,* 30, 351—354, 1954.

50. **Lehrer, W. P., Jr., Wiese, A. C., Harvey, W. R., and Moore, P. R.,** Effect of frozen storage and subsequent cooking on the thiamin, riboflavin, and nicotinic acid content of pork chops, *Food Res.,* 16, 485—491, 1951.

51. **Farkas, D. F. and Lazar, M. E.,** Osmotic dehydration of apple pieces: Effect of temperature and syrup concentration on rates, *Food Technol.,* 23, 688—690, 1969.

52. **Finch, R.,** Fish protein for human foods, *CRC Crit. Rev. Food Technol.,* 1, 519—580, 1970.

53. **Hieu, T. C. and Schwartzberg, H. G.,** Dehydration of shrimp by distillation, *AIChE Symp. Ser.,* 69 (132), 70—80, 1973.

54. **Brennan, J. G. and Priestly, R.J.,** Foam-spray drying using a centifugal atomizer, *Proc. Biochem.,* 7, 25—26, 1972.

55. **Hertzendorf, M. S. and Moshy, H. J.,** Foam drying in the food industry, *CRC Crit. Rev. Food Technol.,* 1, 25—70, 1970.

56. **von Loesecke, H. W.**, *Drying and Dehydration of Foods,* Reinhold Publishing, New York, 1955.
57. **Desrosier, N. W.**, Principles of food preservation by drying, in *The Technology of Food Preservation,* Desrosier, N. W., Ed., AVI Publishing, Westport, Conn., 1959, 132—170.
58. **Brooker, D. B., Bakker-Arkema, F. W., and Hall, C. W.**, *Drying Cereal Grains,* AVI Publishing, Westport, Conn., 1974.
59. **Van Arsdel, W. B., Copley, M. J., and Morgan, A. I., Jr.**, *Food Dehydration,* Vol. 1 and 2, 2nd ed., AVI Publishing Westport, Conn., 1973
60. **Charm, S. E.**, *Fundamentals of Food Engineering,* 2nd ed., AVI Publishing, Westport, Conn., 1971.
61. **Williams-Gardner, A.**, *Industrial Drying,* Leonard Hill, London, England, 1971.
62. **Masters, K.**, *Spray Drying,* CRC Press, Boca Raton, Fla., 1972.
63. **Labuza, T. P.**, Effects of dehydration and storage, *Food Technol.* 27, 20—26, 1973.
64. **Bluestein, P. M. and Labuza, T. P.**, Effects of moisture removal on nutrients, in *Nutritional Evaluation of Food Processing,* 2nd ed., Harris, R. S. and Karmas, E., Eds., AVI Publishing, Westport, Conn., 1975, 289—323.
65. **Lee, S. H. and Labuza, T. P.**, Destruction of ascorbic acid as a function of water activity, *J. Food Sci.,* 40, 370—373, 1975.
66. **Chace, E. M.**, Present status of food dehydration in the United States, in *Proc. Inst. Food Technol.,* Garrard Press, Champaign, Ill., 1942, 70—89.
67. **Kaufman, V. F., Wong, F., Taylor, D. H., and Talburt, W. F.**, Problems in production of tomato juice powder in vacuum, *Food Technol.,* 9, 120—123, 1955.
68. **Henshall, J. D.**, Fruit and vegetable products, *Proc. Nutr. Soc.,* 32, 17—22, 1973.
69. **Thomas, M. and Calloway, D.**, Nutritional value of dehydrated food, *J. Am. Diet. Assoc.,* 39, 105—116, 1961.
70. **Karmas, E., Thompson, J. E., and Peryam, D. B.**, Thiamine retention in freeze-dehydrated irradiated pork, *Food Technol.* 16(3), 107—108, 1962.
71. **Calloway, D. H.**, Dehydrated foods, *Nutr. Rev.* 20, 257—260, 1962.
72. **Harris, R. S. and von Loesecke, H. W.**, *Nutritional Evaluation of Food Processing,* John Wiley & Sons, New York, 1960. Reprinted by AVI Publishing, Westport, Conn., 1971.
73. **Hein, R. E. and Hutchings, I. J.**, Influence of processing on vitamin-mineral content and biological availability in processed foods, in *Nutrients in Processed Foods,* American Medical Association Publishing Sciences Group, Acton, Mass., 1974, 59—68.
74. **Rowe, D. M., Mountrey, G. J., and Prudent, I.**, Effect of freeze-drying on the thiamine, riboflavin, and niacin content of chicken muscle, *Food Technol.,* 17, 1449—1450, 1963.
75. **Miller, C. F., Guadagni, D. G., and Kon, S.**, Vitamin retention in bean products: cooked, canned, and instant bean powders, *J. Food Sci.,* 28, 493—495, 1973.
76. **Klose, A. H., Jones, G. I., and Fevold, H. L.**, Vitamin content of spray dried whole egg, *Ind. Eng. Chem. Anal. Ed.,* 35, 1203—1205, 1943.
77. **Hartman, A. M. and Dryden, L. P.**, *Vitamins in Milk and Milk Products,* American Dairy Science Association, Champaign, Ill., 1965.
78. **Hauge, S. M. and Zscheile, F. P.**, Effect of dehydration on the vitamin A content of eggs, *Science,* 96, 536, 1942.
79. **Denton, C. A., Cabell, C. A., Bastron, H., and Davis, R.**, The effect of spray-drying and the subsequent storage of the dried product on the vitamin A, D, and riboflavin content of eggs, *J. Nutr.,* 28, 421—426, 1944.
80. **Della Monica, E. S. and McDowell, P. E.**, Comparison of beta carotene content of dried carrots prepared by three dehydration processes, *Food Technol.,* 19, 141—143, 1965.
81. **Wanner, R. L.**, Effects of commercial processing of milk and milk products on their nutrient content, in *Nutritional Evaluation of Food Processing,* Harris, R. S. and von Loesecke, H. W., Eds., John Wiley & Sons, New York, 1960, 173-196. Reprinted by AVI Publishing, Westport, Conn., 1971.
82. **Kon, S. K.**, Nutritional effects on milk of chemical additives and processing, *Fed. Proc.,* 20, 209—216, 1961.
83. **Lampert, L. M.**, *Modern Dairy Products,* Chemical Publishing, New York, 1970.
84. **Kon, S. K.**, *Milk and Milk Products in Human Nutrition,* FAO Nutr. Studies 17, Food Agriculture Organization, United Nations, Rome, 1959.
85. **Kon, S. K. and Thompson, S. Y.**, Measurement of vitamins in the control of milk processing, *Milchwissenshaft,* 12, 166—172, 1957.
86. **Kon, S. K.**, *Milk and Milk Products in Human Nutrition,* FAO Nutr. Studies 27, Food Agriculture Organization, United Nations, Rome, 1972.
87. **Pederson, C. S., Mack, G. L., and Athawes, W. L.**, Vitamin C content of sauerkraut, *Food Res.,* 4, 31—45, 1939.
88. **Camillo, L. J., Hoppert, C. A., and Fabian, F. W.**, An analytical study of cucumbers and cucumber pickles, *Food Res.,* 1, 339—352, 1942.

89. Hesseltine, C. W., A millenium of fungi, food, and fermentation, *Mycologia,* 57, 149—197, 1965.

90. Pederson, C. S., *Microbiology of Food Fermentations,* AVI Publishing, Westport, Conn., 1971.

91. Steinkraus, K. H., Hand, D. B., VanBuren, J. P., and Hackler, L. R., Pilot Plant Studies on Tempeh. Proc. Conf. Soybean Products for Proteins in Human Food, U.S. Department of Agriculture, Agric. Res. Serv. Rep. 71—22, 1961.

92. Roelofsen, P. A. and Talens, A., Changes in some B vitamins during molding of soybeans by *Rhizopus oryzae* in the production of tempeh kedelee, *J. Food Sci.,* 29, 224—225, 1964.

93. Murata, K., Ikehata, H., and Miyamoto, T., Studies on the nutritional value of tempeh, *J. Food Sci.,* 32, 580—586, 1967.

94. Hayashi, S., Manufacture of natto, *Soybean Dig.,* 17, 30—31, 1957.

95. Sano, T., Feeding studies with fermented soy products (natto and miso) in *Meeting Protein Needs of Infants and Children,* National Academy of Sciences, National Research Council Publ. 843, 1961.

96. Chang, I. C. and Murray, H. C., Biological value of the proteins and the mineral, vitamin, and amino acid content of soymilk and curd, *Cereal Chem.,* 26, 297—306, 1949.

97. Miller, C. D., Denning, H., and Bauer, A., Retention of nutrients in commercially prepared soybean curd, *Food Res.,* 17, 261—267, 1952.

98. Daun, H., Effects of salting, curing, and smoking on nutrients of flesh foods, in *Nutritional Evaluation of Food Processing,* 2nd ed., Harris, R. S. and Karmas, E., Eds., AVI Publishing, Westport, Conn., 1975, 355—381.

99. Cutting, C. L., Influence of drying, salting, and smoking on the nutritive value of fish, *Conf. Fish Nutr. Working Papers* (Washington, D.C.), United Nations Publishing Service, New York, 1971.

100. Tarr, H. L. A., The effects of commercial processing on the nutrient composition of meat, poultry, and fish products, in *Nutritional Evaluation of Food Processing,* Harris, R. S. and von Loesecke, H. W., Eds., John Wiley & Sons, New York, 1960, 261—304. Reprinted by AVI Publishing, Westport, Conn., 1971.

101. Tarr, H. L. A., Changes in nutritive value through handling and processing procedures, in *Fish as Food,* Vol. 2, Borgstrom, G., Ed., Academic Press, New York and London, 1962, 235—266.

102. Sorasuchart, T., Rep. Technol. Res. Concerning Norwegian Fish Ind., 5, No. 7, 1971.

103. Lawrie, R. A., *Meat Science,* Pergamon Press, London, 1966.

104. Brissey, G.E. and Goeser, P. A., Aging, curing, and smoking of meats, in *Fundamentals of Food Processing Operations. Ingredients, Methods, and Packaging,* Heid, J. L. and Joslyn, M. A., Eds., AVI Publishing, Westport, Conn., 1967, 566—600.

105. Bard, J. and Townsend, W. E., Meat curing, in *The Science of Meat and Meat Products,* 2nd ed., Price, J. F. and Schweigert, B. S., Eds., W. H. Freeman, San Francisco, 1971, 452—483.

106. Rice, E. E., Beuk, J. F., and Fried, J. F., Effect of commercial curing, smoking, storage, and cooking operations upon vitamin content of pork hams, *Food Res.,* 12, 239—246, 1947.

107. Hoagland, R., Hankins, O. G., Ellis, N. R., Hiner, R. L., and Snider, G. G., Composition and nutritive value of hams as affected by method of curing, *Food Technol.,* 1, 540—552, 1947.

108. Jackson, S. H., Crook, A., and Drake, T. G. H., The retention of thiamine, riboflavin, and niacin in cooking pork and in processing bacon, *J. Nutr.,* 29, 391—403, 1945.

109. Newmark, H. L., Osadca, M., Araujo, M., Gerenz, C. N., and DeRitter, E., Stability of ascorbate in bacon, *Food Technol.,* 28(5), 28—31, 1974.

110. Draudt, H. N., The meat smoking process: A review, *Food Technol.* 17, 1557—1598, 1963.

111. Cutting, C. L., Smoking, in *Fish as Food,* Part 1, Vol. 3, Borgstrom, G., Ed., Academic Press, New York, 1965, 55—105.

112. Garbatov, V. M., Krylova, N. N., Volovinskaya, V. P., Lyaskovskaya, Yu. N., Bazarova, K. I., Khlamova R. I., and Yakovleva, G. Ya., Liquid smokes for use in cured meats, *Food Technol.,* 25(1), 71—77, 1971.

113. Schweigert, B. S., McIntire, J. M., and Elvehjem, C. A., The retention of vitamins in pork hams during curing, *J. Nutr.,* 27, 419—424, 1944.

114. Cort, W. M., Effects of treatment with chemical additives, in *Nutritional Evaluation of Food Processing,* 2nd ed., Harris, R. S. and Karmas, E., Eds., AVI Publishing, Westport, Conn., 1975, 383—392.

115. Williams, R. R., Waterman, R. E., Keresztesy, J. C., and Buchman, E. R., Studies of crystalline vitamin B$_1$. III. Cleavage of vitamin with sulfite, *J. Am. Chem. Soc.,* 57, 536—537, 1935.

116. Sistrunk, W. A. and Cash, J. N., Ascorbic acid and color changes in summer squash as influenced by blanch, pH, and other treatments, *J. Food Sci.,* 35, 645—648, 1970.

117. Aylward, F. and Haisman, D. R., Oxidation systems, *Adv. Food Res.,* 17, 1—76, 1969.

118. Bolin, H. R. and Stafford, A. E., Effect of processing and storage on provitamin A and vitamin C in apricots, *Food Sci.,* 39, 1034—1036, 1974.

118a. International Atomic Energy Agency, Food Irradiation, Proc. Symp. Karlsruhe, Vienna, Austria, June 6—10, 1966.

118b. International Atomic Energy Agency, Radiation Preservation of Food, Proc. Symp., Bombay, 1972, Vienna, Austria, 1973.

118c. Joint Committee on Atomic Energy, Congress of the U.S., Hearings on National Food Irradiation Research Program, U.S. Government Printing Office, Washington, D.C., 1956, 1960, 1962, 1963, 1965, 1966, and 1968.

119. Ley, F. J., The use of irradiation for the treatment of various animal feed products, *Food Irradiat., Inf.*, 1, 8—22, 1972.

120. Thomas, M. H., unpublished data, U.S. Army Natick Laboratories, Natick, Mass., 1972.

121. Coates, M. E., Fuller, R., Harrison, G. F., Lev, M., and Suffolk, S. F., A comparison of the growth of chicks in the Gustafson germ-free apparatus and in a conventional environment, with and without dietary supplements of penicillin, *Brit. J. Nutr.*, 17, 141—150, 1963.

122. Josephson, E. S., Thomas, M. H., and Calhoun, W. K., Effects of treatment of foods with ionizing radiation, in *Nutritional Evaluation of Food Processing*, Harris, R. S. and Karmas, E., Eds., AVI Publishing, Westport, Conn., 1975, 393—411.

123. Thomas, M. H. and Josephson, E. S., Radiation preservation of foods and its effect on nutrients, *Sci. Teacher*, 37, 59—63, 1970.

124. Brooke, R. O., Ravesi, E. M., Gadbois, D. F., and Steinberg, M. A., Preservation of fresh unfrozen fishery products by low-level radiation, *Food Technol.*, 18, 1060—1064, 1964, and 20, 1479—1482, 1966.

125. Vakil, U. K., Nutritional and wholesomeness studies with irradiated foods: India's program, in *Radiation Preservation of Food (Proc. Symp. Bombay, 1972.* International Atomic Energy Agency, Vienna, 1973, 673—702.

126. Heiligman, F., Rice, L. J., Smith, L. W., Jr., Thomas, M. H., Kelly, N. J., and Wierbicki, E., Irradiation Disinfestation of Flour. Storage Studies of Irradiated Flour, Presented at 33rd Annu. Meet., Inst. Food Technol., 1973.

127. Wenkham, N. S. and Moy, A. P., Nutritional composition of irradiated fruit. I. Mango and papaya, Ann. Rep. 1, AE C Rep. UH-235-P-5-4, Hawaii Univ. Coll. Trop. Agric., June, 1967 to May, 1968, 126—135.

128. Dennison, R. A. and Ahmed, E. M., Effects of low level irradiation on the preservation of fruit: A 7-year summary, *Isot. Radiat. Technol.*, 9, 194—200, 1971 and 1972.

129. Kuzin, A. M. and Abdurakhmanov, A., Postradiation intensification of carotenogenesis in carrots, *Proc. Sci. Technol. Conf. Util. Ionizing Radiation*, Natl. Econ., Issue 3, Prioks Book Printing Office, Tula, USSR, 1970, 109—117.

130. Kung, H., Gaden, E. L., and King, C. G., Vitamins and enzymes in milk. Effect of gamma radiation on activity, *J. Agric. Food Chem.*, 1, 142—144, 1953.

131. Sheffner, A. L. and Spector, H., Action of ionizing radiations on vitamins, sterols, hormones, and other physiologically active compounds, in *Radiation Preservation of Food*, U.S. Army Quartermaster Corp., U.S. Government Printing Office, Washington, D.C., 1967.

132. Richardson, L. R., Woodworth, P., and Coleman, S., Effect of ionizing radiation on vitamin K, *Fed. Proc.*, 15, 924—926, 1956.

132a. Anon., Statement on wholesomeness of irradiated foods by the Surgeon General, Department of the Army, in Radiation Processing of Foods: Hearings before the Subcommittee on Research, Development, and Radiation of the Joint Committee on Atomic Energy, Congress of the U.S., June 9—10, U.S. Government Printing Office, Washington, D.C., 1965.

133. Reber, E. F., Raheja, K., and Davis, D., Wholesomeness of irradiated foods. An annotated bibliography, *Fed. Proc.*, 25, 1530—1579, 1966.

134. Karel, M. and Heidelbaugh, N. D., Effects of packaging on nutrients, in *Nutritional Evaluation of Food Processing*, 2nd ed., Harris, R. S. and Karmas, E., Eds., AVI Publishing, Westport, Conn., 1975, 412—462.

135. Kramer, A., Storage retention of nutrients, *Food Technol.*, 28(1), 50—58, 1974.

136. National Canners Association, *Retention of Nutrients during Canning*, National Canners Association, Washington, D.C., 1955.

137. Loy, H. W., Jr., Haggerty, J. F., and Combs, E. L., Light destruction of riboflavin in bakery products, *Food Res.*, 16, 360—364, 1951.

138. Kanninen, W. H. and Hardy, W. L., The retention of riboflavin in commercially wrapped enriched breads, paper presented at 15th annual meeting, Inst. Food Technol., Columbus, Ohio, 1955.

139. Birdsall, J. J. and Teply, L. J., Effects of packaging on partially baked rolls: observations on the retention of riboflavin, moisture, and flavor, *Food Technol.*, 11, 608—610, 1957.

140. Morgareidge, K., The effect of light on vitamin retention in enriched white bread, *Cereal Chem.*, 33, 213—220, 1956.

141. Stephens, L. C. and Chastain, M. F., Light destruction of riboflavin in partially baked rolls, *Food Technol.*, 13, 527—528, 1959.

142. Sattar, A. and DeMan, J. M., Effect of packaging material on light induced quality deterioration of milk, *Can. Inst. Food Sci. Technol. J.*, 6(3), 170—174, 1973.

143. Bauernfeind, J. C. and Allen, L. E., Vitamin A and D enrichment of nonfat dry milk, *J. Dairy Sci.*, 46(3), 245—254, 1963.

144. Cox, D. H., Coulter, S. T., and Lunberg, W. O., Effect of NDGA and other factors on stability of added vitamin A in dry and fluid milks, *J. Dairy Sci.*, 40, 564—570, 1957.

145. Bauernfeind, J. C. and Pinkert, D. M., Food processing with added ascorbic acid, *Adv. Food Res.*, 18, 219—315, 1970.

146. Deuel, H. J., Jr. and Greenberg, S. M., A comparison of the retention of vitamin A in margarines and in butter based upon bioassays, *Food Res.*, 18, 497—503, 1953.

147. Marusich, W., DeRitter, E., and Bauernfeind, J. C., Provitamin A activity and stability of β-carotene in margarine, *J. Am. Oil Chem. Soc.*, 34, 217—221, 1957.

148. Bratley, C. O., Loss of ascorbic acid (vitamin C) from tangerines during storage on the market, *Proc. Am. Soc. Hortic. Sci.*, 37, 526—528, 1939.

149. Harding, P. L., Effects of simulated transit and marketing periods on quality of Florida oranges, *Food Technol.*, 8, 311—312, 1954.

150. Scott, L. E. and Kramer, A., Physiological changes in asparagus after harvest, *Proc. Am. Soc. Hortic. Sci.*, 54, 357—366, 1949.

151. Allison, R. M. and Driver, C. M., The effect of variety, storage, and locality on the ascorbic acid content of the potato tuber, *J. Food Sci. Agric.*, 4, 386—396, 1963.

152. Ezell, B. D. and Wilcox, M. S., Loss of carotene in fresh vegetables as related to wilting and temperature, *J. Agric. Food Chem.*, 10, 124—126, 1962.

153. Smith, H. W., The use of carbon dioxide in the transport and storage of fruits and vegetables, *Adv. Food Res.*, 12, 95—146, 1963.

154. Wright, R. C., Rose, D. H., and Whiteman, T. M., The commercial storage of fruits, vegetables, and florist and nursery stocks, Agric. Handb., No. 66, U.S. Department of Agriculture, 1963.

155. Mapson, L. W., Factors in distribution affecting the quality and nutritive values of foodstuffs. Loss of nutrients during the transport and distribution of fruits and vegetables, *Chem. Ind. (London)*, 25—28, 1952.

156. Salunkhe, D. K. and Wu, M. T., Effects of low oxygen atmosphere storage on ripening and associated biochemical changes of tomato fruits, *J. Am. Soc. Hortic. Sci.*, 98(1), 12—149, 1973.

157. Continental Can Company Research Staff, New facts about packaging and storing dehydrated food, *Food Ind.*, 16. 171, 267, 366, 458, 635, 702, 815, 903, and 991; 17, 147, 1944—1945.

158. Legault, R. R., Hendel, C. E., and Talburt, W. F., Retention of quality in dehydrated vegetables through in-package desiccation, *Food Technol.*, 8, 143—148, 1954.

159. Wong, F. F., Dietrich, W. C., Harris, J. G., and Lindquist, F. E., Effect of temperature and moisture on storage stability of vacuum-dried tomato juice powder, *Food Technol.*, 10, 97—100, 1956.

160. Daoud, H. N. and Luh, B. S., Packaging of foods in laminate and aluminum film combination pouches. IV. Freeze-dried red bell peppers, *Food Technol.*, 21(3A), 21A—25A, 1967.

161. Rice, E. E. and Robinson, H. E., Nutritive value of canned and dehydrated meat and meat products, *Am. J. Public Health*, 34, 587—592, 1944.

162. VanArsdel, W. B., Copley, M. J., and Olson, R. L., *Quality and Stability of Frozen Foods. Time-Temperature Tolerance and Its Significance*, Interscience, New York, 1969.

163. Davis, L. G., Below zero temperatures important for vitamin retention in frozen foods, *Food Can.*, 16(4), 24, 1956.

164. Dubois, C. W. and Kew, T. J., Storage temperature effects on frozen citrus concentrates, *Refrig. Eng.*, 59, 772—775, 1951.

165. Huggart, R. L., Harman, D. A., and Moore, E. L., Ascorbic acid retention in frozen concentrated citrus juices, *J. Am. Diet. Assoc.*, 30, 682—684, 1954.

166. Volz, F. E., Gortner, W. A., and Delwiche, C. V., The effect of desiccation on frozen vegetables, *Food Technol.*, 3, 307—313, 1949.

167. Gutschmidt, J. and Wolodkewitsch, N., Effect of drying on frozen fruits and vegetables, *Kaeltetechnik*, 2, 49—55, 1950.

168. Bunnell, R. H., Keating, J., Quaresimo, A., and Parman, G. K., Alpha-tocopherol content of foods, *Am. J. Clin. Nutr.*, 17, 1—10, 1965.

169. Cook, B. B., Morgan, A. F., and Smith, M. B., Thiamin, riboflavin, and niacin content of turkey tissues as affected by storage and cooking, *Food Res.*, 14, 449—458, 1949.

170. Morgan, A. F., Kidder, L. E., Hunner, M., Sharokh, B. K., and Chesbro, R. M., Thiamin, riboflavin, and niacin content of chicken tissues as affected by cooking and frozen storage, *Food Res.*, 14, 439—448, 1949.

171. Hartzler, E., Ross, W., and Willet, E. L., Thiamine, riboflavin, and niacin content of raw and cooked pork from grain-fed and garbage-fed pigs, *Food Res.*, 14, 15—24, 1949.

172. Bauernfeind, J. C. and Cort, W. M., Nutrification of foods with added vitamin A, *CRC Crit. Rev. Food Technol.*, 4, 337—375, 1974.

173. Singh, R. P., Heldman, D. R., and Kirk, J. R., Kinetic analysis of light-induced riboflavin loss in whole milk, *J. Food Sci.*, 40, 164—167, 1975.

174. Singh, R. P., Heldman, D. R., and Kirk, J. R., Kinetics of quality degradation: ascorbic acid oxidation in infant formula during storage, *J. Food Sci.*, 41, 304—308, 1976.

175. Lee, Y. C., Kirk, J. R., Bedford, C. L., and Heldman, D. R., Kinetics and computer simulation of ascorbic acid stability of tomato juice as functions of temperature, pH, and metal catalyst, *J. Food Sci.*, 42, 640—644, 1977.

176. Lachance, P. A., Effects of food preparation procedures on nutrient retention with emphasis upon food service practices, in *Nutritional Evaluation of Food Processing*, 2nd ed., Harris, R. S. and Karmas, E., Eds., AVI Publishing, Westport, Conn., 1975, 463—528.

177. Lachance, P. A. and Erdman, J. W., Jr., Effects of home food preparation practices on nutrient content of foods, in *Nutritional Evaluation of Food Processing*, 2nd ed., Harris, R. S. and Karmas, E., Eds., AVI Publishing, Westport, Conn., 1975, 529—567.

178. Bowers, J. A., Fryer, B. A., and Engler, P. P., Vitamin $B_6$ in pork muscle cooked in microwave and conventional ovens, *J. Food Sci.*, 39, 426—427, 1974.

179. Baldwin, R. E., Korschgen, B. M., Russell, M. S., and Mabesa, L., Proximate analysis, free amino acid, vitamin, and mineral content of microwave cooked meats, *J. Food Sci.*, 41, 762—765, 1976.

180. Ziprin, Y. A. and Carlin, A. F., Microwave and conventional cooking in relation to quality and nutritive value of beef and beef-soy loaves, *J. Food Sci.*, 41, 4—8, 1976.

181. DeRitter, E., Osadca, M., Scheiner, J., and Keating, J., Vitamins in frozen convenience dinners and pot pies, *J. Am. Diet. Assoc.*, 64, 391—397, 1974.

# TRADITIONAL CASSAVA AND SORGHUM TECHNOLOGY AND ITS EFFECT ON MINERAL FOOD VALUE

## A. Joseph

## INTRODUCTION

In spite of the diversity of plants found in Africa, south of the Sahara; due essentially to different ecological conditions, we can identify two main types of foods — the sorghums and millets and the tubers.

Of all starchy foods, the cassava root occupies an important place in the food of the people of the guinean and equatorial regions of Africa. It is the staple food of many of these countries. In southern Togo, more than 90% of the meals are prepared from cassava, accounting for a calorie intake of 30 to 50%, depending on the season and the ethnic group.[1] In the Congo, cassava root generates an estimated 1000 to 1500 calories of energy per capita a day.[2] The same is true of southern Cameroon where cassava is by far the most consumed staple food; 24 to 88% of the calories in the food come from cassava.[3-5] Numerous other African peoples live exclusively on this root, especially in Nigeria,[6] Zaïre, and Madagascar.[7]

As far as African tropical cereals are concerned, they follow climatic zones fairly strictly; above the tenth parallel they constitute the basis of all human food; south of isohyetal 1000, sorghum is dominant. Human consumption of millet and sorghum absorbs more than 80% of the production in the developing countries, while in developed countries it is insignificant. Details of the major categories of use are shown in Table 1.

In the special case of Cameroon, average daily consumption per capita is 450 g (1550 cal) for northern Cameroon, where total production varies between 275,000 and 550,000 tons, depending on the year, for a population of 1,600,000.[8] Between 1966 and 1968, consumption was 374,000 tons distributed as follows: human food; 86.1%, beverage and industry; 1.9%, seeds and losses; 12.0%.

Thus, we see the importance in African food of cassava and sorghum as the two basic items of foodstuffs. In all cases this food is characterized by its monotony. In fact, people in forest areas eat what are essentially poor starchy foods from the point of view of accepted nutritional principles. More importance is attached to bulk than to plastic quality, while in the Sudanese and Sahelian zones, the basic dish is sorghum or millet. These foodstuffs which are eaten during almost every meal supply about 80% of the calories.

The excess carbohydrates associated with the low protein content of cassava, and the qualitative deficiencies of proteins and vitamins A, C, and $B_2$ in sorghum, are not the only specific nutritive characteristics of these amyloids. The mineral contents of these foods will be discussed here.

The importance of minerals in animal feed and human food needs no further proof; much work has been done on the consequences of mineral deficiency in food. The simpler the meal, the greater the risks of mineral deficiency, which is very often the case in equatorial Africa.

It is also known that the ability of minerals to meet minimum daily requirements is dependent upon the hazards of intestinal absorption.

Taking into account the fact that foodstuffs of plant origin are generally poor in mineral content (potassium excepted), we felt it was necessary to carry out a systematic study of the mineral composition of these foodstuffs, and to place special emphasis on the evolution of certain minerals in relationship to food prepared traditionally. The

Table 1
DISTRIBUTION OF THE CONSUMPTION OF MILLET
AND SORGHUM BY CATEGORY OF USE

| Use | Developed countries | Developing countries | Total all countries |
|---|---|---|---|
| Human food | 1.1 | 82.5 | 53.3 |
| Animal feed | 95.8 | 7.7 | 39.4 |
| Beverages and industry | 1.6 | 2.3 | 2.0 |
| Seeds and losses | 1.5 | 7.5 | 5.3 |

*Note:* Average for 1966—1967; 1968—1969 in percent.

From Arnould, J. P., and Miche, J. C., *Agronomie Tropicale*, 26, 865, 1971. With permission.

amount of phytate phosphorus in these same foodstuffs was studied simultaneously; it is very widespread in the plant kingdom and its role in the formation of hardly soluble or insoluble salts in the digestive tract is well known. Thus, phytate phosphorus represents a diminished source of phosphorus and accounts for a reduction in the coefficient of digestive use of certain mineral substances useful to the body, especially calcium, magnesium, iron, and zinc.

The aim of this study was to gain a better knowledge of traditional cassava and sorghum technological processes in Cameroon, and to see their effect on the mineral composition and the phytate phosphorus content of their derivatives.

## EXPERIMENTS AND RESULTS

### Analysis Techniques

In order to determine the quantity of minerals in the foodstuffs, a trial sample of 1 g was burned in an oven at 530 to 550°C for 8 hr. The silicon dioxide was then rendered insoluble, first by 5 m$l$ of HCl and then by a 10% solution of $HNO_3$.

The quantities of Ca, K, and Na were determined by flame photometry using an Eppendorf® photometer. The total quantity of phosphorus was determined by the vanadate method and that of phytate phosphorus by Holt's colorimetric method.[9] The analysis of each sample was done on three trial tests.

### Cassava

The various stages in the preparation of cassava are summarized in Figure 1, which was culled from a study carried out in 1970.[10] The forms directly edible are indicated in boxes. The effect of the technological processing of cassava on the content of mineral substances and phytate phosphorus was shown in another study.[11] The results of that study are given here, again in brief.

#### Meduame-Mbong

Fragments of peeled cassava root are boiled in water for about 1 hr. The result is an edible product which, when washed in a lot of water becomes *meduame-mbong* (see Table 2).

In general, cooking and, above all, prolonged washing, causes a considerable decrease in the amount of mineral matter. On the contrary, a substantial increase in calcium and a very big increase in sodium is found in the final product. The mineral substances brought in by the water used for washing are likely to be responsible for this.

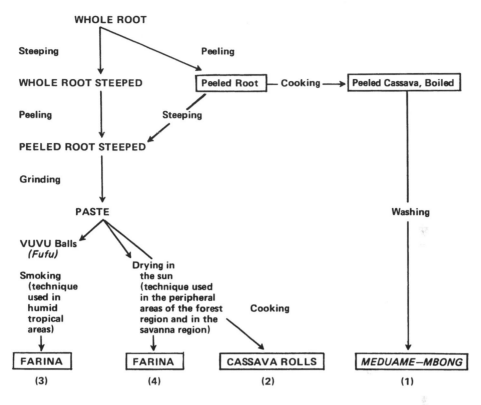

FIGURE 1. Traditional cassava-root technology.[10]

### Table 2
### PREPARATION OF MEDUAME-MBONG

| | Ashes (g) | Total phosphorus (mg) | Phytate phosphorus (mg) | Ca (mg) | K (mg) | Na (mg) |
|---|---|---|---|---|---|---|
| Peeled raw cassava (for 100 g of dry matter) | 2.02 | 210.5 | 88.1 | 34.5 | 658.7 | 7.2 |
| Percentage decrease (−) or increase (+) each time cooked | −18.3 | −9.1 | −35 | −2.9 | −12.4 | +8.3 |
| Percentage increase or decrease for each prolonged washing | −83.7 | −64.1 | −37.4 | +26.5 | −95.1 | +169.2 |

The drop in the amount of phytate phosphorus is the same for both stages of the preparation. It must however, be emphasized that in spite of the high percentage of phytate phosphorus in the final product (52% of total phosphorus), the phospho to calcic ratio, even though small (0.61), gives this foodstuff a better balance if peeled raw cassava is compared to boiled cassava.

### Cassava Rolls

Grinding the steeped peeled root on a millstone (steeping is a process aimed at elim-

## Table 3
## PREPARATION OF CASSAVA ROLLS

| | Ashes (g) | Total phosphorus (mg) | Phytate phosphorus (mg) | Ca (mg) | K (mg) | Na (mg) |
|---|---|---|---|---|---|---|
| Whole root (for 100 g of dry matter) | 1.98 | 70.2 | 32.0 | 48.3 | 483.3 | 6.0 |
| **Percentage Decrease or Increase in Whole Root** | | | | | | |
| Fresh roll | −58.1 | −39.5 | −100 | −42.7 | −45.4 | + 288.3 |
| 8-day roll | −64.6 | −45.6 | −100 | −48.2 | −48.2 | + 321.7 |

## Table 4
## PREPARATION OF CASSAVA BALLS

| | Ashes (g) | Total phosphorus (mg) | Phytate phosphorus (mg) | Ca (mg) | K (mg) | Na (mg) |
|---|---|---|---|---|---|---|
| Whole root (for 100 g of dry matter) | 1.98 | 70.2 | 32.0 | 48.3 | 483.3 | 6.0 |
| **Percentage Decrease or Increase in Whole Root** | | | | | | |
| 15-day ball | −76.3 | −58.1 | −100 | −52.2 | −59.8 | + 23.3 |
| 30-day ball | −75.8 | −58.7 | −100 | −55.9 | −60.2 | + 8.3 |

inating the toxic heteroside of bitter varieties by leaving the root in water for a number of days) produces a paste which is rolled and tied in leaves. This roll is cooked for about 2 hr in a pot lined with leaves (Table 3). It is eaten hot or cold and can be kept for 4 to 7 days.

Cooking and storage increase the nutritive losses considerably. These losses are even greater when the roll is preserved. It is possible that some mineral substances migrate from the paste towards the leaves enveloping the roll, becoming stronger and stronger as it dries during preservation. The very high percentage of sodium can only come from an external source during the grinding of the steeped, peeled cassava on the millstone. The percentage of phytate phosphorus during the experiment is very high: there are 8.5 mg/100 g of dry matter, or 25% of total phosphorus in steeped peeled cassava, and nothing in the final product. This drop can be ascribed to progressive hydrolysis. The phospho to calcic ratio remains unchanged at 0.69 for the whole root and 0.65 for the cassava roll.

*Cassava Balls or "Fufu"*

The paste obtained from the steeped, peeled root is molded into balls, wrapped in leaves and tied. Drying is done on wattles built above the fireplace in the kitchen. Proper dehydration requires a period of about 15 days. Preservation by this method of drying varies from several weeks to several months.

When the ball is removed from its envelope, it is scraped before consumption in order to eliminate the blackish film formed during smoking. When reduced into farina and put into hot water, the result is a thick mash which is the edible form.

As shown in Table 4, mineral losses are high. These are due to the hydrosoluble

## Table 5
## PREPARATION OF SUN-DRIED FARINAS

| | Ashes (g) | Total phosphorus (mg) | Phytate phosphorus (mg) | Ca (mg) | K (mg) | Na (mg) |
|---|---|---|---|---|---|---|
| Whole root (for 100 g of dry matter) | 1.98 | 70.2 | 32.0 | 48.3 | 483.3 | 6.0 |
| | | Percentage Decrease or Increase in Whole Root | | | | |
| Unsieved farina | −61.6 | −52.4 | −82.5 | −59.6 | −60.4 | −15 |
| Sieved farina | −56.1 | −53.4 | −89.6 | −57.3 | −61.1 | −18.3 |

substances in the paste which migrate towards the periphery during smoking and then to the scraping that takes place prior to consumption. This migration of mineral substances, caused by the disappearance of water, is crucial for prolonged dessication. In fact, the decrease of the calcium content in the paste is greater in a 30-day ball than in a 15-day ball. The sodium content remains positive. The presence of phytate phosphorus was not detected in the farinas. The phospho to calcic ratio markedly improved 0.80 in a 15-day ball.

*Sun-Dried Farinas*

The humid paste is spread out on the roadsides or on mats and left in the sun. It is gathered in the form of dry matter. When ground and sieved, it is used to prepare mashes. Table 5 shows that, as in the other preparations, losses are substantial. They are the same for both sieved and unsieved farinas. The percentages of phytate phosphorus remain low (between 10 and 17% of total phosphorus in the final product). The phosphotocalcic ratio is about 0.60.

*Effect of the Method of Drying and Steeping*

There are some differences between sun-drying and smoking. Losses in ashes and total phosphorus are higher in the cassava ball. On the contrary, farinas that are sun-dried are richer in phytate phosphorus and have a lower phospho-calcic ratio.

Steeping can take place before or after peeling the root. Losses appear to be much greater when peeling precedes steeping. The external and internal layers that are removed during peeling appear to play a protective role against the loss of nutrients. It must be pointed out that the inner skin is strongly mineralized; the calcium content is about 210 mg/100 g of dry matter, and the phosphotocalcic ratio is higher than 2.5. On the other hand, sun-dried farinas from wholly steeped cassava have a low phosphotocalcic ratio (0.51) and a higher percentage of phytate phosphorus (about 35% of total phosphorus).

## Sorghum

The role of traditional sorghum technology on its nutritive value was discussed in a 1972 study.[12] The major stages in the preparation of sorghum farinas and *kourou* are briefly described here.

The grain is quickly rinsed in water, put into a wooden mortar, and pounded moderately for a few minutes to remove the husks. During winnowing, the housewife separates the husked grain from the lighter chaff. The husked sorghum is quickly dried and then is either crushed by pounding vigorously in a wooden mortar (traditional grinding) or grinding mechanically.

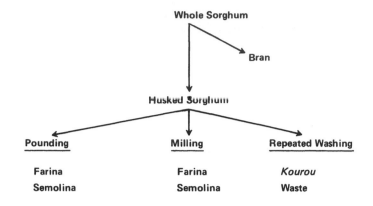

FIGURE 2.    Schematic representation of the preparation of farinas and kourou.

### Table 6
### PREPARATION OF FARINA AND SEMOLINA

#### Traditional Grinding

| | Ashes (g) | Total phosphorus (mg) | Phytate phosphorus (mg) | Ca (mg) | K (mg) | Na (mg) |
|---|---|---|---|---|---|---|
| Whole sorghum (for 100 g of dry matter) | 1.78 | 335 | 194 | 12.8 | 361 | 5.7 |

#### Percentage Decrease or Increase in Whole Grain

| | | | | | | |
|---|---|---|---|---|---|---|
| Semolina | −82 | −87.5 | −83.5 | −43.3 | −78.4 | −19.3 |
| Fresh farina | −34.8 | −32.2 | — | −7.8 | −44.9 | +3.5 |
| Sun-dried farina | −50 | −37.9 | −30.4 | −18.7 | −49 | −17.5 |

Sieving separates the farina derived from mechanical grinding from the semolina and, in the case of traditional grinding, from the broken grains. The broken grains are again pounded to reduce them to farina and semolina.

Several operations are involved in the preparation of kourou. These include the soaking of the husked sorghum, draining off the water, and grinding the grain on a fixed stillmill. The solid residue of the aqueous suspension is mixed with water and then is ground several times. The water is then collected and drained through a piece of cloth or sieved. The residue is made up of bran and semolina. The sieved suspension is decanted with a farina called *kourou.*

To be preserved, farinas and kourou are left to dry in the sun either on the ground or on mats. The farinas and the semolina can be used in preparing pastes or mashes; kourou, however, is prepared only as a mash. A schematic representation of the preparation of farinas and kourou is shown in Figure 2.

*Traditional Grinding*

Traditional pounding results in substantial losses in mineral substances from farina and semolina. There are more losses in semolina than in farina. There are also phytate phosphorus losses, but the percentage of phytate phosphorus in farina and semolina remains high (between 65 and 70% of total phosphorus). The phospho to calcic ratio of 0.15 for semolina is three times higher than the ratio for corresponding farina (Table 6).

### Table 7
### PREPARATION OF SEMOLINA AND FARINA

#### Mechanical Grinding

| | Ashes (g) | Total phosphorus (mg) | Phytate phosphorus (mg) | Ca (mg) | K (mg) | Na (mg) |
|---|---|---|---|---|---|---|
| Whole sorghum (for 100 g of dry matter) | 1.78 | 335 | 194 | 12.8 | 361 | 5.7 |

#### Percentage Decrease or Increase in Whole Grain

| | | | | | | |
|---|---|---|---|---|---|---|
| Semolina | −19.1 | −21.8 | — | +32 | −27.4 | −26.3 |
| Fresh farina | −51.7 | −52.5 | — | −9.4 | −46.4 | −15.8 |

### Table 8
### PREPARATION OF KOUROU

| | Ashes (g) | Total phosphorus (mg) | Phytate phosphorus (mg) | Ca (mg) | K (mg) | Na (mg) |
|---|---|---|---|---|---|---|
| Whole sorghum (for 100 g of dry matter) | 1.78 | 335 | 194 | 12.8 | 361 | 5.7 |

#### Percentage Decrease or Increase in Whole Grain

| | | | | | | |
|---|---|---|---|---|---|---|
| Semolina | −93.8 | −89.6 | −85.6 | −73.4 | −94.2 | −3.5 |
| Fresh kourou | −84.8 | −83.3 | −81.4 | −56.2 | −95.6 | −19.3 |
| Sun-dried kourou | −91.1 | −81.5 | −81.4 | −76.6 | −95 | −15.8 |

*Grinding on a Mechanical Mill*

Compared to whole grain, losses are still high. However, it is necessary to highlight the appreciable increase of calcium in semolina and fewer losses in the farina. Semolina is generally richer than farina. The phospho to calcic ratio is very low in both farina and semolina (Table 7).

The difference observed in the semolina and farina from the two types of grinding is clear: in the case of grinding on a mechanical mill, the farina is poorer than the semolina; while farina obtained from traditional grinding is richer than corresponding semolina. Such a great deficiency suggests to us that traditionally ground semolina is likely to contain a greater quantity of grain endocarp.

*Preparation of Kourou*

Since the preparation of kourou involves repeated grinding and washing, losses are highest compared to farinas and semolinas obtained from pounding and mechanical grinding (Table 8). In spite of the advantageous decreases in phytate phosphorus, its amount in kourou and semolina is considerable: 64% of total phytate phosphorus in fresh kourou and 80% in semolina. The phospho to calcic ratio is very low. Semolina shows greater deficiency compared to kourou.

*Comparison of the Various Farinas and Semolina*

Kourou is more deficient in mineral substances, compared to other farinas. Farina ground traditionally is least affected by the preparation process. Kourou semolinas

## Table 9
## MINERAL COMPOSITION OF CASSAVA DERIVATIVES[a]

| Description | Ashes (g) | Total phosphorus (mg) | Phytate phosphorus (mg) | Ca (mg) | K (mg) | Na (mg) |
|---|---|---|---|---|---|---|
| Meduame-mbong | 0.27 | 68.7 | 35.9 | 42.4 | 28.4 | 21 |
| Fresh cassava roll | 0.83 | 42.5 | 0 | 27.7 | 263.8 | 23.3 |
| Fufu (15 days) | 0.47 | 29.4 | 0 | 23.1 | 194.1 | 7.4 |
| Sun-dried farina (sieved) origin: cassava peeled and steeped | 0.87 | 32.7 | 3.3 | 20.6 | 188 | 4.9 |
| Sun-dried farina (sieved) origin: whole cassava steeped | 1.83 | 57 | 18.8 | 29.2 | 449.8 | 6.2 |

[a]    For 100 grams of dry matter.

and semolinas ground traditionally, both of which are very poor, have practically the same amount of mineral substances; only semolina ground mechanically seems to be better balanced.

### The Effect of Drying

The only reason for drying farinas is to be able to preserve them and use them as the need arises. In spite of the few differences observed between fresh farina and sun-dried farina, it is dangerous to deduce that drying leads to an increase or decrease in the mineral substances under review, especially as there are numerous forms of contamination (e.g., dust and soil).

### Discussion

A substantial decrease in most of the mineral substances was observed during the various methods of preparation (Table 9). In the case of cassava, the varying values obtained for ash content and the main minerals make it difficult to compare these preparations qualitatively. In fact, the variations in each case correspond to different methods of preparation: peeling, steeping, cooking, washing, grinding, and scraping.

Substantial losses in minerals, in terms of the whole root, still must be noted. Sodium, however, is an exception; its results are positive, except for sun-dried farinas obtained from peeled and steeped cassava.

In general, grinding on a stillmill enriches the paste with minerals, unlike the preceding stage, but this is quickly lost during later processes such as scraping the ball, drying, and sieving the farina.

Of all these preparations, only meduame-mbong from beginning to end, is enriched with calcium, and the water used to wash it seems to be responsible for the increase. Meduame-mbong and sun-dried farinas from steeped whole cassava aside, the low phytate phosphorus content or its total absence should not affect the nutritive value of corresponding rations.

When the cassava is steeped, fermentation takes place, and the degree of this fermentation is, among other things, dependent upon the humidity conditions during the preparation of the foods. In the case of tropical foods, fermentation and a moderate temperature enhance the hydrolysis of most of the phytate phosphorus. Its absence in cassava rolls and in fufu is perhaps due to the activation of enzymatic systems. On the other hand, cooking to a boil may destroy the phytases and the dephytinization of

## Table 10
## MINERAL COMPOSITION OF SORGHUM DERIVATIVES[a]

| | Traditional grinding | | | Mechanical | | Preparation of kourou | | |
| | Fresh farina | Sun-dried farina | Semolina | Fresh farina | Semolina | Fresh kourou | Sun-dried kourou | Semolina |
|---|---|---|---|---|---|---|---|---|
| Ashes (g) | 1.16 | 0.89 | 0.32 | 0.86 | 1.44 | 0.27 | 0.16 | 0.11 |
| Total phosphorus (mg) | 227 | 208 | 42 | 159 | 262 | 56 | 62 | 35 |
| Phytate phosphorus (mg) | — | 135 | 32 | — | — | 36 | 36 | 28 |
| Ca (mg) | 11.8 | 10.4 | 6.6 | 11.6 | 16.9 | 5.6 | 3.0 | 3.4 |
| K (mg) | 199 | 184 | 78 | 190 | 262 | 16 | 18 | 21 |
| Na (mg) | 5.9 | 4.7 | 4.6 | 4.8 | 4.2 | 4.6 | 4.8 | 5.5 |

[a] For 100 grams of dry matter.

the final product could only decrease further. This is the case with boiled cassava and meduame-mbong.

The fact remains that the mineral substances we get from cassava-based diets are theoretically lower than needed. But people in tropical forest areas naturally eat some leaves, especially those of cassava. When pounded, these leaves are cooked with a few palm nuts. The biological value of these leaves is well-known and their richness in calcium and phosphorus may compensate for the imbalance in the rest of the meal.

As for sorghum, it is possible to compare the various derivatives from the point of view of their chemical composition and nutritional value (Table 10). Husking and subsequent reduction to farina and semolina lead to substantial losses in mineral salts.

Of all these preparations, traditionally ground semolina and especially kourou seem to be the poorest. In fact, it is the preparation of kourou that accounts for the greatest damage to the nutrients of the original sorghum. The steeping and repeated washing of the grain and its derivatives are likely to be responsible for this.

The fresh farina obtained from mechanical grinding has a composition very similar to farina derived from pounding; the latter type, however, has a slight edge over the former. Only semolina derived from mechanically ground sorghum is, of greater interest, from the point of view of mineral content.

The effect of technological processing on the ability of the grain to meet the calcium needs of an active adult was studied. It appears that for 450 g of dry-processed sorghum (the average daily consumption per capita for all northern Cameroon) 6% of the minimum daily requirement is derived if the grain is pounded traditionally; 7% comes from the derivatives of the mechanically ground grain; and only 1% from kourou. The effects of the method of processing sorghum on the nutritional value of the consumer's usual ration are clear.

Even in the most favorable cases, however, the ability of the grain to supply theoretical calcium needs of an active adult is very doubtful. It would be interesting to study the way the body adapts itself to such small amounts of mineral substances.

## REFERENCES

1. Perisse, J., The food of the rural population of TOGO, *Ann. Nutr. Aliment.,* 16, 1—58, 1962.
2. Bascoulergue, P. and Bergot, J., Rural food in Middle Congo, Joint Service for the Campaign against the Major Endemic Diseases, Imprimerie, Protat Freres, Macon, France, 1959.
3. Gabaix, J., The Standard of Living of the People in the Cocoa Zone of Central Cameroon, Cameroonian Ministry of Economic Affairs and Planning and SEDES, Paris, 1966.
4. Masseyeff, R., Bergeret, B., Cambon, A., Pierme, M. L., and Bebey-eyidi, R., Surveys on Food in Cameroon, Office de la Recherche Scientifique et Technique Outre-Mer, I. Evodoula, 1958; II. Batouri, 1958; III. Golompui, 1959; IV. Douala, 1961, Yaounde.
5. Winter, G., The Standard of Living of the Adamaoua People, the Department of Statistics of Cameroon and Office de la Recherche Scientifique et Technique Outre-Mer, 1964.
6. Oke, O. L., Chemical studies on some Nigerian foodstuffs, *Trop. Sci.,* 8, 23—27, 1966.
7. Francois, P. J., The Budgets and Food of the Rural Households of Madagascar in 1962, Malagasy Ministry of Finance and Trade and the Secretariat of State for Foreign Affairs in charge of Cooperation (France), C.I.N.A.M. and I.N.S.E.E., Madagascar, 1962.
8. Department of Statistics, Socio-Economic Studies on North-Cameroon, Ministry of Economic Affairs, Yaounde.
9. Holt, R., Studies on dried peas. I. The determination of phytate phosphorus, *J. Sci. Food. Agr.,* 6, 136—142, 1955.
10. Favier, J. C., Chevassus-agnes, S., and Gallon, G., Traditional cassava technology in Cameroon. Effects on food value, *Ann. Nutr. Aliment.,* 25, 1—59, 1971.
11. Joseph, A., The effects of traditional cassava technology on the percentage of mineral substances and phytate phosphorus, *Ann. Nutr. Aliment.,* 27, 125—139, 1973.
12. Favier, J. C., Chevassus-agnes, S., Joseph, A., and Gallon, G., Traditional sorghum technology in Cameroon. Effects of grinding on food-value, *Ann. Nutr. Aliment.,* 26, 221—250, 1972.

# EFFECT OF PROCESSING ON NUTRITIVE VALUE OF FOOD: TRACE ELEMENTS*

### John T. Rotruck

## INTRODUCTION

With the recognition of the requirement for trace elements by humans, it becomes increasingly important to determine their levels in foods and to assess the effects of processing on trace element levels in foods. Unlike the major dietary nutrients and the vitamins, extensive compilations of trace element levels in foods have not been made, with iron being the sole exception. This lack of data prevents a detailed analysis of the effects of processing on trace element levels; however, the limited data have been compiled and discussed. In order to appropriately consider the topic, it is necessary to include sections on analysis and variability of elements in foodstuffs.

Although the data presented in this paper are important in determining nutritional status, they are clearly of limited value if considered alone. For example, significant loss of a trace element from a single food or class of foods due to processing may have little effect on the intake of this element, if this food or class of foods is an unimportant source of the element in question. To calculate accurate trace element intakes clearly, the trace element contents of most dietary constituents must be known. In addition, the presence of a trace element in foods does not necessarily mean the element is bioavailable. (Bioavailability is discussed in a separate section of this volume.)

## DEFINITION OF TRACE ELEMENTS

It is difficult to clearly delineate between the so-called trace elements and the major elements. However, those elements that usually occur in concentrations which can be expressed in $\mu g/g$ or $\mu g/ml$ are usually regarded as trace elements.[1] Evidence is available to suggest that 14 trace elements are essential for animals. These elements are iron, iodine, copper, zinc, manganese, cobalt (only as a constituent of vitamin $B_{12}$ for nonruminant animals), molybdenum, selenium, chromium, nickel, tin, silicon, fluorine, and vanadium.[1] It is possible that other trace elements will eventually be added to this list. Because of these considerations, this chapter is not restricted to the required trace elements, but will consider all trace elements for which data are available.

## ANALYSIS OF TRACE ELEMENTS

Over the last several years, great progress has been made in analytical techniques for trace elements. Neutron-activation analysis, emission spectrometry, and atomic-absorption spectroscopy are the most widely used modern methods for analyzing trace elements in foodstuffs.[2] Many techniques utilizing these basic analytical tools have been created. However, such a variety of methods results in severe problems in comparing trace element concentrations determined by different methods.

A recent study which involved a complete analyses of a soybean meal illustrates some of these problems. The following methods were compared: atomic absorption spectrometry, flameless atomic absorption spectrometry, neutron activation, spark emission spectrometry, inductively coupled plasma atomic emission spectrometry, spark source mass spectrometry, colorimetric, fluorescence, and wet chemical. The analyses were conducted in six different laboratories. The multielement techniques in-

* Manuscript submitted April 1, 1977.

cluded neutron activation, spark and inductively coupled spectrometry, and spark source spectrometry.

The single element techniques yielded good agreement for elements in the concentration range from 0.1 to 50%. However, the data for the trace elements showed considerable dispersion. For example, the concentration range using single element techniques varied by factors of 100 for arsenic, 20 for mercury, and 2 for iron. Other trace elements such as zinc, manganese, copper, and chromium varied by ±10 to 20%. Osborn[3] reported that the results from neutron activation and inductively coupled plasma atomic emission compared favorably with the single element techniques. Spark source mass spectrometry and spark atomic emission produced much less acceptable results.

Even for the best available techniques this study shows considerable variability in trace elemental analyses. Osborn[3] concluded that the quality of the results is related not only to the technique used, but also to the skill of the individual laboratory.

Thus, it is obvious that the variety of techniques used for trace element analysis can create serious difficulties if comparisons are to be made; e.g., trace element concentrations in diets from different areas, or for determining processing effects. It is clear that differences in methodology can lead to incorrect conclusions.

To help remedy these problems, the World Health Organization Committee on Trace Elements in Human Nutrition has made several recommendations.[1] The most important of these recommendations are as follow: a reference laboratory should be designated to furnish standard samples. Matrix effects should be tested including such biological materials as blood, serum, milk, animal meat, leafy vegetables, and grain. In addition, the increasing interest in plant protein products suggests that standards of this material should be included. These reference samples should be analyzed by two different methods to certify their trace element content. The standards should then be used to verify the method chosen by individual laboratories.

## STABILITY OF TRACE ELEMENTS

Unlike vitamins, trace elements are not lost due to acid or alkaline treatment, or exposure to air, oxygen, or light. Some minerals may be oxidized by oxygen, and this may affect their bioavailability. However, specific data addressing this question are not presently available.[4] A problem shared by selenium and chromium is their volatility at elevated temperatures. Higgs et al.[5] have presented evidence suggesting that selenium can be volatilized from some foods during cooking. I am not aware of any experiments that demonstrate volatilization of chromium during cooking or processing.

## VARIABILITY OF TRACE ELEMENTS IN FOODSTUFFS

Variability of trace mineral levels among samples of the same type of food is high. In plants and vegetables this variability is thought to be due to such things as genetics, agricultural practices, variations in the soil content of various elements, soil fertility and pH, and environmental factors and plant maturity. Similarly, the dietary content of trace elements in animal foods can greatly influence the elemental concentrations of tissues.[4,6] Since variability appears to be typical for most elements and many foods, I have considered a few typical examples. The reader is directed to the excellent book by Underwood, *Trace Elements in Human and Animal Nutrition,* for references on individual elements not considered here.[6]

Zook and Lehman[7] determined the levels of several trace elements in fruits. The elements included aluminum, boron, copper, iron, and manganese. The authors report that cobalt, chromium, zinc, molybdenum, and selenium were not detectable or were below the detectable limits of their spectrographic technique. These investigators report extensive variation of manganese, boron, copper, and aluminum content among lots of fruits produced in a specific geographical region. Within a producing area manganese varied tremendously. For example, manganese in bananas grown in Ecuador and Jamaica ranged from 55 to 1022 $\mu$g/100 g and 38 to 888 $\mu$g/100 g, respectively. Strawberries grown in Beltsville, Md., ranged from 320 to 3048 $\mu$g/100 g. In general, this study showed larger and more frequent variation within a producing area than it did between geographical areas.

In a study of element content in fresh vegetables from different geographic areas, Hopkins and Eisen[8] reported similar data. Marked differences between different geographical areas were again found for manganese in carrots and celery, as well as for other vegetables. Copper and manganese showed statistically significant variations between the means of individual lots of sweet corn grown on the same farm.

Kirkpatrick and Cothin[9] determined the concentration of chromium, cobalt, copper, iron, manganese, nickel, and zinc in cured meat samples. They report the following averages and range for each of the trace elements (all data are ppm):

| Element | Average concentration | Range (n.d. = not detectable) |
|---------|----------------------|-------------------------------|
| Chromium | 0.06 | n.d.—1.27 |
| Cobalt | 0.06 | n.d.—0.41 |
| Copper | 0.73 | n.d.—1.80 |
| Iron | 16.6 | 4.0—52.4 |
| Manganese | 0.26 | 0.01—1.15 |
| Nickel | 0.14 | n.d.—1.04 |
| Zinc | 24.2 | 6.9—56.6 |

These differences probably reflect the mineral intake by animals prior to slaughter. For a more comprehensive discussion on the relationship between trace element intake and tissue concentrations of trace elements, the reader is advised to consult Underwood.[6]

The results of these studies lead me to conclude that intercomparisons of analysis for different samples cannot be validly made for most elements, and the effect of processing on trace element levels in food should be conducted on samples that have first been shown to be uniform. Unfortunately, sufficient attention has not been given to the variability of trace elements in foods, thus, invalidating much of the existing data. Experimenters should not only verify their analytical method, but also employ sampling techniques that insure uniformity, report the precise identification of the sample including species, variety, and origin of the foodstuff, and include a precise description of any processing or preparation effects studied.

## EFFECT OF MILLING ON TRACE ELEMENTS

The loss of minerals due to milling of wheat is the best known processing effect on trace minerals. The milling effect is due to the removal of the germ and outer bran layers. However, milling does not affect all minerals to the same extent, nor does it remove all minerals. The data for individual minerals are presented in Table 1.[10-13]

The iron content of cereals is greatly reduced by removal of the germ and bran, since iron is concentrated in the germ and bran. A large part of the iron can be restored through supplementation, and this is reflected in the higher level of iron seen in white bread made from enriched flour. Refining of wheat to flour also results in a significant loss of copper. Similarly, manganese, zinc, and cobalt are lost during milling. The percent loss of these minerals is 75.6% for iron, 67.9% for copper, 88.5% for manganese, 77.7% for zinc, and 67.9% for cobalt.

Table 1
EFFECT OF MILLING ON TRACE ELEMENT LEVELS IN
WHEAT

| Element | Wheat | White flour | White bread | Germ | Millfeeds | Loss in flour (%) |
|---|---|---|---|---|---|---|
| Manganese | 46 | 6.5 | 5.9 | 137.4 | 64—119 | 85.8 |
| Iron | 43 | 10.5 | 27.3[a] | 66.6 | 47—78 | 75.6 |
| Cobalt | 0.026 | 0.003 | 0.022 | 0.017 | 0.07—0.18 | 88.5 |
| Copper | 5.3 | 1.7 | 2.3 | 7.4 | 7.7—17.0 | 67.9 |
| Zinc | 35 | 7.8 | 9.7 | 100.8 | 54—130 | 77.7 |
| Molybdenum | 0.48 | 0.25 | 0.32 | 0.67 | 0.7—0.83 | 48.0 |
| Chromium | 0.05 | 0.03 | 0.03 | 0.07 | 0.07 | 40.0 |
| Selenium | 0.63 | 0.53 | — | 1.1 | 0.46—0.84 | 15.9 |
| Cadmium | 0.26 | 0.38 | — | 1.11 | 0.92—1.11 | |

*Note:* Manganese, iron, cobalt, copper, zinc, and molybdenum levels for wheat flour, white bread, and germ were taken from Czerniejewslei et al.[10] The chromium data for these samples is from Schroeder et al.[11] The selenium data for these samples is taken from Schroeder et al.[12] The cadmium data is from Schroeder et al.[13] The mill feeds data originally appeared in references 11—18 by Schroeder et al. I am uncertain whether these data were collected on samples from the same source.

[a]    The increased level of iron in bread reflects enrichment.

Table 2
EFFECT OF PROCESSING ON TRACE ELEMENT
LEVELS IN RICE AND CORN[11-18]

| | Chromium | Manganese | Cobalt | Copper | Zinc |
|---|---|---|---|---|---|
| Rice, unpolished | 0.16 | 2.8 | 0.16 | 4.10 | 6.5 |
| Rice, polished | 0.07 | 1.5 | 0.10 | 3.04 | 1.6 |
| | 75 | 45 | 38 | 26 | 75 |
| Corn, dry | 0.18 | 4.70 | 0.36 | 1.80 | 18.2 |
| Corn meal | 0.08 | 2.05 | 0.87 | 2.13 | 9.0 |
| Corn starch | 0.05 | 0.34 | 0.55 | 1.25 | 0.8 |
| Corn oil | 0.12 | 1.00 | 0.15 | 2.21 | 1.6 |

Although molybdenum is concentrated to some degree in the bran and germ of wheat which is removed during milling, the extent of concentration is not as great as for those elements previously mentioned. The concentration of chromium in the bran and germ closely resembles molybdenum, with losses of molybdenum during milling measured at 48.0% and chromium at 40.0%.

There is a relatively small depletion of cadmium as a result of milling, thus it appears to be more evenly distributed throughout the wheat seed. Selenium is not appreciably affected by milling as the loss is only 15.9%. The effects of milling on the other trace elements have not been studied.

## EFFECT OF PROCESSING ON TRACE ELEMENT LEVELS IN RICE, CORN, AND SUGAR

Trace element levels in rice and corn products are shown in Table 2. Polishing rice causes a 75% loss of chromium and zinc. Losses of manganese, cobalt, and copper

Table 3
EFFECT OF PROCESSING ON TRACE ELEMENT LEVELS IN
SUGAR[11-18]

| | Chromium | Manganese | Cobalt | Copper | Zinc | Molybdenum |
|---|---|---|---|---|---|---|
| Sugar cane | 0.10 | 1.75 | 0.03 | 1.00 | 0.5 | 0.13 |
| Raw sugar | 0.30 | 1.18 | 0.40 | 3.35 | 8.7 | 0.0[a] |
| Molasses | 1.21 | 4.24 | 0.25 | 6.83 | 8.3 | 0.19 |
| White sugar | 0.02 | 0.13 | < 0.05 | 0.57 | 0.2 | 0.0[a] |

[a] These levels are reported as 0.0, but probably should be reported as nondetectable.

due to polishing are much less, ranging from 45% to 26%. Thus, there are significant losses of at least some trace elements during processing of rice.

It would appear from the data on corn products that there is very little loss of trace elements to nonconsumed products, although there is a substantial redistribution of trace elements during corn processing. The effects of processing on trace element levels of corn products are variable. Corn meal contains about one half the chromium and zinc that dry corn contains, whereas corn meal contains higher levels of cobalt and copper than dry corn. Corn starch contains much less chromium, manganese, and zinc than dry corn. However, cobalt levels are slightly higher in corn starch as compared to dry corn. Copper levels are slightly lower in corn starch as compared to dry corn.

Corn oil contains much of the original copper and chromium present in dried corn. Manganese and cobalt levels in corn oil were 21% and 42% of dry corn. The concentration of zinc in corn oil was only about 9% of that in dry corn.

Trace element levels in sugar cane, raw sugar molasses, and white sugar are shown in Table 3. The data show an increase in the concentration of trace elements in molasses as compared to sugar cane. Chromium, manganese, copper, zinc, and molybdenum levels are less in white sugar as compared to molasses, sugar cane, or raw sugar. Cobalt levels are lower in white sugar than molasses. The data do not allow a comparison of cobalt levels in white sugar and sugar cane.

It is clear from these data that raw sugar and molasses are better sources of trace elements than white sugar. However, as I emphasized earlier, one cannot determine from this data whether there is an appreciable effect on trace element intakes by humans.

## SOYBEAN PROTEIN PROCESSING

Trace mineral contents of soybeans and soybean-protein preparations are shown in Table 4. These data were compiled from a number of sources and may not be strictly comparable; however, some trends do emerge. Unlike milling of wheat or polishing of rice, soybean processing does not appear to cause large losses of trace elements with the exception of silicon. In fact, several trace elements including iron, zinc, aluminum, strontium, and selenium are concentrated since the soybean protein is more highly processed to increase the protein content. It would appear likely that these elements are bound to the protein fraction, and thus, follow the protein through processing. Other minerals like manganese, boron, copper, molybdenum, iodine, and barium are variable, and no discernible trend emerges. However, there do not appear to be large losses of these minerals. Silicon shows large losses and probably reflects soil associated with the soybeans. The methods were too insensitive to detect effects of soybean processing on chromium concentration.

Table 4
MINERAL CONTENT OF SOYBEANS AND DERIVED
PRODUCTS

| Mineral | Soybeans[a] | Defatted soybean protein meal[b] | Soybean protein concentrate[b] | Soybean protein Isolates[b] |
|---|---|---|---|---|
| Iron | 80 | 65 | 100 | 167 |
| Manganese | 28 | 25 | 30 | 25 |
| Boron | 19 | 40 | 25 | 22 |
| Zinc | 18 | 73 | 46 | 110 |
| Copper | 12 | 14 | 16 | 14 |
| Barium | 8 | 6.5 | 3.5 | 5.7 |
| Silicon | — | 140 | 150 | 7 |
| Molybdenum | — | 3.9 | 4.5 | 3.8 |
| Iodine | — | 0.09 | 0.17 | 0.10 |
| Aluminum | — | 7.7 | 7.7 | 18 |
| Strontium | — | 0.85 | 0.85 | 2.3 |
| Chromium | — | < 1.5 | < 1.5 | < 1.5 |
| Selenium | — | 0.065[c] | 0.091[c] | 0.137[c] |

[a]    Data from Beeson.[19]
[b]    All data except selenium levels are from Centra Soya Technical Bulletin.[20]
[c]    Data from Ferretti and Levander.[21]

## THE EFFECTS OF CANNING, LEACHING, BOILING, STEAMING, CURING, AND COOKING ON TRACE ELEMENT LEVELS

Although canning, boiling, or cooking in water might be expected to leach minerals out of foods, there is little data available to evaluate this hypothesis. Analyses by Schroeder[11] have shown mineral differences between canned foods and their raw counterparts; however, it is not clear whether these analyses were conducted on the same source of foods. Schroeder[11] reported that canned spinach lost 81.7% of the manganese, 70.6% of the cobalt, and 40.1% of the zinc found in raw spinach. Canned beans lost 60% of the zinc, and canned tomatoes lost 83.8% of the zinc found in the raw counterparts. Canned carrots, beets, and green beans lost 70%, 66.7% and 88.9%, respectively, of the cobalt found in the raw foods. However, canned beets gained manganese by 226.8% and zinc by 60.0% when compared to their raw counterparts. These effects are probably due to metallic contamination.

A study comparing the effects of steaming and boiling shows higher levels of iron in steamed vs. cooked vegetables.[22] The average loss of iron in several vegetables due to boiling was 48.0%. The average loss of iron in these same vegetables subjected to steaming was 21.3%. It is probable that steaming would also result in better retention of other trace elements; however, no data is available.

Although it has been reported[13] that processed or cooked foods tend to contain less selenium than raw foods, the studies have not been carefully controlled and probably do not compare samples from the same source. Higgs et al.[5] conducted an excellent controlled study to determine the effect of cooking on the selenium content of food. Precautions were taken in sampling to insure uniformity. In addition, the various heating and cooking treatments were carefully described and conducted on the same sample.

The results of Higgs et al.[5] show that the major sources of selenium in the American diet (meats, seafoods, eggs, and cereal products) do not lose appreciable amounts of selenium when cooked by most ordinary methods. Some vegetables, such as asparagus and mushrooms which contain relatively high levels of selenium, show significant losses of selenium when cooked. This effect is apparently due to the presence of volatile selenium compounds in the vegetables. Higgs et al.[5] concluded that most usual cooking practices will not appreciably alter selenium intake.

The iron content of processed meats is similar per unit of protein to that of unprocessed meat.[23] In addition, there are no obvious effects of the traditional cooking methods on the iron content of meats.[23]

## SUMMARY

The best known processing effect on trace elements is that due to milling. In addition, refining of sugar and rice results in losses of at least some of the trace elements. Although it might be expected that processes such as canning, boiling, or cooking would leach minerals out of food, data demonstrating this effect is not extensive. Unlike milling of wheat and refining of sugar and rice, soybean-protein processing does not cause major losses of trace elements. In fact, some trace elements tend to be concentrated as a function of soybean processing. The concentrations of at least some of the trace elements appear to parallel the increase in protein concentration that occurs during soybean-protein processing.

Knowledge of the trace element content of foods is presently insufficient to allow extensive consideration of the effect of processing on trace element content in foods. Comparative data based on raw and processed samples from the same raw material are rarely available. Much of the existing data have limited use for several reasons: possible inaccuracies in analytical methods; lack of uniformity in sampling technique and analytical method; lack of precise identification of the species, variety, and origin of the foodstuff; and imprecise information regarding exact processing and preparation effects. Sound studies considering all of these variables are needed, in order to better assess the effect of processing on trace element levels in foods.

## ACKNOWLEDGMENTS

I am grateful to Barbara Beimisch for her assistance in searching the literature and to Wanda Hixson for her help in acquiring the necessary papers. Special thanks go to Dee West for her aid in preparing the manuscript.

## REFERENCES

1. World Health Organization Tech. Rep.No. 532, Trace Elements in Human Nutrition, Geneva, 1975, 5—65.
2. **Winefordner, J. D.**, Comparison of Spectroscopic Methods, in *Chemical Analysis*, Vol. 46, Winefordner, J. D., Ed., John Wiley & Sons, New York, 1976, 419—433.
3. **Osborn, T. W.**, Elemental composition of soybean meal and interlaboratory performance, *J. Agric. Food Chem.*, 25, 229—232, 1977.
4. **Harris, R. S. and Karmas, E.**, *Nutritional Evaluation of Food Processing*, AVI Publishing, Westport, Conn., 1975, 3.
5. **Higgs, D. J., Morris, V. C., and Levander, O. A.**, Effect of cooking on selenium content of foods, *J. Agric. Food Chem.*, 20, 678—680, 1972.

6. Underwood, E. J., *Trace Elements in Human and Animal Nutrition,* 3rd ed., Academic Press, New York, 1971.

7. Zook, E. and Lehmann, J., Mineral composition of fruits, *J. Am. Diet. Assoc.,* 52, 225—231, 1968.

8. Hopkins, H. and Eisen, J., Mineral elements in fresh vegetables from different geographic areas, *J. Agric. Food Chem.,* 7, 633—638, 1959.

9. Kirkpatrick, D. C. and Cothin, D. E., Trace metal content of various cured meats, *J. Sci. Food Agric.,* 26, 43—46, 1975.

10. Czerniejewski, C. P., Shank, C. W., Bechtel, W. G., and Gradley, W. B., The minerals of wheat, flour, and bread, *Cereal Chem.,* 41, 65—72, 1964.

11. Schroeder, H. A., Losses of vitamins and trace minerals resulting from processing and preservation of foods, *Am. J. Clin. Nutr.,* 24, 562—573, 1971.

12. Schroeder, H. A., Balassa, J. J., and Tipton, I. H., Essential trace elements in man: molybdenum, *J. Chronic Dis.,* 23, 481—499, 1970.

13. Schroeder, H. A., Frost, D. V., and Balassa, J. J., Essential trace elements in man: selenium, *J. Chronic Dis.,* 23, 227—243, 1970.

14. Schroeder, H. A., Balassa, J. J., and Tipton, I. H., Abnormal trace elements in man: chromium, *J. Chronic Dis.,* 15, 941—964, 1962.

15. Schroeder, H. A., Balassa, J. J., and Tipton, I. H., Essential trace elements in man: manganese. A study in homeostasis, *J. Chronic Dis.,* 19, 545—571, 1966.

16. Schroeder, H. A., Nasan, A. P., and Tipton, I. H., Essential trace elements in man: cobalt, *J. Chronic Dis.,* 20, 869—890, 1967.

17. Schroeder, H. A., Nasan, A. P., Tipton, I. H., and Balassa, J. J., Essential trace elements in man: zinc. Relation to environmental cadmium, *J. Chronic Dis.,* 20, 179—210, 1967.

18. Schroeder, H. A., Nasan, A. P., and Tipton, I. H., Chromium deficiency as a factor in atherosclerosis, *J. Chronic Dis.,* 23, 123—142, 1970.

19. Beeson, K. C., United States Department of Agriculture Misc. Publ., The mineral composition of crops with special reference to the soils in which they were grown, 369, 1941, from Harris, R. S. and Karmas, E., *Nutritional Evaluation of Food Processing,* AVI Publishing, Westport, Conn., 1975, 161.

20. Tech. Serv. Bull. Central Soya Co., Chicago, from Harris, R. S. and Karmas, E., *Nutritional Evaluation of Food Processing,* AVI Publishing, Westport, Conn., 1975, 161.

21. Ferretti, R. J. and Levander, O. A., Selenium content of soybean food, *J. Agric. Food Chem.,* 24, 54—56, 1976.

22. Cooking for Profit, 1965, 15, from Harris, R. S. and Karmas, E., *Nutritional Evaluation of Food Processing,* AVI Publishing, Westport, Conn., 506.

23. Watt, B. K. and Merrill, A. L., Composition of Foods; Raw, Processed, Prepared, United States Department of Agriculture, Agricultural Handbook 8, Washington, D.C., revised December, 1963.

# THE MAILLARD REACTION

## J. Adrian*

## INTRODUCTION

In a series of papers published between 1912 and 1917, L. C. Maillard[310-315] showed a reaction of organic chemistry occurring between sugars and amino acids (proteins). Maillard's work contained the original explanation in food technology of the nonenzymatic browning phenomena. Although other writers during the same period had supposed the existence of such a reaction,[273,291] only Maillard systematically studied the causes, factors and manifestations. He also foresaw some of the consequences in the analytical and food-industry fields. Thus his name is still connected with this kind of reaction.

Maillard's papers were ignored for several decades, probably because at that time, food technologies were little developed and nutritional sciences were still at their beginning. For example, thiamin had been known for only a year in 1912. Methionine and threonine remained unknown. Only after World War II was Maillard's work and modifications undergone by industrially treated foodstuffs shown to be connected with the reactions between sugars and amino acids. It has been proven that nearly all food industries are more or less affected by the Maillard reaction. Some, such as the sugar or milk industries, are concerned about reactions between these components, because the resultant brownings depreciate the value of food products. Both dairy products and sugar require perfect whiteness to obtain maximum commercial values. In other industries, processing includes a roasting phase that provokes a Maillard reaction. The reaction generates colorations and flavors that increase the value of the foodstuffs treated. The producers of the following food products rely — consciously or unconsciously — on the Maillard reaction: biscuits, bread, cookies, malt, beer, chocolate, peanuts, etc.

From a nutritional point of view, the Maillard reaction damages any foodstuff because of the amino acid destruction which occurs upon heating as well as by prolonged storage, especially when the conservation is carried out in unfavorable conditions. Milk powders lose a large part of their protein efficiency when lactose has reacted with whey proteins. In the same way, fermentation of molasses is difficult after the development of the Maillard reaction.

Thus, for different reasons, food technologists study the manifestations of the reaction between sugars and amino acids. This reaction also draws the attention of chemists who try to define the mechanisms and factors that condition its evolution, whereas nutritionists and physicians are concerned about the physiological consequences of the Maillard reaction. Because this reaction has provoked widespread interest, it is no surprise that hundreds of published works have dealt with the Maillard reaction, of which different aspects have been reviewed.[7,85,113,131,132,216,217,435,436] After recalling the essentials of amino acid-destruction mechanisms, this report will deal mainly with the nutritional and biological consequences of the sugar-amino acid reaction.

## ANALYTICAL CONSIDERATIONS

The analysis of heated products in which the Maillard reaction has developed requires particular precautions. The usual methods of analysis may produce results that do not reflect the efficiency in the animal.

---

\* Translated by Nicole Adrian.

## Sugar Determination

After heating the determination of the total reducing power cannot be validly used to measure the quantity of reducing sugars. Caramelization and the Maillard reaction generate different reducing substances. In extreme cases, the "non-sugar" reducing power represents two thirds of the total reduction, e.g., in the premelanoidins of glucose-glycine[23] (Figure 1). In such cases the reducing sugars cannot be further measured from their reducing properties; more specific analytical methods, such as the chromatographic or enzymatic methods, must be used that measure molecules with perfectly defined structures.

A question remains concerning the metabolizable energy of sugars combined with amino acids or carbohydrate derivatives formed in the course of caramelization. The determination of intact sugars supplies the minimum quantity of biological energy substances. The real efficiency may be superior to this value as long as the organism can benefit from the modified molecules.

## Amino Acid Determination and Measurement of Protein Efficiency

The amino acid determination aims at two different purposes: to determine the total quantity of amino acids contained in a sample and to realize the percentage of their availability.

In the first case the sample must undergo a drastic chemical hydrolysis (HCl $6N$, for 10 to 25 hr at 110 to 130°C). Theoretically, the result gives the total of the amino acids present, regardless of their form. The measure of the available fraction is realized by different methods which will be described in this chapter. The results easily allow classification of products according to the intensity of applied-heat treatments.

The relationship between the two kinds of analysis can be briefly summed up as follows: the available amino acid is equal to the total amino acid minus the blocked and destroyed amino acid. In most nontransformed foodstuff production, the amino acids are always in available form. In this case, the determination of total amino acids satisfactorily corresponds to the measured efficiency in the animal. Rare exceptions to the rule exist; the best known deals with the efficiency defect of methionine in raw soybean.

When food products have undergone a technological process, the analytic methods must be carefully chosen. The meaning of the result with each method has to be determined.

### Total Amino Acid Determination

In theory a drastic acid hydrolysis sets free the available and blocked forms of the amino acids with the exception of the destroyed fraction, which cannot be regenerated by this method. Thus, chemists have ascertained that the first stages of the Maillard reaction are reversible; the amino acids which have combined with sugars can be recovered. In a product that has undergone the Maillard reaction, the measurement of total amino acids gives a value superior to the quantity of amino acids endowed with nutritional activity.

In practice the situation is complex, as can be seen by the behavior of the blocked lysine. Contrary to classical theories, the N-substituted lysines are partially hydrolyzable by the chlorhydric acid: 49.5 ± 2.6% in 6 $N$· HCl medium.[165] Thus, the total lysine corresponds to the available fraction plus half of the blocked form. The other half, which cannot be regenerated chemically, becomes two fifths furosine and one fifth pyridosine in the course of chemical hydrolysis.[165]

Some ε and α N-substituted lysines that react with ninhydrine according to intensities different from those of free amino acids can remain in the hydrolysate. The former have a maximum absorbance at 565 nm, the latter at about 515 nm.[386] These forms

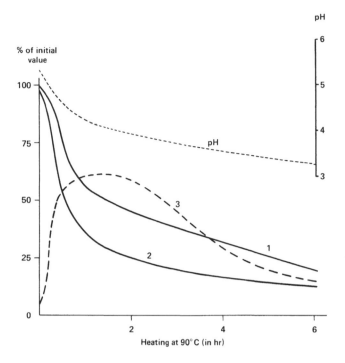

FIGURE 1. Evolution of the glucose-glycine premelanoidins as a function of heating intensity. 1 = glycine; 2 = glucose; 3 = nonsugar reducing power. (From Adrian, J., Frangne, R., Petit, L., Godon, B., and Barbien, J., *Ann. Nutr. Aliment,* 20, 257, 1966. With permission.)

interfere in the colorimetric determination of the total lysine. The difficulty of precisely specifying this interference leads to the questionable applicability of colorimetric determination of total amino acids when the products are heated.

*Determination In Vitro of Available Amino Acids*

The measurement of the amino acid fraction that is available for organisms is particularly useful from the nutritional point of view; especially with respect to lysine, which selectively undergoes the detrimental effects of heat treatments. A successful chemical method, which can distinguish the lysine fraction whose $\varepsilon$-amino groups are available, utilizes the amino acids reaction with fluoro,2,4,dinitrobenzene (FDNB).[278,425,459] Carpenter and Ellinger[84,86,87] have applied this principle to the particular case of $\varepsilon$-NH$_2$ lysine.

In this method, the protein sample is exposed to the action of FDNB. The reactant is combined with the $\varepsilon$-NH$_2$ groups of lysine which have not been blocked by sugar. The sample is then hydrolyzed in 6 $N$ HCl; the DNP amino acids other than DNP lysine are eliminated by ether extraction. Finally, the $\varepsilon$-dinitrophenyllysine (DNP lysine) is colorimetrically determined at 435 nm. The separation of the DNP lysine on an Amberlite® CG-120 column improves the method and makes it more specific.[254,374,433]

The method can be applied to most food products,[83,88,90] particularly to those which have a high percentage of lysine.[500] On the other hand, discrepancies with biological methods have been recorded in highly heated products[41,61,336] and also in vegetal matters that are rich in carbohydrates. In fact, in the course of chemical hydrolysis of the sample, a fraction of DNP lysine may be destroyed by carbohydrates that become reducing substances reacting with the DNP lysine. The pentoses are greatly responsible because they produce furfurals in acidic media.[65,83,90,196,250,298,520]

For materials that contain no carbohydrates, the result must be multiplied by a factor from 1.05 to 1.10 to compensate for the loss of DNP lysine.[65,84] With cereals and leguminous plants and seeds, the multiplication factor ranges from 1.15 to 1.35.[65,250] The reaction with carbohydrates is minimized by hydrolysis of the sample in large volumes of 6 $N$·HCl and by the addition of thiodiglycolic acid.[298] Using the Silcock method,[441] the available lysine can be indirectly estimated by determining the total lysine and the fraction that does not react with the fluorodinitrobenzene. Miscellaneous trials have not shown significant differences between the two methods.[338,380]

Enzymatic and microbiological methods have a value, which is sometimes underestimated, for the estimation of available amino acids. The principle of these methods is to submit the sample to an enzymatic proteolysis by means of papain,[89,169,170] trypsin,[250] pepsin and papain,[170] pepsin and pancreatin,[332] or by realizing a complete proteolytic digestion.[171,178] The biological activity of the amino acid contained in the digestate is then measured by means of a microorganism (*Lactobacillus, Leuconostoc,* or *Streptococcus*) according to classical methods.

In view of the enzyme-resistant character of linkages between sugars and amino acids in the Maillard reaction,[59,107,108,116,134,148,195,223,233,266,333,440,470,480] enzymatic hydrolysis can set free only the unblocked forms of amino acids. The measure of an enzymatic proteolysis, however, must be done in a particular way to be perfectly valid. In fact, compared with a control product, a heated sample gives a percent of solubilized nitrogen nearly unchanged in enzymatic digestate. On the other hand, the composition of the solubilized fraction shows great differences; the rate of free amino acids is decreased, and the rate of soluble blocked forms or soluble peptides is increased.[171,176,178]

Consequently, it is impossible to keep as a simple criterion the percent of solubilized nitrogen, but it is indispensable to search for the rate of free or available amino acids contained in the enzymatic digestate. This operation can be realized by microbiological methods that offer the advantage of measuring the totality of available forms (free amino acids and available oligopeptides). Moreover, these methods can record the effects of an eventual heat-labile inhibitor.[250] They also offer the advantage of reacting only to isomers endowed with biological activity. Thus, it is possible to detect the isomerizations resulting from the heat treatments.

## Determination In Vivo of Protein Efficiency

The in vivo techniques are based on the constitution of a basal diet greatly deficient in the amino acid concerned but without secondary limiting factors. For example, the measurement of available lysine requires a diet deficient in lysine; the wheat or gluten proteins are retained. They are supplemented with isoleucine, methionine, threonine, valine, etc., so that only the lysine deficiency remains. The diets receive increased quantities of lysine in the free state or in the form of a heated product. The comparison between the two series allows calculation of the percent of available lysine given in the form of foodstuff.

The criteria are variable, including PER, biological value or nitrogen retention, NPU, free amino acid in blood serum or muscle, etc. All these measurements are frequently used in nutrition; it is not necessary to detail them here. However, the result of an experiment on an animal depends on controlled conditions, and the lysine destruction in a foodstuff does not necessarily diminish the biological efficiency. For example, if a small amount of the heated product is added to a lysine-deficient diet, blocking or destruction of its lysine is immediately perceived and all damage caused by heating is thus made apparent. If the heated product is the only source of protein in the ration, the situation becomes more complex. If the lysine is the primary limiting factor, its loss will be noticed as above. If the limiting factor is another amino acid, the lysine destruction can be perceived only when its deficiency becomes greater than

## Table 1
### ESTIMATION OF LYSINE BY DIFFERENT TECHNIQUES[530]

| | Control fish meal | | Heated fish meal (74 hr at 130°C) | |
| --- | --- | --- | --- | --- |
| | Lysine (g/16 g N) | Percent of total lysine | Lysine (g/16 g N) | Percent of loss |
| Total lysine | 7.18 | 100 | 6.94 | 4 |
| Available lysine | | | | |
| Chemical methods | | | | |
| Carpenter | 6.56 | 91 | 3.56 | 46 |
| Silcock | 7.01 | 98 | 5.34 | 24 |
| Biological methods | | | | |
| Rat (growth) | 6.68 | 93 | 1.03 | 85 |
| Rat (carcass) | 5.94 | 83 | 0.90 | 85 |
| Chick (growth) | 7.34 | 103 | 1.62 | 78 |

From Walz, O. P. and Ford, J. E., *Z. Tierphysiol. Tierernaehr. Futtermittelkd.*, 30, 304, 1973. With permission.

that of the limiting factor of the untreated foodstuff. Consequently, according to the experimental conditions, a given heat treatment can be judged either damaging or not damaging to the nutritional value.

Another criterion, particularly sensitive in the case of the Maillard reaction, is the measure of the digestibility in vivo of the lysine. For example, when the lysine digestibility is 87% in the control foodstuff, it falls to 50% in the same product when it has undergone a heating.[54]

### Validity of the Results

Diverse analytical principles succinctly explained have a tendency to express the same fact under different conditions. Thus, protein efficiency must be proportional to the amount of available amino acids and inversely proportional to the degree of blocking and destruction of amino acids. When a series of heatings of increasing intensity is applied to the same food product, correlations appear among the diverse measurements. Examples have been given using milk powders. The PER (y) is significantly connected with the rate of lysine deterioration (x) as the regression line shows:[330]

$$y = -56.9 + 1.89 \, x$$

Likewise, the amount of unavailable lysine (y) correlates with the importance of the lysine destruction (x). The equation is[332]

$$y = -9.03 + 2.1 \, x$$

In the case of milk powder, the unavailable lysine is about twice the destroyed amount.

When comparisons are established between in vivo and in vitro methods, the results concerning industrial products are in agreement in most cases. Nevertheless, if the treatments undergone have been drastic, disagreements may appear.

In the case of experimentally heated fishmeal, 4% of lysine is destroyed and 45% is unavailable, according to Carpenter's method. For animals, however, the unavailable lysine reaches about 80% (Table 1). The efficiency is twice as weak as the results of the measurement of available lysine would suggest. The situation is comparable when the quality of protein-enriched cookies is determined by other means (Table 2).

Table 2
## EFFECT OF A STRONG INDUSTRIAL BAKING ON COOKIES SUPPLEMENTED WITH PROTEIN FOODS[17]

| | | Loss of protein supplement after baking (%) | | | |
|---|---|---|---|---|---|
| | | Lysine | | Methionine | |
| Cookies with addition of 2 g/kg lysine in form of | PER | Total | In vitro digestible | Total | In vitro digestible |
| Peanut oil meal | 50 | 21 | 25 | 2 | (+16) |
| Fish meal | 58 | 23 | 28 | 0 | 36 |
| Skim milk powder | 99 | 44 | 70 | 2 | 38 |

In all cases, the decrease in PER is greater than the decrease in amino acids, both total and in vitro-digestible. The use of proteins by the animal is always inferior to the predicted efficiencies, even when the predictions are based on the enzymatic hydrolyzable fractions of amino acids.

In conclusion, the in vitro methods give information on the relative intensity of the Maillard reaction and on the inactivation of amino acids. The methods do not provide sufficient precision to predict the protein efficiency of the heated products. The recorded discrepancies are attributable to the toxic and antinutritional properties of substances formed during the heating (premelanoidins).

## MECHANISMS OF AMINO ACID DESTRUCTION

In the course of heating, amino acids are subject to different types of degradation and destruction, which can be classified as follows:

1.  Destructions occur without any intervention of exterior agents. Losses are provoked by decarboxylation and condensation phenomena. These reactions have a nonenzymatic character because they are produced at high temperatures.
2.  Amino acids are easily combined with reducing sugars at room temperature and even more easily combined during heating. The Maillard reaction is a complex phenomenon that makes the amino acids unavailable and eventually causes them to disappear. It is responsible for a selective destruction of lysine and basic amino acids that is very detrimental to protein efficiency. The Maillard reaction also causes the formation of substances endowed with antiphysiological properties when the animal receives them at high concentrations. It is a nonenzymatic reaction that is mainly responsible for nonenzymatic browning in foodstuffs.
3.  During the development of the Maillard reaction, amino acids can be directly destroyed without previous blocking because of a reaction between reductones and amino acids. This operation does not require the intervention of sugars but does require the intervention of their degradation products or the intervention of other natural biochemicals such as ascorbic acid, pyruvic acid, etc. The mechanism responsible for the operation is the Strecker degradation; although it is prejudicial from a nutritional point of view because of the destruction of amino acids, it is beneficial from the sensory point of view by creating appreciated flavors.

### Reactions Among Pure Amino Acids
When amino acids are heated in a pure medium, i.e., in the absence of sugars, they

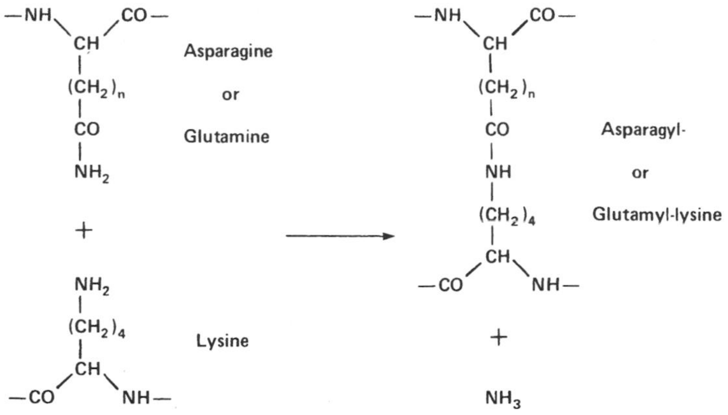

FIGURE 2. Mechanism of the condensation between asparagine or gluta-mine and lysine.

can undergo diverse reactions. The first-identified reaction is a decarboxylation that supplies the amine corresponding to the initial amino acid.[97] The existence of intera-mino acid condensations has been supposed for a long time.[151] More precisely, the possibility of a condensation between lysine and aspartic and glutamic acids has been advanced by means of a pure protein.[147] The bovine-plasma albumin undergoes the following evolutions when it is heated in pure medium:[56]

1. Cystine is the amino acid that is most deteriorated by heating. It decomposes in methylmercaptan, dimethylsulfide, dimethyl disulfide, and hydrogen sulfide. In parallel, a weak increase of methionine is detected, which could indicate that a fraction of the destroyed cystine has become methionine. The same observation has just been made in the course of a technological process of peanut-oil meal.[13] The decomposition products of cystine may play a role in lysine destruction.
2. A liberation of ammonia is observed, sometimes followed by a liberation of $CO_2$. They correspond to deamination and decarboxylation phenomena.
3. Losses of aspartic acid, threonine, serine, and basic amino acids occur in the case of strong heating.
4. The loss of lysine is proportional to the rate of ammonia emitted and the amount in amide N of the protein.

From these observations, it seems clear that a reaction of the amide groups of glu-tamine and asparagine is possible. The scheme of this reaction is shown in Figure 2.

In addition to amino acid destruction, the heating of pure proteins can lead to block-ing and chemical rearrangement of the protein molecule, which makes it resistant to proteolytic, in vitro digestions. This phenomenon has particularly been observed after a treatment in alkaline medium.[266]

The diverse reactions that occur in a pure medium can occur in a more complex medium, e.g., in the presence of sugars, parallel to the Maillard reaction. The eventual cystine loss will be the consequence of the mechanisms that have been described.

## The Maillard Reaction

The chemistry of the Maillard reaction is very complex and many points remain little known. Classically, it occurs between an aldose or a ketose of a sugar and an amino group of an amino acid. It can be extended to various aldehydes and ketones, e.g., those originating from the oxidation of fatty acids to various amines or even to am-monia.

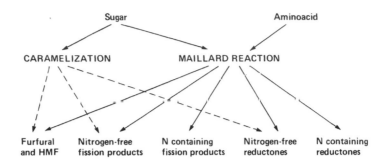

FIGURE 3.    Possible imbrications between caramelization and Maillard reaction.

Some authors have tried to describe the diverse stages of this reaction and have attempted to build a general scheme.[77,131,216,436,493] However, a point must not be forgotten even if the reaction is artificially divided in isolated sets. In practice, the different stages are developed simultaneously and consequently interference exists between them.

The point must be made that the term "melanoidins"[464] precisely defines the insoluble residue, dark or black, that corresponds to the ultimate stage of the Maillard reaction. It is sometimes wrongly used to designate the soluble, colored molecules produced by this reaction. The term "premelanoidin"[408] is reserved for the entire amount of soluble compounds and colorless and colored products, formed during the reaction. Since the former constitute the precursors of the latter, it would be difficult to justify a chemical distinction between these two categories.

Another point is essential for the comprehension of the Maillard reaction: when an amino acid and a sugar are in the presence of each other, an interaction between these two components provokes a Maillard reaction. Simultaneously, however, the sugar undergoes a heat degradation (caramelization or similar phenomenon) without the interference of the amino acid. This explains why products of the Maillard reaction and caramelization are mixed in the reaction medium. Both of these operations produce many molecules that are identical, or nearly so, and only studies with radioactive isotopes can determine the exact origin of premelanoidins, e.g., furfural and reductones are produced both by the degradation of sugar and by the Maillard reaction. The imbrications possible between caramelization and the Maillard reaction are shown in Figure 3. Regardless of their origin, they can react with amino acids and participate in the Maillard reaction.

A fundamental difference exists in considering the Maillard reaction according to a chemical or nutritional point of view. The products obtained during the first stages of the reaction are hydrolyzable chemically, the initial sugar and amino acid can be regenerated even after several stages of reaction. On the contrary, as early as the first stage, the additional compound is nutritionally unavailable. These distinctions are very important. For the chemist, the Maillard reaction begins by a series of reversible reactions; for the nutritionist, the reaction is irreversible in any case.

### Scheme and Chemistry of the Reaction
### The General Hodge Scheme

The classical Hodge scheme[216] shows a number of the diverse mechanisms included in the Maillard reaction. A first stage leads to the Amadori rearrangement products (aminoketose) or Heyns rearrangement products (aminoaldose). Up to this stage, the reaction follows only one direction. From this point, there are several possibilities; the products, formed according to different mechanisms, show mutual interference.

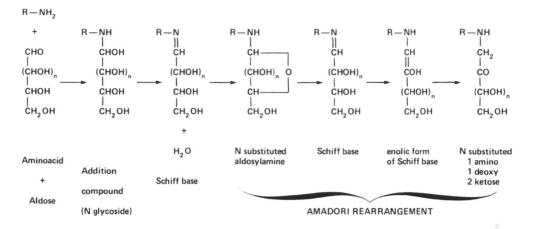

FIGURE 4. Beginning of the Maillard reaction between an aldose and an amino acid.

The Maillard reaction is artificially divided from the stages of aminoketoses or aminoaldoses, as follows:

1. A strong dehydration generates furfural and HMF. These very unstable substances react with many other molecules. They combine particularly with N-containing components to give aldimines, aldols, and polymers.
2. After a moderate dehydration, reductones and dehydroreductones appear. They are also very unstable reducing molecules that react in different ways. The more characteristic method is to develop a Strecker degradation by combination with still-intact amino acids.
3. A fission produces small molecules that may or may not contain nitrogen. These compounds will be found again in diverse reactions. They will be able to take part in the Strecker degradation in the formation of aldimines, ketimines, and soluble polymers.

The products formed in different ways[216] polymerize and insolubilize by producing a precipitate of N-containing melanoidins. Apart from the Strecker degradation, most stages of the Hodge scheme are not completely characteristic of the Maillard reaction. Analogous mechanisms and products of the same nature, comparable but not identical and necessarily nitrogen free, meet each other during the sugar degradation.

First, the beginning of the Maillard reaction will be described as far as the formation of aminoketoses and aminoaldoses, whose process is well established. Some of the mechanisms in the ulterior stages of the Maillard reaction will then be mentioned, especially to reveal the diversity of substances constituting the premelanoidins.

### Aldose Behavior and the Amadori Rearrangement

The first compound of the aldose-amino acid reaction is an additive component, a N glycoside. As early as this stage, the amino acid "blocked" by the sugar is lost in the nutritional field. It then undergoes dehydration and becomes a Schiff base and aldosylamine (Figure 4).

This product is spontaneously converted by isomerization according to a mechanism applicable to all molecules bearing a N substitution on the first carbon.[493] The mechanism is called "Amadori rearrangement"; it leads to a stable isomer: 1-amino-1-deoxy-2-ketose (aminoketose).[26,217,219,344,388] Thus, the initial aldose occurs again at the state of ketose after this rearrangement. In the course of the reaction of a reducing sugar-

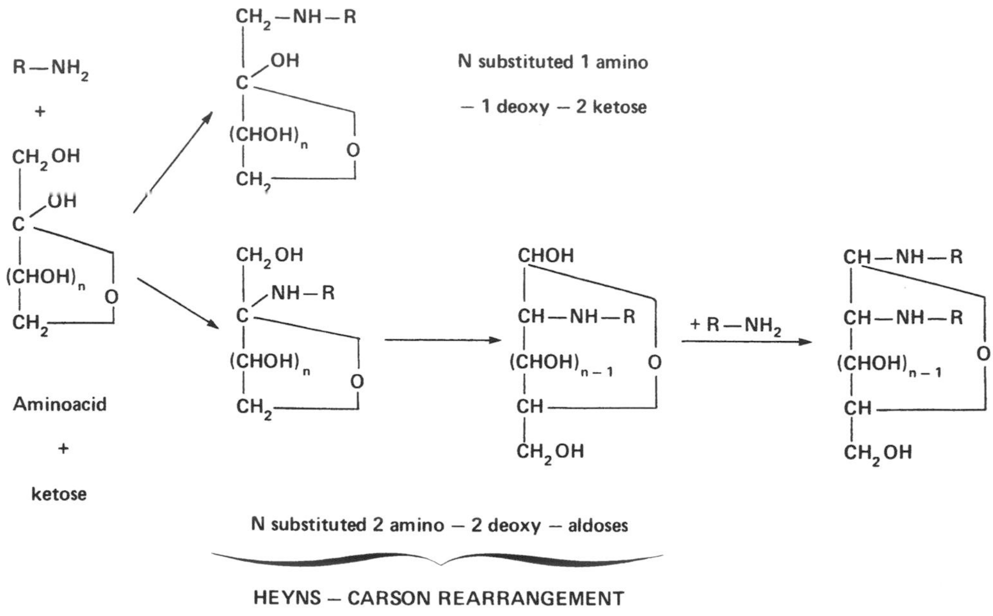
CH2—NH—R
OH
C
(CHOH)n
O
CH2
N substituted 1 amino
– 1 deoxy – 2 ketose
R—NH2
+
CH2OH
OH
C
(CHOH)n
O
CH2
Aminoacid
+
ketose
CH2OH
NH—R
C
(CHOH)n
O
CH2
CHOH
CH—NH—R
(CHOH)n – 1
O
CH
CH2OH
+ R—NH2
CH—NH—R
CH—NH—R
(CHOH)n – 1
O
CH
CH2OH
N substituted 2 amino – 2 deoxy – aldoses
HEYNS – CARSON REARRANGEMENT

FIGURE 5. Beginning of the Maillard reaction between a ketose and an amino acid.

glycine system, the energy of activation is about 26 kcal during the induction phase, fluorescence production, and premelanoidin formation.[399,434,494]

### *Ketose Behavior and the Heyns Rearrangement*

A process of reaction between fructose and ammonia has been established.[210,212] It shows a narrow relationship to the beginnings of the aldose-amino acid reaction in regards to addition compound, Schiff base, etc. The Amadori rearrangement cannot assure the isomerization of the 2-amino sugars, however; consequently, it does not occur with the fructose. In the latter, a different mechanism assures the transformation of ketosylamine; it is known as "Heyns rearrangement" although two teams have described it nearly simultaneously.[92,93,208,214,215] The fructose turns to 2-amino-2-deoxy-glucose or mannose, i.e., it generates an aminoaldose.

Nevertheless, it is also possible to obtain a fixation of the amine on the first carbon and to form 1-amino-1-deoxy-fructose as it is explained in Figure 5. These products of the Heyns rearrangement can still react with a new amino acid which will fix itself on the first carbon.[92]

### *Survey of Following Mechanisms*

After the aminoketose and aminoaldose formation, the Maillard reaction becomes considerably more complicated, and various mechanisms can be developed from the products of the two previously described rearrangements. Some processes have been more deeply studied and a synthesis is presented below. The exact conditions of melanoidin polymerization and insolubilization do not seem to be clearly elucidated.

**Formation of the unsaturated aldimines** — These molecules play a very important part in the Maillard-reaction development because they take part in the fluorescence formation, browning, etc.[493] Some $\alpha$- , $\beta$-unsaturated aldimines are produced from aldoses as well as from ketoses but by different processes including dehydration reactions. These components can comprise one or several unsaturated linkings and one or several imine groups as is illustrated in Figure 6.

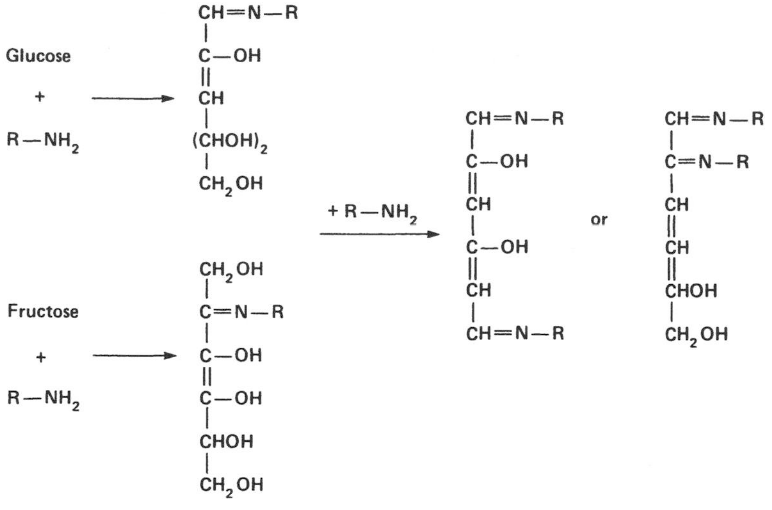

FIGURE 6.   Examples of unsaturated aldimines formed from aldoses or from ketoses. Reprinted from Song, P. S. and Chichester, C. O., *J. Food Sci.,* 31, 914, 1966. Copyright© by Institute of Food Technologists. With permission.

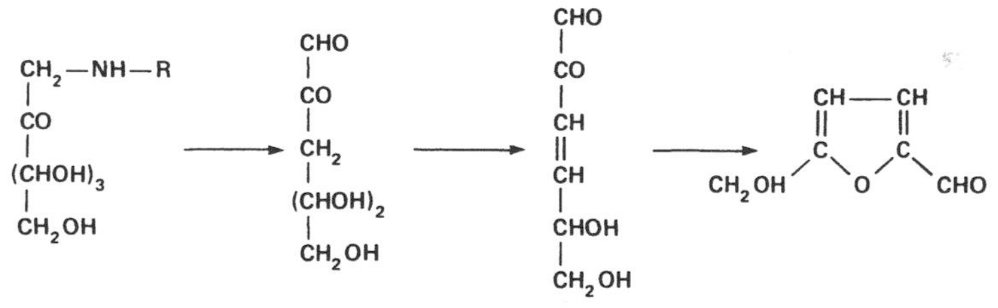

FIGURE 7.   Main stages of the formation of osuloses and HMF from amino ketoses.[33,36,253]

**Formation of osuloses and HMF** — The products of Amadori rearrangement can lose their nitrogen fraction and become osuloses[33,36] that in turn can become hydroxymethyl-furfural (HMF), especially in acid media (Figure 7). These operations confirm the numerous imbrications between caramelization and the Maillard reaction as mentioned in Figure 3. Here, also, dehydration stages take place in the processes of osuloses and HMF formation.

**Formation of reductones** — In addition to the reductones that may come from direct degradation of the sugar (Figure 8), others are also formed from the Maillard reaction that may or may not contain nitrogen.[35,484,485] Figure 8 shows the main stages of this production. This process is responsible for a reducing power and for an important acidification that especially produces acetic acid. The reductones constitute the preparatory stage to the Strecker degradation.

*Produced Molecules*

Whereas the analysis of unsoluble melanoidins is easily realized, and their composition seems to be constant, such is not the case for the considerable amount of soluble

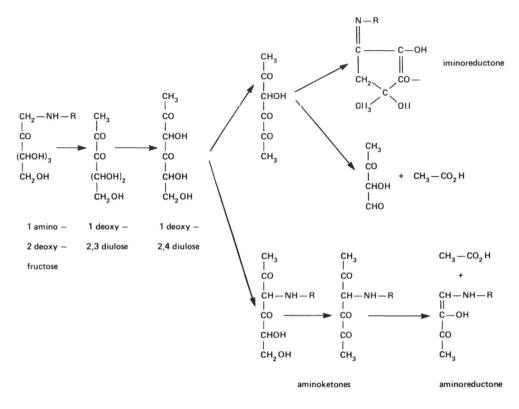

FIGURE 8.    Main stages of the formation of reductones from amino ketoses.[35,484,485]

substances or premelanoidins that appear in the course of the Maillard reaction. It is certainly possible to detect several hundred kinds of molecules in a medium where a Maillard reaction evolves. In fact, at least five categories of components exist simultaneously or successively.

- Those that come directly from the degradation of sugar
- Those that come directly from the decomposition of some amino acids, especially the S-containing amino acids and tryptophan
- Those that are specifically produced by the sugar-amino acid reaction
- Those that are the result of interferences between the different segments of the Maillard reaction
- Those that originate from interactions between the phenomena of the caramelization and those of the Maillard reaction

Nearly a hundred compounds have been isolated after a heat degradation of sugar; most of them (volatiles) are very reactive. In particular, about 30 aldehydes and ketones and some 30 furan compounds, etc.,[152] exist. It is easy to imagine the multiplicity of substances that can be revealed in a medium including amino acids and sugars by considering the diverse activities of the Maillard reaction.

Recently, 45 volatile components have been identified in a pentane-ether extract of the cysteine-ribose heated mixture,[350] and 26 peaks appeared by subjecting a dichloromethane extract of a Maillard-reaction mixture to the gas-chromatography method.[211] Another method, using the gas-liquid chromatography, has just been proposed for the identification of Amadori rearrangement products.[540]

These new methods of fractionation will allow future establishment of an inventory

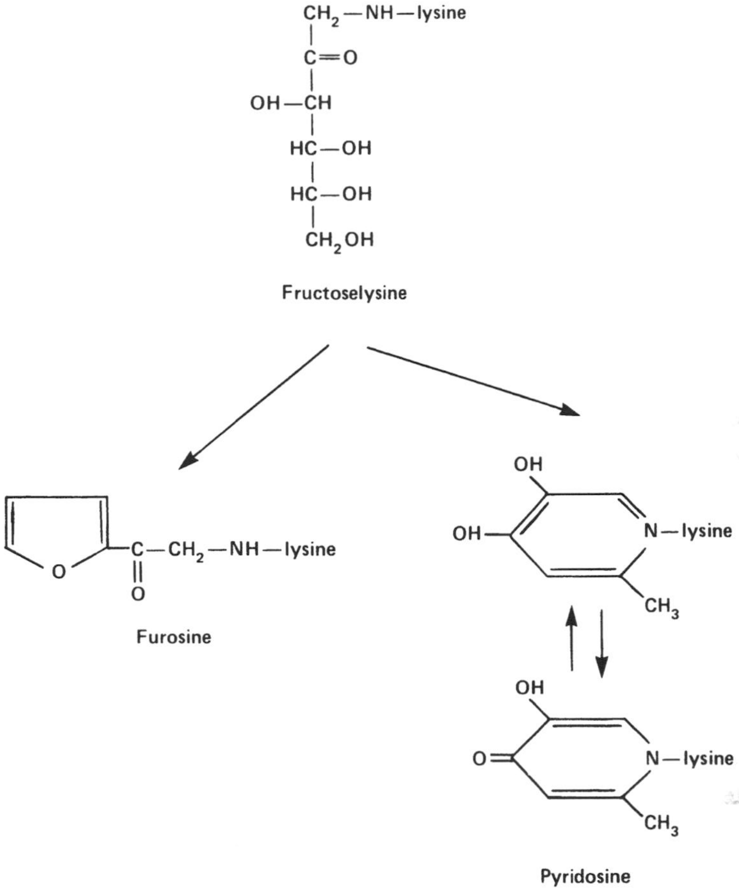

FIGURE 8A

of Maillard reaction products; this is impossible today. Nevertheless, some constituents of premelanoidins will be mentioned in this chapter, e.g., those that emit a fluorescence, are UV absorbing, bear a chromophore group, have reducing properties, or are acidic (see Physico-Chemical Manifestations), are produced during the Strecker degradation (see Degradation Chemistry), and those that have psychosensor properties (see Flavors Produced by the Maillard Reaction). The Amadori rearrangement products have become the object of physiological researches, especially the aminoketoses obtained from glucose and essential amino acids (see Metabolism of Degraded Nitrogen). Two substances that are easily formed in milk powders by reaction between lysine and lactose or lactulose are furosine and pyridosine. The furosine is distinctly more abundant and represents half of the lysine lost in heated milk powders.[69,137,138,144,165-167,209,503]

*Responsible Physical Factors*

The Maillard reaction depends on three physical factors: moisture, pH, and the sum of applied temperature, duration and intensity. Although the actions of pH and moisture are comparatively easy to define, heat action remains difficult to determine; it appears that different heat conditions are responsible for Maillard reactions of different types.

## Table 3
## EFFECT OF TEMPERATURE ON AMINO GROUPS OF TREATED CASEIN IN THE PRESENCE OF FURALDEHYDE[423]

| Temperature (°C) | Percent of blocking after 10 min |
|---|---|
| 4 | 0.002 |
| 25 | 0.025 |
| 40 | 0.300 |
| 60 | 1.0 |
| 80 | 5.5 |
| 100 | 100.0 |

From Pokorny, J., Tai, P. T., and Janicek, G., *Z. Lebensm. Unters. Forsch.*, 151, 36, 1973. With permission.

### Role of Temperature

According to Maillard[310] the reaction is "violent at 150°C, comparatively quick at 100°C, and can be observed after some days at 37°C and even below." This reaction effectively occurs at room temperature; numerous examples show its existence during the storage of food products. It is also manifest at high temperatures such as those during the cooking of bread and biscuits. The reaction is highly activated by an elevation of temperature, as Table 3 proves.

The part played by temperature, however, differs according to the chosen criterion. If the disappearance rate of amino groups is retained, equivalent losses are obtained after a brief treatment of high intensity or after a weak heating applied for a longer period of time. The amino acid loss seems to be proportional to the applied-heat sum and is independent of the operation conditions. Thus, in a mixture of β-lactoglobulin and lactose, the same loss of lysine is observed after a heating for 4 hr at 96°C and after 4 days at 55°C.[181]

If the reaction is estimated according to other criteria, heat action becomes more complex. The exact character of the reaction seems to depend more on the temperature reached than on the quantity of applied heat or heat duration. Thus, glucose-glycine premelanoidins heated for 1 hr at 90°C or 9 hr at 70°C have many identical characteristics (browning, loss of glycine, rate of reducing substances, pH) but the former has an UV absorbance twice as significant as the latter. This indicates that the exact nature of formed molecules is different at 70°C and at 90°C.[407] Likewise, the development of the Strecker degradation — measured by the emission of $CO_2$ — is independent of colored-substances production: at 56°C the Maillard reaction produces a strong browning with a weak emission of $CO_2$; at 100°C the operation provokes inverse manifestations. For the same coloration, the production of $CO_2$ is about five times more intense than at 56°C.[495]

### Role of Moisture

The intensity of the Maillard reaction greatly depends on the hydration of the medium. To achieve its maximum activity, the relative humidity must be included between 50 and 70%, i.e., the product must contain approximately 10 and 15% water. These observations result from many studies and concern the rate of amino-acid loss as well as the production of fluorescent substances or browning.

The Maillard reaction evolves slowly in very diluted media[88,118,294,376,437,473,541] and is considered as nonexistent in the absence of moisture.[63,200,525] Even under these conditions, however, it can evolve. In the absence of moisture, characteristic substances of the Maillard reaction are formed and are detected, e.g., by UV absorbance. According to Figure 9, these molecules are present in comparable amounts after a heating for 2

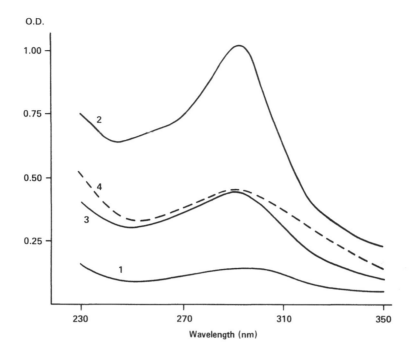

FIGURE 9. UV spectra of glucose-alanine premelanoidins as a function of relative humidity. 1 = 2 hr at 100°C with 0% HR; 2 = 2 hr at 100°C with 15% HR; 3 = 2 hr at 100°C with 73% HR; 4 = 6 hr at 100°C with 0% HR.[52]

hr at 100°C with 73% of R.H. and after 6 hr with 0% of R.H. In anhydrous or very weakly hydrated media, the Maillard reaction would develop by means of water due to the first operations of dehydration (Schiff bases), which would allow a certain mobility to the reactants. The water then exercises an autocatalytic action on the Maillard reaction.[52,294]

If, on the contrary, the hydration of the medium is important, the reaction is lessened because of the water present. In fact, it represents an inhibition factor of dehydration operations that take place in the course of the reaction.

This explains the apparently contradictory action of water on the development of the Maillard reaction. It sometimes acts favorably as a physical support of reactants. It may, however, act detrimentally as a chemical inhibitor of certain stages of the reaction.[52,294]

In practice, the moisture rate is a very important factor for the stability of foodstuffs; they must be as free of moisture as possible. In milk powders, the humidity must be less than 3% so that conservation is not accompanied by a reaction between lactose and protein.[23] It is the same with cod fillets, which lose resistance to the heat if they contain 2 to 3% moisture and are strongly damaged if they contain 11% water.[88]

*Role of pH*

The intensity of the Maillard reaction generally increases with the elevation of the pH. Most authors limit it to an interval between pH 3 and pH 9 or 10.[276,507,551] In more acid or alkaline media, sugar degradation without interference of amino acids tends to dominate; the probability of a Maillard reaction becomes all the more reduced.[222,442,531,551] Nevertheless, even in pH levels that are very remote from neutrality, there are reactions between sugars and amino acids, which explains why it is not possible to fix set limits to this type of reaction.

The amino acids are ampholyte molecules, i.e., they behave like cations in acid media (inferior to pH 1) and like anions in alkaline media (superior to pH 1). At pH 1, they are zwitterions. The following structures show the cationic, zwitterionic, and anionic forms, respectively.

$$^+H_3N-CH-COOH + OH^- \qquad ^+H_3N-CH-COO^- \qquad H_2N-CH-COO^- + H^+$$
$$\qquad\quad | \qquad\qquad\qquad\qquad\quad | \qquad\qquad\qquad\quad |$$
$$\qquad\quad R \qquad\qquad\qquad\qquad\quad R \qquad\qquad\qquad\quad R$$

The reactivity of amino groups is stronger when the amino acid is in anionic form, i.e., when the pH is superior to the pH 1 value.[426,493] This value depends on the amino-acid character; it is low for the diaminoacids (pH 3 for the aspartic and glutamic acids) and high for the basic amino acids (pH 10 for lysine and arginine). In theory, the diaminoacids are less susceptible than the diacids to the Maillard reaction in acid media.

Figure 10A shows the general behavior of amino acids according to pH after heating in presence of glucose (for 6 hr at 120°C). The case of lysine and phenylalanine has been chosen as an example. Apart from some exceptions, the amino acids are more stable as acidity becomes stronger; this justifies the hydrolysis of proteins in 6 $N$ HCl medium. Amino acids become sensitive when the pH occurs near neutrality and present a great fragility in the weakly alkaline pH. In the strongly alkaline pH, they are more stable, but they racemize in these conditions.[3,16]

In strongly acid media (6 $N$ HCl), amino acids are very stable except for methionine (and tryptophan). The stability of methionine heated in the presence of reducing sugars goes through a maximum that corresponds to 1 $N$ HCl (Figure 10B).

In strongly alkaline media, threonine is fragile, even in the absence of carbohydrates. The presence of reducing sugars considerably accelerates the loss of this amino acid (Figure 10C).

Although these functions of amino acids occur in remote conditions of the pH zone where the Maillard reaction dominates, they are dependent on a direct or secondary action of sugars and amino acids. The main exception to the behavior described is relative to tryptophan.[5] This amino acid is extremely sensitive to the presence of reducing sugars, in acid as well as in alkaline media (Figure 10D). Tryptophan is easily destroyed in acid media, and even a heating for 1 hr at 120°C in a medium that is weakly acid greatly damages it (Figure 10E). Because its behavior in the alkaline zone is comparable to that of other amino acids, tryptophan offers the best stability to neutrality (Figure 10D). In the absence of a reducing sugar, it is perfectly stable regardless of the pH value. It is then the Maillard reaction (or oxidant substances) that is responsible for the particular sensitivity of the tryptophan.

The alkaline media are responsible for a racemization of amino acids in regards to the action of the pH. In the course of different heat treatments, these observations have been made. When a racemization occurs, its consequence cannot be revealed by physicochemical methods. Biological or microbiological methods to discover this phenomenon are indispensable.

### Role of Atmosphere

The Maillard reaction is considered a nonoxidative mechanism; consequently, the absence or presence of oxygen must not modify the evolution. This has been verified many times.[88,252,284,376,448] Maillard himself[311] determined that the atmosphere nature (oxygen, hydrogen, nitrogen, or vacuum) had no influence on the intensity of perceptible phenomena of the reaction.

However, the browning intensity is often affected by the atmosphere. Oxygen fre-

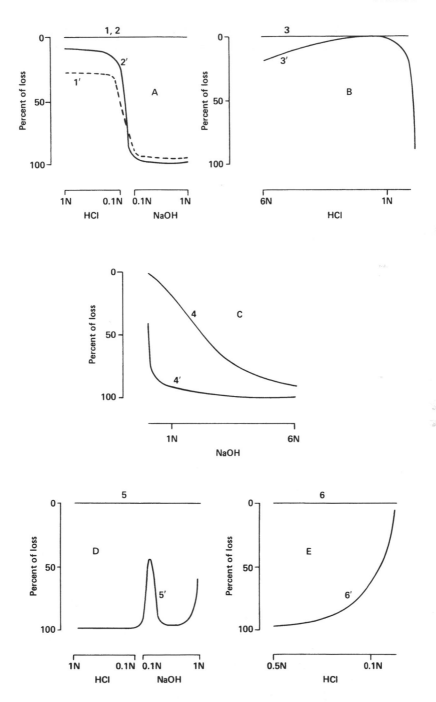

FIGURE 10. Evolution of amino acid solutions heated with or without glucose at various pH. A = General case; B = Case of methionine; C = Case of threonine; D and E = Case of tryptophan. 1, 2 = pure phenylalanine or lysine; 1′ = phenylalanine + glucose; 2′ = lysine + glucose; 3 = pure methionine; 3′ = methionine + glucose; 4 = pure threonine; 4′ = threonine + glucose; 5, 6 = pure tryptophan; 5′, 6′ = tryptophan + glucose. Figures A, B, C, D represent a heating for 6 hr at 120°C; Figure E represents a heating for 1 hr at 120°C.[3,16]

quently tends to increase the coloration,[88,286,525,533] but this action depends on complex factors in which amino acids do not necessarily interfere.[64] Therefore, this possible action of oxygen on browning shows the apparent contradictions that result in estimating the intensity of a Maillard reaction from observations based either on browning or on amino acid destruction.

### Responsible Chemical Factors

Since the Maillard reaction occurs between an aldehyde or ketone and an amine, it particularly occurs between sugars and amino acids. Nevertheless, carbohydrates are not the only products that can supply aldehydes and ketones necessary to the reaction.

In fact, all amino acids and proteins present a nearly comparable sensitivity to the Maillard reaction. They are the passive elements that undergo the sugar action. The rate and especially the nature of the sugars are the primary elements that determine the reaction intensity. The reaction can lead to amino acid and sugar blocking or destruction. The distinction between the two states derives from chemical considerations. The former forms are recoverable by chemical hydrolysis but not the latter. The two categories are lost nutritionally, however, because of their enzyme-resistant characteristic of formed linkages (see Amino Acid Determination and Measurement of Protein Efficiency).

### Sugars

Although the Maillard reaction initially is an isomolecular reaction between a sugar and an amino acid, the loss of the former is always greater than that of the latter (Figure 1). In cocoa-bean roasting 90% of the free sugars are lost, while more than one half of the free amino acids remains intact.[446] In a glucose-glycine isomolecular solution of premelanoidins, sugar losses are 63% when only 44% glycine is destroyed.[24] Theoretically, in the latter case the Maillard reaction is only responsible for the destruction of 44% of glucose. The supplementary part of the destruction would then be the consequence of a mechanism foreign to the Maillard reaction, such as caramelization. Briefly, two thirds of the loss of glucose might be attributable to a reaction with glycine, and one third attributable to a caramelization or to an analogous phenomenon.

As has already been determined, the nature of the carbohydrates is the primary influence on the Maillard reaction; the protein or amino acid nature has only a moderate influence on this reaction.

To react with an amino acid, a sugar must contain an aldehyde or ketone group. Thus, sugars such as sorbitol, mannitol, or glycerol do not provoke a reaction.[16.424] This particularity justifies their wide use in pharmaceutical industries when a sterilization must be carried out without producing a Maillard-reaction product. Likewise, the polymerized carbohydrates (cellulose and starch) do not participate in the Maillard reaction because of the absence of a free-reducing group.[226]

Sugar reactivity is comparable whether the retained criterion is coloration, amino acid loss, or sugar destruction. It depends mainly on three factors: chain length, stereochemical configuration, and sugar-protein nature.

The most important is chain length; the shorter it is, the greater is the sugar reactivity.[5.16.75.177.289.424.456.498] Thus, at isomolecular concentrations in standardized conditions, sugars produce the following losses in lysine: disaccharides, 16%; hexoses, 42%; and pentoses, 66%.

Among isomer sugars, the stereochemical configuration partially determines their reactivity.[16.75.177] Table 4 compares the reactivity with lysine of different disaccharides, hexoses, and pentoses. In regards to the disaccharides, lactose and maltose have comparable reactivities that are relatively important. Inversely, trehalose reacts very weakly. Among the hexoses, galactose appears the most reactive, whereas levulose and rhamnose are considered less reactive.[177.213.424.498] Differences also appear in the activity of different pentoses. Ribose is the most reactive isomer, followed by xylose and then

## Table 4
### INFLUENCE OF THE SUGAR NATURE ON THE LOSS OF LYSINE CONTAINED IN LACTALBUMIN AND SOYBEAN GLOBULIN[177]

| | Loss of lysine (%) | | |
| --- | --- | --- | --- |
| | Lactalbumin | Globulin | Mean |
| **Trisaccharides** | | | |
| Raffinose | 38 | 6 | — |
| **Disaccharides** | | | |
| Lactose | 37 | 33 | 35 |
| Maltose | 32 | 31 | 32 |
| Sucrose | 56 | 5 | — |
| Trehalose | 10 | 2 | — |
| Mean | 39 | 18 | |
| **Hexoses** | | | |
| Galactose | 72 | 72 | 72 |
| Mannose | 69 | 59 | (64) |
| Sorbose | 62 | 66 | 64 |
| Fucose | 66 | 60 | 63 |
| Rhamnose | 65 | 56 | (60) |
| Glucose | 64 | 54 | (59) |
| Levulose | 47 | 47 | 47 |
| Mean | 64 | 59 | |
| **Pentoses** | | | |
| Ribose | 85 | 89 | 87 |
| Xylose | 84 | 88 | 86 |
| Arabinose | 81 | 86 | 84 |
| Mean | 83 | 88 | |

*Note:* 0.5 g of protein plus 1.0 g of sugar in 10 m*l* of water, heated for 5 hr at 120°C.

by arabinose.[3,289,424] For example, although ribose destroys 79% of an amino acid mixture, xylose only destroys 61% under the same conditions.

The reactivity of different isomers seems to be an independent biochemical constant of the experimental conditions; classification of sugars is identically recognized by all authors regardless of the conditions and chosen criteria. These reactivities condition the behavior of various foodstuffs that have undergone a technological process. For example, starchy foods are sensitive only after a conversion of starch into maltose. Dairy products are always sensitive if they contain lactose and if it is hydrolyzed, because galactose is the most reactive of the hexoses. Animal products can also undergo a Maillard reaction if their nucleic acids have been degraded and have generated free ribose. This has been seen in fish meal.

A sugar does not have an absolute degree of reactivity; its behavior depends on the state and nature of its accompanying protein. Table 4 gives some examples of coupled sugar-proteins that condition the intensity of the Maillard reaction.[177,381] The more characteristic cases are as follows:

- Raffinose destroys six times more lactalbumin lysine than globulin lysine.
- Sucrose and trehalose provoke lysine losses four to five times more important with lactalbumin.
- Small molecules (hexoses and pentoses) present a reactivity comparable with the two proteins.

It is possible that sugar behavior is in relation to the stereochemical configuration of proteins. If the protein has a dense structure, the disaccharides have more difficulties in reaching the amino groups of the lysine. Consequently, it tends to be less reactive. The reactivity of levulose and glucose is also different according to the nature of amino groups that are present in the medium.[381]

The sugar nature also conditions the premelanoidin composition. The presence of hexose is interpreted by a formation of HMF without production of furfural; the pentoses produce furfural and HMF mixture.[292] Isomer sugars also influence the proportions of some premelanoidin elements, e.g., levulose produces from two to three times more acetaldehyde, propionaldehyde, 2-methyl propanal, and 3-methyl butanal than glucose. Acrolein does not come from levulose.[95]

### Lipids

The Maillard reaction is usually defined as a combination of reducing sugars and amino acids. In food technology, sugars are the main effective cause of amino acid destruction. Nevertheless, besides sugars many molecules that bear functional groups −CHO or −CO generate a Maillard reaction.

Thus, oxidation products of lipids and oxidizable substances are involved in this type of reaction by the intermediary of their aldehydes and their ketones.[236] For example, the oxidative derivatives of the tocopherols that have diketones can react with the amino acids in two diverse ways, by creating a Maillard reaction or a Strecker degradation[422] (Figure 11).

As the unsaturated aldehydes are more reactive with amino acids,[78] the oxidation products of polyenoic fatty acids preferably combine with proteins.[31,272,502] The main observations are also carried out with lipids, particularly unsaturated and easily oxidizable lipids, such as corn oil,[369] soybean oil,[249] safflower oil,[486] and fish oils[419,420,454,486] or lecithins.[76]

The reaction intensity, in any case, is proportional to the degree of autooxidation or thermal oxidation of these lipids.[249,418,420] The unoxidized lipids, even polyenoic lipids like the fish oils, play no part in the Maillard reaction. In biochemistry and nutrition, the lipid-protein reaction is exactly the same as the sugar-protein reaction in that there is always a browning. If a Strecker degradation occurs by itself, the amino acids are decarboxyled,[486] whereas in the case of the Maillard reaction, the main recorded facts are the following:[502,546,547]

- Decrease of the available lysine
- Decrease of the digestibility in vitro and in vivo of protein and lipid fractions
- Decrease of the biological value
- Reduction of animal growth and hepatic troubles

Such observations are recorded with egg albumen treated in presence of linoleate during 1 week at 50°C with 80% relative humidity. These are conditions that are favorable to the Maillard-reaction development.[546]

### Other Origins of Aldehydes and Ketones

In biological substrates, carbonyl compounds except sugars and lipids produce Mail-

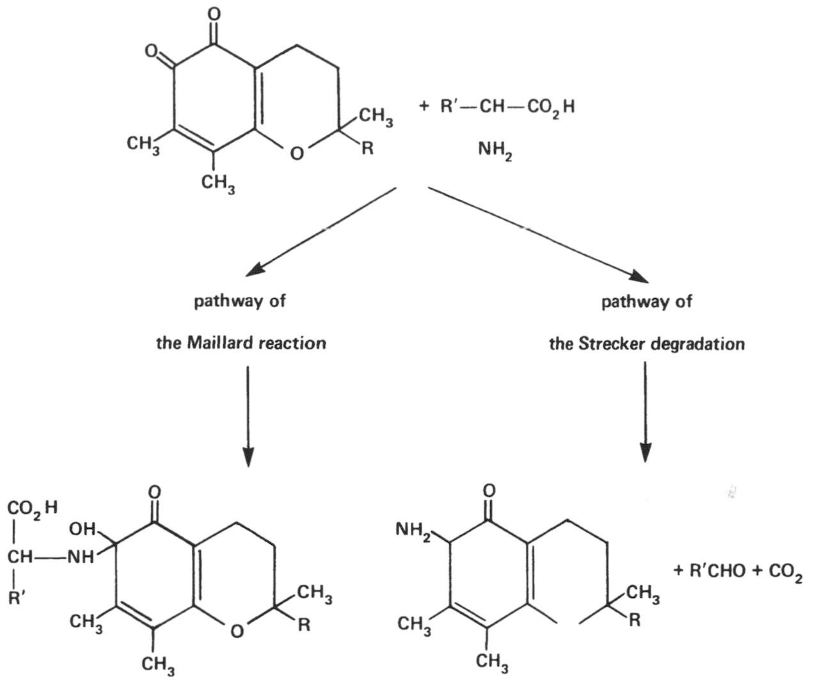

FIGURE 11. Possible reactions between tocopherols and amino acids. (From Pokorny, J., Luan, N. T., and Janicek, G., *Z. Lebensm. Unters. Forsch.*, 152, 65, 1973. With permission.)

lard reactions. Even if this eventuality does not always have important practical consequences, it must not be neglected. It particularly shows the complexity and possible interferences between caramelization, oxidation, Maillard reaction, and Strecker degradation.

For example, products of sugar-heat degradation such as furfural, 5 HMF, and other aldehydes react with amino acids according to the Maillard reaction.[189,421,477] Likewise, aldehydes formed in the course of the Strecker degradation have the possibility of reacting with amino acids that are still available for the Maillard reaction. The reaction can take place from formaldehyde,[175] acetal,[342] propional,[281] etc. This possibility of reaction shows the autocatalytic character of the Maillard reaction and of amino acid destruction. This property also appears when the fission products formed by the Maillard reaction are examined. Among them, many molecules bear aldehyde or ketone groups that in their turn produce blocking or destruction of the amino acids. This can be the case with pyruvic acid, diacetyl, etc.

When a medium contains products of this kind, a Maillard reaction can be developed without direct interference of sugars; such a situation can exist in diverse foodstuffs, mainly in cheese. Ascorbic acid is an important precursor of nonenzymatic browning in fruit and fruit juices.[102] Because the browning occurs in acid media, vitamin C has a greater tendency to provoke a Strecker degradation than a Maillard reaction.

Finally, numerous aldehydes are able to react with amino acids. For example, gossypol (found in cottonseed) reacts with lysine and makes it unavailable.[106,297,323] The list of all these molecules is very large. In particular cases, the Maillard reaction can be partly attributed to them even if sugars usually constitute the main agent responsible for this reaction.

### Amino Acids and Proteins
Unavailability of the Blocked Amino Acids

The first compounds of the Maillard reaction are characterized by enzyme-resistant linkages. The amino acids thus linked to the sugar cannot be enzymatically hydrolyzed; however, a chemical hydrolysis can break the link and regenerate the initial components, sugar, and amino acids (see Amino Acid Determination and Measurement of Protein Efficiency). These amino acids are said to be "blocked" or "unavailable". This distinguishes them from those further involved in the reaction and irrecoverable by means of chemical hydrolysis that are "destroyed" or "lost".

It is possible to distinguish these two types of mechanisms according to the context in which the heat treatment occurs. If the sample is not easily adapted to an intense Maillard reaction, it is possible to obtain an important rate of blocking lysine, but the rate of destroyed lysine won't necessarily be high. An example of this category is observed when a soybean protein is heated alone without any addition of sugar. The traces of present reducing sugars are enough to make unavailable a large lysine fraction, but the reaction does not go further. This blocking can also be attributable to the interamino acid-condensation phenomena.[141]

|  | Heating temperature of the soybean protein (°C) | | | | | |
|---|---|---|---|---|---|---|
| Form of lysine | Control | 95 | 115 | 125 | 140 | 160 |
| Blocked (%) | 0 | 6 | 13 | 16 | 28 | 68 |
| Destroyed (%) | 0 | 5 | 5 | (0) | 9 | 28 |

If the medium is favorable to the development of a Maillard reaction, lysine evolution will not end at the blocking stage but will continue until the amino acid is destroyed. Under such conditions, the greatest part of the destroyed amino acid cannot be recovered by chemical hydrolysis. A solution of glucose-lysine, heated at 120°C for variable durations, demonstrates the low percentage of blocked amino acid.[16]

|  | Percent of lysine in form of: | | |
|---|---|---|---|
| Duration of autoclaving (hr) | Available (by direct determination) | Blocked (supplement found after an acid hydrolysis) | Destroyed (not found again) |
| 1 | 91 | 9 | 0 |
| 2 | 80 | 3 | 17 |
| 4 | 57 | 1 | 42 |
| 10 | 40 | 3 | 57 |

The enzyme-resistant properties of Maillard reaction products and the proofs of amino acid unavailability are treated in the sections on Amino Acid Determination and Measurement of Protein Efficiency and Metabolism of Degraded Nitrogen.

Protein-Bound Amino Acids

Proteins do not exist that are insensible to the Maillard reaction, unless they are insoluble in water. Except for keratins, for example, all proteins are sensitive to the action of reducing sugars when the biochemical context is favorable to the development of the Maillard reaction.

In a protein, the α-amino groups of amino acids are strongly linked to the carboxylic group of close amino acids. Heat treatments and chemical reactions have little probability of reaching these α-amino groups. The more available molecules for the Maillard

## Table 5
## LOSS OF AMINO ACIDS DURING ROASTING OF FOODSTUFFS AT 150°C[6,20]

| Foodstuff | Loss of amino acids (%) | | | | Loss lysine/loss methionine |
|---|---|---|---|---|---|
| | Lysine | Methionine | Threonine | Valine | |
| Yeasts | 9 | 4.5 | — | — | 2.0 |
| Algae (*Spirulina*) | 18.5 | 4.5 | — | — | 4.0 |
| Fish meal | 21 | 14 | 6 | 1 | 1.5 |
| Wheat meal | 35 | 10 | 0 | 1 | 3.5 |
| Cotton oil meal | 44 | 3 | 9 | 0 | 14.5 |
| Peanut oil meal | 51 | 12 | 0 | 5 | 4.5 |
| Skim milk | 95 | 11 | 27 | 11 | 8.5 |
| | | | | | |
| Mean | 49 | 11 | 8 | 3 | |

reaction are the terminal amino acids of the chains and the molecules that have a second amino group in free state. The selective loss of basic amino acids has often been observed when a protein is exposed to the action of reducing sugars.[6,20,68,85,277,279,462]

When a casein-glucose mixture loses 8% of its amino N by heating, the destruction of histidine reaches 17%; that of arginine, 22%; and that of lysine, 46%.[67,140] The latter is essentially due to the amount of the free ε-amino group of lysine. In casein, the quantity of the ε-amino group in free state is 50 times higher than the quantity of the free α-amino group. Since the two lysine amino groups show a comparable reactivity with reducing sugars, the blocking of the ε-amino group is responsible for the most serious consequences in the nutritional field.[278]

Among the three basic amino acids only lysine is essential for the organisms. Thus, the behavior of this amino acid in the course of heat treatments and during all the industrial processes is really primary for the nutritionists.

In reality, two series of basically independent phenomena occur in the course of a heat treatment. On the one hand, protein undergoes amino acid degradations and destructions that particularly affect the S-containing amino acids (see Reactions Among Pure Amino Acids). Apparently, the Maillard reaction is not directly implicated by these destructions. On the other hand, lysine blocking and destruction depend directly on reducing sugars.

Thus, the relationship of "loss of lysine/loss of methionine" or "loss of lysine/loss of cystine" tends to indicate the nature of the phenomena that occur in the course of a heating. The higher this value is, the more dominant the Maillard reaction is, and vice versa. This connection provides the first information relative to the reactivity of carbohydrates present in the sample.

Table 5 interprets the evolution of some foodstuffs during roasting at 150°C. On the average, lysine is five times more often damaged than methionine and ten times more often lost than other essential amino acids; these relationships can be considered as valid values for most food products. From the relationship "loss of lysine/loss of methionine", yeasts and fish meals seem to be relatively immune to the risk of a Maillard reaction. Inversely, skim milk and cotton meal undergo an intense Maillard reaction during heat treatments.

According to Table 5, diverse protein-bound amino acids — other than the basic amino acids — undergo losses of variable intensity during heating. Thus, because of the Maillard reaction, methionine included in the soybean is unavailable for the chick.[226] Likewise, tryptophan of this feed product is blocked by the Maillard reaction.[151] In the casein also, besides the basic amino acids, the S-containing amino acids and tyrosine can be destroyed by the presence of the reducing sugar.[277]

Briefly, in the case of a protein or an undegraded foodstuff, the Maillard reaction selectively destroys lysine and other basic amino acids. Comparatively important losses of S-containing amino acids are frequently registered although it is not presently possible to determine the part of sugar response in these destructions.

Nutritionally, when a Maillard reaction is applied to a protein, a small fraction of the protein N is destroyed, but the principal amino acid balance is modified. This phenomenon is the most serious consequence of the reaction. In any case, the deficit in lysine tends to deepen selectively, and any protein submitted to a sufficient Maillard reaction could be limited primarily by lysine, regardless of its initial amino acid balance. This concept will be experimentally checked with some foodstuffs in the sections on Milk Products and Leguminous Seeds and Oil Meals.

### Protein-Bound Lysine

The behavior of protein-bound lysine tends to depend on the nature of the protein in which it is included. A significant relationship exists between the rate of lysine in protein and the percent of lysine destroyed by the Maillard reaction. The regression line between the rate of lysine in proteins (x) and the percent of lysine destruction (y) is[21,177]

$$y = 9.01 + 2.99 \, x$$

In practice, albumins will tend to undergo important losses during reaction with sugars, because they are generally rich in lysine. On the contrary, lysine-poor cereal proteins appear to be more resistant to the Maillard reaction.[177] By extrapolating the facts, it is possible to consider, *a priori,* that the Maillard reaction is more detrimental for animal-origin productions than for vegetable-kingdom foodstuffs because the rate in lysine is usually higher in the first case than in the second. This partly explains why dairy products offer a great sensitivity to heat treatments. Whey proteins are very rich in lysine and are very reactive in the presence of lactose. The lysine loss of $\beta$-lactoglobulin is superior to that of casein; the difference is about 40%.[177,180,266]

### Free Amino Acids

When free amino acids are in the presence of a sugar, Maillard-reaction effects do not manifest selectively to any greater extent on basic amino acids but do manifest regularly on all amino acids, regardless of their structure. The free diamino acids, in particular, do not undergo a blocking or destruction rate double that of other amino acids. The facts are confirmed by the unavailability rate of different essential amino acids treated in the presence of glucose at 120°C.[3] The mean percents of available amino acids retained after heating are phenylalanine, 57%; methionine, 62%; lysine, 69%; isoleucine, 73%; threonine, 78%; and valine, 80%.

Nevertheless, the amino acid structure weakly conditions its reactivity with reducing sugars. According to the above values, the stereochemical configuration partially determines amino acid behavior. In fact, the most fragile structures (phenylalanine, methionine, and lysine) do not bear any substitution on the $\beta$-carbon; this supposes an easy attack by the sugar. The most resistant (isoleucine, threonine, and valine) bear a methyl or hydroxyl group on the $\beta$-carbon that can impede the action of the sugar molecule. Information relating to amino acid reactivity as a function of amino group position has apparently not been established as has been done for the browning phenomena (see Browning).

## Table 6
## CONSEQUENCES OF THE MAILLARD REACTION IN
## LYSINE-XYLOSE-AMINO ACID MEDIA[22]

| Components[a] | pH | Coloration (520 nm) | Unavailable lysine (%) | Unavailable amino acids (%)[b] |
|---|---|---|---|---|
| Lysine (unheated) | 6.7 | 0 | 0 | |
| Lysine-xylose | 3.7 | 0.04 | 30 | |
| Lysine-xylose-valine | 3.9 | 0.105 | 52 | 8 |
| Xylose-valine | | | | 15 |
| Lysine-xylose-arginine | 5.0 | 0.27 | 13 | 42 |
| Xylose-arginine | | | | 29 |
| Lysine-xylose-cystine | 3.3 | 0.02 | 11 | 2 |
| Xylose-cystine | | | | 0 |

[a] Lysine (0.04 $M$), xylose (0.5 $M$), and other amino acids (0.2 $M$) in a buffered solution, heated for 1 hr at 120°C.
[b] Valine, arginine, or cystine.

### Lysine in the Presence of Other Free Amino Acids

When a Maillard reaction is developing between lysine and sugar, the free amino acid presence tends to modify either protein-bound or free lysine behavior[22] (Table 6). Of 14 amino acids, 8 intensify lysine loss, only 1 (glycine) is without effect, and 4 save lysine by reducing its destruction rate (arginine, cystine, glutamic, and aspartic acids). *A priori*, it is not possible to connect this action of the diverse amino acids with their chemical structure or properties.

The catalytic loss of lysine attributable to most amino acids (mainly valine and threonine) is not the inverse of the preserving action of some amino acids, but is derived from different mechanisms. Both phenomena tend to happen under different conditions. The autocatalytic destruction of lysine attributable to valine or threonine occurs when the Maillard reaction is at its beginnings and the biochemical context is favorable to the reaction. Under these conditions, valine or threonine can double the lysine loss. This supplementary quantity of disappeared lysine is not only blocked but is destroyed. This indicates that valine and threonine strongly intensify the Maillard reaction and, more probably, the Strecker degradation:

| | Percent of lysine in form of: | | |
|---|---|---|---|
| | Unavailable | Blocked | Destroyed |
| Lysine + lactose | 37 | 0.5 | 35.5 |
| Lysine + lactose + valine or threonine | 65 | 1.5 | 63.5 |

These mechanisms of the added amino acids appear in Table 6 which offers the cases of valine, arginine, and cystine.[22]

**Valine** — This amino acid acts by competition with lysine. In medium lysine-xylose-valine, valine destruction is decreased by the presence of lysine, and lysine loss is increased by valine. Valine then seems to direct xylose preferentially towards lysine, resulting in increased lysine destruction. Valine and other amino acids that have the same effect act especially at the beginning of the Maillard reaction.

**Arginine** — This amino acid also acts by competition with lysine, but the situation is the inverse of that observed in the valine case. Xylose affinity is stronger for arginine than for lysine. Arginine then appears to catch sugar for its own benefit and lysine indirectly becomes protected.

**Cystine** — Cystine appears to act quite differently from other amino acids by inhibiting the Maillard reaction; it precociously acidifies the medium that brakes the reaction development. Cystine inhibits the formation of colored-substances, regardless of heating duration. These actions occur without a notable degradation of cystine, although it is weakly soluble in water.

### Amino Acids of the Proteolysates

When a mixture of protein-bound and free amino acids (autolysates, proteolysates) is exposed to a Maillard reaction, amino acid reactivity differs from theoretical forecasts. Mixed amino acid behavior is different both from that of a protein-bound amino acid and that of a free amino acid.[21] This conclusion becomes apparent after the comparison of (1) intact protein, (2) complete autolysate of the protein, i.e., its equivalent in amino acids at a free state, and (3) partial proteolysate, composed of two thirds intact protein and one third its equivalent in free amino acids (Table 7).

In the intact protein, lysine-selective destruction is confirmed. Its loss rate is approximately 20 times higher than that of methionine. In the complete autolysate, various amino acids are more uniformly damaged by the Maillard reaction; the lysine loss becomes only three times superior to that of methionine. This is due to an increase of methionine destruction and to decreased lysine loss. In the partial proteolysate, amino acid reactivity is distinctly reinforced; the amino-N destruction is doubled and amino acid losses are always heavier. The increase of losses concerns amino acids contained in the protein-bound fraction as well as those that are in free state. Protein-bound lysine always supports specifically the reducing sugar action. Moreover, all other amino acids are significantly more damaged than when they are either in free or protein-bound state. The sensitivity of methionine is particularly high in the partial proteolysate. It confirms the catalytic effects of most free amino acids on the Maillard reaction intensity. From the comparison established in Table 7, it is possible to estimate the nutritional repercussions of the Maillard reaction according to its application to an intact protein, a complete autolysate, or a partial proteolysate.

In the case of an intact protein, the Maillard reaction may deeply modify the amino acid balance because of the selective destruction of basic amino acids. In all cases, a lysine deficiency may occur or may be reinforced. In a complete autolysate, the nutritional consequences are less prejudicial. In fact, all amino acids tend to be destroyed in close proportions, and the amino acid balance is not sensibly disturbed. The partial proteolysate represents the more damaged form; the lysine selective destruction is maintained at a level nearly as high as in the intact protein, and all other amino acids are strongly damaged.

In practice, the intermediary state between the intact proteins and the free amino acids is not desirable when the partially degraded foodstuffs risk exposure to a Maillard reaction.

### Physicochemical Manifestations

The Maillard reaction is included in nonenzymatic browning reactions. It produces an important browning that is the main manifestation for many food technologists. However, the Maillard reaction generates other repercussions in the physicochemical field; fluorescence and UV absorbance appear first, then browning appears. At the same time, acid substances and reducing molecules are formed. At a certain stage of the reaction, a gaseous emission occurs, followed by reinforcement of coloration without acid formation. This is the Strecker degradation (see The Strecker Degradation). The reaction ends with the formation of a black precipitate of melanoidins.

Sugar caramelization offers many points analogous to the Maillard reaction, concerning the physicochemical evolution of the medium; however, the situations actually

## Table 7
## MANIFESTATIONS OF THE MAILLARD REACTION ACCORDING TO THE DEGREE OF THE SUBSTRATE PROTEOLYSIS[21]

| | Percent of loss | Percent of difference with |
|---|---|---|
| | **Intact protein** | |
| Amino-N | 6.5 | |
| Lysine | 56.5 | |
| Methionine | 3 | |
| Valine | 4 | |
| | **Complete autolysate** | **Intact protein** |
| Amino-N | 7 | +8 |
| Lysine | 18 | −65 |
| Methionine | 6.5 | +115 |
| Valine | 5 | +25 |
| | **Partial proteolysate** | |
| Amino-N | 13 | |
| Lysine | 42 | |
| Methionine | 16 | |
| Valine | 8 | |
| | | **Complete autolysate** |
| **Protein-bound fraction** | | |
| Amino-N | 14 | +100 |
| Lysine | 26 | +45 |
| Methionine | 17 | +160 |
| Valine | 10 | +100 |
| | | **Intact protein** |
| **Free amino acid fraction** | | |
| Amino-N | 12 | +85 |
| Lysine | 50 | −11 |
| Methionine | 15 | +400 |
| Valine | 7 | +75 |

*Note:* Experimental conditions: intact protein = 2 g of protein (lactalbumin, soybean globulin, or glutenin); complete autolysate = 2 g of protein-equivalent in the form of a free amino acid mixture; partial proteolysate = 1.3 g of protein plus 0.7 g of the amino acid mixture; diluted in 12 m$\ell$ of water and addition of 0.6 g of xylose with autoclaving for 10 hr at 100°C.

differ (Table 8). The amino acids involve appearance of a molecule that cannot be formed simply by sugar degradation. They also modify the quantities of formed substances by favoring some reactions and inhibiting others. The residue obtained at the end of the Maillard reaction also differs from the precipitate formed by caramelization. The latter is obligatorily devoid of nitrogen, whereas the degraded forms of amino acids are fixed with the melanoidin.

Generally, the most reactive amino acids (basic amino acids) are those that tend to give the most intense physical repercussions (fluorescence, browning, etc.).[357,360] However, the nitrogen residues that go through the insoluble melanoidins essentially derive from amino acids that are fragile in the acid media (methionine and tryptophan).[3,5,16,455]

Table 8

## COMPARISON AMONG THE MAIN PHYSICOCHEMICAL MANIFESTATIONS OF THE MAILLARD REACTION, THE STRECKER DEGRADATION, AND CARAMELIZATION

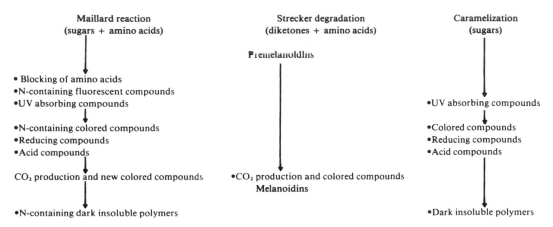

### Fluorescence

This phenomenon is one of the very first manifestations of the Maillard reaction: it clearly occurs before browning formation.[182,279,345,375,382,397,505] Fluorescence quickly develops through a maximum intensity, and then decreases as the browning reactions become important. In some cases, fluorescence has nearly disappeared by the time that coloration occurs.[382]

Fluorescence is a specific mechanism of the Maillard reaction, i.e., the presence of the amino acid is indispensable for its formation.[382] Like all phenomena produced by this reaction, fluorescence is favored by temperature and alkalinity.[399,499] Fluorescence has a maximum at a wavelength of 450 nm.[362] It is so characteristic of the Maillard reaction that it has been proposed as a criterion for the determination of amino acid spots produced by the paper chromatography method.[483]

The fluorophores derive from dehydration mechanisms such as the Schiff base formation, which is composed of unsaturated and N-containing substances.[79,81,99] Fluorescence is linked to an imine structure in conjunction with an electron-donating group. The following formulae of fluorophores have been proposed:[1,99,318]

$$-N=CH-CH=N-CO_2H-CH_2-N=CH-CH_2-CH_2-NH-CO_2H-CH_2-N=CH-CH=CH-OH$$

The fluorescent, colorless compounds are narrowly linked to the chromophores that are ulteriorly developed in the Maillard reaction; the two substances are cationic molecules,[362] and a linear relationship exists between the abilities of fluorescence and browning.[1] It is probable that the colored compounds come from a polymerization phenomenon of fluorescent precursors.[81,397] The two groups of molecules are not necessarily identical, however, and the conversion does not occur either every time or automatically.[182,382,510]

The bisulfite action does not inhibit fluorescent elements but does impede their conversion into colored pigments; in the presence of bisulfite, the Maillard reaction supplies a weak browning intensity but provokes a fluorescent product accumulation.[382] These observations emphasize the filial connection existing between the production of fluorescent compounds and the colored molecules. They also explain why the bisulfites inhibit browning without significantly reducing amino acid loss. These additives do not inhibit the initial phase of the Maillard reaction, i.e., blocking and the nutritional loss in amino acids, but only inhibit the conversion of fluorescent components. This action of the bisulfites also reinforces the distinction that must be established between the phenomena leading to browning and nutritional loss.

## UV Absorbance

Caramelization and the Maillard reaction produce molecules absorbed in UV in the region of 250 to 300 nm.[98,182,357,362,397,406] In acid media or in the presence of excess glucose, the molecule mainly responsible for UV absorbance is 5 HMF, which absorbs strongly at 285 nm and weakly at 228 nm. Levulinic acid, which absorbs at 265 nm, is a degradation product of 5 HMF.[428,487,543]

At the time of a Maillard reaction, the situation is more complex and many peaks are registered. On the one hand, different amino acids, heated in the presence of the same sugar, produce distinct UV spectra, whose only common point is a peak situated at about 280 to 300 nm. On the other hand, the same amino acids produce a great variety of peaks when treated with different sugars. These observations show amino acid responsibility in the production of UV-absorbing substances and the diversity of reactions generated according to the sugar nature. In the field, the amino acid and the sugar have the same importance. However, physicochemical conditions where the Maillard reaction occurs do not determine the characteristics of the UV-absorbing molecules; they only determine the quantity of substances formed (Figure 9C).

A peak has been observed by different authors[98,397,406] and has been studied further. Its wavelength is 296 nm; for that reason it is called the "296 peak".[406] Its molecular weight is 327; its gross formula is $C_{11}H_{15}O_8N$. The molecule has a ketone group, an hydroxyl group, and one or several alcohol groups; it must be unsaturated.

This colorless compound, deriving from an early stage of the Maillard reaction, contributes ulteriorly to the observed browning. In fact, the "296 peak" produces a colored reaction in the presence of an amino acid. This observation is the direct proof that the Maillard reaction is not fundamentally a browning reaction. The coloration develops only after the appearance of the earliest products of the reaction; they act as precursors of colored substances. The amino acid loss has an autocatalytic progression; the first degradation products of the Maillard reaction (nitrogenous compounds) react with new, intact amino acids.

## Browning

When the Maillard reaction reaches a certain intensity, it is accompanied by increasing coloration, which ranges from yellow to dark brown and even to black, although the early compounds are colorless.[182,279,289,382,417,534] Coloration can be developed without any amino acid, however. During caramelization, it derives from pH action and from the temperature on the sugars.[131,469] Coloration remains weak in acid media and intensifies in neutral and alkaline media.[439] Glucose develops coloration with a maximum at pH 8.0 (Figure 12).

The amino acid presence tends to increase the phenomenon in variable proportions according to experimental conditions. The coloration of glycine-glucose premelanoidins follows an evolution parallel to that of glucose solutions (Figure 12), which reveals the existence of a link between the two browning types. This amino acid effect is due to the formation of UV-absorbing precursors of colored substances. The facts are complex. For some, browning development is more dependent on amino acid concentration than on that of the sugar.[79] For others under other conditions, the colorations are increased weakly, if at all, by the presence of amino acids.[98,469]

All authors agree, however, that the action of amino acids relates to the connected unsaturated carbonyl compounds that are formed at the beginning of the reaction (including imine groups)[79,94] and are responsible for the fluorescence appearance. Thus,

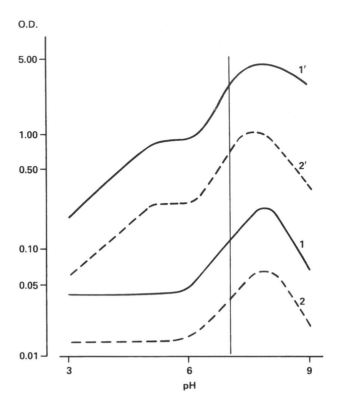

FIGURE 12.    Evolution of browning in buffered solutions of glucose
(1 and 2) and of glucose — glycine (1′ and 2′) as a function of the
pH. 1 = solution of glucose; 1′ = solution of glucose — glycine,
measurement at 430 nm; 2 = solution of glucose; 2′ = solution of
glucose — glycine, measurement at 520 nm.[14]

many observations link amino acid activity to furfural presence,[188,253,307,439,511,512,544,548]
to that of reductones,[98,403,425,534] or, more generally, to that of molecules with high
degrees of unsaturation.[439] More precisely, osuloses (aminoketose degradation products) develop coloration by reaction with amino acids.[32,33] Indirectly, the Amadori
rearrangement products are confirmed in their roles as coloration precursors.

Coloration is probably the result of polymerization phenomena of substances that
initially appeared. Diverse colored compounds correspond to an identical chemical
structure whose degree of polymerization seems to be the only variable between
them.[349]

In short, the chromophores have certain chemical characteristics. The following formula has been attributed to them:[216] $-CH=CH-CH=CH-$, or the following reactional
groups:[94,435] $-CH=CH-$, $-OH$, $C=O$, and $CH=N-$. It is also possible that the sugar
chain has several imine groups as well as unsaturated linkages.[493]

$$CH-C-CH=CH-CHOH-CH_2OH \qquad CH-COH-CH=CH-CHOH-CH_2OH$$

with N and N below (bonded to R and R′), and on the right N and NH below (bonded to R and R′).

Amino acids act according to their nature. As coloration is favored by an elevation
of pH, the neutral or acidic amino acids have little effect on coloration intensity. Inversely, the basic amino acids considerably reinforce pH action on the sugar at pH 6

Table 9
THE EFFECT OF VARIOUS AMINO ACIDS ON THE
BROWNING OF A GLUCOSE SOLUTION

| | Structure of the amino acid | | |
| Amino acid | Number of carbon atoms | Position of the amino groups | Absorbance at 500 nm |
| --- | --- | --- | --- |
| Glucose only | | | 0.64 |
| α-Alanine | 3 | α | 0.77 |
| β-Alanine | 3 | β | 2.00 |
| α-Aminobutyric acid | 4 | α | 1.00 |
| γ-Aminobutyric acid | 4 | γ | 2.30 |
| Norvaline | 5 | α | 1.07 |
| δ-Aminovaleric acid | 5 | δ | 1.88 |
| Ornithine | 5 | α-δ | 3.07 |
| Norleucine | 6 | α | 1.21 |
| Lysine | 6 | ε | 4.10 |

Reprinted from Lento, H. G., Jr., Underwood, J. C., and Willits, C. O., *Food Res.*, 23, 68, 1958. Copyright© by Institute of Food Technologists. With permission.

or above.[537] They then act according to chain length and amino group position. Coloration is favored by long chains and by moving between the amino and carboxylic groups. The latter has an inhibiting action on amino group reactivity.[269,285] The most intense colorations are obtained with ω amino acids, with four carbon atoms and six carbons.[517] Table 9 shows the double action of amino acids on browning development.

It is important to determine that the blocking and destruction of the amino acid depend on mechanisms different from those that check the first stages of coloration. The amino acids are not directly implicated in the early reactions that lead to colored molecules. For these reasons, the coloration measure is not a valid criterion for estimating the reaction intensity between sugars and amino acids.[7,182,537] The nutritional consequences of the Maillard reaction are not fundamentally linked to browning intensity.

The part of mineral elements provides an obvious proof; they often modify browning intensity without having any influence on amino acid evolution. Mineral ions can act on browning: (1) directly by chemical reactions that they provoke, and (2) indirectly by interactions with the medium, particularly with its pH. The pH can maintain mineral ions in an ionized state or can insolubilize them, which will condition their chemical reactivity. Only systematic experimentation under severe conditions would determine the part of these elements in browning phenomena.

It is presently known that phosphates tend to increase coloration[79,174,251,356,358,359,361,504] without accelerating lysine destruction.[16] The part of phosphates is due mainly to direct action on the sugars, i.e., phosphates increase browning by an accelerated degradation of sugar; this phenomenon is independent of the Maillard reaction. Borates also increase coloration.[361] In acid media, copper, iron, and zinc reduce both browning and blocking of amino acids. In weakly alkaline medium, copper increases browning without affecting the loss rate of amino acids.[119,341] In the same way, cobalt tends to weaken color in acid solution and has no effect in neutral medium.[241] The ferrous and ferric ions increase coloration, especially in association with phosphates.[64,79,390] Calcium and magnesium decrease browning.[76,358]

All of these observations still remain fragmentary; the part and conditions of ion action in the field of nonenzymatic browning cannot be determined at this time. However, except for the stannous ion, no mineral element seems to significantly inhibit lysine destruction.[2,16]

## Acidity

The Maillard reaction is always followed by medium acidification. Figure 1 supplies an example showing heating of a viscous mixture of glycine-glycose for 6 hr at 90°C; this causes the pH to change from 5.3 to 3.3. The fall is rapid at the beginning and continues more slowly. The important decrease registered in early stages is parallel to amino group utilization and fluorescence development.[79]

This acidification is the result of several mechanisms. When amino acids are blocked by sugar, the carboxylic group acidity is no longer "buffered" by the amine; it appears freely. The N-glycosylamines are stronger acids than the free amino acids.[335] Moreover, the degradation of the sugar itself and the Maillard reaction produce numerous acid molecules that greatly lower the pH. In particular, there is a formation of levulinic, pyruvic, lactic, and formic acids, according to the pH and mechanisms involved.[152,524,527]

## Nonsugar Reducing Power

Initially, sugar is the only reducing element in the experimental pattern submitted to the Maillard reaction. It quickly disappears during heating, whereas the total reducing power only decreases slowly (Figure 1). Thus, reducing compounds are formed during the Maillard reaction[135,321] in simple experimental mixtures; glucose can represent less than 20% of the reducing power of the medium.[407,512]

The antioxidative properties of these molecules protect the premelanoidins against oil rancidity; at the concentration of 0.5% their antioxygen power is comparable to that of 0.01% of NDGA.[179,316]

The nonsugar reducing substances are abundant in the early premelanoidins and then tend to decrease (Figure 1). Schematically, they are composed of two compound categories. Some are glucose-like substances, measurable by cuprometric or ferricyanide methods. They essentially correspond to the aminoketoses (formed by the Amadori rearrangement) that show very strong reducing properties, whereas the N-substituted glycosylamines have only a weak reducing power.[93,188,216,409,437] The aminoaldoses (produced by the Heyns rearrangement) have a reducing power comparable to that of glucose.[436] In a parallel way, reducing molecules result from both the Maillard reaction and sugar degradation, e.g., furfural and HMF. Some are ascorbic acid-like substances that react with 2,6 dichlorophenolindophenol. This group of reducing compounds is formed later and includes reductones that derive from the sugar degradation in the same manner as from the Maillard reaction. Their reducing power disappears as the Strecker degradation develops.

## Melanoidins

The Maillard reaction ends by the insolubilization of "melanoidins," according to the term coined by Schmiedeberg.[464] It differs from precipitate obtained at the end of the sugar-heat degradation by a significant proportion of nitrogen.

The quantity of melanoidins is proportional first to the sugar amount and then to the medium acidity. The amino acid nature influences both the rate and the composition of residue. In aqueous media, glycine-glucose mixtures give melanoidins containing between 3.5 and 6.0% of nitrogen.[125,135,314] Gross formulae have been proposed:[136,542] $C_{67}H_{76}O_{32}N_5$ or $C_{12}H_{13}O_4N_2CH_2-CO_2H$.

Among the essential amino acids, tryptophan and phenylalanine favor the melanoidin insolubilization, whereas lysine tends to inhibit the precipitate formation.[3,5] The amino acids intervene more strongly in acid media. Under these conditions, for each

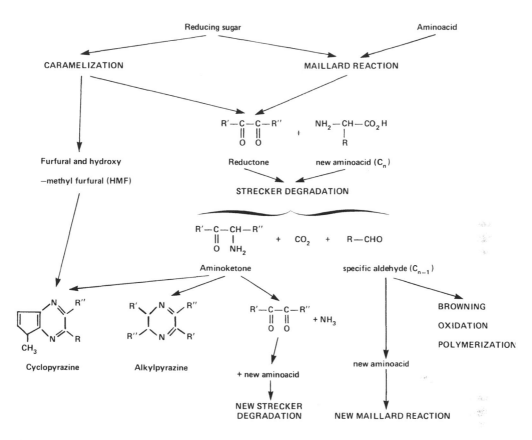

FIGURE 13. Mechanism of the Strecker degradation (oxidative decarboxylation of amino acids) and its consequences: formation of organoleptic molecules and autocatalytic losses of amino acids.

1% of lysine nitrogen fixed by the melanoidin residue, the residue fixes 2.5% of isoleucine and valine, 4.5% of threonine, 7.5% of phenylalanine, and 18% of the methionine. But, it is well-established that the degradation products of tryptophan constitute the main source of melanoidin nitrogen: the precipitate contains all of the destroyed tryptophan nitrogen in acid media.[3,5,110,187,455]

## The Strecker Degradation

In 1862, Strecker[501] observed that alloxan could decompose alanine into acetaldehyde and carbon dioxide. This reaction called the "Strecker degradation", can be applied to amino acids exposed to the diketone — or reductone — action.

### Degradation Chemistry

An overall view of the Strecker degradation is given in Figure 13. It consists in a transamination and an oxidative decarboxylation of the amino acid with production of $CO_2$. The aldehyde formed from the amino acid is a specific molecule of that operation. The active reductones or diketones in this field are numerous. They correspond to the general formula: $- CO - (CH=CH)_n - CO -$ where n is equal to 0, 1, or 3. These molecules can be $\alpha$-keto-aldehydes. $\alpha$-keto-lactones, $\alpha$-keto-acides, or 1,2,diketones. Some examples[465,466] of diketones include (n = 0) pyruvic acid, diacetyl, alloxan, isatin, dehydroascorbic acid, phenylglyoxylic acid, phenylpyruvic acid; (n = 1) anthraquinone, naphtaquinone, indigo, vitamin K; (n = 3) coerulignone. Aldehydes include glyoxal, methylglyoxal, phenylglyoxal, pyruvaldehyde, and aromatic aldehydes.

Table 10

SPECIFIC ALDEHYDES GENERATED BY
THE STRECKER DEGRADATION[259, 368, 430]

| Amino acid | Aldehyde |
| --- | --- |
| Alanine | Acetal |
| Glutamic acid | Butanal or crotonal |
| Cysteine | Ethanal or propanal |
| Glycine | Methanal |
| Isoleucine | 2-Methyl butanal or isobutyraldehyde |
| Leucine | 3-Methyl butanal or isovaleraldehyde |
| Methionine | Methional or propanal |
| Norvaline | Butanal |
| Ornithine | Pyrroline |
| Phenylalanine | Phenylacetal |
| Proline | Pyrroline |
| Serine | Glyoxal or glycol aldehyde |
| Threonine | 2-Hydroxy propanal |
| Valine | 2-Methyl propanal |

These reductones are formed during the Maillard reaction, as well as in the course of the sugar degradation.[8,152,524,526,536] The initial sugar nature conditions the Strecker degradation activity: e.g., fructose allows a greater specific aldehyde production than glucose.[95] This difference may result from the ability of the sugars to produce reductones, precursors of the Strecker degradation. Reductones can exist in nature (vitamin C, vitamin K), or result from enzymatic reactions (pyruvic acid, etc.), or from the degradation of certain molecules (dehydroascorbic acid).[270]

In practice, all the amino acids may be degraded by this mechanism. This generates specific aldehydes; conversions are given in Table 10. The carbon dioxide production is the other specific manifestation of the Strecker degradation: 90% of the $CO_2$ derives from the decarboxylation of the amino acids.[8,496,542] Figure 14 confirms the $CO_2$ origin, whose production is strictly parallel to the lysine destruction and is the direct consequence of it.

Nevertheless, in the absence of amino acids, and at pH 7, the action of a sugar on carboxylic acids also provokes the formation of carbon dioxide, tartric, citric, and lactic acids being the most active molecules.[288] That is why, even in defined and simple conditions, the $CO_2$ production tends to exceed the predicted theoretical quantity that would correspond to the amount of amino acid destroyed.[8,104]

In a parallel way to the amino acid decarboxylation, the Strecker degradation is accompanied by intense dehydration; according to Maillard,[311] for each $CO_2$ molecule produced, 12 water molecules were produced. However, it is possible that these two phenomena occur simultaneously, during the Strecker degradation, even if the dehydration does not depend on this mechanism.

The Strecker degradation intensity decreases with the acidity of the medium.[104] If the value of 1 is given to the quantity of $CO_2$ produced at pH 7, it is 1.04 at pH 6, 0.64 at pH 5, 0.44 at pH 4. The acidity developed during the Maillard reaction constitutes an inhibitory factor towards the Strecker degradation.

This operation does not provoke any medium acidification, but strongly develops its coloration.[8,287,416,496,534,542] The browning formed during this reaction is narrowly linked to the carbon dioxide production and to the amino acid decarboxylation: it is attributed to an aldehyde reaction that derives from the amino acid decomposition.[342,389]

All the characteristic manifestations of a Strecker degradation appear when reduc-

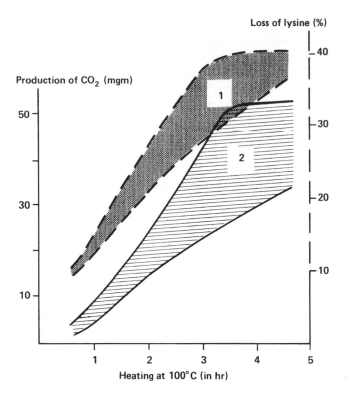

FIGURE 14.   Destruction of lysine (broken line) and production of $CO_2$ (heavy line) in a lysine-xylose solution with or without premelanoidins. The striped surface is bounded by a lower line which corresponds either to the loss of lysine or to the production of $CO_2$ in lysine-xylose pure solution. The upper line corresponds to the same values in presence of premelanoidins. The striped surface 1 shows the increase of lysine losses in presence of premelanoidins and surface 2 shows the increase of $CO_2$ production under the same conditions. (From Adrian, J., *Ann. Nutr. Aliment,* 27, 299, 1973. With permission.)

tones or their precursors are added to a reactive medium. In this case, the degradation mechanism is added to that of the Maillard reaction that is normally developed during the heating.[8]

|  | Solution of lysine — xylose (Maillard reaction only) | Solution of lysine — xylose + premelanoidins (Maillard reaction plus Strecker degradation) |
|---|---|---|
| $CO_2$ production (mg/g of lysine) | 18.8 | 34.6 |
| Loss of lysine (%) | 24.4 | 31.8 |
| pH | 3.60 | 3.55 |
| Browning (590 nm) | 0.21 | 0.34 |

In practice, $CO_2$ production is revealed in milk powders when stored in defective conditions,[202,203] or during the heating of foodstuffs kept in shut containers.[287,295] The fact is important with tomato or plum concentrates: in such products, rich in carboxylic acids, a $CO_2$ fraction probably comes from a direct interaction between sugars and organic acids.

*Autocatalytic Destruction of Amino Acids*

The Strecker degradation has several consequences in the biochemical and nutritional fields. One favorable result is the formation of flavors that are appreciated by the consumer (see Flavors Produced by the Maillard Reaction). An unfavorable consequence is the autocatalytic mechanism of amino acid destruction, signaled by Maillard[314] observing that "the glycine and glucose reaction goes on even at 15°C after beginning at high temperature".

When a medium includes reductones, each reductone molecule can cause a continual disappearance of amino acids; Figure 13 explains the process. In the first stage, every reductone destroys an amino acid molecule: this is due to the Strecker degradation. The initial reductone can then be regenerated and consequently begin again an identical reaction with a new amino acid. Simultaneously, the aldehyde formed from the decarboxylated amino acid can generate a Maillard reaction, i.e., blocking and destroying an amino acid, and ultimately producing new reductone. Thus, the amino acid destruction will be able to go on indefinitely.

The facts confirm this theory: when a medium contains reductones or their precursors, the browning and the amino acid destruction are greatly increased.[8,80] For example, the premelanoidins accelerate the lysine destruction by provoking its decarboxylation (Figure 14). They act by favoring the Strecker degradation only. A Maillard reaction would block the lysine, but would not entail its decarboxylation. It can be ascertained that successive heat treatments provoke a cumulative effect on the rate of amino acid losses. This cumulative action is more marked as the conditions are less adapted to a Maillard reaction: e.g., in the case of brief heatings or of products resistant to heat effects.

A product which is very susceptible to the Maillard reaction (milk powder) will have no aggravated lysine loss by the presence of premelanoidins (reductones or their precursors) whereas a resistant foodstuff (soybean protein) will undergo increased lysine destruction due to premelanoidins, primarily when the conditions are less adapted to a Maillard reaction. In the same way, the effect of a premelanoidin addition is more destructive as the heating duration is shorter, i.e., the installation of a Maillard reaction is less easy.[8] These facts illustrate the autocatalytic character of premelanoidin on the Maillard reaction development and the Strecker degradation.

The action of these reductones can be considerable in a technological process. If a milk sterilization makes 18% of lysine unavailable, the same treatment carried out after addition of caramelized glucose or the addition of glucose-glycine premelanoidins will increase the blocking of lysine to 42%, i.e., the addition of heated products multiples by 2½ the damage to milk during sterilization. Therefore a moderate heat treatment will be weakly prejudicial when it is applied to an unheated foodstuff. The heat treatment will cause greater damage if it is applied to a sample containing Maillard reaction products which have already undergone a heat treatment. The caramel addition of milk is a demonstrative illustration.

## PHYSIOLOGICAL PROPERTIES OF SOLUBLE PREMELANOIDINS

The Maillard reaction not only causes amino acid destruction, but forms substances which affect the food efficiency as well as the metabolism: the numerous molecules formed during the Maillard reaction can be deleterious to the nutritional and physiological properties. This problem has been neglected for a long time in favor of the phenomena causing amino acid loss. Experiments and observations have shown that among premelanoidins certain nonidentified molecules can impede nutritional utilization of the foodstuff or have toxic effects upon animals and microorganisms. Numerous experiments have displayed discrepancies between the results of the in vitro assays and the values recorded with the animal, which correspond to the real availability.

If the Maillard reaction could be reduced solely to amino acid destruction, appropriate addition of amino acids in heated products would entirely restore the resulting protein deficiency. This restoration does not take place in highly damaged foodstuffs, however, which leads us to conclude that substances reducing food efficiency may have been formed; amino acid supplementation restores the food value to that of a slightly heated product, but is not effective after a drastic Maillard reaction. For example, after casein has reacted with glucose, the PER falls from 2.6 to 0.7, but can only be raised again to 2.2 when lysine and methionine are added.[432] Supplementation of heated milk powders shows similar results.[14,69]

Other observations show a fall in nitrogen digestibility, or in the liberation in vitro of amino acids by enzymatic proteolysis. It cannot be explained by lysine blocking or destruction, and even less so with respect to other amino acids. An early study describes the problem: amino acid sensitivity to the Maillard reaction is brought out when soybean oil meal is heated at 120°C for 4 hr. The percentage of amino acids destroyed is 52% for lysine and 2% for methionine. Proteolysis on the same sample indicates that digestible lysine is reduced by 72% and methionine by 42%.[440] Poor reactivity of methionine during the Maillard reaction does not explain such low enzymatic proteolysis.

Other researches indicate a conflict between results obtained on animals and the amount of available or digestible amino acids. In cotton oil meal, biological efficiency decreases by 50% when available lysine has diminished by 30%.[41] Meats losing 15% of their lysine and 35% of their methionine show a 50% fall in the NPU.[121] A fish meal losing 53% of its FDNB lysine has a measured efficiency with the chick that is only 2% of that of the control sample.[336] The FDNB method has also been shown to differ with measurements on the rat in the case of autoclaved egg albumen: when the FDNB method shows 60% of available lysine remaining, the rat assay shows only about 20% of lysine.[61] The fraction of amino acids which is digestible in vitro is always greater than the PER value. This is especially evident in the case of peanut oil meal or fish meal. Since methionine is the primary limiting factor in these two foodstuffs, heat treatment should only slightly modify the PER because of the stability of this amino acid during heat treatment. However, when digestible methionine decreases by 4% and digestible lysine by 49%, the PER decreases to 74% of its original value.[176]

| | Loss after roasting (%): | | |
| --- | --- | --- | --- |
| | Digestible lysine | Digestible methionine | PER |
| Peanut oil meal | 49 | 4 | 74 |
| Fish meal | 12 | 5 | 33 |
| Milk powder | 74 | 23 | 85 |

Analogous phenomena are observed during the manufacture of protein cookies, supplying 2 g of lysine per kg: the PER is always less than the amino acids which are digestible in vitro, i.e., those that have not reacted with sugars. For example, the PER of the peanut cookie is reduced by 50% during cooking whereas the fall in total and digestible lysine is only 20 to 25%; the same holds true for other types of cookies (Table 2).

These metabolic perturbations also appear when the Maillard reaction consequences are applied to casein: the amino acids show a greater decrease in the blood plasma than the decrease in digestibility in the same amino acids. This difference is particularly clear for methionine, lysine, and threonine.[68,140,141]

On the whole, everything points out a disturbance in the protein efficiency of foods subjected to a Maillard reaction: the remaining proteins seem to be rendered less available.

### Metabolism of Degraded Nitrogen

There is a distinction between the metabolism of the products of interamino acids condensation and that of the Maillard reaction products.

The glutamyl lysine has a growth-promoting value that is equal to the lysine, i.e., the condensation products are available for organisms,[329,528] although the digestive enzymes cannot release lysine from this peptide linkage. This type of compound is highly resistant to attack in the lumen of the gut.[38,414] It has been advanced that the dipeptide hydrolysis takes place within the intestinal wall;[528] it can also occur by means of kidney enzymes.[282,385]

The situation is totally different for the products of the Maillard reaction. Indeed, the links that block the amino acids have no peptide nature. The metabolic differences between the lysine that is heat damaged without a Maillard reaction intervention and the lysine that is blocked by this reaction appear in the comparison below. The data results from subjecting egg albumen to heat treatment, either in the absence of sugar traces, or after addition of glucose. In the first case, the lysine is condensed with aspartic or glutamic acids; in the second case, it has been blocked by the glucose.[519]

|  | Metabolism of radioactive lysine in heated egg albumen | |
|---|---|---|
| Percent of lysine recovered in: | Heating without glucose (condensation) | Heating with glucose (Maillard reaction) |
| Feces | 32.2 | 73.6 |
| $CO_2$ | 10.6 | 3.2 |
| Urine | 0.8 | 2.8 |
| Retained (by difference) | 56.4 | 20.4 |

By working with pure premelanoidins, it appears that a large percentage of their degraded nitrogen is able to pass through the intestinal wall. A fraction of absorbed nitrogen is eliminated by the urinary system and a fraction is retained by the animal, though it cannot be used for metabolism. If animals receive a nitrogen-free diet, the degraded nitrogen of glycine-glucose premelanoidins has a true digestibility of 71.4% and a true retention of 48.3%.[19] In the same way, a large percentage of the unavailable lysine can go through the intestinal wall, even at the small intestine.[72] This high digestibility has to be connected with that of caramelized sugar, which also has a digestibility of between 70 and 85%.[191]

The degraded nitrogen of premelanoidins remains unavailable, even if it is retained. Its presence is detrimental to the organism because the presence of premelanoidins in a nitrogen-free diet aggravates the weight loss of the animal: −1.36 g/day weight loss against a −1.13 g/day weight loss in the control diet.[19] This situation is substantially confirmed by studies of the metabolism of the Amadori rearrangement products, which reveal inefficient use in most cases[69] but no evidence of toxic properties. This is the case with fructose tryptophan,[506] fructose leucine,[461] fructose lysine,[329] or fructose methionine.[223] These compounds are generally absorbable, probably by means of a passive diffusion, in the cecum or in the large intestine.

The digestive flora favor the digestibility of substance. Indeed, the administration of antibiotics, or the cecumectomy, reduces the absorption rate of the 1-amino-1-deoxy-2-ketoses,[371,461,506] or increases their toxicity.[14] The absorbable fraction is unavailable for the animal: less than 1.5% is incorporated in the liver[461] and approxi-

Table 11
METABOLISM OF PROTEIN-BOUND LYSINE IN
CONTROL AND HEATED PROTEINS[55,172,429]

| | Control protein | Heated protein |
|---|---|---|
| General metabolism | | |
| FDNB lysine (% of total) | 85 | 13 |
| % of recovered lysine in | | |
| Fecal elimination | 14 | 66 |
| Urinary elimination | 1 | 14 |
| Urinary elimination (mg/day) | | |
| Free lysine | 4.5 | 15.3 |
| Peptide lysine | 3.0 | 20.3 |
| Portal vein plasma ($\mu$mol/10 m$\ell$) | | |
| Total lysine | 9.0 | 9.9 |
| Free lysine | 3.7 | 2.8 |
| Bound lysine | 5.3 | 7.1 |
| Peptide lysine | 4.9 | 4.6 |
| Blocked lysine | 0.5 | 2.6 |

mately 1% is recovered in the expired air.[506] The urine contains an appreciable percentage of 1-amino-1-deoxy-2-ketoses.

However, these substances are not completely devoid of biological efficiency, even if the organism cannot use the amino acid molecule contained in these components. Enzymatic systems, other than those of digestive tract, can realize the hydrolysis of Amadori rearrangement products: *Leuconostoc mesenteroides* use the 1-methionine-1-deoxy-2-fructose as source of methionine with an efficiency of 80% compared with methionine.[223] Likewise, the amino group of fructose glycine can constitute a source of basic nitrogen for the rat.[195] Perhaps, the blocking of an amino acid by the Maillard reaction is prejudicial only when it is an essential nutrient, which will only be subjected to the enzymatic systems of the digestive tract.

Table 11 supplies additional information, relative to the metabolism of the blocked lysine. A great part is present in an unabsorbable form; it signifies that the soluble polymers that are formed after the Amadori rearrangement reach too large a size to be able to pass through the intestinal membrane.

The analysis of portal vein plasma is interesting because it cautions against erroneous interpretations: the recovery rate of total lysine is not inferior in animals that receive the blocked lysine, which can entail false conclusions. The lysine repartition in the plasma is different in the two lots (Table 11): in the control lot, a higher percentage of the free and peptide forms are recovered, whereas the ingestion of blocked lysine is responsible for an appreciable percentage of blocked lysine in the plasma. In this case, a part of the plasma lysine is unavailable for the organism. Only the determination of the available lysine form of the plasma has a biological signification. These facts illustrate the absorbability of unavailable forms of amino acids.

They are eliminated by the urinary system: after ingestion of blocked lysine, the urine contains three times more free lysine and seven times more bound lysine when the animal receives the blocked forms of lysine. The kidney passes molecules containing amino acids in combined form.[55,172,429] It is possible that the kidney hydrolyzes some peptides, which would lead to an increase of free amino acids in the urine.

So, the degraded nitrogen of premelanoidins is absorbable and partially retained and provokes an increase of nitrogen disposal through the urinary system. Such an evolution interferes with the protein-N metabolism and causes interpretation errors when the digestibility and the retention of nitrogen diet are established.

The energy utilization of the sugar fraction of the Maillard reaction products is not determined at the present time. It is probably low. Indeed, in industrial molasses, a fraction of nonsugar reducing substances, attributable to the Maillard reaction, is unfermentable and reduces the alcohol production.[460]

### Manifestations of Heated Nitrogenous Products

Various observations support several conclusions about the toxicity of products formed in the course of the Maillard reaction.

#### $LD_{50}$ of Heated Products

The determination of the intraperitoneal toxicity to the mouse of mixtures composed of 1 part of amino acid and 3 parts of glucose, indicates that a heating for 10 min at 160°C increases the toxicity from a value greater than 20 g/kg of living weight to values ranging from 4 to 11 g. The lysine and tryptophan premelanoidins develop the strongest toxicity, the lysine glucose heated mixture having an $LD_{50}$ of 4.15 g/kg, and tryptophan-glucose of 6.1 g/kg.[268] This observation has worrying consequences in reason of the particular sensitivity of lysine and tryptophan throughout the course of the Maillard reaction: these amino acids have the strongest probability of destruction, and generating premelanoidins that will be the most toxic.

Likewise, ribonucleic acids see their toxicity rise after a heating, with or without an addition of glucose. The $LD_{50}$ increase after heat treatment of ribonucleic acid alone demonstrates that the contained ribose is sufficient to create a reaction with the amino acids, a reaction that is obviously favored by a glucose addition.[274]

In a more direct way, the toxicity of Maillard reaction products has been revealed by injecting into the mouse diverse forms of reductones having N-substitutions: according to the exact nature of the reductone, the $LD_{50}$ rises from 1200 to 300 mg/kg. An oral administration in the rat produces the typical symptoms of superexcitability, elevation and nodding of the head, and whirling.[27]

The furfural, another Maillard reaction product, has been linked to diverse pathological and toxic states.[438] It is also possible to connect the toxic character of the premelanoidins to their depressive action on the ponderal evolution of animals.[19]

#### Anatomical and Histological Modifications

The ingestion of heated foodstuffs which have undergone a Maillard reaction involves modifications concerning particularly the liver and the cecum. The direct responsibility of the premelanoidins in these phenomena has been established.

In a ration containing Maillard reaction products, a liver disorder, a type of necrosis without hypertrophy, has been described by different workers. Animals receiving dried skim milk powder show a hepatic necrosis proportional in intensity to the severity of the heat treatment. The two factors are so strongly linked that the necrosis can be used as a sensitive test for determining the heat treatment of milk.[162-164] However, in this case, the Maillard reaction is not the only responsible factor for the necrosis; it is caused, at least partially, by an unavailability of the selenium contained in the milk.

With other foodstuffs, the premelanoidin responsibility is more obvious. A study was made on the repercussions of drying meat with glycosylamines. The results show the responsibility of the Maillard reaction products because the phenomena occur only if glycosylamines are added to the meat before drying.[154-156] The liver is slightly hypertrophied. Mainly it offers two kinds of lesions: (1) early necrotic lesions with hemorrhagic symptoms and corresponding to acute intoxication; and (2) later cirrhotic-like lesions which correspond to subacute intoxication.

In another way, the Maillard reaction products tend to create a cecal hypertrophy, which has important repercussions for the animal. This hypertrophy is a basic phenomenon, that appears every time the diet contains substances undegraded by intestinal

Table 12
PHYSIOLOGICAL PROPERTIES OF GLYCINE-
GLUCOSE PREMELANOIDINS AS A FUNCTION
OF THE RAT STRAINS[14]

| | Difference with the control diet (%) | | |
| --- | --- | --- | --- |
| | Wistar | Sherman | Sprague-Dawley |
| Growth | −34 | −14 | −8 |
| PER | −21 | −12 | −8 |
| In % of living weight | | | |
| Cecum with contents | + 146 | + 108 | + 70 |
| Empty cecum | + 57 | + 32 | + 15 |
| Kidney | + 51 | + 22 | −3 |
| Liver | + 6 | −1 | 0 |

enzymes, but hydrolyzable by the enzymatic systems of the cecal flora: this occurs after ingestion of lactose, uncooked potato starch, xylose, etc.

In the particular case of premelanoidin, the cecal hypertrophy is responsible for a certain degree of degradation of these substances, a transformation which favors their absorption and reduces their toxicity.[14,519] Moreover, the intensity of the degradation in the cecum determines: (1) the repercussions that the premelanoidins will have on the nutrition efficiency of the diet (growth, PER, etc.); and (2) the absorption rate of the molecules which are unmetabolizable and which will create a kidney hypertrophy. So, indirectly, the cecum development is responsible for the kidney hypertrophy.

On the whole, the degree of cecal hypertrophy of the rat constitutes a sensitive indicator of the repercussions that will be generated by the premelanoidins: the Wistar strain appears to be very sensitive to these heat products because it is able to attack them intensely, which facilitates their absorption. On the contrary, the Sprague-Dawley strain is only weakly sensitive because the premelanoidins seem little degraded in the cecum and, in consequence, pass less easily through the intestinal membrane (Table 12).

*Allergy Phenomena*

The Maillard reaction can have a certain responsibility in allergy phenomena; the allergy to the milk proteins illustrates it. The $\beta$-lactoglobulin in the native state has a weak allergic character which develops quickly at the beginning of a Maillard reaction. The allergen has a maximum reactivity when about 25% of the lysine is blocked by lactose and when the fluorescence is multiplied by seven, i.e., when the Maillard reaction has reached the Amadori rearrangement stage.[58] If the heat treatment continues, the reactivity tends to decrease again. That is why, in the case of allergy to $\beta$-lactoglobulin, the first preventive measure consists in eliminating the pasteurized milk — whose heating corresponds to the beginning of a Maillard reaction. It is necessary to replace it by milks which have not undergone heating or more intense treatment (e.g., evaporated milk).

For the moment, the Maillard reaction seems to be implicated only in the case of allergy due to the $\beta$-lactoglobulin; it is not possible to say precisely if this situation is exceptional or represents an illustration of a general rule.

## Effects of Premelanoidins on Metabolism

The Maillard reaction products are endowed with antienzymatic properties that particularly concern the hydrolysis of carbohydrates and proteins; there is also a strong presumption that the premelanoidins disturb the calcium metabolism. Though in this

## Table 13
## EFFECT OF PREMELANOIDINS ON IN VITRO PROTEOLYSIS WITH PEPSIN, TRYPSIN, AND EREPSIN[19]

| Recovered lysine in digestate (%) | Modalities of the proteolysis | | |
| --- | --- | --- | --- |
| | Protein | Protein with premelanoidins | Difference (%) |
| Total digestate | 90 | 92 | +2 |
| Free amino acid | 74 | 63 | −15 |
| Soluble peptides | 16 | 29 | +81 |

field the observations are still incomplete, they confirm that the elaborated products during the heat treatments can reduce the efficiency of nutrients that remain undamaged after a heating.

The premelanoidins seem responsible for decreased malt activity.[550] An alcohol-soluble fraction of premelanoidins, in the same way, reduces the action of the salivary amylase on the starch.[117] The result is that the starchy foods are less easily hydrolyzed when they have undergone a roasting.

The situation is more complex and perhaps less immediately perceptible in the protein field. At first, the Maillard reaction compounds present an enzyme-resistant character, and the decrease in enzymatic proteolysis has been attributed to this fact.[57,108,148,195,223,233,333,440,470,480] In another way, the proteins still intact are less adapted to the proteolysis when they are in presence of premelanoidins. In vitro, the premelanoidin presence modifies the nature of hydrolyzed products: the rate of free amino acids is decreased but the quantity of soluble peptides is greatly increased.[19,171] It is possible that the molecules incompletely hydrolyzed correspond to peptides and also to blocked forms of amino acids, absorbable by the animal but not metabolizable and eliminated by the urinary system.

In the soluble digestate, since the rate of amino acids remains unchanged, the determination of nitrogen or solubilized amino acids can be misleading (Table 13). To measure the precise effect of the premelanoidins, it is necessary to determine the amount of free amino acid in the digestate. This particularly occurs in the case of methionine. It would explain some observations done with the animal, which show an important decrease in the methionine efficiency in the heated foodstuffs although this amino acid exhibits little tendency towards blocking during the Maillard reaction.

In vivo, the premelanoidin activity impedes the protein efficiency when animals receive 3.8 g of degraded nitrogen per kg of diet: the digestibility, like the biological value, of the casein is significantly affected in these conditions (Table 14). Thus, in presence of premelanoidins, the retention of nitrogen by the animal is decreased in significant proportions, reaching 43% in the case of the experiment mentioned in Table 14. Such a situation can lead to a status of nitrogen deficiency, which has appeared with the gestant rat.

When these animals receive a well-balanced diet, with 16% of casein, the premelanoidins (3.8 g of degraded nitrogen per kg of diet) decrease the female fertility by 26%, double the number of stillborn young and multiply by five the intrauterine resorptions. Finally, even though the experimental litters are less numerous, the weight and the growth of the young remain inferior to that of control diet.[25] These diverse manifestations illustrate a nutritional status deficient in protein in spite of a diet covering — in theory — the requirements. They clearly illustrate the antinutritional, or perhaps toxic, properties of the Maillard reaction products.

## Table 14
### NITROGEN BALANCE OF CASEIN IN THE PRESENCE OF PREMELANOIDINS[19]

|  | Casein diet | Casein + premelanoidins diet | Difference (%) |
|---|---|---|---|
| Daily growth of rat (g) | 1.85 | 0.95 | −49 |
| Metabolism of casein |  |  |  |
| Ingested (mg N/day) | 210.6 | 171.0 | −19 |
| Retained (mg N/day) | 93.0 | 52.95 | −43 |
| Digestibility | 90.8 | 82.3 | −10 |
| Biological value | 48.6 | 37.6 | −23 |

The same glycine-glucose premelanoidins modify the calcium metabolism and probably have an influence on the development of the osseous tissue. When these premelanoidins are introduced in a diet rich in calcium (0.9%), hypercalcification troubles are strongly attenuated. This fact is not attributable to the natural acidity of the premelanoidins because it also occurs in the premelanoidins neutralized with soda.[15]

|  | Number of rats | Percent of rats presenting calculi in | | | Calcium in kidney (mg per two kidneys) |
|---|---|---|---|---|---|
|  |  | Bladder | Ureter | Kidney |  |
| Control diet | 12 | 59 | 25 | 8 | 0.62 |
| Premelanoidins | 23 | 48 | 8 | 0 | 0.32 |
| Neutralized premelanoidins | 23 | 26 | 0 | 0 | 0.32 |

This phenomenon is the probable consequence of a partial insolubilization of the calcium by the premelanoidins and of a lesser intestinal absorption of this component.

The Maillard reaction also contributes to reduce the efficiency of the diet calcium: its intestinal absorption is facilitated by the presence of amino acids and, especially, of lysine.[532] By blocking and selectively destroying this amino acid, the Maillard reaction suppresses one of the factors favoring calcium efficiency. For these diverse reasons, heated foodstuffs are known to provoke problems with calcium metabolism and calcification of the osseous tissue[71,264] and the teeth.[299] In the latter case, the tooth decay (caries) is proportional to the intensity of heat treatment. Foodstuffs rich in calcium, like the milk powders, can thus become cariogenic after a drastic heating.[46,300] This result certainly comes from a modification of the physical status of the calcium, but also from the action of the Maillard reaction that develops during the treatment.

### Effects of Premelanoidins on Animals

The soluble premelanoidins have the physiological properties that have just been described. It is certain that this field is far from entirely known today and that new manifestations will be discovered in the near future.

The described properties are more attributable to Maillard reaction products than to sugar caramelization products, i.e., they are the consequence of the amino acids present in the medium. As an example, by treating in the same conditions a glucose solution and a glucose-glycine solution, the PER decrease is, respectively, 3% and 18%.[23]

The effect of the premelanoidins on the nutritional efficiency depend on three main factors: (1) the stage of the Maillard reaction to which the premelanoidins correspond; (2) the nature of the initial constituents of the Maillard reaction; and (3) the quantity of premelanoidins introduced in the diet.

*Activity as a Function of the Maillard Reaction Stage*

The first colored compounds are more active physiologically than those that are formed at a later stage: the insoluble melanoidins are practically inert physiologically.[23,24,339] When a Maillard reaction produces insoluble melanoidins after 10 hr of heating, the effects of the premelanoidins are the following:

|  | Differences with the control diet (%): | | | |
|---|---|---|---|---|
|  | First assay | | Second assay | |
| Duration of heating (hr) | Growth | PER | Growth | PER |
| 1 | − 27 | − 26.5 | − 42 | − 24 |
| 4 | − 24 | − 22.5 | — | — |
| 6 | − 15.5 | − 11.5 | — | — |
| 9 | — | — | − 22 | − 13 |
| 15 | — | — | + 2 | + 1 |

It is impossible at the present time to precisely state the activity of earliest uncolored Maillard reaction products, such as the Amadori rearrangement products, in comparison with the colored molecules that represent the result of a first operation of polymerization.

*Activity as a Function of the Premelanoidin Nature*

In most experiments, the used premelanoidins are formed from a mixture of glycine and glucose, in equimolar ratio. This type of premelanoidin is far from being the most active physiologically. The premelanoidin activity depends on the sugar nature and on the amino acid nature. Their part corresponds precisely to their reactivity in the Maillard reaction (see Sugars and Amino Acids and Proteins). In short, the most reactive molecules are those that supply the most physiologically active premelanoidins. Isomolecular mixtures of glycine and various sugars, heated in identical conditions, will form premelanoidins of different intensity: if the physiological activity of disaccharide premelanoidin is 1, then that of hexose premelanoidin is 1.75 and that of pentose premelanoidins is 3.25.[14] Moreover, premelanoidins from isomer sugars have variable properties: when the sorbose-glycine premelanoidins cause a PER decrease of 13%, the decrease is 27% with xylose-glycine, and 39% with arabinose-glycine premelanoidins.

In the same way, the amino acid nature conditions the premelanoidin properties. It must be emphasized that the lysine premelanoidins are three times more reactive than the glycine premelanoidins. This observation must be connected with the $LD_{50}$ of lysine premelanoidins (see Allergy Phenomena) and with lysine selectivity during the Maillard reaction: the probability of obtaining premelanoidins from lysine after the heat treatment of a foodstuff is very high.

If sugars and amino acids which are each particularly reactive are associated, their effects become cumulative and the premelanoidins obtained can become extremely detrimental. The following example illustrates the effect of the premelanoidin initial constituents on the physiology of the rat.[14]

| | Difference with the control diet (%) | |
|---|---|---|
| Nature of premelanoidin constituents | Growth | PER |
| Glucose-glycine | − 7 | − 9 |
| Glucose-lysine | − 21 | − 12 |
| Xylose-glycine | − 21 | − 19 |
| Xylose-lysine | − 65 | − 39 |

*Activity as a Function of Utilized Doses*

At slight doses (8.5 to 50 mg degraded nitrogen per kg of diet), premelanoidins have basically favorable effects that stimulate consumption, thanks to their flavor. In the most favorable cases, intake increases by 40%, causing an average weight augmentation of 25%. This influence is quite transient, for after 6 weeks of experiment, the ingestion tends to become comparable to that of the control ration. Premelanoidins act differently at high doses (1.5 to 3.8 g of degraded nitrogen per kg of diet): they reduce the PER in proportions ranging from 20% to 40%, about the glucose-glycine premelanoidins, without significantly modifying intake, which only tends to decrease in some experiments.

The PER fall varies in time, reaching a maximum about the 4th week of the experiment, then tends to lessen. It has a more lasting effect on appetite, however, than minimal doses. After 6 weeks the PER of glucose-glycine premelanoidin diet is 30% lower than that of the control diet. This retards animal growth in high proportions.[23]

## Effect of Premelanoidins on Microorganisms

The development of microorganisms has been shown to be sensitive to premelanoidin action. Results obtained by various observations confirm that premelanoidins affect cellular metabolism, comparable to toxicity phenomena in animals. According to dispersed observations, the sterilization of media culture is sufficient to generate substances that sometimes favor the microbial growth[220,444] and sometimes inhibit it.[305,523]

More specific studies have been undertaken with pure glucose-glycine premelanoidins. Their action depends highly on both the dose used and on the heating stage to which they correspond. The factors conditioning their activity seem to be more numerous than those which produce effects on animals: according to heating time, a mixture of glucose-glycine activates or inhibits the growth and metabolism of a strain.

Generally speaking, the early Maillard reaction products are favorable, whereas premelanoidins obtained later have inhibiting effects. In yeast, inhibition significantly decreases the assimilation of the various nitrogen compounds, as well as both carbon dioxide and biomass production.[234,408,444,478,479] The first Maillard reaction products equally increase aspergilli growth, while simultaneously lessening citric acid production. Late premelanoidins inhibit the growth.[237]

In yeast and aspergilli, these substances partly owe their effects to their function as pyruvic acid decarboxylase activators.[238,239] Premelanoidin action must be comparable if not identical in myceliums, for they have a synergy with thiamin.[234] Lactobacilli behave differently from other microorganisms and are less sensitive to these compounds: only the late Maillard reaction products reduce the growth.

In addition to their effects on the kinetics of cellular development, premelanoidins can modify cellular structure. In myceliums, they increase the proportion of vesiculous cells as well as the number of nuclei in cells.[234] As a consequence, soluble Maillard reaction products show physiological activity, both in animals and microorganisms. A certain relationship exists between the action conditions of premelanoidins in diverse organism categories. Thus, the xylose-lysine premelanoidins, which have been shown to be highly prejudicial to the rat, are also those which strongly inhibit bacteria, yeast, and mold growth.[271]

## FOODSTUFF BEHAVIOR

A Maillard reaction development can be seen during heat treatment as well as during conservation at room temperature, or in tropical conditions. The fact has been observed many times with milk powders,[60,137,144,202-204,367,463] egg powders,[181,248,399,499,505] and with diverse foodstuffs.[49,381] This proves that the amino acid destruction under the influence of the Maillard reaction depends on the received heat quantity and not on the heat application conditions.

Two essential rules condition the foodstuff behavior during a technological treatment or during a storage. In technology, the medium wherein the heat is applied is a primary influence on the likelihood of occurrence of the Maillard reaction. Generally, all heat treatments in wet media (autoclaving, parboiling, water boiling) show only a weak probability of generating a Maillard reaction. On the contrary, the drier the atmosphere where the treatment takes place (roasting, toasting), the higher is the reaction risk. These two types of operation are separated by the moisture rate and by the heat intensity. The former are carried out at moderate temperatures (about 100 to 120°C), whereas the latter occur in more drastic conditions (about 130 to 250°C according to the process).

There are no proteins and foodstuffs fundamentally resistant to the Maillard reaction: if the physicochemical context is adapted to this reaction, any protein matter will be affected. That is to say that the Maillard reaction depends mainly on the type and the quantity of reducing sugars and carbohydrates, various physicochemical factors, etc. That is why, in the natural context, some foodstuffs are highly sensitive and others resistant, although the behavior of all the proteins is nearly the same when the medium favors the Maillard reaction. A hierarchy of various foodstuffs arises from Figure 15, based on the lysine evolution of some products in the course of a roasting at 150°C: the milk powder is exceptionally sensitive because of its high percentage of lactose and also the strong reactivity of whey proteins: inversely, the yeast is remarkably resistant by reason of a low percentage of reducing sugars and a buffered natural acidity.

### Milk Products

Milk constitutes a favorable biochemical medium for the Maillard reaction because of its high amount of lactose and of the presence of whey proteins among the most reactive. Because of this, the milk powders, and even more, the whey powders and all the byproducts containing both lactose and whey proteins offer an extreme sensitivity to the Maillard reaction. The milk products constitute the best substrate for reaction studies, since all the manifestations and consequences of the Maillard reaction appear with great intensity after heat treatment or storage in bad conditions.[11,203] The same phenomena could also appear in other foodstuffs, but only after a drastic heating. It is rare to obtain the manifestations of the Maillard reaction so clearly with products other than the milk products. The only factors that can reduce the intensity of this reaction are dilution in the case of liquid milk, the acidity of some derivatives, the strong dehydration of the powders, or the fractionation of diverse components: delactozation, deproteinization, etc.

### Manifestations of the Maillard Reaction

Table 15 gives a comprehensive view of milk powder evolution during a Maillard reaction. Its physical manifestations in the milk product are

1.  A fluorescence, whose origin is very complex in the case of milk products, but whose part, at least, is attributable to the early stages of a lactose amino acid reaction.[240,510]
2.  A browning, whose intensity depends on the severity of the heat treatment, or the storage conditions of milk products.[74,393,509] Obviously, this browning is partially the consequence of a lactose caramelization and partially the manifestation of a reaction between sugar and milk proteins.[251,393,427]

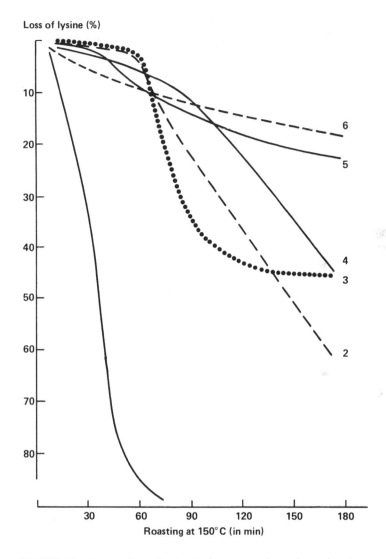

FIGURE 15. Destruction of lysine during an experimental roasting. 1 = milk powder; 2 = peanut oil meal; 3 = cotton oil meal; 4 = wheat flour; 5 = fish meal; 6 = dried yeast (Torula). (From Adrian, J. and Frangne, R., *Ind. Aliment Agric.*, 87, 393, 1970. With permission.)

3.   An acidification, also the mark of a lactose degradation, linked to the development of a Maillard reaction.[190,392,393,467]
4.   A reducing power, also derived primarily from the lactose thermolysis, but also from the Maillard reaction.[395,509] Among the substances formed, 5 HMF is an early sign of deleterious changes in the milk powders.[410]
5.   A decrease in solubility, linked to the intensity of the Maillard reaction. It is particularly proportional to the available lysine diminution.[143]

When the casein or the milk proteins are subjected to a Maillard reaction, the amino acid balance is deeply transformed: the characteristic fact is a quick and selective decrease of the lysine, which is blocked and destroyed; the last fraction generating the furosine and pyridosine. The other essential amino acids, methionine included, are practically stable during the heatings. Among the nonessential amino acids, the basic

## Table 15
## EVOLUTION OF A SPRAY SKIM MILK POWDER AFTER STORAGE IN NITROGEN FOR 60 DAYS AT 37°C, WITH 7.3% OF MOISTURE[202]

|  | Fresh powder | Stored powder |
|---|---|---|
| Color (Lovibond yellow and red units) | 0.5 | 2.2 |
| pH of reconstituted milk | 6.73 | 6.50 |
| Reducing power (ferricyanide value) | 0.9 | 16.0 |
| Solubility at 20°C, (%) | 99.0 | 70.0 |
| Free amino-N content (% initial value) | 100 | 36 |
| Reducing sugar combined with protein (mg lactose/g protein) | 6.0 | 49.0 |
| $CO_2$ produced (mg/100 g powder) | — | 5.8 |
| True nitrogen digestibility | 91.2 | 86.0 |
| Biological value | 84.5 | 67.5 |
| Biological value with added lysine | 76.4 | 80.1 |
| Flavor of reconstituted milk | Palatable | Nauseating, caramelized, gluey |

Reprinted by permission from Henry, K. M., Kon, S. K., Lea, C. H., Smith, J. A. B., and White, J. C. D., *Nature*, 158, 348. Copyright© 1946 MacMillan Journals Ltd.

## Table 16
## EVOLUTION OF LYSINE AND PROTEIN EFFICIENCY IN AN OVERHEATED MILK POWDER

| Percent of protein | Control milk powder | Overheated powder | Percent of control |
|---|---|---|---|
| Lysine | 8.9 | 5.8 | 65 |
| Available lysine | 6.6 | 2.2 | 33 |
| Furosine | 0.5 | 5.3 | 1060 |
| Other essential amino acids |  |  | ≥94 |
| Cystine | 1.0 | 0.8 | 80 |
| PER |  |  |  |
| Milk powder | 100 | 17 |  |
| Milk powder + 0.28% of lysine |  | 89 |  |

From Ebersdobler, H. and Dümmer, H., *Z. Tierphysiol. Tierernaehr. Futtermittelkd.*, 28, 224, 1971. With permission.

molecules are strongly damaged; a cystine destruction is sometimes observed.[68,128,139,176,431,432,450] Table 16 emphasizes the specific character of the lysine disappearance during a heating of milk powder.

This phenomenon has important nutritional repercussions, which do not necessarily appear in experiments upon animals. The milk proteins, especially the whey proteins, are characterized by a lysine excess in comparison with amino acid requirements.[9] At the beginning of a Maillard reaction (Figure 16, segments A and B), the lysine loss will not be apparent if milk constitutes the only protein source in the diet: the PER remains unchanged because it is always limited by the methionine deficiency whose value remains stable.[68,265] Under these conditions, only a decrease in nitrogen digestibility indicates that the milk has undergone a detrimental heat treatment.[68,108,201,309,468,472,481] The effects of the Maillard reaction appear clearly if the milk

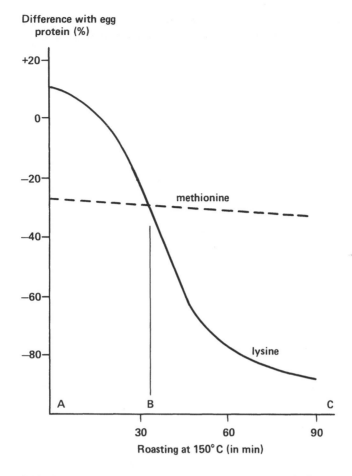

FIGURE 16. Amino acid balance of skim milk powder during an experimental roasting. (From Adrian, J., *Ann. Nutr. Aliment*, 21, 129, 1967. With permission.)

is used in a small amount for supplementation of a cereal diet, deficient in lysine.

If the heating is more drastic, the lysine destruction reaches such an extent that this amino acid becomes the primary limiting factor of milk proteins, replacing methionine in this role (Figure 16, segments B and C). This permutation of the limiting factor is easily obtained in the case of dairy products after experimental heatings for 20 to 30 min at 140 or 150°C,[6,192,330] or after autoclaving a milk concentrate for 15 min at 120°C,[265] or with a scorched roller dried powder,[330,521] or with a casein heated at 85°C with 15% of moisture[432] or, simply, with a milk powder kept in no severe conditions of stability.[202]

From the B point (Figure 16), the protein value quickly falls, paralleling the destruction of the primary limiting factor (lysine). The milk quickly loses its nutritional essence. In the extreme cases, the methionine does not appear even as secondary limiting factor[432] thus emphasizing its good stability in the course of the Maillard reaction when applied to a dairy product. In some cases, the detrimental effect of heating cannot be inhibited by a lysine addition.[116]

*Occurrences in Industrial Processes*

Milk constitutes a biochemical complex sensitive enough to the Maillard reaction that the usual handling and treatment provokes a lysine deterioration. This is observed both during the stabilization operation (heating or drying) and during the storage. The remarkable stability of some forms of dairy products (sterilized and condensed milks, milk powders, etc.) make the storage possibilities very important; it follows that the risk of a Maillard reaction is greater during the storage than during the stabilization process.

### Stabilization by Heating

Apart from the HTST and the UHT processes, which do not have practical biochemical effects,[10] all operations responsible for the beginning of a Maillard reaction translate the blocking and destruction of a small fraction of lysine. The destruction is variable with the treatment and has the following approximate values:[70,120,124,328,331,398,492]

| Commercial form of milk | Lysine deterioration (%): | |
|---|---|---|
| | Total lysine | Available lysine |
| Pasteurized | 3—5 | 2—4 |
| Sterilized (120°C) | 7—11 | 11—16 |
| Evaporated | 5—12 | 28—43 |
| Sweetened condensed | 19 | 3—42 |

The sterilized or evaporated milks have undergone a Maillard reaction of sufficient intensity that their protein efficiency is slightly decreased, when it is measured on the animal.[109,193]

### Stabilization by Drying

A severe preheating for 30 min at 74°C before a spray drying is responsible for a decrease in nitrogen utilization by the very young calf.[481] However, it has not been proved that the effects observed derive exclusively from the Maillard reaction which develops during the preheating. It is recognized that the spray drying per se does not develop a sufficient temperature to block the milk lysine. Conversely, roller drying is a brutal operation and generally prejudicial when it is applied to the milk, which involves a blocking and a destruction of its lysine.[60,144,221,302,412,516,521] In reality, the intensity of the Maillard reaction developed in the course of roller drying is variable and depends on the industrial conditions.[139,221,332,521] A heating excess provokes a considerable aggravation of the Maillard reaction effects. The example, below, illustrates the autocatalytic character of this reaction.[139]

| Roller-drying conditions | | Lysine (percent in proteins) | |
|---|---|---|---|
| Temperature of roller (°C) | Duration of contact (sec) | Total | Available |
| 116 | 4 | 8.9 | 6.6 |
| 120 | 7.5 | 5.8 | 2.2 |

### Storage

In liquid milks, the risk of a Maillard reaction remains low because of the dilution. Sterilized milk kept for 6 months at 38°C nevertheless shows a nitrogen digestibility and a biological value slightly less than the fresh product.[228] In evaporated milk, which has already undergone a heating and a concentration, the Maillard reaction occurs more easily and after 8 years of storage, two thirds of its lysine is blocked.[516]

In milk powders, the probability of a lactose-protein reaction is far greater.[60,202,204,231,260] Table 15 gives an example. The Maillard reaction intensity is narrowly linked to the milk powder moisture: below 3%, the powder is practically inert, from a chemical point of view; between 7 and 15% of moisture, the reaction reaches its maximum intensity.[127,137,143,144,203,260,367] One must add that the hygroscopic character of lactose is responsible for the propensity of the milk powder — and with greater intensity, the whey powder — to rehydrate from atmospheric moisture. This property raises the problem of milk powder packing.

The moisture rate at which the Maillard reaction becomes important is that point where the lactose, normally in an amorphous state, becomes crystalized: after 53 months of storage at 20°C, the loss of available lysine remains less than 5% if the lactose is still amorphous; it rises to between 30 and 45% in the powders where moisture has allowed a crystalization of the lactose.[231,232]

## Fish Products

Fish and its derivatives constitute a particular case in the field of the Maillard reaction. *A priori,* conditions are not favorable to this reaction and fish should be classified among the resistant foodstuffs. In fact, the biochemical and technological conditions present an unfavorable environment to the amino acids: (1) fish contains lipids rich in polyenoic acids, very unstable substances that rapidly form peroxides and create oxidative reactions which result in aldehydes and ketones; and (2) the post-mortem phenomena increase the pH by producing volatile bases while simultaneously they provoke the beginning of a hydrolysis that releases hexoses and pentoses, creating oligopeptides or even free amino acids. These molecules are all available to initiate a Maillard reaction. The muscles of chill-stored codling contain from 0 to 3 mg % of free pentoses and from 0 to 33 mg % of free hexoses according to the conditions of storage[246] and, more generally, the flesh of fish of various species contains from 16 to 64 mg % of free reducing sugars.[355] In fraction acid-soluble, the amount of sugars is really higher, ranging from 12 to 92 mg % for the pentoses and from 46 to 556 mg % for the hexoses according to the species.[363] Among these free sugars, there is ribose, derived from nucleic acid degradation, especially during the spawning season, whose reactivity with the amino acids has been emphasized and to which is attributed a part in browning and Maillard reaction phenomena.[53,183,246,366,511,515]

It is reasonable to suppose that the presence of reducing sugars and that of the oxidation products of lipids can be, jointly or not, responsible for some of the manifestations observed in fish and its derivatives, such as fluorescence, browning, and losses of amino acids, etc., phenomena usually attributed to the Maillard reaction but whose origin is perhaps more complex in the fish case.

This Maillard reaction is made possible by means of oligopeptides and free amino acids. In the herring, the free molecules are at a rate of about 600 mg % of nobbed fish.[227]

When the fish muscle becomes spoiled or during a heating, a fluorescence and a browning can be observed. These physicochemical phenomena are the consequences of a reaction between the sugars and the amino acids, favored by an elevation of pH. In this reaction, the hexoses play a predominant part.[246,363,364] At the same time, the rate of reducing sugars greatly decreases during the browning and constitutes the limiting factor of its intensity; while addition of hexoses or pentoses increases the browning.[91,183,366,378,387,515]

On the other hand, the fluorescent compounds which are formed seem to be identical to those of sugar — amino acid systems.[364,365] The fluorescence — which is one of the earliest stages of the Maillard reaction — constitutes a symptom of fish deterioration, and can be used as a sensitive indicator to determine the freshness of this food product.[379] Even when the Maillard reaction responsibility is so well-established, it is impossible to underestimate the contribution of the fish lipids in the browning development,[355,514] because their intervention can occur in association with or independently of the Maillard reaction.

Two facts seem to coexist concerning the amino acid evolution. The destruction of lysine and some other amino acids can legitimately be attributed to the development of a Maillard reaction. The losses go through a zone of maximum intensity that corresponds to a moisture level between about 5 and 15%.[91] The lysine loss is limited by the quantity of reducing sugars and any sugar addition increases its destruction,[336,337,363] which confirms the sensitivity of the fish proteins to this reaction:

| | Loss of lysine in heated fish meal (%) | |
| --- | --- | --- |
| | Heating without glucose | Heating with glucose |
| Total lysine | 28 | 66 |
| Available lysine | 27 | 64 |

The blocking and destruction of lysine in the course of the fish meal treatment entails a diminution of the nutritional value of this foodstuff, especially noticeable in growing animals or when the fish meal is introduced into the diet for cereal supplementation. This is why fish meal quality is frequently estimated according to the percent of available lysine[167,258,377,489] or according to its pepsin digestibility.[354,377]

Nevertheless, in the fish meals, lysine destruction does not offer the specificity that is usual in the Maillard reaction. The heatings are often accompanied by an important fall of the sulfur-containing amino acids, methionine and cystine,[62,336,337,347,348] and the restoration of these products can be obtained by a supplement of methionine.[6,488] In fact, in the course of fish meal treatment, two mechanisms are superimposed and, probably, show mutual interference: (1) the fish meal, heated only, undergoes a selective loss of cystine (Table 17); and (2) if a Maillard reaction is also developed, it provokes an appreciable destruction of lysine and methionine, without modifying the cystine loss. This latter is probably foreign to the Maillard reaction (see Reactions Among Pure Amino Acids), but can the sulfur-containing amino acids be destroyed, directly or not, by the oxidation products of the fish lipids?

Some signs emphasize this possibility. A defatted product undergoes roasting for 4 hr at 120°C without any serious deterioration: there is no destruction of the basic amino acids, methionine and tryptophan; only the cystine is destroyed, at a rate of 30%.[123] Even the lysine destruction seems to be dependent on the oxidation: the loss in this amino acid is reduced after a defatting or the use of inert atmosphere during heating or storage.[280,281]

In short, fish and the fish derivatives appear to be a very complex case: the more spoiled they are, the more adapted are the conditions to a Maillard reaction. At the same time, an oxidative environment can be easily created because of the fatty acid nature. This contributes, directly or in association with the intermediate products of the Maillard reaction, to the destruction of diverse amino acids, the sulfur-containing amino acids included. For these reasons, it is difficult to set criteria for fish and fish meals during the heat treatment. In practice, their protein quality spreads over a wide range: the nitrogen digestibility ranges from 97 to 47%, the biological value ranges from 82 to 39%, and the NPU ranges from 80 to 18%.[47,371] The Maillard reaction and the oxidation phenomena are primarily responsible for the poor quality of some mak-

### Table 17
### EVOLUTION OF SOME AMINO ACIDS
### DURING AUTOCLAVING OF COD MUSCLE

| | Treatment of cod muscle (% of protein) | | |
|---|---|---|---|
| | Control | Heated with 14% water | Heated with 14% water and 10% glucose |
| Cystine | 1.1 | 0.45 (−59%) | (0.40) (−64%) |
| Methionine | 3.4 | 3.2 (−6%) | 2.85 (−16%) |
| Lysine | 9.0 | 8.4 (−6%) | 6.3 (−30%) |

From Miller, E. L., Hartley, A. W., and Thomas, D. C., *Br. J. Nutr.*, 19, 565, 1965. With permission, Cambridge University Press.

ings of fish meal. In the absence of a high quality process, it is impossible to avoid some product deterioration due to these reactions.

### Meat

Apart from the exceptional case, meat is highly resistant to the Maillard reaction, i.e., after a roasting there are no appreciable nutritional losses. Nevertheless, on the surface of roasted meat, a reaction between the sugars and amino acids can develop.

The stability of meat is the consequence of its biochemical evolution during maturation: the glycogen is largely converted into lactic acid, i.e., there is a simultaneous disappearance of carbohydrates, and acidification, two phenomena that contribute to the inhibition of a Maillard reaction.[401] It follows that the traditional roasting of meat involves neither blocking, nor appreciable destruction of the main amino acids (lysine, methionine, tryptophan).[126,199,296,387,474,490] In these conditions, only a cystine destruction, up to 35%, can be detected.[126] In the case of experimental heatings, this amino acid is also the more damaged.[121] Such a situation is reminiscent of what has just been described about the fish; this particularity does not depend on the Maillard reaction (see Reactions Among Pure Amino Acids).

During roasting, however, the characteristics of this reaction appear on the outermost part: the Maillard reaction is responsible for the browning that occurs during frying,[401,402] and it is also the origin of some volatile compounds (see Aroma of Roasted Meat). The surface coagulation of the proteins creates a screen against heat penetration during roasting, preventing all but a small fraction of the meat from undergoing a Maillard reaction.

If the meat proteins undergo special or experimental heatings, the Maillard reaction can be developed and lead to a lysine deterioration. Thus, the simple coating of meat with wheat flour, i.e., an addition of carbohydrates, entails an appreciable loss of lysine during roasting.[112] The detrimental effects are even more manifest if reducing sugars are added to the meat,[387,471] or if the pH is increased.[471] In the same way, autoclaving for about 20 hr is responsible for a blocking and even for an appreciable destruction of lysine and the sulfur-containing amino acids.[121,199] In this eventuality, the amino acid evolution is comparable to that observed in the fish meals.

### Egg

A Maillard reaction cannot develop strongly in the egg because of its small amount of carbohydrates. However, egg albumen is adapted to this reaction since it contains a small quantity of combined and free sugars and it has an alkaline pH (about 9).

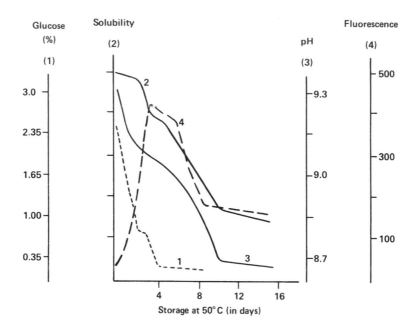

FIGURE 17.    Physicochemical evolution of dried egg albumen during storage. Reprinted with permission from Kline, R. W. and Stewart, G. F., *Ind. Eng. Chem.,* 40, 919, 1948. Copyright 1948 American Chemical Society.

Because of these two factors, the beginning of a Maillard reaction is detectable in dried egg albumen[399,499,505] and in shell eggs.[153] Unless reducing sugars are added,[462,519] the Maillard reaction is limited to the early physicochemical manifestations of the reaction: fluorescence, browning, and acidification, consequences of the quick disappearance of reducing sugars (Figure 17).

### Bread and Cereal Products

Cereal grain is remarkably stable during storage and, theoretically, the meal is also resistant to the Maillard reaction, although lysine losses are detected in unfavorable conditions of storage.[40,247,248] However, most of the processes when applied to wheat flour favor the development of a Maillard reaction. At first, the bread fermentation partially hydrolyzes the starch and proteins. The doughs frequently contain glucose, sucrose or milk powder additions, that add a supplementary amount of reducing sugars. Baking powders increase the alkalinity during the cooking of cereal products and can increase the amino acid losses, such as with thiamin,[383] whereas any acidification (sour milk, etc.) will increase the amino acid stability.[384]

The cooking conditions also influence the Maillard reaction intensity: it is proportional to the heat penetration. For example, the bread crust shields the crumb and impedes a sugar-amino acid reaction in the crumb. Inversely, the porous structure of toast and rusk make these products especially vulnerable to heat effects. In cereal foodstuffs, the Maillard reaction is expressed in two ways: (1) on the whole product, the reaction causes a selective loss of lysine, due to protein-bound lysine; while (2) in the outermost crust, the reaction mainly concerns the amino acids in free state, i.e., it uniformly destroys the whole amino acid.

Considering that the lysine is the primary limiting factor of all the cereals, the Maillard reaction will first induce a deficiency of the limiting factor and, consequently, a decrease of protein quality. When the cooking is done in pans (English type bread), the heating effects are less intense because the pan constitutes a heat screen. In the

Table 18
TOTAL AND AVAILABLE LYSINE IN VARIOUS
BAKED PRODUCTS

| | Total lysine (% proteins) | Available lysine | |
|---|---|---|---|
| | | Percent of total lysine | Percent of proteins |
| White wheat flour | 2.05 (100) | 97 | 2.00 |
| Crumb bread | 2.33 (114) | 98 | 2.30 |
| Crust bread | 1.61 (78) | 75 | 1.20 |
| Rusk or toast | 1.25 (61) | 70 | 0.87 |
| Roasted bread crumbs | 1.81 (88) | 67 | 1.20 |
| Fruit cake | 2.95 (144) | 80 | 2.35 |
| Butter-biscuit | 1.70 (83) | 71 | 1.20 |
| Gingerbread | 1.23 (60) | 25 | 0.31 |

From De Vuyst, A., Vervach, W., Charlier, H., and Jadin, V., *Le Lait*, 52, 444, 1972. With permission.

bread, the natural lysine fall is about 10%[73,100,205,301,449] and that of the free added lysine is between 15 and 30%.[145,146,449] The PER of the bread has an average value of 23% less than that of the flour.[101,184,304,317,457]

In the bread crust, the situation is different: the Maillard reaction develops strongly and often the factor that limits the intensity is the absence of moisture. That is why, in the baking industries, vapor injections are used in the ovens to favor the Maillard reaction on the surface of the products.[51] In a French type bread (baked without pan), the crust contains about two to three times less free amino acids than the crumb,[346] which demonstrates the intensity of the reaction in this part of the bread.

In other various cereal products, the reaction intensity is variable, the two main responsible factors being (1) the addition of reducing sugars that aggravate the consequences of baking;[100,145,146,184,457] and (2) the structure and the dimensions of the baked product, which determine the depth of heat penetration. Table 18 shows some examples of lysine unavailability in baked products. In some cases (crumb, bread, fruit cake), additions like yeast or milk powder increase the percent of lysine in proteins and could indicate that the Maillard reaction does not occur. In most cases, the reaction destroys an appreciable fraction of lysine and, moreover, blocks a part of remaining amino acid. The bread crust, toast, and also gingerbread are among the more damaged products due to their exposure to the heat, and probably, due to the strong reactivity of the ingredients. It is important to note that the cereal foodstuffs can undergo Maillard reactions in moderate heat conditions, at temperatures much less than those of a cooking oven. The bread kept at 50°C undergoes a lysine destruction of 10% in 3 weeks.[497] The lysine destruction during storage is a continuation of the Maillard reaction initiated by the original cooking; it can illustrate the autocatalytic character of this reaction. This mechanism cannot be invoked to explain the blocking and destruction of lysine in the course of paste drying (Table 19). Although these foods do not undergo degradation by fermentation and the drying is carried out at low temperatures (below 100°C), an appreciable fraction of the lysine is lost. From the nutritional point of view, i.e., in a weakly hydrated medium, the cereal foods present a fairly great sensitivity to the Maillard reaction.

The heat method used influences the development of this reaction. All the works quoted utilized conventional ovens. The use of microwave baking nearly eliminates the nutritional deficiencies detected during the baking of cereals or starchy foods.[101,168]

Table 19
LYSINE DETERIORATION DURING
PASTE DRYING

| Drying conditions | | Deteriorated lysine (%) | | |
|---|---|---|---|---|
| T°C | Duration (hr) | Blocked | Lost | Nutritional detriment |
| 45 | 18 | 16 | 6 | 22 |
| 60 | 10 | 21 | 7 | 28 |
| 70 | 7 | 22 | 7 | 29 |
| 80 | 6 | 35 | 12 | 47 |

From Cubadda, R., Fabriani, G., and Resmini, P., *Quad. Nutr.*, 28(5), 199, 1968. With permission.

Microwave baked bread conserves its lysine in available form, while the lysine of conventionally baked bread loses 25% of its efficiency.

### Leguminous Seeds and Oil Meals

For most of the leguminous seeds, a moderate heat treatment in wet medium is is necessary to destroy the thermolabile factors, which have antidigestive properties, in order that the proteins can reach their maximum efficiency. Even if this treatment type is prolonged, the proteins are very seldom damaged.[4,29,82,194,372,476,508,538]

Apart from some exceptions, these foodstuffs are classified among the products resistant to the Maillard reaction. Peanut oil meal furnishes an illustration: after 1 hr at 150°C in dry or wet media, there is only a blocking of amino acid — which reduces the protein efficiency — but not any amino acid destruction. To achieve an amino acid destruction the heat treatment must be very drastic, e.g., a roasting 2.5 hr at 150°C. Under these conditions, lysine suddenly becomes the primary limiting factor, in the place of methionine: then peanut oil meal loses its nutritional value.[6] This substitution of the limiting factor recalls the changes in milk powder. But, to arrive at the same situation, the peanut oil meal must undergo a treatment four times more intense than the milk powder. The stability of peanut oil meal is attributable to its small percentage of reducing sugars and to the complexity of its polymerized carbohydrates. Their depolymerization seems to interfere only after an intense heating. At this time, reducing molecules appear that easily react with the peanut globulins. The comparison of the curves 1 and 2 in Figure 15 show that from the stage where a Maillard reaction develops, the peanut sensitivity recalls that of milk proteins. These remarks are valid for the whole group of leguminous foodstuffs: their high resistance to the Maillard reaction is essentially due to an absence of reducing sugars. As a corollary, any addition of sugars to these products provokes a rapid lysine fall.[30,147,149,150,476] For all the leguminous seeds, a heat treatment causes not only a blocking or destruction of basic amino acids, but also an important unavailability of cystine.[39,148,149,194,476,508] This has been observed in other foodstuffs also containing globulins. This observation may only be fortuitous. In soybean proteins, there is another mechanism of lysine blocking, other than the Maillard reaction, and described in the section on reactions among pure amino acids. In the absence of sugar (Table 20), an appreciable part of lysine, aspartic, and glutamic acids are blocked but not destroyed, i.e., they are recoverable by chemical hydrolysis. There is a formation of peptide-like bonds between ε-amino groups of the lysine and the free carboxylic groups of glutamic and aspartic acids.[48,150] In the presence of sucrose, a substantial destruction of basic amino acids is added to this phenomenon: it is the classical manifestation of the Maillard reaction. The data of the Table

Table 20
EVOLUTION OF AMINO ACIDS IN SOYBEAN
DURING AN AUTOCLAVING

Amino acid decrease (%)

| Heated medium | Soybean protein only | | Soybean with glucose | |
|---|---|---|---|---|
| | Blocked | Destroyed | Blocked | Destroyed |
| Arginine | 8 | 3 | 55 | 42 |
| Histidine | 10 | 3 | 42 | 10 |
| Lysine | 30 | 3 | 84 | 47 |
| Aspartic acid | 37 | 7 | 34 | 6 |
| Glutamic acid | 24 | 2 | 50 | 3 |
| Cystine | 14 | 9 | 86 | 22 |
| Methionine | 6 | 3 | 41 | 2 |

From Evans, R. J. and Butts, H. A., *Science*, 109, 569, 1949. With permission.

20 emphasize the imbrications between the mechanisms likely to lead to an amino acid unavailability during heat treatment.

Among the oil meals, the cotton seed manifests a high sensitivity to heating; it is damaged even in industrial processes. Thus, the screw process provokes an available lysine loss of about 15% and a food efficiency diminution of about 35%.[41] In the same way, an autoclaving (20 min at 120°C) decreases the PER by 25%.[322] In addition, the storage conditions of oil meals can generate a lysine fall, after a prolonged duration in an unfavorable medium.[30,48,49]

## Food Microorganisms

The food yeasts (*Candida, Saccharomyces*) are the products most resistant to the Maillard reaction (Figure 15). Their lysine is remarkably stable during experimental heatings, whether they take place in wet or in dry media (Table 21). In the course of industrial drying processes, the yeast proteins are never damaged by the heat: *Candida utilis* can undergo a preheating (plasmolysis) of 35 min at 80°C, followed by a roller drying (7.5 sec on a cylinder at 175°C) without damage to either its protein efficiency or the availability of its lysine and methionine.[18] However, this stability is not characteristic of all food microorganisms: the spirulina algae lysine is clearly more sensitive than that of the yeast, mainly during the roastings (Table 21).

However, this stability is not characteristic of all food microorganisms: the spirulina algae lysine is clearly more sensitive than that of the yeasts, mainly during the roastings (Table 21).

The heat stability of the yeast proteins is due to three factors:

1. A very weak quantity of soluble reducing sugars (on an average, below 5%), which limits the possibilities of a sugar-amino acid reaction. It is sufficient to add a sugar, like xylose, to make the yeast proteins highly reactive and multiply the lysine destruction by five.
2. The yeast proteins buffered acidity (about pH 6.2) contributes to maintain them at a pH at which the Maillard reaction is inhibited. If the samples are placed at pH 9.0, the lysine loss is slightly increased, which confirms that the more important factor is the low percentage of reducing sugars. Indeed, if at pH 9, the heat is applied in presence of xylose, the yeasts become very sensitive to the Maillard reaction and their lysine is rapidly destroyed.

## Table 21
## EVOLUTION OF LYSINE IN FOOD MICROORGANISMS DURING EXPERIMENTAL HEATINGS[20]

| | Lysine loss (%) | | | |
|---|---|---|---|---|
| | Product only | Plus 11% of xylose | At pH 9 | Plus 11% of xylose and pH 9 |
| **Autoclaving (5 hr at 120°C)** | | | | |
| Yeasts | | | | |
| All samples | 9.0 | 59.0 | | |
| Hardly autolyzed samples | 8.0 | 59.0 | | |
| Weakly autolyzed samples | 14.0 | 60.0 | | |
| Spirulina algae | 18.5 | 65.5 | | |
| Oil meals | 24.5 | 73.0 | | |
| **Roasting (1 hr at 150°C)** | | | | |
| Yeasts | | | | |
| All samples | 12.5 | | 18.0 | 74.0 |
| Hardly autolyzed samples | 10.0 | | | |
| Weakly autolyzed samples | 19.0 | | | |
| Spirulina algae | 32.0 | | 38.0 | 75.0 |
| Oil meals | 14.5 | | 15.0 | 74.0 |

3.   The lysine loss depends on the autolysis intensity of the yeasts: the more auto-lyzed the yeast is before drying, the higher are the amounts of free sugars and free amino acids, and consequently the greater is the Maillard reaction probability.

So, the percent of lysine in free state (x) is linked to the rate of lysine destruction (y), by the following equations:[21] for a roasting of 1 hr at 150°C

$$y = 8.88 + 0.66 \, x$$

and for a roasting of 3 hr at 150°C

$$y = 12.30 + 1.30 \, x$$

For that reason, the yeast cultivated on gas oil offers a fairly remarkable stability during heat treatment because it undergoes a purification phase that practically elimi-nates all the free amino acids and reducing substances.[96] It must be emphasized that in the yeasts during the experimental heatings, the methionine destruction is generally half of that of the lysine.[18,20] Considering the remarkable stability of lysine, this does not signify that the yeast methionine has, in absolute, a particular sensitivity during the heatings.

### Nutritional Consequences

The Maillard reaction modifies the protein quality of foodstuffs. This fact can make a protein food ineffective for a special use: it has been shown that the addition of a scorched milk product cannot supplement a cereal diet effectively. As the various cat-egories of foodstuffs have heat behaviors very different from each other, the damage caused by a particular treatment will be itself more or less important according to the food product nature: when 17% of yeast lysine is destroyed, the loss is 24% for fish meal, 42% for wheat flour, 60% for peanut oil meal, and it's total for a milk powder (Figure 15).

For that reason, the protein efficiency of a foodstuff does not depend on its initial protein value, but on its behavior during the heat processes. Table 2 demonstrates that the addition of skim milk powder to cookies is ineffective nutritionally, whereas the use of peanut oil meal or fish meal is recommended because of their satisfying heat stability.[17]

|  | PER | |
|---|---|---|
|  | Raw mix | Cookies strongly cooked |
| Control cookies | 1.09 | 0.19 |
| Iso-lysine cookies |  |  |
| Peanut cookies | 1.76 | 0.87 |
| Fish meal cookies | 1.63 | 0.69 |
| Milk cookies | 2.10 | 0.02 |

Because of the cumulative effects of successive heatings, a particular treatment has repercussions that will depend on two factors: (1) the intensity of the heating itself; and (2) the presence in the medium of the Maillard reaction products derived from previous heatings. These are precursors of the Maillard reaction and, particularly, of the Strecker degradation, and will accelerate the heat effects autocatalytically. Thus, making biscuits with a same percentage of milk powder, the nutritional value of the finished products will be different according to the drying process (spray or roller drying). In a roller drying powder, the process will damage the milk lysine and, more-over, the powder brings products of the Maillard reaction to the mix, which will intensify the cooking effects. On the whole, the 'roller drying milk biscuit' is clearly inferior to the 'spray drying milk-biscuit'.[14]

|  | Raw mix (with spray drying) | Cookies with milk powder | |
|---|---|---|---|
|  |  | Spray dried | Roller drying |
| Rat growth (grams per day) | 3.0 | 2.1 | 1.1 |
| PER | 2.74 | 1.39 | 1.04 |

The heating consequences largely depend on the biochemical context of the proteins. Even by choosing the most resistant foodstuffs, a sugar addition (galactose, glucose, lactose, etc.) or a pH increase (addition of baking powder, alkaline salts, etc.) modifies the protein behavior and intensifies the Maillard reaction. The rate of lysine destruction may be multiplied by six after a sugar addition and an alkalinization.

The destruction generated by a Maillard reaction cannot be totally annulled by restoring the amino acid balance. First, the operation is difficult because the rate of unavailability of each amino acid must be measured precisely. Then, even if the balance is restored, the protein efficiency remains slightly inferior to that of unheated product. The fact has been observed after experimental roastings. The same discrepancy is directly observed in the products that have undergone a strong Maillard reaction. The in vivo measure of protein efficiency is always inferior to the amino acid fraction remaining available after the heat treatment.

These distortions are the consequences of the physiological activities of the Maillard reaction products. They reduce to hydrolytic mechanisms during digestion, they particularly decrease the nitrogen utilization, and they may cause toxicity. Briefly, the premelanoidins formed during the Maillard reaction prevent a satisfying efficiency of the undegraded nutrients remaining after heating.

## FLAVORS PRODUCED BY THE MAILLARD REACTION

Industrial heat treatments develop flavors that are often highly appreciated by the consumer.* Among the more appetizing aromas, many come from the Maillard reaction, more precisely from the Strecker degradation: the flavor of fresh bread crust, of roasted cocoa, and of roasted peanuts are characteristic examples.

These flavors take a particular place in the aroma category: they are not really natural aromas, nor synthetic aromas. It is possible to classify them as technological aromas. Then, they practically escape any legal definition because the obtaining conditions are impossible to codify.

The production of these flavors during food processing depends on a certain number of conditions and factors.[12,218,259,445] The food products must undergo an intense heat treatment in a weakly hydrated medium (roasting) to develop a Maillard reaction and, also, a Strecker degradation. Moderate baking in an hydrated medium (autoclaving) rarely leads to the mechanisms that develop the flavors. Thus, the bread crust flavor is essentially attributable to a Strecker degradation developed during the baking, whereas the flavor of the bread crumb reflects the appearance of other mechanisms, occurring in the course of bread fermentation. The crumb has not been cooked intensely enough to ensure significant biochemical modifications of the dough products.

The food products must contain sugars and amino acids in a free state or in the form of oligosaccharides and oligopeptides: the flavor formation is only initiated by these substances. Generally, the amount of free amino acids is the factor that limits the aroma production. That is why, in food processing, the products are frequently submitted to a preliminary phase during which a fermentation — spontaneous or provoked — is developed. It is accompanied by amylolytic and proteolytic activities which increase the quantity of reactants available for the aroma formation. The addition of proteolytic systems, resulting in a larger proportion of oligopeptides and free amino acids, will be expressed by an increase in the amount of carbonyl compounds during the last roasting.[242]

In the absence of any preliminary operation, aroma production will be less. It seems that this defect can be compensated for by an appropriate amino acid addition. If such a use is developed, it would open many perspectives to the technologists. On one hand, it would allow correction of products from low commercial quality lots; and on the other hand, it would allow modification of the industrial processes without entailing an obvious diminution of the sensorial quality.

Every food product seems to contain free amino acids in highly variable amounts. *A priori,* those that predominate are responsible for the resulting flavors. In the products which usually undergo roasting, free amino acids found in high proportion are the following:

| Potato | Peanut | Beef | Cocoa bean |
|---|---|---|---|
| Asparagine | Alanine | Valine | Leucine |
| Glutamine | Phenylalanine | Glycine | Alanine |
| Valine | Asparagine | Leucine | Phenylalanine |
| Aminobutyric acid | Arginine | | Valine |

---

* The flavor is composed of the sensations perceived by the taste and by the smell. The first sensation (taste) is the effect of nonvolatile compounds perceived as bitter, acid, sweet, or salted. The second sensation (aroma) is the effect of volatile molecules on the olfactory system.

   The flavors developed during roastings are principally due to aromas (production of volatile molecules) and secondly to tastes.

## Table 22
### AROMAS PRODUCED DURING HEATINGS OF MIXTURES COMPOSED OF ONE AMINO ACID AND ONE SUGAR[37,44,133,207,218,244,360,453,539]

| Nature of amino acid | Aroma |
| --- | --- |
| Alanine | Caramel, nutty, malt, malt-coffee |
| Aminobutyric acid | Caramel, maple syrup, walnut, nuts, burnt sugar |
| Arginine | Bready, popcorn, buttery, burnt sugar |
| Aspartic acid | Caramel, rock candy |
| Cysteine | Meaty, overboiled or rotten egg, burnt horn |
| Cystine | Crispy pastry, smoky, burnt turkey skin, burnt |
| Glutamic acid | Caramel, chocolate, butterscotch, chicken broth, baked ham, charred meat, old wood, burnt sugar, chicken tray, chicken manure |
| Glycine | Caramel, baked potato, beef broth, burnt candy, smoky, burnt |
| Histidine | Corn bread, bready, buttery, burnt sugar |
| Isoleucine | Malty, apple, fruity, crust, musty, dried linseed oil, burnt chocolate, burnt cheese |
| Leucine | Sweet chocolate, toasted, bready, baked potato, cheesy, malt, malt-coffee, burnt cheese |
| Lysine | Bready, baked sweet potato, rotten raw potato, fried potato, stale potato, corn syrup, boiled meat, frying butter, burnt fried potato, burnt wet wood |
| Methionine | Potato, boiled-potato, overcooked sweet potato, cabbage, chopped cabbage, overcooked cabbage, bean soup, broth, beany, leek, harsh horseradish, cheese-broth, burnt wood |
| Phenylalanine | Caramel, sweet caramel, violets, lilac, rose, hyacinth, perfume, chocolate, roasted nuts, almonds, honey, rancid caramel, dirty dog |
| Proline | Bakery, cracker, crust, toast, very roasted wheat flour, cooked bread, potato, mushroom, burnt egg |
| Serine | Maple syrup, vaguely breadlike |
| Threonine | Chocolate, maple syrup |
| Tryptophan | Fried oil, burnt hair |
| Tyrosine | Caramel, rose, violets, lilac, perfume |
| Valine | Apple, fruity, sweet chocolate, bread, rye bread, malt-coffee, yeasty, protein hydrolysate |

In a simplified way, every amino acid tends to give a dominant or characteristic flavor, when heated in the presence of sugar. This results from the specific aldehyde production during the Strecker degradation (Table 10). Thus, the glycine produces a flavor of meat broth, proline produces a bread crust aroma, etc. However, according to the sugar nature and mainly according to the heat intensity and conditions, the same amino acid can be at the origin of many flavors. Table 22 enumerates the flavors obtained by heating a sugar and an amino aicd in simple conditions. Under these circumstances, lysine is able to produce flavors of bread, potato, meat, and beans. This variability of aromas shows the multitude of factors attending the production of volatile molecules during the heatings.

The particular responsibility of the Strecker degradation has been demonstrated by heating an amino acid directly with a reductone (isatin), i.e., by avoiding the development of a Maillard reaction. By proceeding in this way, the following aromas have been obtained: malt from alanine, malt-apple from isoleucine, apple from valine, malt from leucine, mushroom from proline, violets from phenylalanine, cheese-broth from methionine, flowers from norleucine and cheddar from norvaline.[257]

When Maillard reaction jointly occurs with a Strecker degradation, three types of flavors are successively perceived as the heat intensifies: (1) at the beginning, a 'caramel' flavor predominates,[360] confirming that the sugars are quickly degraded before the Maillard reaction is clearly developed; (2) then comes the optimum phase during which specific aromas are produced, corresponding to the aldehydes of the Strecker degradation; and (3) if the heating goes on beyond this optimum phase, the aromatic substances evolve rapidly because of their chemical instability and a 'burnt' flavor predominates, whatever the amino acid is.[218] Experimenting with pure products has linked the flavor of 'burnt' or 'smoky' to the ratio between 2-methyl butanal and ethylene sulfide.[405]

The variation and the gradation of flavors is even greater in complex media, as in food products, where flavors coming from amino acid degradation, fatty acid oxidation, and sugar thermolysis interfere with each other. The different molecules formed in these ways play a double part — direct and indirect — in the formation of roasted product flavors. At first, sugar caramelization and heat oxidation of lipids leads to volatile compounds, richly supplied with aromatic properties: they directly create flavors. Then, among these molecules, there are many aldehydes, ketones, and diketones, which react with amino acids according to the Maillard reaction and the Strecker degradation mechanisms. Indirectly, the products of carbohydrates and lipid decomposition contribute to the production of flavors from amino acids. Phenomena of this nature occur during the roasting of meat, peanut, and all food products containing a notable proportion of lipids.

The difficulties of flavor detection and evaluation must be mentioned. Flavor perception first depends on the concentration of volatile molecules.[340] It also depends on the context where the volatiles are situated.[50,370,396] Thus, when the volatile products of a roasted peanut are dissolved in paraffin oil, the response of the sensory evaluation is again 100% 'peanut aroma'. The same extract in aqueous solution gives responses ranging from 'disagreeable' to 'burned' or 'overroasted peanut'.[263]

Even if it is not possible to attribute a flavor to only one factor, for some roasted foodstuffs, flavor development is the unquestionable consequence of a Maillard reaction or a Strecker degradation. Analytical works have even determined the amino acid nature exercising the main responsibility in the production of the flavor. Some demonstrative examples are described below. It is possible that in other food products, the Strecker degradation occupies a place in the flavor observed after a heating.

### Aroma of Bread Crust

Bread flavor is composed of a great variety of volatile substances.[351-353] The flavor of the crust particularly comes from products formed by the Maillard reaction and the Strecker degradation.[105,242,244,259] It can be determined immediately that the crumb and the crust flavors are completely different and that their origin is also different. The crumb flavor comes especially from products formed by enzymatic action during the kneading and the fermentation, e.g., fatty acids,[122] which are not modified during baking. The crust flavor results from a double phenomenon: the yeast activity produces simple molecules (sugars, amino acids) which play the part of aroma precursors, i.e., they are transformed into aromatic substances during the crust roasting. This reaction decomposes fatty acids[320] and carbohydrates,[152,353,482] but principally allows many sugar-amino acid reactions. They lead to a number of substances, both volatile and not, that are the main agents of the crust flavor.[243,451]

After fermentation, the dough contains an appreciable quantity of maltose, that comes from the starch hydrolysis. It may eventually include a small amount of sucrose. It also has amino acids, sometimes at a level superior to that of the initial flour (lysine,

Table 23
EVOLUTION OF SOME AMINO ACIDS RESULTING FROM FERMENTATION
AND BAKING OF BREAD

| | Flour ($\mu$ mole %) | Dough (flour = 1) | | Crumb ($\mu$ mole %) | Bread | |
|---|---|---|---|---|---|---|
| | | | | | Crust (crumb = 1) | |
| | | Unfermented | Fermented | | Unfermented | Fermented |
| Glycine | 4.1 | 2.88 | 2.56 | 12.8 | 0.60 | 0.07 |
| Alanine | 14.35 | 6.06 | 1.60 | 31.2 | 1.03 | 0.07 |
| Glutamic acid | 8.85 | 8.10 | 5.28 | 53.9 | 0.18 | 0.02 |
| Proline | 4.65 | 4.65 | 3.67 | 19.5 | 0.45 | 0.02 |
| Lysine | 2.40 | 13.50 | 10.65 | 21.25 | 0.46 | 0 |
| Arginine | 2.10 | 3.15 | 7.25 | 16.25 | 0.03 | 0 |
| Tyrosine | 3.10 | 1.92 | 0.16 | 0.90 | — | — |
| Phenylalanine | 3.30 | 1.78 | 0.05 | 1.60 | — | — |
| Leucine | 5.55 | 1.56 | 0.31 | 3.90 | 0.70 | 0.07 |
| Isoleucine | 4.15 | 1.60 | 0.38 | 2.50 | 0.81 | 0.07 |

From El-Dash, A. A. and Johnson, J. A., *Cereal Chem.*, 47, 247, 1970. With permission.

arginine, glutamic acid, proline), sometimes in lesser quantities (tyrosine, phenylalanine, leucines) (Table 23). These variations reflect both a certain consumption of free amino acids by the yeast and, at the same time, a certain production during the fermentation.[130,303,346]

During the crust baking, various processes happen simultaneously. The maltose reacts with free amino acids and, at the same time, it is partially transformed into hexoses. These react at a higher level in the crust than in the crumb. In dry matter, the bread crumb contains 4.3 g of maltose and the crust 0.85 g; the crumb only contains about 0.05 g each of glucose and fructose, whereas the crust contains about 0.15 g of each.[114] This conversion of disaccharide into hexoses has also been observed during the peanut roasting.

The sugars are caramelized in the crust by giving furfural and HMF.[292,293] After addition of sugars to a dough, the crust often holds ten times more furfural than the crumb and five times more HMF. Generally, the sucrose and the hexoses tend to increase the amount of HMF more than that of the furfural; the pentoses (arabinose, xylose) furnish comparable quantities of furfural and HMF.[292,293] These observations do not totally correspond to theoretical predictions.

The free amino acids disappear from the crust in great proportions, whereas they appear little touched in the crumb.[130,292,303,346] The crust retains 20 times less amino acids, in the free state, than the crumb.[130] The rate of destruction of total amino acids is 45% in the crust and 11% in the crumb.[186] According to Table 23, the basic amino acid proline and glutamic acid disappear nearly totally from the crust of fermented bread, i.e., their derivatives may be at the origin of the crust flavor.

In the crust of unfermented bread, the free amino acids are clearly less touched. This fact signifies that in such products the rate of reducing sugars remains insufficient to provoke a maximum Maillard reaction. The main interest of the fermentation seems to be the starch hydrolysis and the maltose formation rather than the flour proteolysis. The reducing sugar rate remains the limiting factor of the Maillard reaction, if the mix contains neither sucrose nor lactose addition. If there is a sugar addition, the quantity of free amino acids can become the limiting factor of this reaction.

In the crust, the Maillard reaction goes as far as the Strecker degradation, since the bread presents specific aldehydes that are absent from the dough and preferments:

formaldehyde, propionaldehyde, isobutyraldehyde, crotonaldehyde, phenylacetalde-hyde, methional.[244] An addition of valine to the dough multiplies by eight the quantity of isobutyraldehyde in the crust, but only by two that of the crumb. In the same way, the isoleucine multiplies by three the rate of isovaleraldehyde without a similar increase in the crumb.[458] These results confirm that the crust and crumb evolution are distinct and that only the crust flavor is attributable to Strecker degradation substances, and secondly to Maillard reaction phenomena.

The production of these aldehydes and other volatile molecules is proportional to the baking duration, i.e., to the heat sum applied to the crust.[320,452,513] After a baking of 30 min, the bread contains 1.75 mg% of total aldehydes, after a baking of 4 hr, this value reaches 2.65 mg. The sensory value of bread follows the same evolution; it seems to be parallel to the percentage of some aldehydes like acetaldehyde, methylbu-tanal, isobutanal, etc.[320] Thus, during the baking, the Strecker degradation constitutes the main origin of the crust flavor. Among the amino acids, lysine and proline degra-dation are the primary agents of this flavor. The pyrroline and the pyrrolidone coming from the proline (Figure 18) possess the characteristic aroma of bread and cracker.[207,262] It is also possible to obtain 2-acetyl-1,4,5,6,tetrahydropyridine from this amino acid, which has a very strong flavor of cracker and crust.[229,230,539]

The crust flavor rapidly evolves after cooking: in 4 days, the amount of acetalde-hyde, isobutanal, acetone, and methyl butanals is reduced by half.[293,320,539] This reduc-tion results from a diffusion of volatile molecules and their chemical transformation. In the crust, the quantity of aldehydes decreases by about 55% in 7 days; during this time, part diffuses toward the atmosphere and part toward the crumb: the amount of carbonyl compounds in the crumb doubles by the second and third day after baking, and then decreases.[293] On the other hand, the sensorial loss also comes from the chem-ical instability of the volatile compounds and their oxidation. For example, the proline derivatives, which are less volatile than others, develop a characteristic stale odor on oxidation.[116]

Various methods exist to reinforce the crust flavor. Some, like papain and protease, improve the color and flavor of the crust by increasing the hydrolytic effects of the yeast.[129,242,346] Other methods include a growing trend towards the addition of free amino acids and flavor enhancers, especially when the time of fermentation and en-zymic hydrolysis is reduced.[259] Naturally, such methods cannot be considered without the previous agreement and favorable opinion of the Public Health Service.

### Aroma of Roasted Cocoa

The flavor of roasted cocoa bean is the result of a large number of volatile sub-stances, of which more than 300 have been identified. Among them are 54 esters, 37 acids, 34 hydrocarbons, 31 pyrazines, 30 ketones and 30 alcohols, 25 aldehydes, 15 furans, 10 pyrrols, etc.[255] Certainly, some of these products come from a Strecker degradation occurring in conditions reminiscent of those described apropos of the bread crust.

The bean roasting is preceded — in most cases — by a phase of complex fermenta-tion. It particularly takes place in acid medium and has the technological aim of the elimination of the external membranes of the bean: it is called a 'demucilagination'.[443] All the authors recognize the importance of this operation for the subsequent devel-opment of the aroma during the roasting.[115,255,446] It provokes the augmentation of reducing sugars and of free amino acids. According to the varieties and the treatments, the grain before the roasting contains from 9 to 16 mg% of free amino acids[411] and from 8.6 to 18.6 mg% of reducing sugars.[255]

These differences are an important factor in flavor and commercial value of co-coas.[115,255,446] The free amino acid quantities often seem to be the limiting factor of

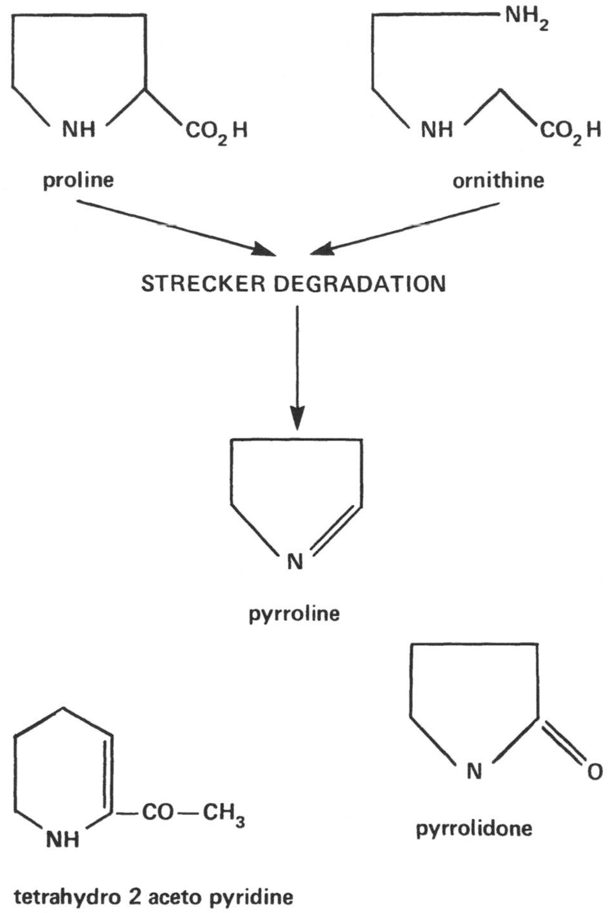

FIGURE 18.   Degradation products of proline and ornithine.[230,259]

aroma production during the roasting. In the course of roasting, the reducing sugars are three times more likely to disappear than the amino acids.[411] An analysis of the reaction shows that 6% of the sucrose and the bulk of the glucose and fructose are lost, whereas 49% of the free amino acids and 4% of those contained in the oligopeptides have reacted with the sugars.[343]

Among these amino acids, phenylalanine, tyrosine, threonine, leucine and, probably, lysine undergo important losses and their degradation products play a primary role in the cocoa flavor.[115,343,411] They are destroyed by a Strecker degradation and converted into isovaleraldehyde, phenylacetaldehyde, acetaldehyde, etc.[115] Moreover, many alkylpyrazines are formed, in amounts ranging from 0.70 mg% for the Ghana varieties to 0.14 mg% for the Tabasco varieties.[255] The production of these molecules largely depends on the previous fermentation phase of the bean: if it has been fermented, it generates more than 0.8 mg% of pyrazines after a roasting of 45 min; if it hasn't been fermented, the amount remains below 0.4 mg.[255,522] These pyrazines are a consequence of the Strecker degradation (Figure 13). They occur in many roasted products and constitute an element of their flavor. Besides the cocoa, they can be detected in peanuts, potatoes, potato chips, coffee,[263] and sesame seeds.[319,491] Pyrrole compounds have also been detected in the cocoa aroma.[522]

Other studies have extracted a concentrate of cocoa aroma[343] as well as a bitter agent contained in this product. It is 5-methyl-2-phenyl hexanal; this molecule is attributed

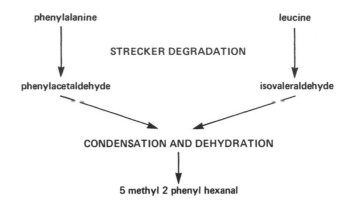

FIGURE 19.    Strecker degradation. Reprinted with permission from
Van Pragg, M., Stein, N. S., and Tibbets, M. S., *J. Agric. Food
Chem.*, 16, 1005, 1968. Copyright 1968 American Chemical Society.

to a condensation reaction between two specific aldehydes formed by the Strecker degradation[522] (Figure 19).

### Aroma of Roasted Peanut

Peanut roasting is distinct from the operations described earlier by the absence of previous fermentation (except as a mishap during harvesting) which permits augmentation of the precursors of bread and cocoa aromas. Nevertheless, as in cocoa and other roasted products, the number of carbonyl compounds is extremely high in the roasted peanut: more than 320 molecules have been identified as against 60 in the unroasted bean.[42,66,67,325] The obtained flavor is 'one of the most desirable and universally enjoyed flavors'.[324]

The roasting development of this bean must both favor the precursor production and create the reactions leading to volatile molecules. The unroasted grain is characterized by a high rate of sucrose (4%) and a very small amount of hexoses (0.2%).[23a,103,198,326,373] During the roasting, an appreciable fraction of sucrose disappears, whereas the hexoses remain nearly constant, and even sometimes can be doubled: there is a fission of the sucrose into hexoses, which furnishes the elements necessary to a Maillard reaction. On the other hand, the roasting produces many derivatives of fatty acids, that play a double part in the flavor formation: they act directly by themselves, but it is possible that they supplement the aldehydes, becoming available for the Maillard reaction. The unroasted grain also contains free amino acids, at various concentrations (Table 24).

The origin of the peanut flavor will partially depend on genetic factors, and also on the harvesting methods and the factors that determine the quantity and the nature of free amino acids. However, in the peanut as well as in the cocoa, it has been demonstrated that peptides can react in the Maillard reaction and participate in flavor formation. In particular, at the end of maturation, a peptide appears in the peanut bean; it contains a high proportion of glutamic acid and phenylalanine and it undergoes a significant destruction during roasting: its amino acid content must be considered as an appreciable contribution to the flavor of roasted peanuts.[326] Among the amino acids responsible for the typical flavor are: aspartic and glutamic acids, histidine, and phenylalanine; inversely, the degradation products of threonine, tyrosine, and lysine tend to give an atypical aroma.[373]

Roasting supplies two categories of products: some are only increased by the heating, others appear only in the roasted bean: these are specific substances of heat treat-

## Table 24
### RELATIONSHIP BETWEEN BIOCHEMICAL COMPOSITION OF UNROASTED PEANUT BEAN AND ITS FLAVOR AFTER ROASTING

| μ mole % | Sample | | | |
|---|---|---|---|---|
| | C1 | C2 | N2 | N1[a] |
| Sucrose | 70 | 137 | 174 | 49 |
| Glucose + fructose | 0.95 | 3.2 | 14.75 | 2.65 |
| Total free amino acids | 43.0 | 27.8 | 6.5 | 19.2 |
| Aspartic acid | 5.0 | 3.1 | 0.9 | 3.2 |
| Glutamic acid | 10.0 | 6.1 | 2.0 | 5.0 |
| Phenylalanine | 2.5 | 0.9 | Tr | 0.8 |
| Histidine | 2.0 | 0.6 | Tr | 1.4 |
| Flavor score (%) | 74 | 66 | 42 | Poor |

[a] The sample N1 is an immature bean. Its weak amount of sucrose confirms earliest harvest.[135]

Reprinted from Cobb, W. Y. and Swaisgood, H. E., *J. Food Sci.*, 36, 538, 1971. Copyright© by Institute of Food Technologists.

ment. Among them are 2-methyl propanal, 2-methyl and 3-methyl butanal, 2,4-pentadianal, 2,4-hexadienal, etc.[66,67] These specific substances are notably products formed in the course of Strecker degradation, like acetaldehyde, isobutyraldehyde, phenylacetaldehyde, methylbutanals, etc.[42,43,198,325] Moreover, the degradation generates pyrazines that participate in the roasted peanut flavor.[198,259,263,324]

The sensory factor seems to be linked to three precise molecules: the flavor is proportional to the ratios: 'methylpropanal/hexanal' and 'methyl butanal/hexanal.'[173] These relations illustrate the complexity of the peanut flavor: it comes both from the degradation products of the amino acids (Strecker degradation) and a decomposition of fatty acids. Different processes of roasting (oven, microwave, coconut oil bath) lead to slightly different sensory values[549] which indicates all the imponderable factors that can modify the biochemical reactions during roasting operations.

### Aroma of Roasted Meat

The flavor of cooked meat has a particularly complex origin, especially when it is roasted. Its elements exhibit a variety of characteristics,[224,225,404,413,415] and come from diverse types of biochemical reactions: (1) heat decomposition of fatty acids, (2) decomposition of amino acids, especially the sulfur-containing amino acids, (3) reactions between sugars and amino acids, (4) eventual reactions between oxidation products of fatty acids and amino acids. The sulfur-containing amino acids produce many substances that participate in the meat flavor; among them: hydrogen sulfide, the methyl, ethyl-, propyl-, and butyl-mercaptans, dimethyl disulfide, etc.[206,284,404]

The possibility of a Maillard reaction is less evident in meat than in other food products. Nevertheless, several authors have concluded that meat flavor development is chiefly a consequence of this reaction. In favor of this theory, meat evolution during maturation must be detailed. On one hand, glycogen is converted into lactic acid; this fact constitutes an inhibiting factor of the Maillard reaction. On the other hand, meat contains a certain number of elements necessary to this reaction and their quantity increases in the course of maturation. There is an augmentation of free amino-N, in parallel to the appearance of free sugars, partially formed from sugar phosphates: the ribose-5-phosphate plays an important part in the sugar-amino acid reaction. It is able to provoke browning of meat, even at room temperature.[545] Glycoproteins also constitute precursors of the roasted flavor.

The Maillard reaction can also be developed by means of the following components, present in meat at the concentration of (in % of wet product): about 140 mg of free amino acids, including alanine, glutamic acid, leucine, valine, phenylalanine, methionine, etc.; about 60 mg of free sugars, including glucose, fructose, ribose (1 mg), and about 1.5 mg of sugar phosphates.[95,308] This composition depends on the degree of maturation of the meat. Among the products detected in the meat flavor, some indisputably depend on sugar thermolysis and the Strecker degradation: acetaldehyde, 3-methyl propanal, 3-methyl- and 2-methyl-butanal, methional, phenylacetaldehyde, and furfural.[225,404] These substances rapidly disappear, even in a product that does not run the risk of oxidation, like canned beef: in 6 months, 83% of the methyl butanals disappear in the cans.[404]

### Aroma of Dairy Products

As in the case of meat, the role of the derivatives of the fatty acids is considerable in the flavors of dairy products. The fact has been particularly noted in the fermented cheeses and in the butter products. Nevertheless, the Maillard reaction or the Strecker degradation is not always foreign to the flavors produced in certain conditions. But, in the field, the flavors developed in dairy products by means of these reactions are generally unfavorable, contrary to what occurs in all other food products. If the Maillard reaction is not at the origin of a 'cooked', 'stale', or 'oxidized' flavor, it more or less contributes to the development of a 'cereal' flavor, noticed in some dry milks.[256] This flavor is proportional to the concentration of HMF, which comes mainly from the degradation of lactose. This supposes a Maillard reaction, developed in parallel:

| Flavor of reconstituted milk | $\mu$mol HMF per liter |
|---|---|
| No criticism | 4.5 |
| Slight cereal | 11.0 |
| Cereal | 14.0 |

In spray dried whey powder, stored for 3 years at 4°C, characteristic products of the Strecker degradation have been identified, such as the pyrazines and the pyrroles, together with those depending on a caramelization, such as maltol or benzaldehyde.[158] About 40 volatile molecules (including pyrazines, pyrroles, pyridines) are also present in the skim milk powders or in lactose-casein mixtures after heating or storage.[159-161] As the casein is a glycoprotein, often with residual traces of lactose, it can develop a Maillard reaction or a Strecker degradation by itself after a heating in a pure medium. Thus, the specific aldehydes of the Strecker degradation are detected in a casein solution, autoclaved for 1 hr at 140°C.[368] However, this does not reveal itself as favorable from a sensory point of view: the flavor of the casein decreases with the duration of storage or with its residual lactose,[529] i.e., when conditions favor the Maillard reaction.

The only dairy derivative where a Strecker degradation is beneficially expressed is fermented cheese: in the course of maturation, the proteolytic activity of the flora produces free amino acids and oligopeptides. These can be the object of a Strecker degradation under the influence of some products of the microbial metabolism, such as pyruvic acid. It is by means of this type of reaction that the aged Cheddar flavor can be attributed to. This flavor is reinforced in the case of toasted cheese.[257]

The dairy products constitute an exceptional case because they can contain molecules specific to the Strecker degradation without the intervention of this mechanism. There exist at least two examples of the presence of methional and that of 3-methyl butanal produced without intervention of the Strecker degradation.

Methional is an important product in the 'sunlight' defect of milk. It comes from a reaction of methionine photolysis, catalyzed by riboflavin.[394] As to 3-methyl butanal, it is detected in dairy products inoculated by *Streptococcus lactis* var. *maltigenes*. All the strains of *S. lactis* deaminate the leucine and provide the $\alpha$-ketoisocaproic acid. But only *S. lactis* var. *maltigenes* converts the formed acid into methyl butanal by decarboxylation.[306] This product of leucine microbial degradation develops a characteristic malty aroma, even at the concentration of 0.5 ppm in the milk.[235]

Even if such examples remain exceptional, they show that the Strecker degradation is not the only mechanism able to transform the amino acids in $C_n$ into aldehydes in $C_{n-1}$ and that the chemical and enzymatic fields are not separated in an absolute way: some molecules may be common to both of these fields.

### Aroma of Coffee

Coffee is roasted with such an intensity that the Maillard reaction stage is passed and that of carbonization is often reached. In this context, the products eventually formed in the course of the Maillard reaction are transformed afterwards and it becomes difficult to measure the role of this reaction in the aroma formed during the roasting.

The coffee bean contains free amino acids, reducing sugars, ascorbic acid, all of which can provoke a Maillard reaction and a Strecker degradation during the storage of the green bean. At the beginning of storage, a simultaneous disappearance of these substances is noted without browning development; then, a second stage occurs during which the quantity of these substances increases, by reason of an hydrolysis of polysaccharides and proteins. At this time, a significant browning occurs. If a bean lot undergoes such an evolution, the sensory quality of the coffee beverage deteriorates.[417] The Maillard reaction that occurs during storage modifies the conditions under which the roasting develops and changes the flavor of the soluble fraction. As in the case of dairy products, a Maillard reaction is unfavorable from a sensory point of view when it develops in the coffee bean.

## CONCLUSION

In the nutritional field, the Maillard reaction is incontestably detrimental because of the lysine unavailability that it causes. Moreover, it is not limited to sugar and amino acid losses. It also generates many substances that have physiological properties, some detrimental (antinutritional, toxic properties), others favorable (flavor). To be ignorant of the unavailability of amino acids or of the properties of premelanoidins can lead to a serious misconception of the reality.

In the technological field, the Maillard reaction is sometimes considered as a disastrous operation because it gives a browning to products appreciated for their whiteness, and sometimes it adds to the value of the food products by creating desirable and pleasurable colorations and flavors.

Should the Maillard reaction be encouraged or instead, opposed? It is difficult to give a complete answer; in fact, the Maillard reaction must be considered for every foodstuff. Cocoa is consumed for its attractive properties and not as a protein food; if a fraction of its amino acids is destroyed during the commercial roasting, the nutritional status of the consumer is not perturbed. The Maillard reaction cannot be considered as prejudicial in this case.

The peanut represents a comparable situation: the roasting greatly improves the value of a foodstuff little appreciated in its unroasted state. The roasted flavor is obtained before any deterioration appears in its nutritional content: the destruction rate of amino acids is negligible and the protein efficiency remains undamaged in roasted peanuts. There, too, the controlled development of a Maillard reaction is justified.

In the cereal products, the Maillard reaction is more criticizable. Most certainly, it gives to the bread crust, toast, cookies, and biscuits an appreciated flavor, but the reaction is accompanied by a substantial diminution of the protein quality and a decrease in the amount of lysine, the primary limiting factor. As the cereal foods constitute an important nutritional element in the diet, a decrease in their protein value is of concern to the consumer.

The dairy products represent an extreme case, where the Maillard reaction causes serious nutritional damage, without any counterpart in sensory effects. The situation is the more serious in that milk constitutes one of the best sources of lysine. After an intense Maillard reaction, the milk falls to the same nutritional value as the soybean or peanut oil meals, according to the heating intensity. These examples demonstrate that the Maillard reaction can be considered as the best, or the worst thing. Aesop has said the same about the tongue.

# REFERENCES

1. Adhikari, H. R. and Tappel, A. L., *J. Food Sci.*, 38, 486—488, 1973.
2. Adrian, J., *Bull. Soc. Chim. Biol.*, 37, 107—121, 1955.
3. Adrian, J., *Ann. Nutr. Aliment.*, 17, 1—35, 1963.
4. Adrian, J., *Ann. Nutr. Aliment.*, 18, 1—18, 1964.
5. Adrian, J., *Ann. Nutr. Aliment.*, 19, 27—45, 1965.
6. Adrian, J., *Ann. Nutr. Aliment.*, 21, 129—147, 1967.
7. Adrian, J., *Ind. Aliment. Agric.*, 89, 1281—1289 and 1713—1720, 1972; 90, 449—455 and 559—564, 1973; *World Rev. Nutr. Diet.*, 19, 71—122, 1974.
8. Adrian, J., *Ann. Nutr. Aliment.*, 27, 299—314, 1973.
9. Adrian, J., *La Valeur Alimentaire Du Lait*, Vol. 1, Maison Rustique, Paris, 1973.
10. Adrian, J., *Ind. Aliment. Agric.*, 91, 1525—1534, 1974.
11. Adrian, J., *Lait*, 55, 24—40 and 182—206, 1975.
12. Adrian, J., *Labo Pharma*, 244, 614—619, 1975.
13. Adrian, J., *Rev. Fr. Corps Gras*, 23, 209—212, 1976.
14. Adrian, J., unpublished data.
15. Adrian, J., and Boisselot-Lefebvres, J., *Cahier Nutr. Diet*, 12, 233—234, 1977.
16. Adrian, J. and Favier, J. C., *Ann. Nutr. Aliment.*, 15, 181—225, 1961.
17. Adrian, J. and Frangne, R., *Ind. Aliment. Agric.*, 86, 801—806, 1969.
18. Adrian, J. and Frangne, R., *Ind. Aliment. Agric.*, 87, 393—399, 1970.
19. Adrian, J. and Frangne, R., *Ann. Nutr. Aliment.*, 27, 111—123, 1973.
20. Adrian, J. and Frangne, R., *Ind. Aliment. Agric.*, 92, 1365—1375, 1975.
21. Adrian, J. and Frangne, R., *Ind. Aliment. Agric.*, 93, 23—28, 1976.
22. Adrian, J. and Frangne, R., unpublished data.
23. Adrian, J., Frangne, R., Petit, L., Godon, B., and Barbier, J., *Ann. Nutr. Aliment.*, 20, 257—277, 1966.
23a. Adrian, J. and Jacquot, R., *Valeur Alimentaire De l'Arachide*, vol. 1, Maisonneuve et Larose, Paris, 1968.
24. Adrian, J., Petit, L., and Godon, B., *C. R. Acad. Sci.*, 255, 391—393, 1962.
25. Adrian, J. and Susbielle, H., *Ann. Nutr. Aliment.*, 29, 151—158, 1975.
26. Amadori, M., *Atti. Accad. Naz. Lincei. Mem. Cl. Sci. Fis. Mat. Nat. Rend.*, 2, 337, 1925; 9, 68, and 226, 1929; 13, 72 and 195, 1931.
27. Ambrose, A. M., Robbins, D. J., and de Eds, F., *Proc. Soc. Exp. Biol. Med.*, 106, 656—659, 1961.

28. Anantharaman, K. and Carpenter, K. J., *Proc. Nutr. Soc.*, 24, 32, 1965.
29. Anantharaman, K. and Carpenter, K. J., *J. Sci. Food Agric.*, 20, 703—708, 1969.
30. Anantharaman, K. and Carpenter, K. J., *J. Sci. Food Agric.*, 22, 412—418, 1971.
31. Andrews, F., Bjorksten, J., Trenk, F. B., Henick, A. S., and Koch, R. B., *J. Am. Oil Chem. Soc.*, 42, 779—781, 1965.
32. Anet, E. F. L. J., *Aust. J. Chem.*, 12, 491—496, 1959.
33. Anet, E. F. L. J., *Aust. J. Chem.*, 13, 396—403, 1960.
34. Anet, E. F. L. J., *Aust. J. Chem.*, 15, 503—509, 1962.
35. Anet, E. F. L. J., *Adv. Carbohydr. Chem.*, 19, 181—218, 1964.
36. Anet, E. F. L. J., *Tetrahedron Lett.*, 31, 3525—3528, 1968.
37. Arroyo, P. T. and Lilliard, D. A., *J. Food Sci.*, 35, 769—770, 1970.
38. Asquith, R. S., Otterburn, M. S., Buchanan, J. H., Cole, M., Fletcher, J. C., and Gardner, K. L., *Biochim. Biophys. Acta*, 221, 342—348, 1970.
39. Badenhop, A. F. and Hackler, L. R., *J. Food Sci.*, 36, 1—4, 1971.
40. Balasubranian, S. C., Ramachandran, M., Viswanathan, T., and De, S. S., *Indian Med. Res.*, 40, 219—234, 1952.
41. Baliga, B. P., Bayliss, M. E., and Lyman, C. M., *Arch. Biochem. Biophys.*, 84, 1—6, 1959.
42. Ballschmieter, H. M. B. and Derckson, A. W., *Fette Seifen Anstrichm.*, 72, 719—721, 1970.
43. Ballschmieter, H. M. B. and Germishuizen, P. J., *Fette Seifen Anstrichm.*, 70, 571—574, 1968.
44. Barnes, H. M. and Kaufman, C. W., *Ind. Eng. Chem.*, 39, 1167—1170, 1947.
45. Batzer, O. F., Santoro, A. T., and Landmann, W. A., *J. Agric. Food Chem.*, 10, 94—96, 1962.
46. Bavetta, L. A. and McClure, F. J., *J. Nutr.*, 63, 107—108, 1957.
47. Bender, A. E. and Haizelden, S., *Br. J. Nutr.*, 11, 42—43, 1957.
48. Ben—Gera, I. and Zimmermann, G., *Nature*, 202, 1007—1008, 1964.
49. Ben—Gera, I. and Zimmermann, G., *J. Food Sci. Technol.*, 9, 113—118, 1972.
50. Bennett, G., Liska, B. J., and Hempenius, W. L., *J. Food Sci.*, 30, 35—43, 1965.
51. Bertram, G. L., *Cereal Chem.*, 30, 127—139, 1953.
52. Bimbenet, J. J., Thesis, University of Paris, 1969.
53. Bissett, H. M. and Tarr, H. L. A., *Poultry Sci.*, 33, 250—254, 1954.
54. Bjarnason, J. and Carpenter, K. J., *Proc. Nutr. Soc.*, 28, 2A—3A, 1969.
55. Bjarnason, J. and Carpenter, K. J., *Br. J. Nutr.*, 23, 859—868, 1969.
56. Bjarnason, J. and Carpenter, K. J., *Br. J. Nutr.*, 24, 313—329, 1970.
57. Bleumink, E., personal communication.
58. Bleumink, E. and Young, E., *Int. Arch. Allergy Appl. Immunol.*, 81, 1136—1149, 1968.
59. Block, R. J., Jones, D. B., and Gersdorff, C. E. F., *J. Biol. Chem.*, 105, 667—668, 1934.
60. Bock, H. D. and Wünsche, J., *Nahrung*, 9, 131—135, 1965.
61. Boctor, A. M. and Harper, A. E., *J. Nutr.*, 94, 289—296, 1968.
62. Boge, G., *J. Sci. Food Agric.*, 11, 362—365, 1960.
63. Boggs, M. N. and Fevold, H. L., *Ind. Eng. Chem.*, 38, 1075—1079, 1946.
64. Bohart, G. S. and Carson, J. F., *Nature*, 175, 470—471, 1955.
65. Booth, V. H., *J. Sci. Food Agric.*, 22, 658—665, 1971.
66. Brown, D. F., Senn, V. J., Dollear, F. G., and Goldblatt, L. A., *J. Am. Oil Chem. Soc.*, 50, 16—20, 1973.
67. Brown, D. F., Senn, V. J., Stanley, J. B., and Dollear, F. G., *J. Agric. Food Chem.*, 20, 700—706, 1972.
68. Brüggemann, J. and Erbersdobler, H., *Z. Tierphysiol. Tierernaehr. Futtermittelkd.*, 24, 55—67, 1968.
69. Brüggemann, J. and Erbersdobler, H., *Z. Lebensm. Unters. Forsch.*, 137, 137—143, 1968.
70. Budny, J., Chodkowska, B., and Rutkowski, A., *Przem. Spozyw.*, 18, 153—157, 1964.
71. Bujard, E., Mauron J., and Bujard, E., *Arch. Anat. Histol. Embryol.*, 47, 241—272, 1964.
72. Buraczewska, L., Buraczewski, S., Raczynski, G., and Zebrowska, T., *Rocz. Nauk. Roln. Ser. B*, 94, 123—134, 1974.
73. Bürke, R. P., *S. Afr. Agric. Sci.*, 3, 633—641, 1960.
74. Burton, H., *J. Soc. Dairy Technol.*, 18, 58—65, 1965.
75. Burton, H. S., and McWeeny, D. J., *Nature*, 197, 266—268, 1963.
76. Burton, H. S. and McWeeny, D. J., *Nature*, 197, 1086—1087, 1963.
77. Burton, H. S. and McWeeny, D. J., *Chem. Ind.*, 11, 462—463, 1964.
78. Burton, H. S. McWeeny, D. J., and Biltcliffe, D. O., *J. Sci. Food Agric.*, 14, 911—920, 1963.
79. Burton, H. S., McWeeny, D. J., and Biltcliffe, D. O., *J. Food Sci.*, 28, 631—639, 1963.
80. Burton, H. S., McWeeny, D. J., and Biltcliffe, D. O., *Chem. Ind.*, 10, 693—695, 1963.
81. Burton, H. S., McWeeny, D. J., Pandhi, P. N., and Biltcliffe, D. O., *Nature*, 196, 948—950, 1962.
82. Buss, L. W. and Goddard, V. R., *Food Res.*, 13, 506—511, 1948.

83. Butterworth, M. H. and Fox, H. C., *Br. J. Nutr.,* 17, 445—452, 1963.
84. Carpenter, K. J., *Biochem. J.,* 77, 604—610, 1960.
85. Carpenter, K. J., *Nutr. Rev.,* 43, 423—451, 1973.
86. Carpenter, K. J. and Ellinger, G. M., *Proc. Biochem. Soc.,* 61(3), 11, 1955.
87. Carpenter, K. J. and Ellinger, G. M., *Poultry Sci.,* 34, 1451—1452, 1955.
88. Carpenter, K. J., Ellinger, G. M., Munro, M. I., and Rolfe, E. J., *Br. J. Nutr.,* 11, 162—173, 1957.
89. Carpenter, K. J., Lea, C. H., and Parr, L. J., *Br. J. Nutr.,* 17, 151—169, 1963.
90. Carpenter, K. J. and March, B. E., *Br. J. Nutr.,* 15, 403—410, 1961.
91. Carpenter, K. J., Morgan, C. B., Lea, C. H., and Parr, L. J., *Br. J. Nutr.,* 16, 451—465, 1962.
92. Carson, J. F., *J. Am. Chem. Soc.,* 77, 1881—1884, 1955.
93. Carson, J. F., *J. Am. Chem. Soc.,* 77, 5957—5960, 1955.
94. Carson, J. F. and Olcott, H. S., *J. Am. Chem. Soc.,* 76, 2257—2258, 1954.
95. Casey, J. C., Self, F., and Swain, R., *J. Food Sci.,* 30, 33—34, 1965.
96. Champagnat, A. and Adrian, J., *Pétrole et Protéines,* Vol. 1, Doin, Paris, 1974.
97. Chatelus, G., *Bull. Soc. Chim. Fr.,* 2523—2532, 1964.
98. Chichester, C. O. Stadtman, F. H., and Mackinney, G., *J. Am. Chem. Soc.,* 74, 3418—3420, 1952.
99. Chio, K. S. and Tappel, A. L., *Biochemistry,* 8, 2821—2827, 1969.
100. Clark, H. E., Howe, J. M., Mertz, E. T., and Reitz, L. L., *J. Am. Diet. Assoc.,* 35, 469—471, 1959.
101. Clarke, J. A. K. and Kennedy, B. M., *J. Food Sci.,* 27, 609—616, 1962.
102. Clegg, K. M., *J. Sci. Food Agric.,* 15, 878—885, 1964.
103. Cobb, W. Y. and Swaisgood, H. E., *J. Food Sci.,* 36, 538—539, 1971.
104. Cole, S. J., *J. Food Sci.,* 32, 245—250, 1967.
105. Collyer, D. M., *Bakers Dig.,* 38, 43—54, 1964.
106. Conkerton, E. J. and Frampton, V. L., *Arch. Biochem. Biophys.,* 81, 130—134, 1959.
107. Cook, B. B., Fraenkel-Conrat, J., Singer, B., and Morgan, A. F., *J. Nutr.,* 44, 217—235, 1951.
108. Cook, B. B., Morgan, A. F., Singer, B., and Parker, J., *J. Nutr.,* 44, 63—81, 1951.
109. Cook, B. B., Morgan, A. F., Weast, E. O., and Parker, J., *J. Nutr.,* 44, 51—61, 1951.
110. Cristol, P., Monnier, P., and Marot, R., *Bull. Soc. Chim. Biol.,* 24, 1412—1417, 1942.
111. Cubadda, R., Fabriani, G., and Resmini, P., *Quad. Nutr.,* 28, 199—208, 1968.
112. Czeremski, K. and Jarzabek, A., *Przem. Spozyw.,* 18, 714, 1964.
113. Danehy, J. P. and Pigman, W. W., *Adv. Food Res.,* 3, 241—290, 1951.
114. Daniels, D. G. H., *J. Sci. Food Agric.,* 22, 136—139, 1971.
115. Darsley, R. R. and Quesnel, V. C., *J. Sci. Food Agric.,* 23, 215—225, 1972.
116. Davis, R. M., Rizzo, P., and Smith, A. H., *J. Nutr.,* 37, 115—126, 1949.
117. Dechezleprêtre, S. and Guilbot, A., *Cah. Nutrit. Diet.,* 3(3), 39—45, 1968.
118. De Lange, P. and Van den Mijll Dekker, L. P., *Nature,* 173, 1040—1041, 1954.
119. Deschreider, A. R., *Rev. Ferment. Ind. Aliment.,* 9, 25—34, 1954; 9, 111—116, 1954.
120. De Vuyst, A., Vervach, W., Charlier, H. and Jadin, V., *Lait,* 52, 444—453, 1972.
121. Donoso, G., Lewis, O. A. M., Miller, D. S., and Payne, P. R., *J. Sci. Food Agric.,* 13, 192—196, 1962.
122. Drapron, R., and Beaux, Y., *C. R. Acad. Sci.,* 286, 2598—2600, 1969.
123. Dubrow, D. L. and Stillings, B. R., *J. Food Sci.,* 35, 677—680, 1970.
124. Dulcino, J. and Lontie, R., *Proc. 7th Coll. prot. biol. fluids,* Bruges, 1959, 99—104.
125. Du Toit, M. M. S. and Page, H. J., *J. Agric. Sci.,* 22, 115, 1932.
126. Dworschak, E., *Z. Lebens. Unters. Forsch.,* 143, 167—174, 1970.
127. Dworschak, E. and Hegedüs, M., *Acta Aliment. Budapest,* 3, 337—347, 1974.
128. Eggum, B. O., Nielsen, H. E., and Rasmussen, F. L., *Z. Tierphysiol. Tierernaehr. Futtermittelkd.,* 27, 18—23, 1970.
129. El—Dash, A. A., *Bakers Dig.,* 45(12), 26—31, 1971.
130. El—Dash, A. A. and Johnson, J. A., *Cereal Chem.,* 47, 247—259, 1970.
131. Ellis, G. P., *Adv. Carbohydr. Chem.,* 14, 63—134, 1959.
132. Ellis, G. P. and Honeyman, J., *Adv. Carbohydr. Chem.,* 10, 95—168, 1955.
133. El'Ode, K. E., Dornseifer, T. P., Keith, E. S., and Powers, J. J., *J. Food Sci.,* 31, 351—358, 1966.
134. Elred, N. R. and Rodney, G., *J. Biol. Chem.,* 112, 261—165, 1946.
135. Enders, C., *Kolloid Z.,* 85, 74, 1938.
136. Enders, C. and Theis, K., *Brennst. Chem.,* 19, 360—365, 1938; 19, 402—407, 1938; 19, 439—449, 1938.
137. Erbersdobler, H., *Milchwissenschaft,* 25, 280—284, 1970.
138. Erbersdobler, H. and Bock, G., *Naturwissenschaften,* 54, 648, 1967.
139. Erbersdobler, H. and Dümmer H., *Z. Tierphysiol. Tierernaehr. Futtermittelkd.,* 28, 224—231, 1971.
140. Erbersdobler, H., Dümmer, H., and Zucker, H., *Z. Tierphysiol. Tierernaehr. Futtermittelkd.,* 24, 136—152, 1968.

141. Erbersdobler, H., Weber, G., and Gunsser, I., *Z. Tierphysiol. Tierernaehr. Futtermittelkd.*, 29, 325—334, 1972.

142. Erbersdobler, H. and Zucker, H., *Z. Tierphysiol. Tierernaehr. Futtermittelkd.*, 19, 244—255, 1964.

143. Erbersdobler, H. and Zucker, H., *Monatsh. Futtermittelkd. Wirtschaft*, 49(7), 1966.

144. Erbersdobler, H. and Zucker, H., *Milchwissenschaft.*, 21, 564—568, 1966.

145. Ericson, L. E. and Larsson, S., *Acta Physiol. Scand.*, 55, 64—73, 1962.

146. Ericson, L. E., Larsson, S., and Lid, G., *Acta Physiol. Scand.*, 53, 85—98, 1961; 53, 366—375, 1961.

147. Evans, R. J., Bandemer, S. L., and Bauer, D. H., *J. Food Sci.*, 26, 663—669, 1961.

148. Evans, R. J. and Butts, H. A., *J. Biol. Chem.*, 175, 15—20, 1948.

149. Evans, R. J. and Butts, H. A., *J. Biol. Chem.*, 178, 543—548, 1949.

150. Evans, R. J. and Butts, H. A., *Science*, 109, 569—571, 1949.

151. Evans, R. J. and Butts, H. A., *Food Res.*, 16, 415—421, 1951.

152. Fagerson, I. S., *J. Agric. Food Chem.*, 17, 747—750, 1969.

153. Feeney, R. E., Clary, J. J., and Clark, J. R., *Nature*, 201, 192—193, 1964.

154. Ferrando, R., *C. R. Acad. Sci.*, 257, 1161—1163, 1963.

155. Ferrando, R., *Bull. Acad. Natl. Med. Paris*, 148, 570—576, 1964.

156. Ferrando, R., Henry N., and Parodi, A., *C. R. Acad. Sci.*, 259, 1237—1238, 1964.

157. Ferreira, M. F., *Bol. Pecu.*, 32, 25—35, 1964.

158. Ferretti, A. and Flanagan, V. P., *J. Dairy Sci.*, 54, 1769—1771, 1971.

159. Ferretti, A. and Flanagan, V. P., *J. Agric. Food Chem.*, 19, 245—249, 1971.

160. Ferretti, A. and Flanagan, V. P., *J. Agric. Food Chem.*, 20, 695—698, 1972.

161. Ferretti, A., Flanagan, V. P., and Ruth, J. M., *J. Agric. Food Chem.*, 18, 13—18, 1970.

162. Fink, H., *Milchwissenschaft.*, 14, 323—325, 1959.

163. Fink, H., *Nahrung*, 7, 277—288, 1963.

164. Fink, H., Schlie, I., and Ruge, U., *Z. Naturforsch.*, 13B, 610—616, 1958.

165. Finot, P. A. and Mauron, J., *Helv. Chim. Acta*, 55, 1153—1164, 1972.

166. Finot, P. A., Viani, R., Bricout, J., and Mauron, J., *Experientia*, 24, 1097—1099, 1968.

167. Finot, P. A., Viani, R., Bricout, J., and Mauron, J., *Experientia*, 25, 134—135, 1969.

168. Fitzpatrick, T. J. and Porter, W. L., *Am. Potato J.*, 45, 103—110, 1968.

169. Ford, J. E., *Br. J. Nutr.*, 16, 409—425, 1962.

170. Ford, J. E., *Br. J. Nutr.*, 18, 449—460, 1964.

171. Ford, J. E. and Salter, D. N., *Br. J. Nutr.*, 20, 843—860, 1966.

172. Ford, J. E. and Shorrock, G., *Br. J. Nutr.*, 26, 311—322, 1971.

173. Fore, S. P., Goldblatt, L. A., and Dupuy, H. P., *J. Am. Peanut Res. Educ. Assoc.*, 4, 177—185, 1972.

174. Fox, M. R. S. and Mickelsen, O., *J. Nutr.*, 68, 289—295, 1959.

175. Fraenkel-Conrat, H. and Mecham, D. K., *J. Biol. Chem.*, 177, 477—486, 1949.

176. Frangne, R. and Adrian, J., *Ann. Nutr. Aliment.*, 163—174, 1967.

177. Frangne, R. and Adrian, J., *Ann. Nutr. Aliment.*, 26, 97—106, 1972.

178. Frangne, R. and Adrian, J., *Ann. Nutr. Aliment.*, 26, 107—119, 1972.

179. Franske, C. and Iwainsky, H., *Dtsch. Lebensm. Rundschau*, 50, 251—254, 1954.

180. Freimuth, U., *Period. Polytech. Budapest*, 17, 19—28, 1973.

181. Freimuth, U. and Trübsbach, A., *Nahrung*, 13, 199—206, 1969.

182. Friedman, L. and Kline, O. L., *J. Biol. Chem.*, 184, 599—606, 1950.

183. Fujimoto, K., Saito, J., and Kaneda, T., *Nippon Suisan Gakkaishi*, 37, 44—47, 1971.

184. Gates, J. C. and Kennedy, B. M., *J. Amer. Diet. Assoc.*, 44, 374—377, 1964.

185. Ginger, I. D., Wachter, J. P., Doty, D. M., and Schweigert, B. S., *Food Res.*, 19, 410—416, 1954.

186. Gorbach, G. and Regula, E., *Fette Seifen*, 66, 920—925, 1964.

187. Gortner, R. A. and Blish, M. J., *J. Am. Chem. Soc.*, 37, 1630, 1915.

188. Gottschalk, A., *Biochem. J.*, 52, 455—460, 1952.

189. Gottschalk, A. and Partridge, S. M., *Nature*, 165, 684—685, 1950.

190. Gould, I. A., *J. Dairy Sci.*, 28, 367—377, 1945.

191. Grafe, as cited by Wahl, P., *Acta Chim. Acad. Sci. Hung.*, 23, 159—177, 1960.

192. Greaves, E. O. and Morgan, A. F., *Proc. Soc. Exp. Biol. Med.*, 31, 506—507, 1933.

193. Gregory, M. E., Henry, K. M., and Kon, S. K., *J. Dairy Res.*, 31, 113—119, 1964.

194. Hackler, L. R. and Stillings, B. R., *Cereal Chem.*, 44, 70—77, 1967.

195. Hagan, S. N., Horn, M. J., Lipton, S. H., and Womack, M., *J. Agric. Food Chem.*, 18, 273—275, 1970.

196. Handwerck, V., Bujard, E., and Mauron, J., *Biochem. J.*, 76, 1—54, 1960.

197. Hannan, R. S. and Lea, C. H., *Biochim. Biophys. Acta*, 9, 293—305, 1952.

198. Hauffpauir, C. L., *J. Agric. Food Chem.*, 1, 668—671, 1953.

199. Heller, B. S., Chutkow, M. R., Lushbough, C. H., Siedler, A. J., and Schweigert, B. S., *J. Nutr.,* 73, 113—116, 1961.
200. Hendel, C. E., Burr, H. K., and Boggs, M. M., *Food Technol.,* 9, 627—629, 1955.
201. Henry, K. M., Houston, J., Kon, S. K., and Thompson, S. Y., *J. Dairy Res.,* 13, 329—339, 1944.
202. Henry, K. M., Kon, S. K., Lea, C. H., Smith, J. A. B., and White, J. C. D., *Nature,* 158, 348, 1946.
203. Henry, K. M., Kon, S. K., Lea, C. H., and White, J. C. D., *J. Dairy Res.,* 15, 292—363, 1948.
204. Henry, K. M., Kon, S. K., and Rowland, S. J., *J. Dairy Res.,* 14, 403—414, 1946.
205. Hepburn, F. N., Lewis, E. W., Jr., and Elvehjem, C. A., *Cereal Chem.,* 34, 312—322, 1957.
206. Herz, K. O. and Chang, S. S., *Adv. Food Res.,* 18, 1—83, 1970.
207. Herz, W. J. and Schallenberger, R. S., *Food Res.,* 25, 491—494, 1960.
208. Heyns, K., Breuer, H., and Paulsen, H., *Chem. Ber.,* 90, 1374—1386, 1957.
209. Heyns, K., Heukeshoven, J., and Brose, K. H., *Angew Chem.,* 80, 627, 1968.
210. Heyns, K. and Koch, W., *Z. Naturforsch.,* 7B, 486—488, 1952.
211. Heyns, K., Koch, H., and Röper, H., N—nitroso Compounds Anal. Form., Proc. Work Conf., 48—54, 1971.
212. Heyns, K. and Meinecke, K. H., *Chem. Ber.,* 86, 1453—1462, 1953.
213. Heyns, K. and Paulsen, H., *Wiss. Veroeff. Dtsch. Ges. Ernaehr.,* 5, 15—42, 1960.
214. Heyns, K., Paulsen, H., and Breuer, H., *Angew. Chem.,* 68, 334—335, 1956.
215. Heyns, K., Paulsen, H., and Schroeder, H., *Tetrahedron,* 13, 247—257, 1961.
216. Hodge, J. E., *J. Agric. Food Chem.,* 1, 928—943, 1953.
217. Hodge, J. E., *Adv. Carbohydr. Chem.,* 10, 169—205, 1955.
218. Hodge, J. E., in *Chemistry and Physiology of Flavors,* Schultz, H. W., Day, E. A., and Libbey, L. M., Eds., AVI Publishing, Westport, Conn., 1967, 465—491.
219. Hodge, J. E. and Rist, C. E., *J. Am. Chem. Soc.,* 75, 316—322, 1953.
220. Hoffmann, C. E., Stokstad, E. L. R., Hutchings, B. L., Dornbusch, A. C., and Jukes, T. H., *J. Biol. Chem.,* 181, 635—644, 1949.
221. Holm, H., *J. Sci. Food Agric.,* 22, 378—381, 1971.
222. Holtermand, A., *Stärke,* 18, 319—328, 1966.
223. Horn, M. J., Lichtenstein, H., and Womack, M., *J. Agric. Food Chem.,* 16, 741—745, 1968.
224. Horstein, J., Crowe, P. E., and Salzbacher, W. L., *J. Agric. Chem.,* 8, 65—67, 1960.
225. Hrdlicka, J., and Kuca, J., *Poultry Sci.,* 44, 27—31, 1965.
226. Hsu, P. T., McGinnis, J., and Graham, W. D., *Poultry Sci.,* 27, 668, 1948.
227. Hughes, R. B., *J. Sci. Food Agric.,* 12, 475—483, 1961.
228. Hugot, D. and Causeret, J., *Ann. Technol. Agric.,* 11, 55—62, 1962.
229. Hunter, I. R., Walden, M. K., McFadden, W. H., and Pence, J. W., *Cereal Sci. Today,* 11, 493—494, 1966.
230. Hunter, I. R., Walden, M. K., Scherer, J. R., and Lundin, R. E., *Cereal Chem.,* 46, 189—195, 1969.
231. Huss, W., *Landwirtsch. Forsch.,* 27, 199—210, 1974.
232. Huss, W., *Z. Tierphysiol. Tierenaehr. Futtermittelkd.,* 34, 60—67, 1974.
233. Iacobellis, M., *Arch. Biochem.,* 59, 199—206, 1955.
234. Impens, X. X., personal communication.
235. Jackson, H. W. and Morgan, M. E., *J. Dairy Sci.,* 37, 1316—1324, 1954.
236. Janicek, G. and Pokorny, J., *Z. Lebensch. Unters. Forsch.,* 145, 142—147, 1971.
237. Jemmali, M., Thesis, University of Paris, Ser. A, No. 942, 1965.
238. Jemmali, M., *C. R. Acad. Sci.,* 264, 2672—2674, 1967.
239. Jemmali, M., Petit, L., and Godon, B., *36th Int. Congr. Ind. Chem.,* 642(11), 28, 1966.
240. Jenness, R. and Coulter, S. T., *J. Dairy Sci.,* 31, 367—381, 1948.
241. Johansen, G. and Nickerson, J. W., *1st Int. Congr. Biochem.,* Cambridge, Abstr. 223, 1949.
242. Johnson, J. A. and El—Dash, A. A., *Bakers Dig.,* 41(10), 74—78, 1967.
243. Johnson, J. A. and El—Dash, A. A., *J. Agric. Food Chem.,* 17, 740—746, 1969.
244. Johnson, J. A., Rooney, L., and Salem, A., *Adv. Chem. Ser.* 56, 153—173, 1966.
245. Johnson, J. A. and Sanchez, C., Flavor Symp. 162nd ACS Annu. Mtg., 1971.
246. Jones, N. R., *Food Res.,* 24, 704—710, 1959.
247. Jones, D. B., Divine, J. P., and Gersdorff, C. E. F., *Cereal Chem.,* 19, 819—830, 1942.
248. Jones, D. B. and Gersdorff, C. E. F., *Cereal Chem.,* 18, 417—434, 1941.
249. Kajimoto, G. and Yoshida, H., *Nippon Nogei Kagaku Kaishi,* 47, 515—522, 1973.
250. Kakade, M. L. and Evans, R. J., *Can. J. Biochem.,* 44, 648—650, 1966.
251. Kass, J. P. and Palmer, L. S., *Ind. Eng. Chem.,* 32, 1360—1366, 1940.
252. Kato, H., *Bull. Agric. Chem. Soc. Jpn.,* 20, 273—278, 1956.
253. Kato, H., *Bull. Agric. Chem. Soc. Jpn.,* 24, 1—12, 1960.
254. Kedenburg, C. P., *Landwirtsch. Forsch. Sonderh.,* 23, 59—62, 1969.

255. Keeney, P. G., *J. Am. Oil Chem. Soc.*, 49, 567—572, 1972.
256. Keeney, M. and Bassette, R., *J. Dairy Sci.*, 42, 945—960, 1959.
257. Keeney, M. and Day, E. A., *J. Dairy Sci.*, 40, 874—876, 1957.
258. Kellenbarger, S., *Poultry Sci.*, 40, 1756—1759, 1961.
259. Kinsella, J. E., *Adv. Food Res.*, 19, 147—213, 1971.
260. Kisza, J., Sobina, A., and Zbikowski, Z., 17th Int. Congr. Dairy, E3, 85—9, 1966.
261. Kline, R. W. and Stewart, G. F., *Ind. Eng. Chem.*, 40, 919—922, 1948.
262. Kobayasi, N. and Fujimaki, M., *Agric. Biol. Chem.*, 29, 1059—1060, 1965.
263. Koehler, P. E., Mason, M. E., and Odell, G. V., *J. Food Sci.*, 36, 816—818, 1971.
264. Koyoumdjisky, E., *J. Nutr.*, 63, 509—522, 1957.
265. Kraft, R. A. and Morgan, A. F., *J. Nutr.*, 45, 567—581, 1952.
266. Krause, W. and Schmidt, K., *Nahrung*, 18, 833—839, 1974.
267. Kretovich, W. L. and Ponomareva, A. N., *Biokhimya*, 26, 237—243, 1961.
268. Krug, E., Prellwitz, W., Schäffner, E., Kiekebusch, W., and Lang, K., *Naturwissenschaften*, 46, 534—535, 1959.
269. Kubota, T., *J. Biochem. Tokyo*, 34, 119—141, 1941.
270. Kurata, T. and Sakurai, Y., *Agric. Biol. Chem.*, 31, 177—184, 1967.
271. Kuwabara, S., Simizu, U., and Yajima, M., *Nippon Nogei Kagaku Kaishi*, 46, 89—93, 1972.
272. Kwon, T. W., Menzel, D. B., and Olcott, H. S., *J. Food Sci.*, 30, 808—813, 1965.
273. Lafar, F., *Z. Oesterr. Ing. Zuckerindust.*, 42, 737, 1913.
274. Lang, K. and Schäffner, E., *Z. Ernaehrungswiss.*, 4, 235—245, 1964.
275. Lea, C. H., unpublished data.
276. Lea, C. H. and Hannan, R. S., *Biochim. Biophys. Acta*, 3, 313—325, 1949.
277. Lea, C. H. and Hannan, R. S., *Biochim. Biophys. Acta*, 5, 433—456, 1950.
278. Lea, C. H. and Hannan, R. S., *Biochim. Biophys. Acta*, 4, 518—531, 1950.
279. Lea, C. H. and Hannan, R. S., *Nature*, 165, 438—439, 1950.
280. Lea, C. H., Parr, L. J., and Carpenter, K. J., *Br. J. Nutr.*, 12, 297—312, 1958.
281. Lea, C. H., Parr, L. J., and Carpenter, K. J., *Br. J. Nutr.*, 14, 91—113, 1960.
282. Leclerc, J. and Benoiton, L., *Can. J. Biochem.*, 45, 471—475, 1968.
283. Ledl, F. and Severin, T., *Chem. Mikrobiol. Technol. Lebensm.*, 2, 155—160, 1973.
284. Legault, R. R., Talburt, W. F., Mulne, A. M., and Bryan, L. A., *Ind. Eng. Chem.*, 39, 1294—1299, 1947.
285. Lento, H. G., Jr., Underwood, J. C., and Willits, C. O., *Food Res.*, 23, 68—71, 1958.
286. Lewin, S., *Biochem. J.*, 63, 14—22, 1956.
287. Lewis, V. M., Esselen, W. B. Jr., and Fellers, C. R., *Ind. Eng. Chem.*, 61, 2587—2591, 1949.
288. Lewis, V. M., Esselen, W. B., Jr., and Fellers, C. R., *Ind. Eng. Chem.*, 61, 2591—2594, 1949.
289. Lewis, V. M. and Lea, C. H., *Biochim. Biophys. Acta*, 4, 532—534, 1950.
290. Lindsay, R. C. and Lau, V. K., *J. Food Sci.*, 37, 787—788, 1972.
291. Ling, A. R., *J. Inst. Brew. London*, 14, 494, 1908.
292. Linko, Y. Y. and Johnson, J. A., *J. Agric. Food Chem.*, 11, 150—152, 1963.
293. Linko, Y. Y., Johnson, J. A., and Miller, B. S., *Cereal Chem.*, 39, 468—476, 1962.
294. Loncin, M., Jacqmain, D., Tutundjian-Provost, A. M., Lenges, J. P., and Bimbenet, J. J., *C. R. Acad. Sci.*, 260, 3208—3211, 1965; *J. Food Technol.*, 3, 131—142, 1968.
295. Luh, B. S. and Chaudhry, M. S., *Food Technol.*, 15, 52—54, 1961.
296. Lushbough, C. H., Porter, T., and Schweigert, B. S., *J. Nutr.*, 62, 513—526, 1957.
297. Lyman, C. M., Baliga, B. P., and Slay, M. W., *Arch. Biochem. Biophys.*, 84, 486—497, 1959.
298. Lyman, C. M. and Thomas, M. C., *J. Assoc. Off. Agric. Chem.*, 48, 858—859, 1965.
299. McClure, F. J., *Science*, 116, 229—231, 1952.
300. McClure, F. J. and Folk, J. E., *J. Nutr.*, 55, 589—599, 1955.
301. McDermott, E. E. and Pace, J., *Br. J. Nutr.*, 11, 446—452, 1957.
302. McDonald, F. J., *Nature*, 209, 1134, 1966.
303. McDonald, J. and Gilles, F., *Bakers Dig.*, 41(2), 45—49, 1967.
304. McGarr Gotthold, M. L. and Kennedy, B. M., *J. Food Sci.*, 29, 227—232, 1964.
305. McKeen, W. E., *Science*, 123, 509, 1956.
306. McLeod, P. and Morgan, M. E., *J. Dairy Sci.*, 39, 1125—1133, 1956.
307. McWeeny, D. J. and Burton, H. S., *J. Sci. Food Agric.*, 14, 291—302, 1963.
308. Macy, R. L., Jr., Naumann, H. D., and Bailey, M. E., *J. Food Sci.*, 29, 136—141, 1964; 29, 142—148, 1964.
309. Mader, I. J., Schroeder, L. J., and Smith, A. H., *J. Nutr.*, 39, 341—355, 1949.
310. Maillard, L. C., *C. R. Acad. Sci.*, 154, 66—68, 1912.
311. Maillard, L. C., *C. R. Soc. Biol.*, 72, 599—601, 1912.
312. Maillard, L. C., *C. R. Acad. Sci.*, 155, 1554—1556, 1912.

313. Maillard, L. C., *C. R. Acad. Sci.*, 156, 1159—1162, 1913.

314. Maillard, L. C., *Ann. Chim. Paris*, 6, 258—317, 1916.

315. Maillard, L. C., *Ann. Chim. Paris*, 7, 113—152, 1917.

316. Maleki, M., *Fette Seifen Anstrichm.*, 75, 103—104, 1973.

317. Maleki, M. and Djazayeri, A., *J. Sci. Food Agric.*, 19, 449—451, 1968.

318. Malshet, V. G. and Tappel, A. L., *Lipids*, 8, 194—198, 1973.

319. Manley, C. H., Vallon, P. P., and Erickson, R. E., *J. Food Sci.*, 39, 73—76, 1974.

320. Markova, J., Honischova, E., and Hampl, J., *Brot Gebaeck*, 9, 166—173, 1970.

321. Markuse, Z., *Rocz. Pzh.*, 7, 395—404, 1956.

322. Martinez, W. H., Beradi, L. C., Frampton, V. L., Wilcke, H. L., Greene, D. E., and Teichman, R., *J. Agric. Food Chem.*, 15, 427—432, 1967.

323. Martinez, W. H., Frampton, V. L., and Cabell, C. A., *J. Agric. Food Chem.*, 9, 64—66, 1961.

324. Mason, M. E., Johnson, B., and Hamming, M. C., *J. Agric. Food Chem.*, 14, 454—460, 1966.

325. Mason, M. E., Johnson, B., and Hamming, M. C., *J. Agric. Food Chem.*, 15, 66—73, 1967.

326. Mason, M. E., Newell, J. A., Johnson, B. R., Koehler, P. E., and Waller, G. R., *J. Agric. Food Chem.*, 17, 728—732, 1969.

327. Mason, M. E. and Waller, G. R., *J. Agric. Food Chem.*, 12, 274—278, 1964.

328. Mauron, J., *Int. J. Vit.*, 34, 96—116, 1964.

329. Mauron, J., *Int. J. Vit. Nutr. Res.*, 40, 209—227, 1970.

330. Mauron, J. and Mottu, F., *Arch. Biochem. Biophys.*, 77, 312—327, 1958.

331. Mauron, J. and Mottu, F., *J. Agric. Food Chem.*, 10, 512—515, 1962.

332. Mauron, J., Mottu, F., Bujard, E., and Egli, R. H., *Arch. Biochem.*, 59, 433—451, 1955.

333. Menden, E. and Cremer, H. D., *Z. Lebensm. Unters. Forsch.*, 104, 105—121, 1956.

334. Micheel, F. and Dijong, I., *Liebigs Ann. Chem.*, 658, 120—127, 1962.

335. Micheel, F. and Klemer, A., *Chem. Ber.*, 84, 212—215, 1951; 85, 1083—1086, 1952; Micheel, F. and Dinkloh, E., *Chem. Ber.*, 84, 210—212, 1951.

336. Miller, E. L., Carpenter, K. J., and Milner, C. K., *Br. J. Nutr.* 19, 547—564, 1965.

337. Miller, E. L., Hartley, A. W., and Thomas, D. C., *Br. J. Nutr.* 19, 565—573, 1965.

338. Milner, C. K. and Westgarth, D. R., *J. Sci. Food Agric.*, 24, 873—882, 1973.

339. Min, L. C., *Diss Abstr. Int.* 1125B, 1975.

340. Minor, L. J., Pearson, A. M., Dawson, L. E., and Schweigert, B. S., *J. Agric. Food Chem.*, 13, 298—300, 1965.

341. Mohammad, A., Fraenkel-Conrat, H., and Olcott, H. S., *Arch. Biochem.*, 24, 157—178, 1949.

342. Mohammad, A., Olcott, H. S., and Fraenkel-Conrat, H., *Arch. Biochem.*, 24, 270—280, 1949.

343. Mohr, W., Röhrle, M., and Severin, T., *Fette Seifen Anstrichm.*, 73, 515—521, 1971.

344. Montgomery, M. W. and Day, E. A., *J. Food Sci.*, 30, 728—732, 1965.

345. Mori, Y. and Kano, M., *Eiyo To Shokuryo*, 27, 255—261, 1974.

346. Morimoto, T., *J. Food Sci.*, 31, 736—741, 1966.

347. Morrison, A. B., *Can. J. Biochem. Physiol.*, 41, 1589—1594, 1963.

348. Morrison, A. B. and Sabry, Z. I., *Can. J. Biochem. Physiol.*, 41, 649—655, 1963.

349. Motai, H. and Inoue, S., *Agric. Biol. Chem.*, 38, 233—239, 1974; Motai, H., *Agric. Biol. Chem.*, 38, 2299—2304, 1974.

350. Mulders, E. J., *Z. Lebensm. Unters. Forsch.*, 152, 193—201, 1973.

351. Mulders, E. J. and Dhont, J. H., *Z. Lebensm. Unters. Forsch.*, 150, 228—232, 1972.

352. Mulders, E. J., Maarse, H., and Weurman, C., *Z. Lebensm. Unters. Forsch.*, 150, 68—74, 1972.

353. Mulders, E. J., Ten Noever de Brauw, M. C., and Van Straten, S., *Z. Lebensm. Unters. Forsch.*, 150, 305—310, 1973.

354. Myklestad, O., Bjornstad, J., and Njaa, L. R., *Fiskeri dir. Nor. Skr. Ser. Teknol. Unders.*, 5(10), 3—15, 1972.

355. Nagayama, F., *Bull. Jpn. Soc. Sci. Fish.*, 26, 1026—1031, 1960.

356. Nagayama, F., *Bull. Jpn. Soc. Sci. Fish.*, 26, 1107—1113, 1960.

357. Nagayama, F., *Bull. Jpn. Soc. Sci. Fish.*, 27, 28—33, 1961.

358. Nagayama, F., *Bull. Jpn. Soc. Sci. Fish.*, 27, 34—37, 1961.

359. Nagayama, F., *Bull. Jpn. Soc. Sci. Fish.*, 27, 158—161, 1961.

360. Nagayama, F., *Bull. Jpn. Soc. Sci. Fish.*, 28, 45—48, 1962.

361. Nagayama, F., *Bull. Jpn. Soc. Sci. Fish.*, 28, 49—54, 1962.

362. Nagayama, F., *Bull. Jpn. Soc. Sci. Fish.*, 28, 165—168, 1962.

363. Nagayama, F., Hiraide, H., and Sano, K., *Bull. Jpn. Soc. Sci. Fish.*, 28, 1188—1191, 1962.

364. Nagayama, F. and Ono, T., *J. Tokyo Univ. Fish.*, 50, 31—36, 1963.

365. Nagayama, F. and Ono, T., *J. Tokyo Univ. Fish.*, 50, 37—41, 1963.

366. Nagayama, F. and Sano, K., *Bull. Jpn. Soc. Sci. Fish.*, 28, 828—832, 1962.

367. Nakanishi, T. and Itoh, T., *Milchwissenschaft*, 21, 635—637, 1966.

368. Nakanishi, T. and Itoh, T., *Agric. Biol. Chem.*, 31, 1066—1069, 1967.
369. Narayan, K. A., Sugai, M., and Kummerov, F. A., *J. Am. Oil Chem. Soc.*, 41, 254—259, 1964.
370. Nawar, W. W., *Food Technol.*, 20, 115—117, 1966.
371. Nesheim, M. C. and Carpenter, K. J., *Br. J. Nutr.*, 21, 399—411, 1967.
372. Neucere, N. J., Conkerton, E. J., and Booth, A. N., *J. Agric. Food Chem.*, 20, 256—259, 1972.
373. Newell, J. A., Mason, M. E., and Matlock, R. S., *J. Agric. Food Chem.*, 15, 767—772, 1967.
374. Nielsen, J. J. and Weidner, K., *Acta Agric. Scand.*, 16, 144—146, 1966.
375. Nikonorow, M. and Przybinska-Karpinska, H., *Rocz. Pzh.*, 11, 23—32, 1960.
376. Olcott, H. S. and Dutton, H. J., *Ind. Eng. Chem.*, 37, 1119—1121, 1945.
377. Olley, J. and Watson, H., *J. Sci. Food Agric.*, 12, 316—326, 1961.
378. Ono, T. and Nagayama, F., *Bull. Jpn. Soc. Sci. Fish.*, 24, 833—836, 1959.
379. Ono, T., Nagayama, F., Yoshikane, T., and Muto, Y., *Bull. Jpn. Soc. Sci. Fish.*, 28, 936—940, 1962.
380. Ostrowski, H., Jones, A. S., and Cadenhead, A., *J. Sci. Food Agric.*, 21, 103—107, 1970.
381. Overby, L. R., Fredrickson, R. L., and Frost, D. V., *J. Nutr.*, 69, 318—322, 1959.
382. Overby, L. R. and Frost, D. V., *J. Nutr.*, 46, 539—550, 1952.
383. Pace, J. K. and Whitacre, J., *Food Res.*, 18, 231—238, 1953.
384. Pace, J. K. and Whitacre, J., *Food Res.*, 18, 245—249, 1953.
385. Paik, W. K. and Benoiton, L., *Can. J. Biochem. Physiol.*, 41, 1643—1654, 1963.
386. Paik, W. K. and Kim, S., *Nature*, 202, 793—794, 1964.
387. Pais de Azevedo, J., Rebelo Abranches, J. A. P. F., and Soares Costa, M. J. D., *Melhoramento*, 15, 91—135, 1962.
388. Palm, D. and Simon, H., *Naturforscher*, 20, 32—35, 1965.
389. Patrick, T. M., Jr., *J. Am. Chem. Soc.*, 74, 2984—2986, 1952.
390. Patron, A., *Fruits Outre Mer*, 5, 201—207, 1950.
391. Pattee, H. E., Beasley, E. O., and Singleton, J. A., *J. Food Sci.*, 30, 388—392, 1965.
392. Patton, S., *J. Dairy Sci.*, 33, 324—328, 1950.
393. Patton, S., *J. Dairy Sci.*, 35, 1053—1066, 1952.
394. Patton, S., *J. Dairy Sci.*, 37, 446—452, 1954.
395. Patton, S., *J. Dairy Sci.*, 38, 457—478, 1955.
396. Patton, S., *J. Food Sci.*, 29, 679—680, 1964.
397. Patton, A. R. and Chism, P., *Nature*, 167, 406, 1951.
398. Payne-Botha, S. and Bigwood, E. J., *Br. J. Nutr.*, 13, 385—389, 1959.
399. Pearce, J. A., *Ind. Eng. Chem.*, 41, 1514—1517, 1949.
400. Pearce, J. A., *Food Technol.*, 4, 416—419, 1950.
401. Pearson, A. M., Harrington, G., West, R. G., and Spooner, M. E., *J. Food Sci.*, 27, 177—181, 1962.
402. Pearson, A. M., Tarladgis, B. G., Spooner, M. E., and Quinn, J. R., *J. Food Sci.*, 31, 184—190, 1966.
403. Pecherer, B., *J. Am. Chem. Soc.*, 73, 3827—3830, 1951.
404. Persson, T. and Von Sydow, E., *J. Food Sci.*, 39, 406—413, 1974.
405. Persson, T., Von Sydow, E., and Akesson, C., *J. Food Sci.*, 38, 682—689, 1973.
406. Petit, L., *Ann. Technol.*, 1, 5—33, 1959.
407. Petit, L., *Ind. Aliment. Agric.*, 81, 905—914, 1964.
408. Petit, L. and Godon, B., *C. R. Acad. Sci.*, 257, 1993—1995, 1963.
409. Pigman, W., Cleveland, E. A., Couch, D. H., and Cleveland, J. H., *J. Am. Chem. Soc.*, 73, 1976—1979, 1951.
410. Pijanowski, E., Kolanecka, H., and Molska, I., *Rocz. Technol. Chem. Zywn.*, 19, 19—35, 1970.
411. Pinto, A. and Chichester, C. O., *J. Food Sci.*, 31, 726—732, 1966.
412. Pion, R. and Rerat, A., *16th Int. Congr. Dairy*, 2, 993—1001, 1962.
413. Pippen, E. L., Fyring, E. J., and Nonaka, M., *Poultry Sci.*, 39, 922—924, 1960.
414. Pisano, J. J., Finlayson, J. S., and Peyton, M. P., *Biochemistry*, 8, 871—876, 1969.
415. Pokorny, J., *Prom. Potravin.*, 21, 262—263, 1970.
416. Pokorny, J., Côn, N. H., and Janicek, G., *Sci. Pap. Inst. Chem. Technol. Prague*, 1972.
417. Pokorny, J., Côn, N. H., Smidrkalova, E., and Janicek, G., *Z. Lebensm. Unters. Forsch.*, 158, 87—92, 1975.
418. Pokorny, J., El-Zeany, B. A., and Janicek, G., *Z. Lebensm. Unters. Forsch.*, 151, 31—35, 1973.
419. Pokorny, J., El-Zeany, B. A., and Janicek, G., *Z. Lebensm. Unters. Forsch.*, 151, 157—161, 1973.
420. Pokorny, J., El-Zeany, B. A., Kolakowska, A., and Janicek, G., *Z. Lebensm. Unters. Forsch.*, 155, 287—291, 1974.
421. Pokorny, J. and Janicek, G., *Z. Lebensm. Unters. Forsch.*, 145, 217—222, 1971.

422. Pokorny, J., Luan, N. T., and Janicek, G., *Z. Lebensm. Unters. Forsch.*, 152, 65—70, 1973.
423. Pokorny, J., Tai, P. T., and Janicek, G., *Z. Lebensm. Unters. Forsch.*, 151, 36—40, 1973.
424. Pomeranz, Y., Johnson, J. A., and Schellenberger, J. A., *J. Food Sci.*, 27, 350—354, 1962.
425. Porter, R. R. and Sanger, F., *Biochem. J.*, 42, 287—294, 1948.
426. Powell, R. C. T. and Spark, A. A., *J. Sci. Food Agric.*, 22, 596—599, 1971.
427. Prahl, L. and Taüfel, K., *Nahrung*, 11, 257—265, 1967.
428. Proctor, B. E., and Goldblich, S. A., *Science*, 109, 519—522, 1949.
429. Raczynski, G. and Buraczewski, S., *Arch. Tierenaehr.*, 25, 151—156, 1975.
430. Ramshaw, E. H. and Dunstone, E. A., *J. Dairy Sci.*, 36, 203—213, 1969.
431. Rao, M. N. and McLaughlan, J. M., *J. Assoc. Off. Anal. Chem.*, 50, 704—707, 1967.
432. Rao, M. N., Sreenivas, H., Swaminathan, M., Carpenter, K. J., and Morgan, C. B., *J. Sci. Food Agric.*, 14, 544—550, 1963.
433. Rao, S. R., Carter, F. L., and Frampton, V. L., *Anal. Chem.*, 35, 1927—1930, 1963.
434. Reynolds, T. M., *Aust. J. Chem.*, 12, 265—274, 1959.
435. Reynolds, T. M., *Adv. Food Res.*, 12, 1—52, 1963; 14, 168—283, 1965.
436. Reynolds, T. M., in *Carbohydrates and Their Roles*, Schultz, H. W., Cain, R. F., and Wrolstad, R. W., Eds., AVI Publishing, Westport, Conn., 1969.
437. Richards, E. L., *Biochem. J.*, 64, 639—644, 1956.
438. Rice, E. W., *Clin. Chem.*, 18, 1550—1551, 1972.
439. Rice, R. G., Kertesz, Z. I., and Stotz, E. H., *J. Am. Chem. Soc.*, 69, 1798—1800, 1947.
440. Riesen, W. H., Clandinin, D. R., Elvehjem, C. A., and Cravens, W. W., *J. Biol. Chem.*, 167, 143—150, 1947.
441. Roach, A. G., Sanderson, P., and Williams, D. R., *J. Sci. Food Agric.*, 18, 274—278, 1967.
442. Roche, M., *Ind. Aliment. Agric.*, 88, 981—983, 1971.
443. Roelofsen, P. A., *Adv. Food Res.*, 8, 225—298, 1958.
444. Rogers, D., King, T. E., and Cheldelin, V. H., *Proc. Soc. Exp. Biol. Med.*, 82, 140—144, 1953.
445. Rohan, T. A., *Food Technol.*, 24, 29—37, 1970.
446. Rohan, T. A. and Stewart, T., *J. Food Sci.*, 30, 416—419, 1965.
447. Rooney, L. W., Salem, A., and Johnson, J. A., *Cereal Chem.*, 44, 539—550, 1967.
448. Rosen, L., Johnson, K. C., and Pigman, W., *J. Am. Chem. Soc.*, 75, 3460—3464, 1953.
449. Rosenberg, H. R. and Rohdenburg, E. L., *J. Nutr.*, 45, 593—598, 1951.
450. Ross, I. and Krampitz, G., *Z. Tierphysiol. Tierernaehr. Futtermittelkd.*, 15, 95—101, 1960.
451. Rothe, M., *Nahrung*, 5, 131—142, 1960.
452. Rothe, M. and Thomas, B., *Nahrung*, 3, 1—17, 1959.
453. Rothe, M. and Voigt, L., *Nahrung*, 7, 50—59, 1963.
454. Roubal, W. T. and Tappel, A. L., *Arch. Biochem. Biophys.*, 113, 5—8 and 150—155, 1966.
455. Roxas, M. L., *J. Biol. Chem.*, 27, 71—93, 1916.
456. Rubenthaler, G., Pomeranz, Y., and Finney, K. F., *Cereal Chem.*, 40, 658—665, 1963.
457. Sabiston, A. R., and Kennedy, B. M., *Cereal Chem.*, 34, 94—110, 1957.
458. Salem, A., Rooney, L. W., and Johnson, J. A., *Cereal Chem.*, 44, 576—583, 1967.
459. Sanger, F., *Biochem. J.*, 39, 507—515, 1945.
460. Sattler, L. and Zerban, F. W., *Ind. Eng. Chem.*, 41, 1401—1407, 1949.
461. Scarbieri, V. C., Amaya, J., Tanaka, M., and Chichester, C. O., *J. Nutr.*, 103, 657—663, 1973.
462. Scarbieri, V. C., Amaya, J., Tanaka, M., and Chichester, C. O., *J. Nutr.*, 103, 1731—1738, 1973.
463. Schiller, K., *Z. Tierphysiol. Tierernaehr. Futtermittelkd.*, 15, 95—101, 1960.
464. Schmiedeberg, as cited by Samuely, F., *Beitr. Chem. Physiol.*, 2, 355, 1902.
465. Schönberg, A. and Moubacher, R., *Chem. Rev.*, 50, 261—277, 1952.
466. Schönberg, A., Moubacher, R., and Mostafa, A., *J. Chem. Soc.*, 70, 176—182, 1948.
467. Schormüller, J. and Andräss, W., *Z. Lebensm. Unters. Forsch.*, 118, 12—22, 1962.
468. Schroeder, L. J., Iacobellis, M., and Smith, A. H., *J. Nutr.*, 49, 549—561, 1953.
469. Schroeder, L. J., Iacobellis, M., and Smith, A. H., *J. Biol. Chem.*, 212, 973—983, 1955.
470. Schroeder, L. J., Iacobellis, M., and Smith, A. H., *J. Nutri.*, 55, 97—104, 1955.
471. Schroeder, L. J., Iacobellis, M., and Smith, A. H., *J. Nutr.*, 73, 143—150, 1961.
472. Schroeder, L. J., Stewart, R. A., and Smith, A. H., *J. Nutr.*, 45, 61—74, 1951.
473. Schwartz, H. M. and Lea, C. H., *Biochem. J.*, 50, 713—716, 1952.
474. Schweigert, B. S. and Guthneck, B. T., *J. Nutr.*, 54, 333—343, 1954.
475. Seaver, J. L. and Kertesz, Z. I., *J. Am. Chem. Soc.*, 68, 2178—2179, 1946.
476. Segal, R., *Ind. Aliment. Agric.*, 87, 703—709, 1970.
477. Sentheshanmuganathan, S. and Hoover, A. A., *Biochem. J.*, 68, 621—626, 1958.
478. Sheikh, N. M., Thesis, University of Paris, Ser. A, No 909, 1960.
479. Sheikh, N. M., Godon, B., and Petit, L., *Ann. Technol. Agric.*, 10, 5—42, 1961.
480. Shemer, M. and Perkins, E. G., *J. Nutr.*, 104, 1389—1395, 1974.

481. Shillam, K. W. G. and Roy, J. H. B., *Br. J. Nutr.*, 17, 171—181, 1963.
482. Shimizu, Y., Matsuto, S., Mizunuma, Y., and Okada, I., *Eiyo To Shokuryo*, 23, 276—280, 1970.
483. Shore, V. G., and Pardee, A. B., *Anal. Chem.*, 28, 1479—1481, 1956.
484. Simon, H., *Chem. Ber.*, 95, 1003—1008, 1962.
485. Simon, H. and Heubach, G., *Chem. Ber.*, 98, 3703—3711, 1965.
486. Sims, R. J. and Fioriti, J. A., *J. Am. Oil Chem. Soc.*, 52, 144—147, 1975.
487. Singh, B., Dean, G. R., and Cantor, S. M., *J. Am. Chem. Soc.*, 70, 517—522, 1948.
488. Smith, R. E. and Scott, H. M., *Poultry Sci.*, 44, 394—400, 1965.
489. Smith, R. E. and Scott, H. M., *Poultry Sci.*, 44, 401—408, 1965.
490. Sokolov, A. A. and Kamal, J. M., *Vopr. Pitan.*, 21, 82—84, 1962.
491. Soliman, M. M., Kinoshita, S., and Yamanishi, T., *Agric. Biol. Chem.*, 39, 973—977, 1975.
492. Soman, U. P. and Ambegaokar, S. D., *J. Nutr. Diet.*, 3(4), 1—4, 1966.
493. Song, P. S. and Chichester, C. O., *J. Food Sci.*, 31, 914—926, 1966.
494. Song, P. S., Chichester, C. O., and Stadtman, F. H., *J. Food Sci.*, 31, 906—913, 1966.
495. Stadtman, F. H., Chichester, C. O., and Mackinney, G., *J. Am. Chem. Soc.*, 74, 194—196, 1952.
496. Stadtman, F. H., Chichester, C. O., and Mackinney, G., *J. Am. Chem. Soc.*, 74, 3194—3196, 1952.
497. Stenberg, R. J. and Geddes, W. F., *Cereal Chem.*, 37, 614—622, 1960.
498. Stepachenko, B. N. and Serbyuk, O. G., *Biokhimya*, 15, 155—164, 1950.
499. Stewart, G. F. and Kline, R. W., *Ind. Eng. Chem.*, 40, 916—919, 1948.
500. Stott, J. A. and Smith, H., *Br. J. Nutr.*, 20, 663—673, 1966.
501. Strecker, A., *Annalen*, 123, 363, 1862.
502. Sugai, M., *Diss. Abstr.*, 20, 3257, 1960.
503. Sulser, H., *Z. Lebensm. Wiss. Technol.*, 6, 66—69, 1973.
504. Tamaki, Y., *J. Chem. Soc. Jpn.*, 56, 460—461, 1953; Kudo, K. and Tamaki, Y., *J. Chem. Soc. Jpn.*, 57, 249—250, 1954.
505. Tanaka, M., Lee, T. C., and Chichester, C. O., *Agric. Biol. Chem.*, 39, 863—866, 1975.
506. Tanaka, M., Lee, T. C., and Chichester, C. O., *J. Nutr.*, 105, 989—994, 1975.
507. Tannenbaum, S. R., *J. Food Sci.*, 31, 53—57, 1966.
508. Tannous, R. I. and Ullah, M., *Trop. Agric.*, 46, 123—129, 1969.
509. Tarassuk, N. P. and Jack, E. L., *J. Dairy Sci.*, 31, 255—268, 1948.
510. Tarassuk, N. P. and Simonson, H. D., *Food Technol.*, 4, 88—92, 1950.
511. Tarr, H. L. A., *Nature*, 171, 344—345, 1953.
512. Täufel, K. and Iwainsky, H., *Biochem. Z.*, 323, 299—308, 1952.
513. Thomas, B. and Rothe, M., *Bakers Dig.*, 34, 50—56, 1960.
514. Toyomizu, M. and Chung, C. Y., *Nippon Suisan Gakkaishi*, 34, 857—862, 1968.
515. Toyomizu, M., Yamazaki, T., and Komori, Y., *Nippon Suisan Gakkaiski*, 34, 853—856, 1968.
516. Tsugo, T., Yamauchi, K., and Yoshino, U., *Nippon Nogei Kagaku Kaishi*, 35, 888, 1961.
517. Underwood, J. C., Lento, H. G., Jr., and Willits, C. O., *Food Res.*, 24, 181—184, 1959.
518. Valera, G., Vidal, C., and Zamora, S., *An. Bromatol.*, 22, 323—329, 1970.
519. Valle—Riestra, J. and Barnes, R. H., *J. Nutr.*, 100, 873—882, 1970.
520. Van Buren, J. P., Steinkraus, K. H., Hackler, L. R., El Rawi, I., and Hand, D. B., *J. Agric. Food Food Chem.*, 12, 524—528, 1964.
521. Van den Bruel, A. M. R., Jenneskens, P. J., and Mol, J. J., *Neth. Milk Dairy J.*, 26, 19—30, 1972.
522. Van Pragg, M., Stein, H. S., and Tibbets, M. S., *J. Agric. Food Chem.*, 16, 1005—1008, 1968.
523. Viswanathan, L. and Sarma, P. S., *Nature*, 180, 1370—1371, 1957.
524. Vodrazka, Z. and Soucek, J., *Biochem. Z.*, 332, 477—487, 1960.
525. Volgunov, G. P. and Pokhno, M. T., *Biokhimya*, 15, 67—74, 1950.
526. Von Euler, H., Hasselquist, H., and Erickson, E., *Ann. Chem.*, 588, 205—210, 1954.
527. Wahl, P., *Acta Chim. Acad. Sci. Hung.*, 23, 159—177, 1960.
528. Waibel, P. E. and Carpenter, K. J., *Br. J. Nutr.*, 27, 509—515, 1972.
529. Walker, N. J., *J. Dairy Res.*, 39, 231—238, 1972.
530. Walz, O. P. and Ford, J. E., *Z. Tierphysiol. Tierernaehr. Futtermittelkd.*, 30, 304—322, 1973.
531. Wanatabe, J., *J. Biochem. Tokyo*, 16, 163, 1932.
532. Wasserman, R. H. and Langemann, F. W., *J. Nutr.*, 70, 377—384, 1960.
533. Webb, B. H., *J. Dairy Sci.*, 18, 81, 1935.
534. Wedzicha, B. L. and McWeeny, D. J., *J. Sci. Food Agric.*, 25, 577—587, 1974.
535. Weissberger, W., Kavanagh, T. E., and Keeney, P. G., *J. Food Sci.*, 36, 877—879, 1971.
536. Wendland, G., *Arch. Pharm. Paris*, 285, 71—79, 1952; 285, 109—120, 1952.
537. Willits, C. O., Underwood, H. G., Jr., and Ricciuti, C., *Food Res.*, 23, 61—67, 1958.
538. Wilson, B. J. and McNab, J. M., *Br. Poultry Sci.*, 13, 67—73, 1972.
539. Wiseblatt, L. and Zoumut, H. F., *Cereal Chem.*, 40, 162—169, 1963.
540. Wolfrom, M. L., Kashimura, N., and Horton, D., *J. Agric. Food Chem.*, 22, 791—795, 1974.

541. Wolfrom, M. L. and Rooney, C. S., *J. Am. Chem. Soc.*, 75, 5435—5436, 1953.
542. Wolfrom, M. L., Schlicht, R. C., Langer, A. W., Jr., and Rooney, C. S., *J. Am. Chem. Soc.*, 75, 1013, 1953.
543. Wolfrom, M. L., Schütz, R. D., and Cavalieri, L. F., *J. Am. Chem. Soc.*, 70, 514—517, 1948.
544. Wolfrom, M. L., Schütz, R. D., and Cavalieri, L. F., *J. Am. Chem. Soc.*, 71, 3518—3523, 1949.
545. Wood, T., *J. Sci. Food Agric.*, 12, 61—69, 1961.
546. Yanagita, T. and Sugano, M., *Eiyo To Shokuryo*, 27, 275—280, 1974.
547. Yanagita, T. and Sugano, M., *Eiyo To Shokuryo*, 27, 281—287, 1974.
548. Yoshihiro, Y., Kuroiwa, S., and Nakamura, M., *J. Chem. Soc. Jpn. Ind. Chem.*, 64, 551—555, 1961.
549. Young, C. T., Young, T. G., and Cherry, J. F., *J. Am. Peanut Res. Educ. Assoc.*, 6, 1, 1974.
550. Zabrodskii, A. G. and Vitkovskaya, V. A., *Tr. Kiev. Fil. Vses. Nauchno Issled. Inst. Spirt. Likero-Vodochn. promsti.*, 4, 37—43, 1958.
551. Zabrodskii, A. G. and Vitkovskaya, V. A., *Tr. Kiev. Fil. Vses. Nauchno Issled. Inst. Spirt. Likero-Vodochn. Promsti.*, 4, 87—95, 1958.
552. Zweig, G. and Block, R. J., *J. Dairy Sci.*, 36, 427—436, 1953.

# EFFECTS OF PROCESSING ON PESTICIDE RESIDUES IN FOODS

## S. J. Ritchey

Several reviews[9,10,13,23,35] have provided an excellent basis for a collation of present knowledge on the effects of processing on pesticide residues in foods. Because "processing" may be a poorly defined term, it has been interpreted as any operation performed on a food, food source, or food product from the point of harvest through consumption. Thus, for purposes of this review, processing includes such operations as washing, peeling or the equivalent, canning, freezing, storage, drying, cooking, and the preparation of foods from an original source.

The effects of processing operations on foods are to cause a reduction in the level of residue. The extensive review by Farrow et al.[9] indicated that operations in a typical canning plant will remove most of the pesticide residues from vegetable crops. Residues which are loosely held on the surface are removed by washing and blanching, but residues which penetrate the tissues are more difficult to remove from the food. The removal of residues from food depends upon numerous factors, including the type of food, the specific pesticide, and the severity of the processing operation. Certain residues such as the chlorinated hydrocarbons are located primarily in the lipid materials of animal products and tend to be retained with the lipids during processing. Residues are found in dried form on plant surfaces or they may be absorbed and bound to the waxy components in the skin of fruits and vegetables. Residues may be translocated to the inner tissues of plants and fruits.

The effects of processing have been organized to indicate the food or product, the process, the specific residue, and the effect expressed as percentage reduction of the residue as a result of the processing treatment in foods from animal sources (Table 1) and from plant sources (Table 2). The original publication and/or the review cited in each table will provide much greater detail for the interested reader.

Table 1

THE EFFECTS OF PROCESSING UPON PESTICIDE RESIDUES IN FOODS
FROM ANIMAL SOURCES

| Food or product | Process | Residue | Percent reduction | Ref. |
|---|---|---|---|---|
| Milk | Preparation of butter, buttermilk, cream, etc. | DDT, lindane | None | 20 |
| | Condensation, sterilization, drying, etc. | Dieldrin, endrin, and heptachlor | None | 21 |
| | Processing, refrigeration, storage (room temp) | Chlordane, dieldrin, DDT, heptachlor, lindane | None | 22 |
| | Spray drying | Chlordane, dieldrin, lindane | 11 27 34 | 22 |
| Milk fat | Molecular distillation (200°C; pressure of 5 × 10⁻⁴ torr) | Aldrin, DDT, heptachlor, lindane | 95—99 | 2 |
| | Freeze drying and mild deodorization | Dieldrin, heptachlor epoxide | None | 15 |
| | Steam deodorization | Dieldrin, heptachlor epoxide | 100 | 15 |
| Bacon | Cooking | Dieldrin | 47—80 | 37 |
| Eggs | Boiling | DDT | None | 26 |
| | | HCH | None | 26 |
| | Freeze drying | Dieldrin | 37 | 38 |
| | | DDT | 44 | 38 |
| | | Lindane | 50—79 | 38 |
| | | PCB | 27 | 17 |
| Chicken | Cooking (baking, frying, steaming) | Aldrin | 21—30 | 29 |
| | Cooking | Chlordane | Slight reduction | 24 |
| | Cooking (baking, frying, steaming) | Dieldrin | 22—42 | 25, 29 |
| | | DDT | 15—18 | 27 |
| | | Endrin | 20—31 | 29 |
| | | Heptachlor | 0—21 | 29 |
| | Cooking (121°C; 3 hr) | Kelthane | None | 24 |
| | Cooking (baking, frying, steaming) | Lindane | 0—60 | 25, 27, 29 |
| | Cooking | Ovex | None | 24 |
| | | Tolodrin | Slight reduction | 24 |

Table 2

THE EFFECTS OF PROCESSING UPON PESTICIDE RESIDUES
IN FOODS FROM PLANT SOURCES

| Food | Residue | Process | Percent reduction | Ref. |
|---|---|---|---|---|
| Bread | Lindane | Baking | 16—25 | 30 |
| Broccoli | Carbaryl | Washing (detergent) | 77 | 9 |
| | | Blanching, washing | 99 | 9 |
| | Parathion | Water wash | None | 9 |
| | | Detergent wash | 30—33 | 9, 19 |
| | | Blanching, washing | 10 | 9 |
| | | Hand washing | None | 19 |
| | | Washing, blanching, freezing | 10 | 9 |
| | Malathion | Washing, cooking | 7—34 | 14 |
| | | Storage (6 months frozen) | 45—77 | 14 |

## Table 2 (continued)
## THE EFFECTS OF PROCESSING UPON PESTICIDE RESIDUES
## IN FOODS FROM PLANT SOURCES

| Food | Residue | Process | Reduction | Ref. No. |
|------|---------|---------|-----------|----------|
| Celery | Parathion | Washing (alkaline hydrogen peroxide) | 20—90 | 35 |
| Cherries | Gordona | Canning | 95 | 5 |
| Corn | Gordona | Husking | 99 | 6 |
| | | Canning | >99 | 6 |
| Grapes | Chlorcholine chloride | Winemaking | None | 33 |
| Green beans | Azodrin® | Washing and blanching | 33—53 | 6 |
| | | Canning | 99 | 6 |
| | Carbaryl | Blanching | 68 | 9 |
| | Carbaryl | Washing, blanching, canning | 73 | 9 |
| | DDT | Blanching | 50 | 9 |
| | DDT | Washing, blanching, canning | 83 | 9 |
| | | Washing, trimming | 9 | 12 |
| | | Washing, trimming, cooking | 63 | 12 |
| | DDT | Washing, blanching, freezing (0°F, 4 months) | 61 | 3 |
| | | Canning | 100 | 3 |
| | Gordona | Washing, blanching | 90 | 6 |
| | | Canning | 99 | 6 |
| | Guthion® | Washing, blanching, freezing (0°F; 4 months) | 86 | 3 |
| | | Canning | 98 | 3 |
| | Malathion | Blanching | 71 | 9 |
| | | Cold water wash | 96 | 19 |
| | | Washing, blanching, and canning | 94 | 9 |
| | Parathion | Neutral soap wash | 52 | 36 |
| Lemon | Guthion® | Washing | 63 | 11 |
| Mustard greens | Parathion | Neutral soap wash | 87 | 36 |
| Orange | Guthion® | Washing | 30 | 1 |
| | | Washing | 84 | 11 |
| Peaches | Gordona | Lye peeling | 99 | 5 |
| Pears | Gordona | Canning and peeling | 98 | 5 |
| Potatoes | DDT | Peeling (home) | 91 | 18 |
| | | Washing (5% lye) and peeling | 94 | 9, 18 |
| | | Washing (15% lye) | 90 | 9 |
| | | Washing, blanching, canning | 96 | 9 |
| | | Washing, commercial | 20 | 18 |
| | | Cooking (in skins) | None | 18 |
| | | Storage (45°F; 6 weeks) | None | 18 |
| Spinach | DDT | Detergent washing | 48 | 9 |
| | | Blanching, washing | 60 | 9 |
| | | Washing, blanching, canning | 91 | 9 |
| | Carbaryl | Washing, blanching, canning | 99 | 9 |
| | | Detergent washing | 87 | 9 |
| | | Blanching, washing | 97 | 9 |
| | Diazinon | Blanching, washing | 60 | 9 |
| | | Water (detergent) washing | None | 9 |
| | Parathion | Blanching, washing | 71 | 9 |
| | | Water washing | 9 | 9 |
| | | Detergent washing | 24 | 9, 19 |
| | | Hand washing (home) | 39 | 19 |
| | | Washing, blanching, canning | 66 | 9 |

## Table 2 (continued)
## THE EFFECT OF PROCESSING UPON PESTICIDE RESIDUES IN FOOD FROM PLANT SOURCES

| Food | Residue | Process | % Reduction | Ref. |
|------|---------|---------|-------------|------|
| Soybeans | DDT isomer | Cooking | 20—80 | 34 |
| | BHC isomer | Cooking | 31—67 | 34 |
| Tomatoes | Azodrin® | Cold wash | 36—77 | 7 |
| | | Hot lye peel | 93 | 7 |
| | Carbaryl | Detergent washing | 97 | 9 |
| | | Washing and peeling | 99 | 9 |
| | | Washing, blanching, canning | 99 | 9 |
| | | Storage (55°F; 7 days) | 30 | 8 |
| | | Cooking | 69 | 8 |
| | | Home canning | 92 | 8 |
| | | Commercial canning and juicing | >99 | 8 |
| | DDT | Water washing | 91 | 9 |
| | | Detergent washing | 73 | 9 |
| | | Washing and peeling | 99 | 9 |
| | | Washing, blanching, and canning | 99 | 9 |
| | | | None | 8 |
| | | Storage (55°F; 7 days) | 85 | 8 |
| | | Cooking | >99 | 8 |
| | | Home canning | >99 | 8 |
| | | Commercial canning and juicing | | |
| | Diazinon | Water detergent | 88 | 9 |
| | Gordona | Washing | 50 | 6 |
| | | Canning | 99 | 6 |
| | | Hand wash | None | 19 |
| | Malathion | Water washing | 36—79 | 16 |
| | | Detergent wash | 90—95 | 9, 19 |
| | | Washing, peeling | 99 | 9 |
| | | Washing, blanching, and canning | 99 | 9 |
| | | | 90 | 8 |
| | | Cooking | None | 8 |
| | | Storage (55°F; 7 days) | >99 | 8 |
| | | Home canning | >99 | 8 |
| | | Commercial canning and juicing | | |
| Tomato juice | Carbaryl | Home canning | 67 | 8 |
| Vegetable oils | Chlorinated pesticide | Commercial processing | Removed by deodorization and hydrogenation | 32 |

# REFERENCES

1. **Anderson, C. A., MacDougall, D., Kesterson, J. W., Hendrickson, R., and Brooks, R. F.,** The effect of processing on Guthion® residues in oranges and orange products, *J. Agric. Food Chem.*, 11, 422, 1963.

2. **Bills, D. D. and Sloan, J. L.,** Removal of chlorinated insecticide residues from milk fat by molecular distillation, *J. Agric. Food Chem.*, 15, 676, 1967.

3. **Carlin, F. A., Hobbs, E. T., and Dahm, P. A.,** Insecticide residues and sensory evaluation of canned and frozen snap beans field sprayed with Guthion® and DDT, *Food Technol.*, 20, 80, 1966.

4. **Carter, R. H., Hubanks, P. E., and Maan, H. D.,** Effect of cooking on the DDT content of beef, *Science*, 107, 347, 1948.

5. **Fahey, J. E., Nelson, P. E., and Ballee, D. L.,** Removal of Gordona from fruit by commercial preparative methods, *J. Agric. Food Chem.*, 18, 866, 1970.

6. **Fahey, J. E., Gould, G. E., and Nelson, P. E.,** Removal of Gordona and Azodrin® from vegetable crops by commercial preparative methods, *J. Agric. Food Chem.*, 17, 1204, 1969.

7. **Fahey, J. E., Nelson, P. E., and Gould, G. E.,** Removal of Azodrin® residues from tomatoes by commercial preparative methods, *J. Agric. Food Chem.*, 19, 81, 1971.

8. **Farrow, R. P., Lamb, F. C., Cook, P. W., Kimball, J. R., and Elkins, E. R.,** Removal of DDT, Malathion and Carbaryl from tomatoes by commercial and home preparation methods, *J. Agric. Food Chem.*, 16, 65, 1968.

9. **Farrow, R. P., Elkins, E. R., Rose, W. W., Lamb, F. C., Ralls, J. W., and Mercer, W. A.,** Canning operations that reduce insecticide levels in prepared foods and in solid food wastes, *Residue Rev.*, 29, 73, 1969.

10. **Geisman, J. R.,** Reduction of pesticide residues in food crops by processing, *Residue Rev.*, 54, 43, 1975.

11. **Gunther, F. A., Carman, G. E., Blinn, R. C., and Barkley, J. H.,** Persistence of residues of Guthion® on and in mature lemons and oranges in laboratory processed citrus "pulp" cattle feed, *J. Agric. Food Chem.*, 11, 24, 1963.

12. **Hemphill, D. D., Baldwin, R. E., Deguzman, A., and Deloach, H. K.,** Effects of washing, trimming and cooking on levels of DDT and derivatives in green beans, *J. Agric. Food Chem.*, 15, 290, 1967.

13. **Kawar, N. S., de Batista, G. C., and Gunther, F. A.,** Pesticide stability in cold-stored plant parts, soils and dairy products, and in cold-stored extractives solutions, *Residue Rev.*, 48, 45, 1973.

14. **Kilgore, L. and Windham, F.,** Disappearance of Malathion residue in broccoli during cooking and freezing, *J. Agric. Food Chem.*, 18, 162, 1970.

15. **Kroger, M.,** Effect of various physical treatments on certain organochlorine hydrocarbons insecticides found in milk fat, *J. Dairy Sci.*, 51, 196, 1968.

16. **Koivistoinen, P., Karinpoa, A., Kononen, M., and Roine, P.,** Malathion residues on fruit treated by dipping, *J. Agric. Food Chem.*, 12, 551, 1964.

17. **Kuhn, M. A., Rao, M. R., and Novak, A. F.,** Reduction of polychlorinated biphenyls in shrimp and eggs by freeze-drying techniques, *J. Food Sci.*, 41, 1137, 1976.

18. **Lamb, F. C., Farrow, R. P., Slkins, E. R., Cook, R. W., and Kimball, J. R.,** Behavior of DDT in potatoes during commercial and home preparation, *J. Agric. Food Chem.*, 16, 272, 1968.

19. **Lamb, F. C. and Farrow, R. P.,** Investigations on the Effect of Preparation and Cooking on the Pesticide Residue Content of Selected Vegetables, National Canners Association Research Federation Report, Washington, D.C., 1967.

20. **Langlois, B. E., Liska, B. J., and Hill, D. L.,** The effects of processing and storage of dairy products on chlorinated insecticide residues. I. DDT and lindane, *J. Milk Food Technol.*, 27, 264, 1964.

21. **Langlois, B. E., Liska, B. J., and Hill, D. L.,** The effects of processing and storage of dairy products on chlorinated insecticide residues. II. Endrin, dieldrin and heptachlor, *J. Milk Food Technol.*, 28, 9, 1965.

22. **Li, C. F., Bradley, R. L., Jr., and Schultz, L. H.,** Fate of organochlorine pesticides during processing of milk into dairy products, *J. Assoc. Off. Agric. Chem.*, 53, 127, 1970.

23. **Liska, B. J. and Stadelman, W. J.,** Effects of processing on pesticides in food, *Residue Rev.*, 29, 61, 1969.

24. **McCaskey, T. A., Stemp, A. R., Liska, B. J., and Stadelman, W. J.,** Residues in egg yolks and raw and cooked tissues from laying hens administered selected chlorinated hydrocarbon insecticides, *Poult. Sci.*, 47, 564, 1969.

25. **Morgan, K. J., Zabik, M. E., and Funk, K.,** Lindane, dieldrin and DDT residues in raw and cooked chicken and chicken broth, *Poult. Sci.*, 51, 470, 1972.

26. **Nikonorow, M. and Zimak, J.,** I. Effect of boiling on contents of and changes in DDT and HCH in eggs, *Rocz. Panstw. Zakl. Hig.*, 26, 153, 1975; as cited in *Food Sci. Abstr.*, 7, 184, 1975.

27. Ritchey, S. J., Young, R. W., and Essary, E. O., The effects of cooking on chlorinated hydrocarbon pesticide residues in chicken tissues, *J. Food Sci.,* 32, 238, 1967.

28. Ritchey, S. J., Young, R. W., and Essary, E. O., Cooking methods and heating effects on DDT in chicken tissues, *J. Food Sci.,* 34, 569, 1969.

29. Ritchey, S. J., Young, R. W., and Essary, E. O., Effects of heating and cooking method on chlorinated hydrocarbon residues in chicken tissues, *J. Agric. Food Chem.,* 20, 291, 1972.

30. Saha, J. G. and Sumner, A. K., Fate of lindane -¹⁴C in wheat flour under normal conditions of bread making, *Can. Inst. Food Sci. Technol. J.,* 7, 101, 1974.

31. Solar, J. M., Liuzzo, J. A., and Novak, A. F., Removal of aldrin, heptachlor epoxide and endrin from potatoes during processing, *J. Agric. Food Chem.,* 19, 1008, 1971.

32. Smith, K. J., Polen, B., Devries, D. M., and Coon, F. B., Removal of chlorinated pesticides from crude vegetable oils by simulated commercial processing procedures, *J. Am. Oil Chem. Soc.,* 45, 866, 1968.

33. Tafuri, F. T., Businelli, M., Scarponi, L., and Giusguiani, P. L., Chlorocholine chloride residue in grapes and their fate in winemaking, *J. Agric. Food Chem.,* 18, 869, 1970.

34. Takeda, M., Otsukf, K., Sekita, H., and Tanobe, H., Analysis of pesticide residue in foods. IX. Effect of cooking on the reduction of organochlorine pesticide residues in rice, red beans and soybeans, *J. Food Hyg. Soc.,* 14, 142, 1973.

35. Thompson, N. P., Reduction of parathion residue on celery, *Residue Rev.,* 29, 39, 1969.

36. Thompson, B. D. and Van Middelem, C. H., The removal of toxaphene and parathion residues from tomatoes, green beans, celery and mustard with detergent washings, *Proc. Am. Soc. Hortic. Sci.,* 65, 357, 1955.

37. Yadrick, M. K., Fank, K., and Zabik, M. E., Dieldrin residues in bacon cooked by two methods, *J. Agric. Food Chem.,* 19, 491, 1971.

38. Zabik, M. E. and Dugan, L., Jr., Potential of freeze drying for removal of chlorinated hydrocarbon insecticides from eggs, *J. Food Sci.,* 36, 87, 1971.

# *Index*

# INDEX

content of Italian cheeses, I: 85
in silage, II: 43, 44, 103, 104
in sweet potato and cassava silage, II: 229
production in animal digestive tracts, II: 120
use in grain storage, II: 118

# C

Cabbage
  ascorbic acid retention in home storage, I: 247
  boiled, nutrient loss in, I: 252
  chopping effect on nutrients, I: 250
  dehydrated
  dehydrated, packaging requirements, I: 501
    flavor retention, I: 152
    packaging requirements, I: 50
    vitamin C retention in storage, I: 292
  drying, thiamin retention in, I: 489
  effect of blanching on vitamins, I: 484
  fermentation, vitamin retention in, I: 489, 491,
      492
  flavor production, I: 146
  freeze-dried, vitamin C retention, I: 54
  irradiation treatment effects, I: 199, 200; II:
      155
  microwave or conventional cooking, vitamin C
      retention, I: 224, 226, 255
  toxic factors, elimination of, II: 363, 364
  trimming loss, I: 250
  vitamin loss, I: 34, 256
Cadavarine, formation in ensilage, II: 104
Cadmium, loss in milling of wheat, I: 524
Caffeic acid, action on in enzymatic browning, I:
    141
Cake, shelf life, I: 249
Calcium
  age affecting absorption, II: 355
  availability affected by ethylene-
      diaminetetraacetic acid, II: 353
  availability in baked goods, I: 254
  content of beet pulp products, II: 248
  content of herring meals, II: 284
  content of milk and cheese, I: 398
  content of milk products, I: 394
  content of molasses, II: 241, 243
  content of shellfish, I: 338, 340
  effect of processing on, II: 358
  effect on browning reaction, I: 559
  excess, effect on nutrient requirements, II: 352
  fortification of cereal products with, I: 481
  interaction with vitamin D and phosphorus in
      rickets, II: 352
  ions, I: 139, 151
  levels in feed, effects of, II: 271
  loss during ensilage, II: 111
  metabolism affected by premelanoidins, I: 569,
      571
  requirement of hens, II: 352
  retention
    in canned peaches, I: 304, 313, 314
    in cooking of vegetables, I: 251, 252

in freeze-drying, I: 50, 59
role in muscle function, I: 91—94, 103, 104
salts, use in reducing cottonseed toxicity, II:
    390
Calcium caseinate, lysinoalanine formation in, I:
    442
Calcium formate as silage additive, II: 53, 108
Calcium hydroxide, use in alkali treatment of
    feeds, II: 65, 75
Calcium oxalate, toxic effects, II: 232
Calcium pantothenate, thermal degradation
    parameters, I: 5
*Calla palustris*, chemical composition, II: 252
Calves, see Cattle
Canadian bacon, broiled, thiamin retention in, I:
    241, 242
Cancer, association of thermally oxidized fats
    with, I: 421
Candy, use of invertage in manufacture, I: 160
*Candida* spp., heat resistance, I: 585
Cane, see Sugarcane
Canned foods
  fish, vitamin content, I: 364, 367, 370
  fruits and vegetables, shelf life, I: 249
  meat storage, nutrient loss in, I: 328—330
  rice, production, I: 476
  storage
    temperature affecting nutrient content, I:
        287—289, 329, 330, 495
    vitamin stability in, I: 495, 497
Canning
  blanching process, I: 16—20, 24, 26
  distribution of nutrients between solid and
      liquid portions of food, I: 24
  effect on nutritive values, I: 13—22
  effect on pesticide residues, I: 611, 612
  effect on trace elements, I: 526
  holding between blanching and processing,
      effect of, I: 20
  home process, of meats, vitamin retention, I:
      245
  loss of nutrients in, I: 4, 7, 11
  of clams, nutritional effect, I: 342—344, 370
  of crab, effect on composition, I: 346, 349
  of fruit, effect on nutrients, I: 15, 303,
      311—316, 320
  of juices, vitamin retention, I: 13
  of meat and fish products, effect on nutritive
      values, I: 21, 245, 325, 430
  of mussels, effect on composition and mineral
      content, I: 350
  of oysters, effect on vitamin content, I: 353,
      370
  of pork, vitamin loss in storage, I: 247, 294
  of root crops, II: 226
  of shrimp, effect on composition and nutrients,
      I: 355, 358, 370
  of vegetables, vitamin retention, I: 16, 17
  process, I: 485
  size of container affecting thiamin retention, I:
      21
  storage effects, I: 22, 25
  studies of nutritional value of canned foods, I:

effect on nutritive value of chick feed, I: 496 II: 405

effect on vitamins, I: 495, 496

forms of processing, I: 182

forms of radiation used, I: 182

lipids affected by, I: 188

of animal foods, vitamin retention in, I: 496

of clams, nutritional effect, I: 342—344

of fish, nutritional effects, I: 376

of meat, nutritional effects, I: 328

of milk, I: 384

of shrimp, effects of, I: 356, 358

physiological effects, I: 203

proteins of various foods affected by, I: 183

protocols for animal feeding studies, II: 145

radiolytic products

in food-chain sequences, II: 153

of amino acids, : 183; II: 147—149

of carbohydrates, II: 147, 148

of lipids, II: 149

of nucleic acids, II: 151

of proteins, I: 183; II: 147—149

of sensory compounds, II: 151

of steroids, II: 151

of vitamins, II: 151

sensory effects, II: 151

specific applications, II: 142, 143

structural effects, II: 152

treatments, II: 141

units of power, II: 141

vitamins affected by, I: 191, 307, 495; II: 347

wholesomeness of treated foods, II: 152, 156

Isobutyric acid, use in grain storage, II: 118

Isoleucine

activity in fermentation of yogurt, I: 63

content of clams, processing effects, I: 342

content of herring meals, II: 285, 294

content of meat processing raw products, II: 273

content of shrimp, processing effects, I: 358

fermentation of wheat affecting, I: 72

loss in heat-treated proteins, II: 333

sensitivity factors, I: 310

Isomeamaranol in sweet potatoes, II: 231

Isovaleric acid, values in processed milo feed, II: 198

## J

Jack beans, toxic factors, elimination of, II: 363, 364

Jet-sploding processing of feeds, II: 411

Juices, see also particular fruit

apple, vitamin C loss in processing, I: 305

canned, I: 249, 287

cranberry, vitamin C loss in processing, I: 304

freeze-dried, retention of carotenoids, I: 55

irradiation treatment, I: 185

loss of ascorbic acid in glucose oxidase treatment for, I: 161

nonenzymatic browning of, role of ascorbic

acid in, I: 548

nutrient retention in canning, I: 13—15

removal of anthocyanins, I: 140

use of enzymes in production, I: 150, 151

## K

Kale

ascorbic acid loss in storage, I: 250

carotene loss in storage, I: 500

effect of blanching on, I: 484

vitamin retention in blanching, I: 32

Keratin content of meal byproducts, II: 272, 275

Ketonic rancidity, II: 169

Ketchup, I: 249, 291

Ketones, Maillard reaction of, I: 535, 546, 548

Kidney beans

canned, shelf life, I: 249

cooking affecting vitamin availability, II: 346

germination, effect on trypsin inhibitor activity, II: 368

heat treatment effect on trypsin inhibitor and hemagglutinating activity, II: 367

irradiation effects, II: 150

toxic factors, elimination of, II: 362, 364

Kourou, preparation, I: 515, 517

Kunitz soybean inhibitor, effect on growth rate, II: 328

## L

Lactase, I: 86, 87, 125

Lactate silage, production, II: 41

Lactic acid

affecting silage intake, II: 112

as end product of silage fermentation, II: 118

content of alfalfa silage, II: 256

content of ensiled aquatic plants, II: 254, 255, 257

in cassava and sweet potato silage, II: 229

production during fermentation, I: 75

production in water-soaked feed, II: 131

role in ensilage, see Silage

role in fermentation process, I: 63

Lactic acid bacteria

as fish silage additive, II: 115

as silage additives, II: 53

role in silage production, II: 41, 42, 46

*Lactobacillus* spp.

fermentation of taro, II: 226

in silage, II: 103

Maillard reaction effects, I: 573

production of lactic acid in water-soaked feed, II: 131

role in yogurt production, I: 63, 392

Lactose

characteristics, I: 86, 87

content in milk, I: 86

conversion to other sugars, I: 87

intolerance, I: 87

freezing, effects of, II: 18
silage, see Silage

# S

*Saccharomyces* spp.
  heat resistance, I: 585; II: 376
  use in pyridoxine retention assay, I: 246
Safflower
  hulls, alkali treatment for digestibility, II: 82
  oil, linoleic acid loss in frying, I: 253
  seed, nutritive composition, II: 215, 218
*Sagittarie* spp., chemical composition, II: 252
Salad dressings, shelf life, I: 249
Salad greens, I: 247, 250
Salad oil, shelf life, I: 249
Salami, vitamin content, I: 493
Salisbury steak in frozen storage, vitamin loss in,
  I: 285, 286
Salmon, see Fish
*Salmonella* spp.
  contamination of feeds, II: 373
  contamination of meat byproducts, II: 271
  contamination of stored concentrates, II: 164
  fumigation effects, II: 380
  heat processing affecting, II: 373—375
  inactivation in storage, II: 382
  irradiation process effects, II: 142, 379, 380
  meat scrap processing to reduce contamination
    by, effect of, II: 8
  pelleting affecting, II: 377
  pet food contamination, II: 379
Salseed cake, effect on water treatment, II: 407
Selting process, I: 492
Saponin, II: 227, 363
Sarcoplasmic reticulum, see Muscles
Sardines, see Fish
Sauerkraut, vitamin loss in processing, I: 491
Sausages, I: 117, 493
Scallops, I: 239, 338, 340
Sea food, see Fish
Sea water, refrigerated, as fish preservative, II:
  286
Selenium
  as essential nutrient, II: 356
  availability in cooked beans, II: 346
  content of soybeans, effect of processing, I:
    526
  content of wheat, loss in milling, I: 524
  cooking effects, I: 526
Serine
  content of clams, processing effects, I: 343
  content of herring meals, II: 285
  content of meat processing raw materials, II:
    274
  content of shrimp, processing effects, I: 358,
    359
  irradiation effects, II: 148
  levels in yogurt, I: 63
Sesame, II: 162, 215
Sex of animals, effect on flavor of meat, I: 115

Sheep
  aquatic plant feed, II: 259, 261
  beet pulp lamb feed, II: 247
  component acids in fat, II: 182
  cottonseed meal feed, heat treatment effects,
    II: 323
  digestibility of soybean protein by lambs, II:
    322
  digestion of alkali-treated straw, II: 86
  digestion of silage mixtures, II: 91
  enzyme supplementation of feed, II: 136
  formaldehyde treatment of silage, effect on
    intake, II: 115
  formic acid treatment of silage, effects of, II:
    110
  growth rate of lambs, silage treatment
    affecting, II: 110
  intake of silage, factors affecting, II: 111, 113,
    115
  meat byproducts of, composition, II: 270
  propionic acid-treated grain as feed, II: 61
  ryegrass feed, effects of freezing, II: 18
  skim milk powder, heat-treated, effect in lamb
    diet, II: 305
  stiff lamb disease, role of raw beans in, II: 346
  urine concentration of sodium associated with
    treated-feed diet, II: 96
  voluntary intake by lambs of feed following
    alkali treatment, II: 87-89, 91
  weight gain, II: 93, 279
  wood production, effect on meat byproducts in
    feed, II: 279
Shelf life of food products, I: 240, 249
Shellfish, see also specific shellfish, I: 338, 340
Shortening, linoleic acid loss in frying, I: 253
Shrimp
  chemical composition and vitamin content, I:
    366, 369
  enzymatic browning, I: 140
  fatty acids of, effect on processing, I: 355, 356
  freeze-dried
    protein quality of, I: 441
    retention of amino acids and proteins, I: 52
    retention of fats and fatty acids, I: 59
    retention of folic acid, I: 57
    retention of niacin, I: 57
    retention of pantothenic acid, I: 58
    retention of pyridoxine, I: 58
    retention of riboflavin, I: 57
    retention of thiamin, I: 56
  frozen storage life, I: 239
  Newburg
    frozen, thiamin retention on reheating, I:
      220, 221, 224, 247
    thiamin content, processing effects, I: 357
  nutritional content, I: 339, 340
  nutrients, processing effects on, I: 358, 370
Silage
  acetate, production, II: 43, 51
  acetic acid
    affecting intake, II: 112
    as buffering constituent, II: 104